Practice of Intramedullary Locked Nails

New Developments in Techniques and Applications

Chief Editors K.-S. LEUNG · G. TAGLANG
R. SCHNETTLER

Co-Editors V. ALT · H. J. T. M. HAARMAN
H. SEIDEL

Ed. Secretary I. KEMPF

Practice of Intramedullary Locked Nails

New Developments in Techniques and Applications

Recommended by
"Association Internationale pour l'Ostéosynthèse Dynamique" (AIOD)

WITH 294 FIGURES AND 20 TABLES

Springer

Chief Editors
Professor Dr. Kwok-Sui Leung
The Chinese University of Hong Kong
Department of Orthopaedics
and Traumatology
Prince of Wales Hospital
Shatin, Hong Kong SAR
Republic of China

Dr. Gilbert Taglang
Centre de Traumatologie et d'Orthopédie
10 Avenue A. Baumann
67400 Illkirch-Graffenstaden
France

Prof. Dr. Dr. Reinhard Schnettler
Universitätsklinikum Gießen
Klinik und Poliklinik für Unfallchirurgie
Rudolf-Buchheim-Str. 7
35385 Gießen
Germany

Co-Editors
Dr. Volker Alt
Universitätsklinikum Gießen
Klinik und Poliklinik für Unfallchirurgie
Rudolf-Buchheim-Str. 7
35385 Gießen
Germany

Professor Dr. H.J.T.M. Haarman
Academisch Ziekenhuis
Department of Surgery
De Boelelaan 1117, P.O. Box 7057
1007 MB Amsterdam, The Netherlands

Dr. Hartmut Seidel
Rewentlowstr. 48
22605 Hamburg, Germany

Ed. Secretary
Professor Dr. Ivan Kempf
AIOD
Rue du Parc, 16
67205 Oberhausbergen, France

ISBN-10 3-642-44414-8
ISBN-13 978-3-642-44414-2
Springer-Verlag Berlin Heidelberg New York

Springer is a part of Springer Science+Business Media
springer.com

Softcover re-print of the Hardcover 1st edition 2006

Editor: Gabriele Schröder
Desk editor: Irmela Bohn
Production: Elke Beul-Göhringer
Cover design: Estudio Calamar, F. Steinen-Broo, Pau/Girona, Spain
Typesetting: K + V Fotosatz GmbH, Beerfelden, Germany

Printed on acid-free paper
24/3151/beu-göh 5 4 3 2 1 0

Preface

During the preparation and publishing of the first two volumes of our textbook, entitled *Practice of Intramedullary Locked Nails*, the editorial team took into account the most recent and then current technical evolutions in the treatment of long bone fractures. Progress, technical advances, and new concepts in bone biology and fracture healing were, as a result, included in some chapters. That is why Volume 2 was entitled *Advanced Techniques and Special Applications* at the time of its publication. Nevertheless, it was felt that this second volume was only a first step in presenting the new techniques and scientific information associated with the biological, biomechanical, instrumentation and technical improvements associated with intramedullary nailing that were then just beginning to be introduced.

The goal of this third volume is to chronicle and present in more details this perpetual evolution. Numerous renowned authors with diverse specialisations kindly helped us to finalise this volume. Our special gratitude goes to all authors, as well as to the staff of the Association Internationale pour l'Ostéosynthèse Dynamique (AIOD) and of the publishing house, Springer-Verlag, with particular recognition of Mrs. Margot Hamm from the AIOD, and Mrs. Gabriele Schroeder from Springer-Verlag.

Prof. Ivan Kempf

Contents

List of Contributors

Volker Alt
Universitätsklinikum Giessen
Klinik und Poliklinik für Unfallchirurgie
Rudolf-Buchheim-Straße 7
35385 Giessen, Germany

George Anastopoulos
Department of Orthopedic Surgery
and Traumatology
Athens General Hospital
154 Messogion Ave.
11527 Athens, Greece

Rainer Baumgart
Klinikum der LMU München
Chirurgische Klinik und Poliklinik
Innenstadt
Nussbaumstraße 20
80336 München, Germany

Thorsten Bechert
Bio-Gate Bioinnovative Materials GmbH
Neumeyer Straße 48
90411 Nürnberg, Germany

Pietro De Biase
Second Orthopaedic Division
Centre of Oncological
and Reconstructive Surgery
Azienda Ospedaliera Careggi
Centro Traumatologico Ortopedico
Largo Palagi 1
50139 Florence, Italy

Peter J. Buecker
Department of Orthopedic Surgery
University of Louisville
Louisville, KY 40292, USA

Volker Bühren
BG – Unfallklinik Murnau
Unfallchirurgie
Prof.-Küntscher-Straße 8
82418 Murnau, Germany

Rodolfo Capanna
Second Orthopaedic Division
Centre of Oncological
and Reconstructive Surgery
Azienda Ospedaliera Careggi
Centro Traumatologico Ortopedico
Largo Palagi 1
50139 Florence, Italy

Lucio Cardador
Hospital do Litoral Alentejano
Servico de Ortopedia
7450-239 Santiago Do Cacém, Portugal

Jean-Michel Clavert
Pediatric Orthopedics Unit
Department of Pediatric Surgery
Hautepierre University Hospital
Strasbourg, France

Kyle F. Dickson
Department of Orthopedic Surgery
Trauma and Adult Reconstruction
William Beaumont Army Medical Center
El Paso, Texas, USA

Achim Elsen
Klinikum Hannover Nordstadt
Klinik für Unfall-, Hand-
und Wiederherstellungschirurgie
Haltenhoffstraße 41
30167 Hannover, Germany

Georges Finidori
Service d'Orthopédie et Traumatologie
Pédiatriques
Groupe Hospitalier Necker – Enfants Malades
149, rue de Sèvres
75015 Paris, France

Jörg Franke
Klinikum Hannover Nordstadt
Klinik für Unfall-, Hand- und Wiederherstellungschirurgie
Haltenhoffstraße 41
30167 Hannover, Germany

Jan Paul Frölke
Trauma Surgery
University Medical Centre Nijmegen
P.O. Box 9101
6500 HB Nijmegen, The Netherlands

Thomas Fuchs
Klinik und Poliklinik für Unfall-, Hand- und Wiederherstellungschirurgie
Westfälische Wilhelms-Universität Münster
Waldeyerstraße 1
48149 Münster, Germany

Jeannot Gaudias
Centre de Traumatologie et d'Orthopédie
10 Avenue A. Baumann
67400 Illkirch-Graffenstaden, France

Philippe Gicquel
Pediatric Orthopedics Unit
Department of Pediatric Surgery
Hautepierre University Hospital
Strasbourg, France

Christophe Glorion
Service d'Orthopédie et Traumatologie Pédiatriques
Groupe Hospitalier Necker – Enfants Malades
149, rue de Sèvres
75015 Paris, France

Christian Hierholzer
BG – Unfallklinik Murnau
Unfallchirurgie
Prof.-Küntscher-Straße 8
82418 Murnau, Germany

T. Hierl
Klinikum der LMU München
Chirurgische Klinik und Poliklinik
Innenstadt
Nussbaumstraße 20
80336 München, Germany

Stefan Hinterwimmer
Klinikum der LMU München
Chirurgische Klinik und Poliklinik
Innenstadt
Nussbaumstraße 20
80336 München, Germany

Martin Hofmeister
BG – Unfallklinik Murnau
Unfallchirurgie
Prof.-Küntscher-Straße 8
82418 Murnau, Germany

Uwe Horas
Chirurgische Klinik II – Unfallchirurgie
Kliniken des Main-Taunus-Kreises
Lindenstraße 10
65719 Hofheim, Germany

Joseph R. Hsu
Department of Orthopedic Surgery
Trauma and Adult Reconstruction
William Beaumont Army Medical Center
El Paso, TX 79920-5001, USA

Frank Kandziora
Zentrum für Muskolo Skeletale Chirurgie der Charité Berlin (CMSC)
Klinik für Orthopädie
Champus Charité Mitte
Schumannstraße 20/21
10117 Berlin, Germany

Claude Karger
Pediatric Orthopedics Unit
Department of Pediatric Surgery
Hautepierre University Hospital
Avenue Molière
67000 Strasbourg, France

Michael Krammer
Klinikum der LMU München
Chirurgische Klinik und Poliklinik
Innenstadt
Nussbaumstraße 20
80336 München, Germany

Kwok-Sui Leung
Department of Orthopaedics and Traumatology
Prince of Wales Hospital
The Chinese University of Hong Kong
Shatin
Hong Kong SAR, Republic of China

T. R. Lewis
Department of Orthopedic Surgery
Scott and White Memorial Hospital and Clinic
Scott, Sherwood and Brindley Foundation
The Texas A&M University System Health
Science Center College of Medicine
Temple, TX 76508, USA

Martin Lucke
Zentrum für Muskolo Skeletale Chirurgie
der Charité Berlin (CMSC)
Klinik für Unfall-
und Wiederherstellungschirurgie
Champus Virchow-Klinikum
Augustenburger Platz 1
13353 Berlin, Germany

Thomas Mückley
Friedrich-Schiller-Universität Jena
Unfall-, Hand- und
Wiederherstellungschirurgie
Erlanger Allee 101
07737 Jena, Germany

Holger Müller-Daniels
Stryker Trauma GmbH
Prof.-Küntscher-Straße 1–5
24232 Schönkirchen/Kiel, Germany

Wolf Mutschler
Klinikum der LMU München
Chirurgische Klinik und Poliklinik
Innenstadt
Nussbaumstraße 20
80336 München, Germany

Justin S. Ogden
Department of Orthopedic Surgery
University of Louisville
Louisville, KY 40292, USA

Robert A. Probe
Department of Orthopedic Surgery
Scott and White Memorial Hospital and Clinic
Scott, Sherwood and Brindley Foundation
The Texas A&M University System Health
Science Center College of Medicine
Temple, TX 76508, USA

Philip Procter
Applied Technology
and Science Technology Group
Stryker Trauma SA
Chemin du Pont-du-Centenaire, 110
1228 Plan-les-Ouates
Geneva, Switzerland

Michael-J. Raschke
Klinik und Poliklinik für Unfall-, Hand-
und Wiederherstellungschirurgie
Westfälische Wilhelms-Universität Münster
Waldeyerstraße 1
48149 Münster, Germany

Wolfgang Roth
St. Elisabeth-Klinik
Chirurgische und Unfallchirurgische Klinik
Kapuzinerstraße 4
66740 Saarlouis, Germany

Dirk Salz
Fraunhofer Institut für Fertigungstechnik
und Angewandte Materialforschung
Wiener Straße 12
28359 Bremen, Germany

Amir Sarvestani
Stryker Navigation
Bötzinger Straße 41
79111 Freiburg, Germany

Gerhard Schmidmaier
Zentrum für Muskolo Skeletale Chirurgie
der Charité Berlin (CMSC)
Klinik für Unfall- und
Wiederherstellungschirurgie
Champus Virchow-Klinikum
Augustenburger Platz 1
13353 Berlin Germany

Reinhard Schnettler
Universitätsklinikum Giessen
Klinik und Poliklinik für Unfallchirurgie
Rudolf-Buchheim-Straße 7
35385 Giessen, Germany

Hartmut Seidel
Reventlowstraße 48
22605 Hamburg, Germany

David Seligson
Department of Orthopedic Surgery
School of Medicine
University of Louisville
Louisville, KY 40292, USA

Cornelia Siemers
Labor für Experimentelle Unfallchirurgie
Kerkrader Straße 9
35392 Giessen, Germany

Andreas Speitling
Applied Technology
and Science Technology Group
Stryker Trauma SA
Chemin du Pont-du-Centenaire, 110
1228 Plan-les-Ouates
Geneva, Switzerland

Jens-Peter Stahl
Universitätsklinikum Giessen
Klinik und Poliklinik für Unfallchirurgie
Rudolf-Buchheim-Straße 7
35385 Giessen, Germany

Richard Stange
Klinik und Poliklinik für Unfall-, Hand-
und Wiederherstellungschirurgie
Westfälische Wilhelms-Universität Münster
Waldeyerstraße 1
48149 Münster, Germany

Peter Steinrücke
Bio-Gate Bioinnovative Materials GmbH
Neumeyer Straße 48
90411 Nürnberg, Germany

Gilbert Taglang
Centre de Traumatologie et d'Orthopédie
10 Avenue A. Baumann
67400 Illkirch-Graffenstaden, France

Peter Thaller
Klinikum der LMU München
Chirurgische Klinik und Poliklinik
Innenstadt
Nussbaumstraße 20
80336 München, Germany

Vicken Topouchian
Service d'Orthopédie et Traumatologie
Pédiatriques
Groupe Hospitalier Necker – Enfants Malades
149, rue de Sèvres
75015 Paris, France

Katja Trinkaus
Labor für Experimentelle Unfallchirurgie
Kerkrader Straße 9
35392 Giessen, Germany

Geert Von Oldenburg
Applied Technology
and Science Technology Group
Stryker Trauma SA
Chemin du Pont-du-Centenaire, 110
1228 Plan-les-Ouates
Geneva, Switzerland

Holger Von Wieding
Applied Technology
and Science Technology Group
Stryker Trauma SA
Chemin du Pont-du-Centenaire, 110
1228 Plan-les-Ouates
Geneva, Switzerland

Michael Wagener
Bio-Gate Bioinnovative Materials GmbH
Wiener Straße 12
28359 Bremen, Germany

Michael Weber
St. Elisabeth-Klinik
Chirurgische und Unfallchirurgische Klinik
Kapuzinerstraße 4
66740 Saarlouis, Germany

Sabine Wenisch
Universitätsklinikum Giessen
Klinik und Poliklinik für Unfallchirurgie
Rudolf-Buchheim-Straße 7
35385 Giessen, Germany

Britt Wildemann
Zentrum für Muskolo Skeletale Chirurgie
der Charité Berlin (CMSC)
Klinik für Unfall-
und Wiederherstellungschirurgie
Champus Virchow-Klinikum
Augustenburger Platz 1
13353 Berlin Germany

Section 1 Introduction

CHAPTER 1.1

Introduction

K.-S. Leung, G. Taglang, R. Schnettler

This is an era of explosion of information and advancement of technologies. The surgical sciences are by no means excluded. Although the basic principles remain mostly unchanged, the applications of new technologies in modern surgical treatment are always appealing. There have been many advances in the treatment of long bone fractures in recent years. These include new materials available, new applied technologies, and advances in the understanding of the pathology and biology of fracture healing. The understanding of this emerging knowledge and the acquiring of the new technologies will keep us up to the modern standards of fracture management. We believe that the present volume of *Practice of Intramedullary Locked Nails* is a timely update of all this information to help our readers to catch up with the rapid advancement in the practice of fracture care.

This book is the third volume of *Practice of Intramedullary Locked Nails,* with special focus on the recent advancement in the understanding of the biology of healing of fractures of the long bones, the emerging technologies that further enhance the minimally invasive nature of closed treatment of fractures and the availability of various surgical techniques in intramedullary fixation. The contributors to this volume are from different well-known trauma centres and they are the pioneer surgeons in the development and practice of intramedullary locked nails.

In this volume, the understanding of fracture healing in a closed treatment is further depicted through molecular biology studies, new systems, new materials and new technology; in particular, the application of computer-aided surgical techniques is discussed thoroughly. The application of new technology in the prevention of infection and the application of intramedullary fixation of fractures in paediatric and adolescent patients are also described.

We believe that the pursuit of perfection in surgical techniques, the joy of acquiring new knowledge and witnessing the improvement in patient care are most satisfying to surgeons. The fundamental requirement of lifelong learning in our profession was also one of the major encouragements to all the contributors of this volume.

Section 2 Advances in Biology and Fracture Healing in Locked Nails

Cellular Aspects of Bone Defect Healing After Implantation of Calcium Phosphate-Based Bone Substitutes

R. Schnettler, V. Alt, J.-P. Stahl, S. Wenisch

Background

The replacement of bone by means of foreign materials was carried out as long ago as prehistoric times. Nowadays autogenous bone grafting is designated as the "golden standard" to fill large osseous defects that result from many causes, such as traumas, tumours, or birth defects. However, its disadvantages such as limited supply of autogenous bone and donor site morbidity have favoured the use of bone substitutes. As these materials are characterised by their unlimited availability without bearing the risk of disease transmission, research on improving bone tissue healing by using bone substitutes of synthetic or biological origin is a field of major interest.

Focus of Interest

Bone substitutes used clinically in orthopaedics, periodontics, oral and maxillofacial surgery as well as in plastic, trauma, and reconstructive surgery comprise a wide variety of materials and have been the focus of interest for the last 80 years. The present review focuses on the frequently used calcium phosphate-based bone substitutes revealing either resorbable or non-resorbable properties. Their excellent biocompatibility due to their close mimicking of the inorganic phase of the natural bone mineral has led to their widespread use in bone reconstructive surgery.

Examination Tools

Before biomaterials can be applied clinically, biocompatibility must be tested, by monitoring osseointegration, degradation, and foreign body reactions. In order to elucidate physicochemical properties of the presently investigated materials, X-ray diffraction and scanning electron microscopy have been used. Bioreactivity has been elucidated by means of comparative histological evaluations with the use of various animal models. Cell-mediated degradation has been studied at the ultrastructural level and immunohistochemically. The results are discussed with special regard to the origin, composition, and general characteristics of inorganic bone substitutes.

Bone Graft Substitutes: Alternatives to Bone Grafting

Bone Substitutes Are Taken into Account

Operative treatment of large bone defects has remained a challenge for orthopaedic surgeons. In about 10% of all reconstructive operations caused by traumatic, resectional, or congenital defects, bone transplants and bone substitute materials are necessary. Allogenic bone material carries the potential risk of transmitting tumour cells and a variety of bacterial and viral infections including those that cause HIV or hepatitis in patients. Additionally, blood group-incompatible bone transplantation can cause the development of antibodies within the ABO system. This bears the risk of the occurrence of morbus haemolyticus neonatorum in the case of later pregnancy. Generally, a more or less distinct histoincompatibility, due to the transfer of immunocompetent lymphatic donor cells, exists in allogenic bone transplantation as well as in the transplantation of solid organs [1]. Therefore, and because of its superior osteogenic potential compared to allogenic transplants, autogenous bone grafting continues to be the "golden standard" in reconstructive surgery. However, as the limited availability of autogenous bone is a major problem for the surgeon and his patient, inorganic implants such as calcium phosphate (CaP)-based bone substitutes of synthetic or biological origin are useful alternatives to autogenous bone grafting [2, 3]. Consequently, during the last decades, there has been a marked increase in the use of biomedical devices. However, when a tissue is exposed to the surface of a medical device, a classic foreign body response is initiated by the surgical procedure itself, followed by the reaction to the material surface [4–6]. At the cellular level the foreign body response is characterised by initial monocyte recruitment and adhesion to implant surfaces that are too large to engulf [6]. The initial adhesion leads to differentiation of monocytes into activated macrophages, which fuse to form inflammatory giant cells or foreign body giant cells [7]. The initial inflammatory response after implantation triggers beneficial effects, such as coagulation, recruitment and activation of neutrophils and macrophages, followed by mesenchymal cell recruitment, proliferation and matrix synthesis. However, the failure to resolve proceeding inflammation leads to chronic inflammatory responses including fibrous encapsulation of the implant. Giant cells are known to be involved in the degradation of bone substitutes [8–10], but they are also regarded to be the central cellular mediators of the chronic inflammatory response to biomedical material implants [11]. Therefore, before a biomaterial can be applied in hospital, its biocompatibility must be tested by monitoring the foreign body reaction. In particular, a better understanding of the mechanisms causing the fusion of macrophages into giant cells as a reaction to material surfaces is a major prerequisite for the prevention of adverse tissue reactions after implantation of bone substitutes.

Calcium Phosphate-Based Bone Substitutes: An Overview

Bone substitutes should have a good local and systemic compatibility, the capability of being substituted by bone and of completely filling any defect. These features require osteoconductive and/or osteoinductive properties of the implant comparable to those of the natural bone. Therefore research in improving bone tissue healing by biological and mechanical approaches is a field of major interest.

Knowledge of the mechanisms concerning bone formation and bone repair, and of the manner by which bone interacts with bone substitutes are the basis of clinical practice in orthopaedic surgery. Nowadays we are in the midst of intensive research that is being focused on the field of cellular and molecular biology. The majority of data provide information about the response of cells to their physiological environment with special regard to the effects of growth factors, cytokines, extracellular matrix proteins, and receptor–cell interactions inducing cellular differentiation and/or transformation.

Currently available bone substitutes show a variety of compositions and properties. Among them, inorganic CaPs are used frequently (Table 2.1.1). These materials include CaP ceramics (hydroxyapatite [HA]: Endobone, Cerabone, Ceros 80; tricalcium phosphate [β-TCP]: Ceros 82), CaP cements (Biobon [α-BSM], Calcibon) or CaP granules (Calcibon), and nanoparticular hydroxyapatite paste (Ostim). Depending on the nature of the interfaces between them and the host bone, these materials are described either as bioinert or bioactive. They undergo processes of dissolution and precipitation resulting in a strong material-bone interface [12–14].

The biocompatibility of HA and the similarities between the crystal structure of HA and bone mineral have led to its widespread use in bone reconstructive surgery [15–18]. The use of low density HA with highly interconnected porosity is different to that of dense HA [19]. The porous structure and its biocompatibility enable the ingrowth of bone into the implant, which promotes mechanically stable and biologically integrated repair [15]. Several bone-bonding mechanisms in different bioactive materials have been discussed [20–22].

By means of scanning electron microscopy the interconnecting pore system of a bone-derived HA ceramic can be visualised (Fig. 2.1.1 a). A close-up of the trabeculae demonstrates the size of the crystals and their tight connection (Fig. 2.1.1 b). Synthetic ceramics are similar in their

Table 2.1.1. Origin and composition of inorganic bone substitutes

Material	Origin	Composition	Porosity	Resorption
Endobon (Biomet-Merck)	Bovine bone	HA	Macroporous	Non-resorbable
Cerabone (AAP-Mebio)	Bovine bone	HA	Macroporous	Non-resorbable
Ceros 80 (Mathys)	Synthetic	HA	Macroporous	Non-resorbable
Biobon (α-BSM, Etex, 26, Biomet-Merck)	Synthetic	HA	In situ curing paste	Resorbable
Calcibon (Biomet-Merck)	Synthetic	HA	In situ curing paste and granules	Resorbable
Ostim (AAP-Mebio)	Synthetic	HA	Non-curing paste	Resorbable

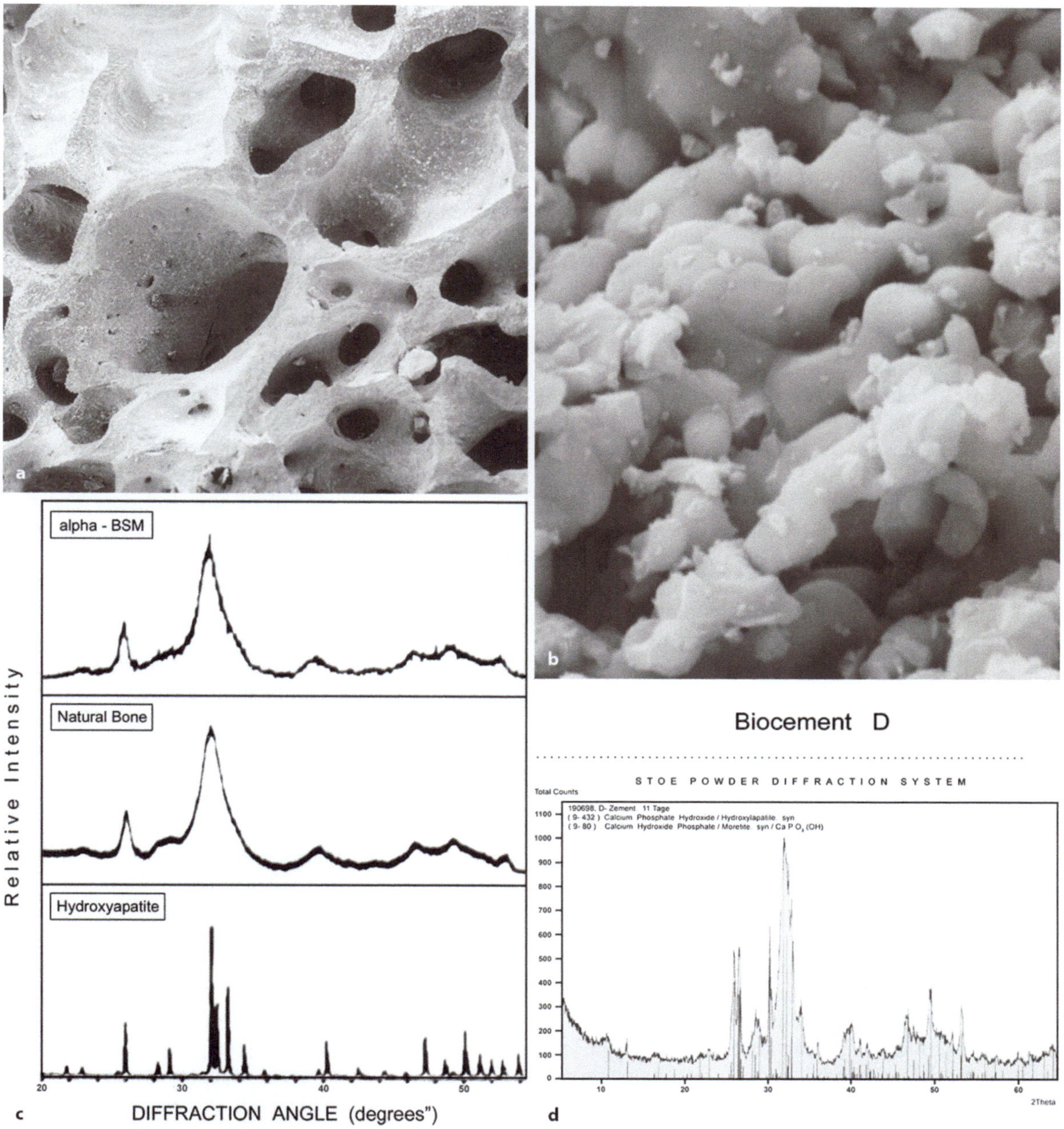

Fig. 2.1.1. **a** Scanning electron micrograph of an HA ceramic derived from bovine bone. **b** Higher magnification of HA crystals, which are tightly connected. Scanning electron microscopy. **c** X-ray diffraction pattern of Biobon, natural bone, and hydroxyapatite. **d** X-ray diffraction pattern of Calcibon

crystal configuration, but differ in size and number of pores.

The dynamic bone–HA interface is one of the most important requirements for the tight junction of ceramics with living tissues by osseointegration [23]. For example, HA derived from bovine cancellous bone (Endobon) offers the dynamic interface between the ceramic and the newly formed bone [24]. It is produced by hydrothermal defatting and calcination of bovine cancellous bone, which has an open "foam-like" trabecular macrostructure [19].

CaP cements consist of particles of different size, which are embedded in a cement matrix. One of their characteristics is that they can be handled easily. Mixing the CaP powder with an accurate amount of sterile saline, water or buffer solution results in a paste that remains formable for hours at room temperature. It hardens in generally less than 20 min at body temperature

(37 °C) and then displays limited solubility. CaP cements can be injected during the operation and fill defects of any size or shape, resulting in an excellent bone-implant contact. Biobon is a fully synthetic microcrystalline hydroxyapatitic bone substitute needing a specific setting reaction, which depends upon conversion of precursor calcium phosphates to a poorly crystalline apatite with a nanocrystalline structure that is virtually identical to normal bone [25, 26]. X-ray diffraction is one of the most important characterisation tools used in solid-state chemistry and material science. It is suitable to determine the composition of different minerals and has been used in two main areas: the fingerprint characterisation of crystalline materials and the determination of their structure. Each crystalline solid has its unique characteristic X-ray powder pattern, which may be used as a "fingerprint" for its identification. Once the material has been identified, X-ray crystallography may be used to determine its structure, crystalline state, interatomic distance and angle. The X-ray diffraction pattern of Biobon in comparison to natural bone is shown in Fig. 2.1.1 c. Although similar to natural bone, HA diffraction peaks are distinctly broader. The X-ray diffraction pattern of Calcibon in contrast to the pattern of synthetic HA can be seen in Fig. 2.1.1 d.

Comparative In Vivo Studies

Materials and Methods

In order to evaluate characteristics such as osseointegration, osteoinduction, biocompatibility, and degradation of CaP-based implants, their biological reactivity has been investigated in various animal models. Cylindrical bone defects were created by using a diamond-coated drill (diamond bone-cutting system) with water irrigation. The sizes of the defects were 9.6 mm diameter and 10 mm depth in miniature pigs, 11 mm diameter and 20 mm depth in sheep, and 5.6 mm and 8 mm in rabbits, respectively. The animals were left in vivo for different periods (Table 2.1.2).

Using the method of Donath and Breuner [27] undecalcified samples were embedded in methyl methacrylate and sawed into 20-µm sections for histological examinations under light microscopy. Subsequently the sections were stained with toluidine blue.

Enzymatic detection of tartrate-resistant acidic phosphatase (TRAP) activity was performed by incubation of the slices in a solution of naphthol AS-BI phosphate (Sigma Chemical) and fast red violet LB salt (Sigma Chemical) in 0.2 M acetate buffer (pH 5.0) containing 50 mM (+) tartaric acid for 20 min at 37 °C. Then the slices were counterstained with haematoxylin.

For immunocytochemistry, decalcified samples of the defect areas were embedded in paraffin and cut on a microtome into 5-µm sections. The sections were treated with xylol, dehydrated in alcohol, and washed in phosphate-buffered saline before they were incubated with primary antibodies against CD44 (Serotec, UK) and CD68 (DAKO, Denmark) for 1 h at room temperature. Further labelling was performed by using biotinylated secondary antibodies (Biologo, Germany) and exposure to the avidin-biotin complex (Vectastain Elite Kit, Vector, Germany). Diamino-benzidine-tetrahydrochloride (Biologo, Germany) or NovaRed (Vector Laboratories, Burlingame, CA) served as chromogens. The specificity of all immunohistochemical procedures was controlled by incubating sections without the primary antibody.

For ultrastructural examinations small samples were postfixed at 4 °C for 24 h in Yellow Fix (4% paraformaldehyde, 2% glutaraldehyde, 0.04% picric acid). After several washes in 0.1 M phosphate buffer (pH 7.2), the non-decalcified specimens were fixed for 2 h in 1% osmium tetroxide (OsO_4), washed carefully and repeatedly in 0.1 M phosphate buffer (pH 7.2), and dehydrated in series in graded ethanol. Subsequently the specimens were embedded in Epon (Serva, Heidelberg, Germany). Polymerisation was performed at 60 °C for 20 h. Thin sections were cut with a diamond

Table 2.1.2. Inorganic bone substitutes and animal model

Material	Species	Model	Follow-up
Endobon (Biomet-Merck)	Miniature pigs	Femoral condyle, press fit	42 days, 84 days
Cerabone (AAP-Mebio)	Rabbits	Femoral condyle, press fit	42 days, 84 days
Ceros 80 (Mathys)	Miniature pigs	Femoral condyle, press fit	42 days, 84 days
Biobon (α-BSM, Etex, 26, Biomet-Merck)	Sheep	Tibial head	42 days
Calcibon (Biomet-Merck)	Sheep	Tibial head	5 days, 10 days, 42 days
Ostim (AAP-Mebio)	Sheep	Tibial head	30 days, 60 days
Ostim (AAP-Mebio)	Rabbits, Miniature pigs	Femoral condyle, press fit	10 days, 20 days, 40 days

knife (45°, Diatome, Switzerland) on an Ultracut (Reichert-Jung, Germany). Semithin sections (1 μm) were stained with Richardson (1% methylene blue, 1% borax, 1% azure II). Ultrathin sections (80 nm) were counterstained with uranyl acetate and lead citrate (Reichert Ultrostainer, Leica, Germany) and examined in a Zeiss EM 109 transmission electron microscope.

In order to study the temporal pattern of bone formation, fluorochrome labelling by means of tetracycline, alizarin complexon, calcein green, and calcein blue was performed at defined moments of the implantation periods.

Results and Discussion

HA Ceramics

The histological response to implants of different chemistry and structure was similar in HA ceramics but differed considerably when resorbable implants were used. In sintered HA ceramics (Fig. 2.1.2 a, b), active areas of bone deposition as well as resorption and remodelling were present. Bone ingrowth started (Fig. 2.1.2 c) from the fifth week onward and was complete after 10 weeks. At this time the bone around the completely integrated implant underwent remodelling caused by osteoclastic (Fig. 2.1.2 d) and osteoblastic activities. Abundant evidence of osteoblastic activity could be seen during the early stages of reconstitution, but particularly at the time when appositional activity was present. Bone ingrowth tended to proceed from the bottom of the defect as well as from the walls. There were no signs of fibrous encapsulation, but in some histological sections aggregations of HA crystallites surrounded by macrophages could be observed (Fig. 2.1.2 e). This phenomenon might have been caused by the implantation procedure. However, due to their porosity, osteoconductive HA implants can undergo a significant degree of degradation and resorption. Apposition of lamellar bone along the implant surfaces could be seen 4–6 weeks after HA ceramic implantation (Fig. 2.1.2 f).

Considering their properties, porous and dense HA implants cause different tissue responses. Ultimately, porosity and interconnectivity of a ceramic are the determining factors for the amount and type of newly formed bone.

All in all, HA ceramics with an interconnective pore system are highly osteoconductive and act as a scaffold for appositional bone formation. When the newly formed bone has grown through all the pores of an osteoconductive material, the implant–bone composite changes its original biomechanical properties.

Calcium Phosphate Cements

By using the sheep tibial head defect model, it became evident that cellular degradation of both CaP cements – Biobon and Calcibon – coincided with the formation of new bone. Bone formation had already occurred 6 weeks after implantation (Fig. 2.1.4 a). In semi-thin sections the close association between osteoblasts, the newly formed bone, and the implant surfaces could be seen (Fig. 2.1.3 a–d). The defect areas, filled either with Calcibon (Fig. 2.1.3 a, b) or Biobon (Fig. 2.1.3 c, d) were characterised by long slender projections of bone marrow forming a circumscribed labyrinth system within the cements. The bone marrow projections contained numerous cells and capillaries. Heterogeneous morphology of the cells was caused by their different stages of maturation and by the presence of different cell types. Bone marrow areas facing the cement surfaces were covered with bands of osteoblasts generating the new bone matrix in the direction of the implants. Due to proceeding centripetal osseous bone ingrowth, which started from the host bone, complete filling of the defects could be seen 48 weeks after implantation (Fig. 2.1.4 c). Fluorescence labelling done at distinct moments of the implantation periods revealed the temporal bone formation pattern. Alizarin red, injected at day 34 and day 38 after implantation, had caused the red-coloured bone shown in Fig. 4 b and d, indicating bone formation from day 34 on. Due to calcein green injections at day 9 and day 5 prior to explantation, green-coloured bone indicated bone formation at later implantation periods (Fig. 2.1.4 b, d).

Regarding the degradation pattern of the CaP cements investigated, multinucleated cells localised along the cement surfaces, and in close vicinity to the osteoblasts, can be seen histologically (Fig. 2.1.3 a–d). Comparative ultrastructural investigations of both implants – Biobon and Calcibon – performed 6 weeks after implantation, showed that the multinucleated cells were osteoclasts (Fig. 2.1.5 a, b), which expressed high levels of TRAP (Fig. 2.1.5 c). These findings are in accordance with investigations documenting that osteoclasts are able to resorb calcium phosphates [28–31]. Recent in vitro experiments have provided additional information regarding the physiological functions of osteoclasts during the degradation of CaP surfaces [31–33]. These studies ascribe a role to osteoclasts in phagocytosis without denying

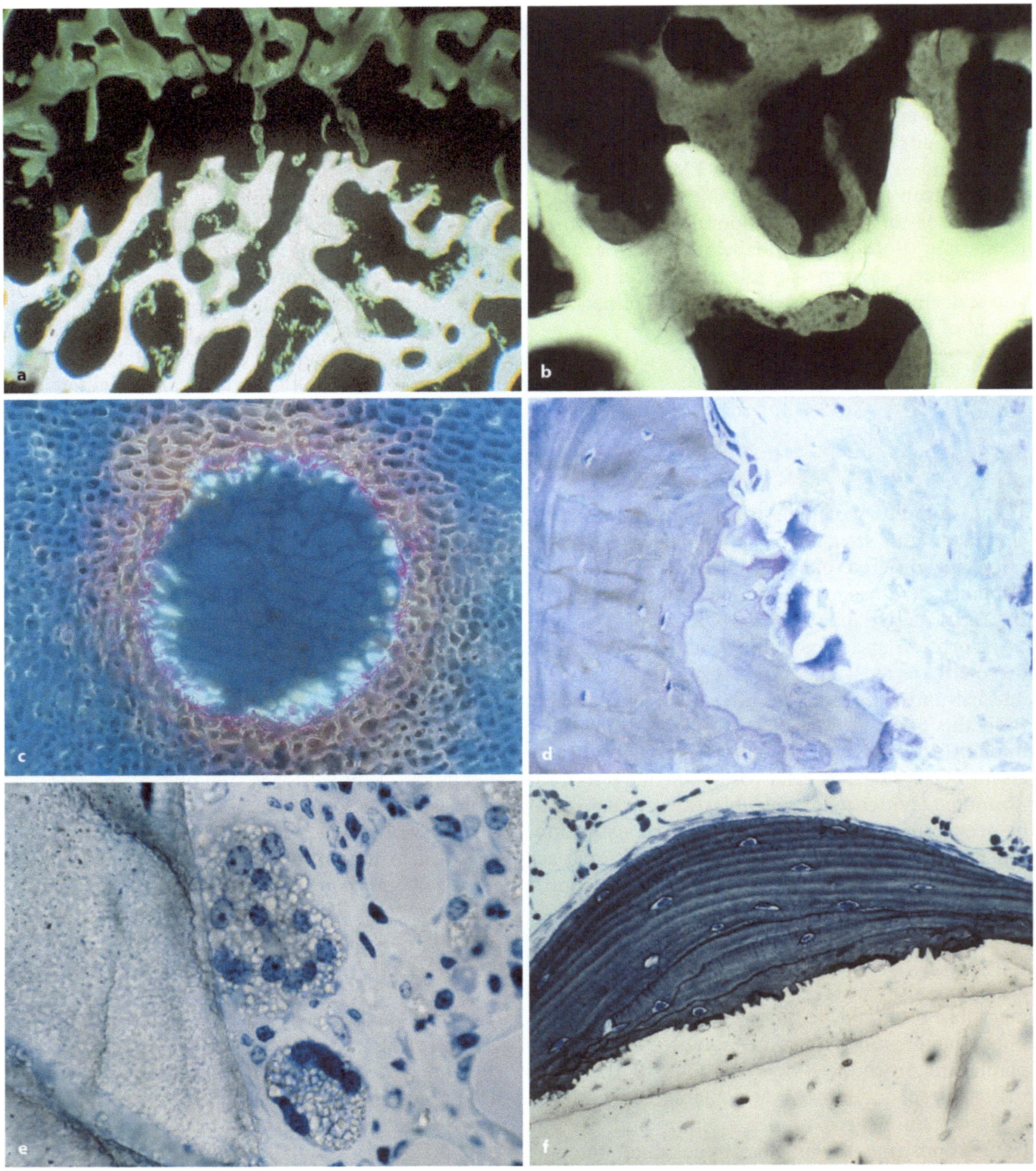

Fig. 2.1.2. a After implantation of bovine bone-derived HA, bone formation can be seen within the interface region as shown by microradiography. b Bovine bone-derived HA revealing areas of bone deposition. Microradiography. c Bone ingrowth has already started 42 days after implantation of an HA ceramic. d The resorption lacunae along the bone surface are caused by resorption activity of osteoclasts. Histological section, toluidine blue, ×125. e HA crystals have been phagocytosed by multinucleated giant cells. Histological section, toluidine blue, ×640. f Lamellar bone formation can be seen along the external ceramic surface 84 days after implantation in the rabbit. Histological section, toluidine blue, ×250

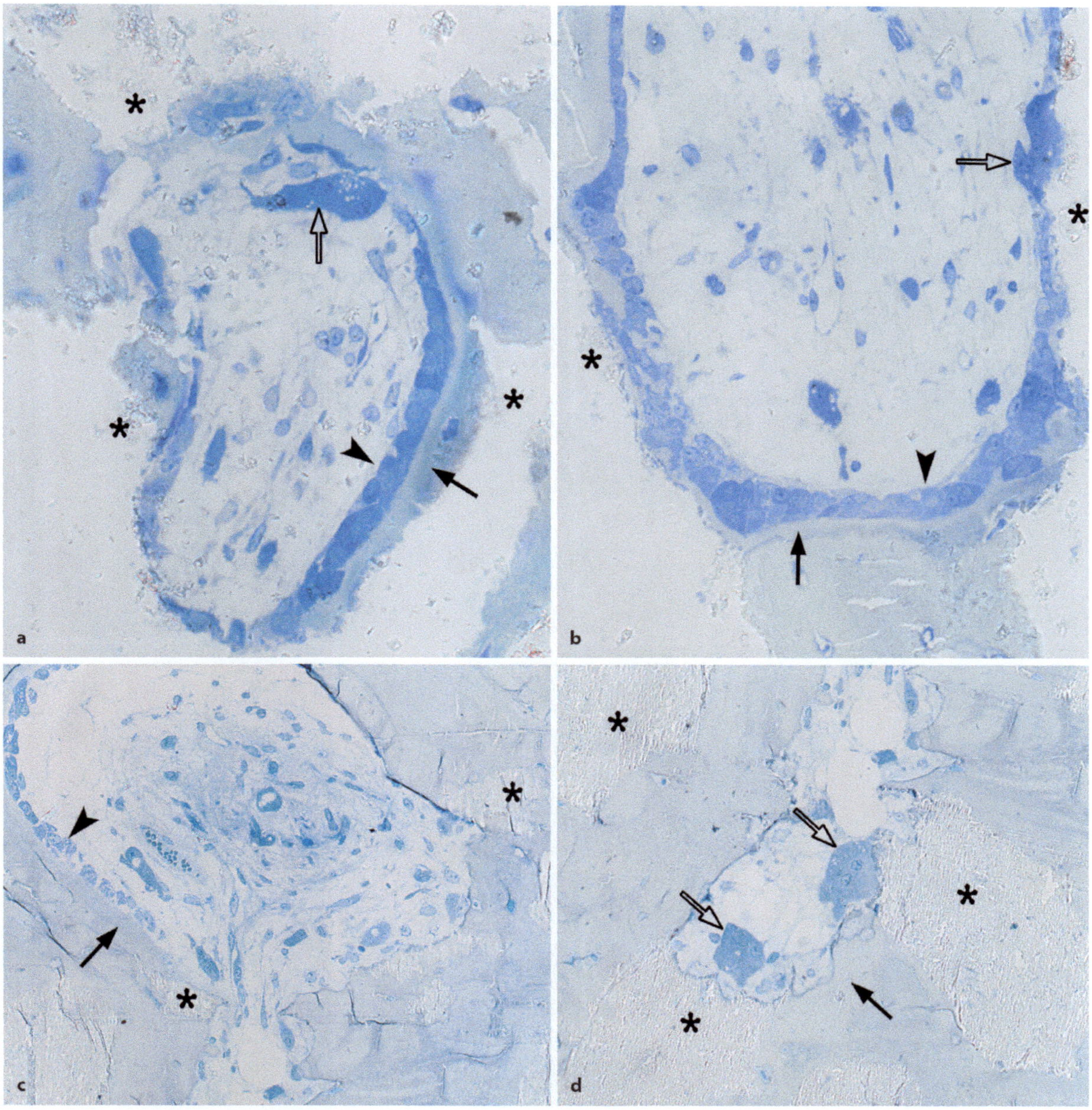

Fig. 2.1.3 a, b. Six weeks after implantation of the CaP cement Calcibon (*asterisks*) into the tibial head defect of sheep, the coincidence of bone formation (*arrows*), mediated by osteoblasts (*arrowheads*), and degradation, due to the activity of osteoclasts (*transparent arrow*), can be seen. Semithin sections, toluidine blue, a ×430, b ×380. c, d Successful bony integration of an implant, as shown in the case of Biobon (*asterisks*) 24 weeks after implantation, requires both osteoblastic (*arrowheads*) and osteoclastic (*transparent arrows* in d) activities. The newly developed bone (*arrows*) is in close contact with the implant surfaces. Semithin sections, toluidine blue, c ×230, d ×250

their resorption capacity. This observation has been confirmed by our in vivo investigation into osteoclast-mediated degradation of Biobon 6 weeks after implantation into tibial head defects of sheep [34].

Successful incorporation of an implant, its degradation, and its subsequent replacement by autologous tissue are dependent upon the cellular responses during the initial and chronic inflammatory phases of healing [35]. The steps toward successful osseointegration and bone healing are mediated by highly interrelated implant characteristics such as surface composition, surface roughness, surface energy, and surface topography [35, 36]. Especially in connection with the factors that govern osteoclastic resorption, the surface characteristics play an important role by influencing the types of cells that attach to the implant [35, 36].

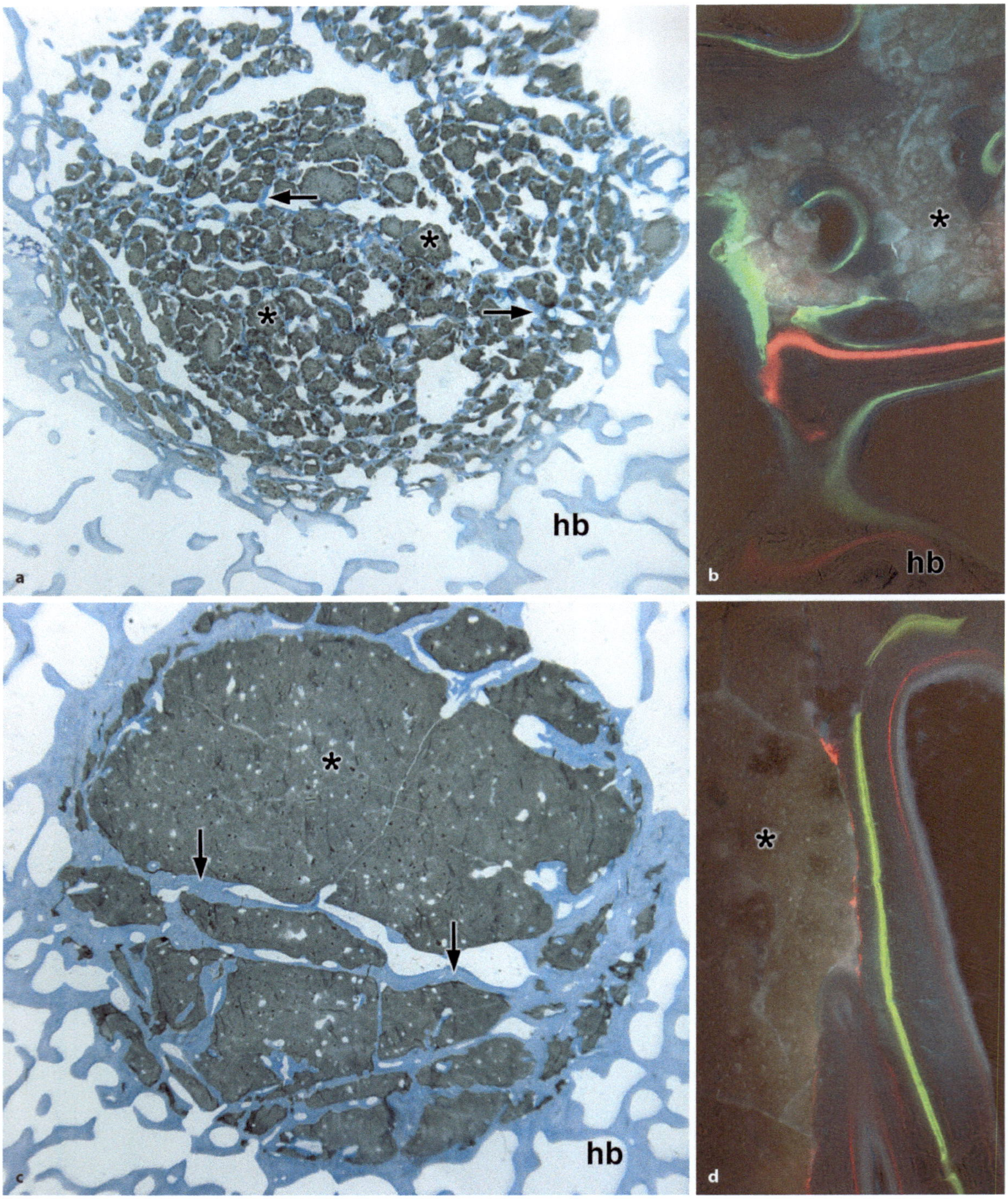

Fig. 2.1.4. a Six weeks after implantation of Biobon into tibial head defects, bone formation has occurred in an osteoconductive manner starting from the bottom and the walls of the defect, as shown histologically after toluidine blue staining (*hb* host bone), ×8.2. b Fluorescence labelling performed at defined moments of the implantation period of Biobon (*asterisks*) reveals the temporal pattern of bone formation, ×86. c Histological overview of the defect area 48 weeks after implantation of Calcibon (*asterisks*) into the tibial head of sheep, toluidine blue, ×8.2. d Due to alizarin and calcein green injections red- and green-coloured bone, formed during distinct implantation periods, can be seen, ×86

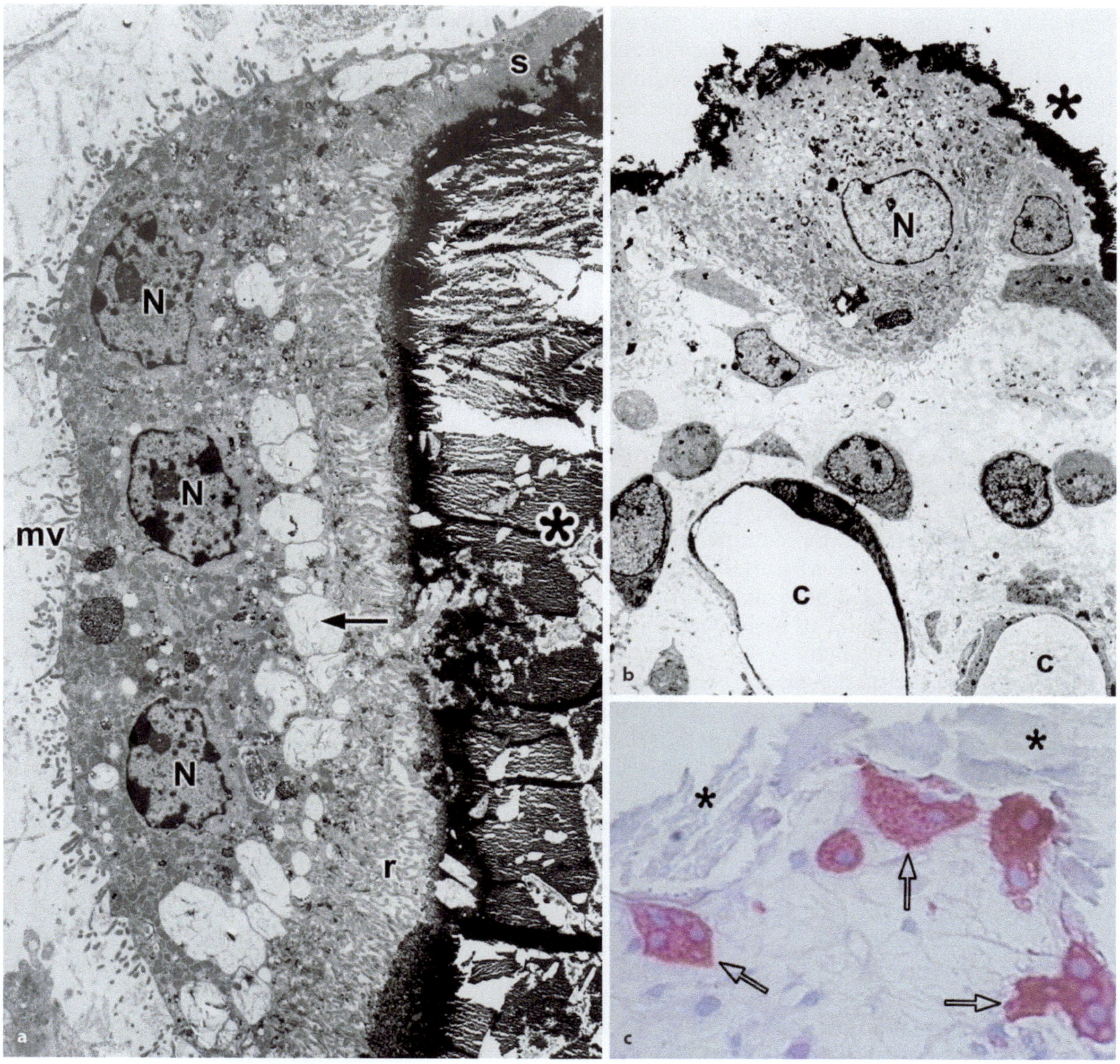

Fig. 2.1.5. a As shown ultrastructurally, osteoclasts can be seen along the cement surface of Biobon (*asterisks*) after 6 weeks of implantation. Osteoclasts are polarised cells that reveal typical morphological features, such as the ruffled border (*r*), facing the cement surface, the basal microvilli (*mv*), and the sealing zone (*s*). The nuclei (*N*) are localised towards the basis of the cell, ×3800. b Ultrastructural overview of an osteoclast adhering at the surface of the CaP cement Calcibon (*asterisk*) after 6 weeks of implantation. Within the underlying tissue, capillaries (*c*) can be seen, ×2155. c Multinucleated cells (*transparent arrows*) localised at the implant (Biobon, *asterisks*) surface express high levels of TRAP. Semithin section counterstained with haematoxylin, ×500

Rough apatitic surfaces appear to be more suitable for osteoclastic attachment than smooth surfaces [37]. Macrophages are supposed to be involved in "cleaning" the surface of dense HA implants from loose implant particles via phagocytosis [36], whereas attachment of osteoclasts to the implant surface is mediated largely by extracellular matrix proteins [35]. Thus, the protein adsorption capability of the implant surface has profound effects on the subsequent attachment of cells [35]. Adhesion of osteoclasts to the implant surface by means of the $\alpha_v\beta_3$ integrin depends upon adsorption of extracellular matrix proteins containing an arginine–glycine–aspartic acid (RGD) binding site sequence such as vitronectin. In addition, the capability of osteoclasts to resorb CaP implants may also be related to the solubility of the implant. In contrast to the CaP used in the present study – displaying minimal solubility [25, 26] – CaP disks in vitro showing high solubility were not resorbed by osteoclasts [38]. This decrease in osteoclastic activity might be caused by environmental changes leading to high extracellular calcium levels, which in turn induce increased intracellular levels in osteoclasts responsible for the decreased podosome assembly and the resorption of osteoclasts [38]. Furthermore, osteoclastic resorption of apatite cements is totally different from that of sintered apatite, possibly because of differences in crystallinity. Although the data documenting the osteoclastic resorption capacity of sintered apatite are still contradictory, it is becoming clear that osteoclastic resorption activity of sintered apatite depends upon numerous parameters such as the method of sintering, sintering temperature, sintering period, porosity, and surface roughness [38]. Moreover, it has been taken into consideration that the appearance of osteoclasts at biomaterial surfaces depends on the length of time after implantation. As shown in Fig. 2.1.5, osteoclasts can be identified at the surfaces of CaP cements 6 weeks after implantation, while giant cells predominate along the surfaces of implanted CaP granules in early periods (e.g. 5 and 10 days after implantation; Fig. 2.1.6). These findings suggest that the presence of macrophage polykaryons and osteoclasts changes in the course of the implantation period, and that the appearance of a certain cell type – either giant cells or osteoclasts – depends strongly on the time period after implantation. The presence of giant cells in early periods is mainly caused by the occurrence of the host-foreign body response, which is a common phenomenon after implantation of any medical device. The foreign body response is initiated by the surgical procedure itself and by the exposure of the host tissue (e.g. bone) to the foreign material (e.g. implant), both of which lead to destruction of tissue integrity [39]. In response to the injury to blood vessel walls, circulating platelets release multiple growth factors, such as the vascular endothelial growth factor, platelet-derived growth factor and transforming growth factor-β (TGF-β), which activate and regulate cellular chain reactions associated with inflammation and healing [40]. In particular, TGF-β leads to chemotaxis of neutrophils and monocytes to the injury site [41], and within 48 h after implantation monocytes are the predominant cell type found at the tissue–implant interface [6]. Initial monocyte adhesion to the implant surfaces leads to differentiation into macrophages [7]. Cross-linking of Fc-receptors on activated macrophages induces the cells to release reactive oxygen species as well as hydrolytic enzymes [42], and to form foreign body giant cells [4–6]. Therefore, the presence of multinucleated giant cells at the surfaces of implants a few days after implantation is a "biological" phenomenon, which must be regarded as a part of the essential host immune response in favour of the restoration of tissue integrity. However, giant cells are also believed to be the central cellular mediators of the chronic inflammatory response to biomedical material implants [7] and have been observed at the implant–tissue interface for periods extending beyond years [43]. Therefore, information regarding the material- and time-dependent presence of adherent macrophages/giant cells at implant surfaces will reduce the risk of implant damage and chronic inflammatory responses after the use of bone substitutes [43, 44]. This, in turn, requires a better understanding of the mechanisms by which mononucleate macrophages adhere to implants, fuse with each other, and differentiate into either osteoclasts or giant cells. Both cell types, although distinct, share the same functional markers and both differentiate by fusion of precursors of the monocyte–macrophage lineage. Although it is well established that osteoclasts differentiate on bone, while giant cells differentiate primarily in chronic inflammatory sites, there is no information concerning the factors governing the differentiation along the distinct pathways. Especially, the mechanism of the fusion of mononuclear precursors into macrophage polykaryons or osteoclasts remains poorly understood. It is thought that the fusion process is based upon cell–cell adhesion, and involves an attachment mechanism as well as a fusion protein, similar to those used by viruses to fuse with host cells [45]. Although the fusion peptide has not yet been identified, increasing evidence suggests that CD44, a cell surface glycoprotein known to play a role in haematopoietic cell–cell adhesion, may control the mononucleate status of macrophages in tissues [45, 46]. This is supported by our results documenting that CD44 expression by macrophages is highly and transiently induced prior to macrophage multinucleation. Ten days after implantation of CaP granules into tibial head defects of sheep, numerous mononucleate macrophages – characterised immunohistochemically by their strong CD68 expression – invaded the defect area (Fig. 2.1.6 a, b). In close vicinity to the implant particles, the macrophages accumulated to form cell clusters (Fig. 2.1.6 c). Clustering is an essential step, because in order to fuse the cells must reach a critical density [45]. The plasma membranes of mononucleate macrophages exhibited a strong CD44 signal, whereas the signal of multinucleated macrophages was weaker. This expression pattern suggested that strong CD44 staining is functionally associated with the onset of cell fusion. Besides, CD44 distri-

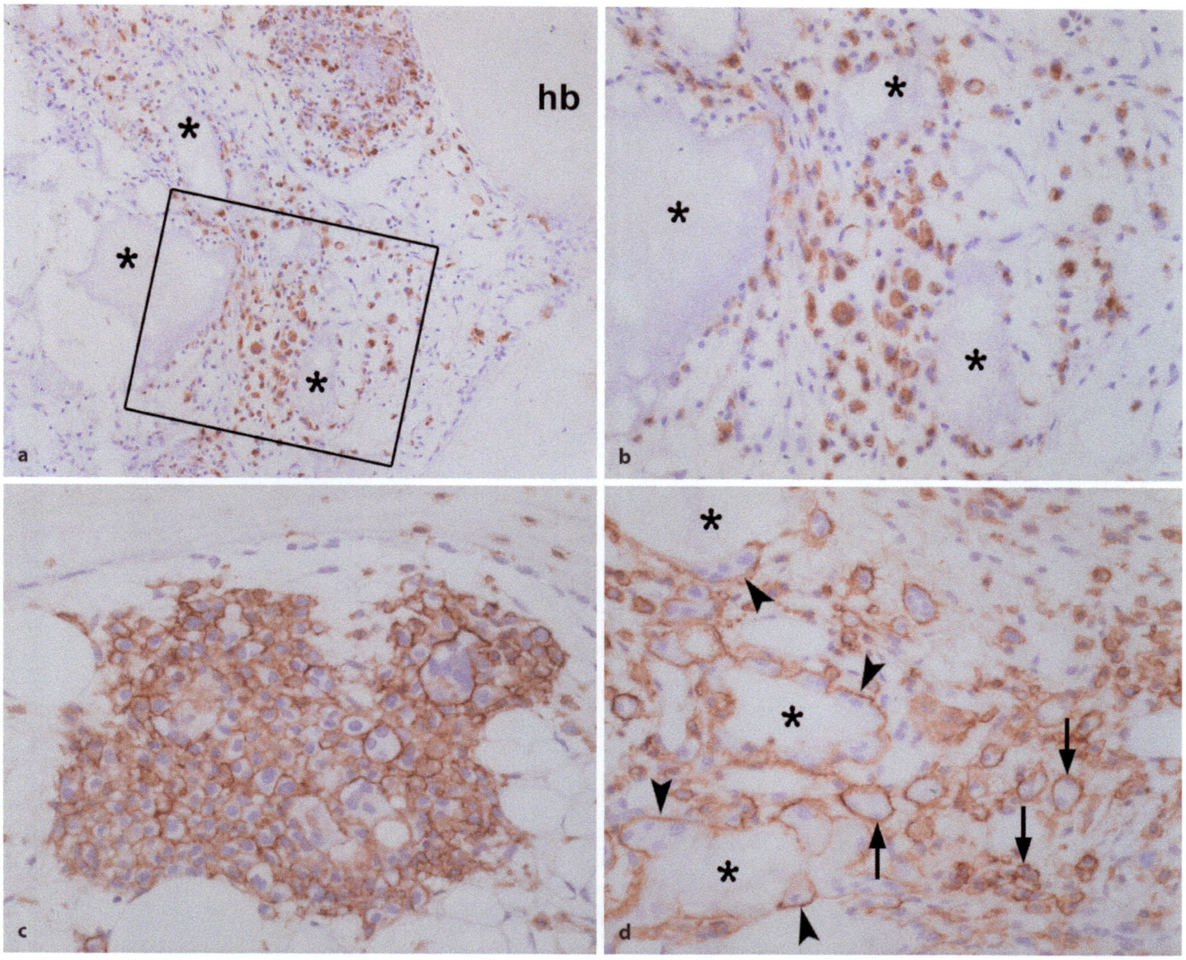

Fig. 2.1.6 a, b. Overview of the tibial head defect area 10 days after implantation of CaP granules (Calcibon). CD68-expressing macrophages are localised in the vicinity of the implant granules (*asterisks*). The boxed area is shown enlarged in b (*hb* host bone), a ×120, b ×250. c CD44-expressing macrophages form cell clusters in order to reach a critical density prior to fusion. Note that the CD44 signal is restricted to the plasma membranes, ×250. d Non-adherent macrophages express CD44 homogenously throughout the entire circumference of the plasma membrane (*arrows*), while macrophages that adhere at the implant (*asterisks*) and have already assumed a multinucleated state, reveal the expression of CD44 only along the basolateral aspects of the plasma membranes (*arrowheads*), ×250

bution along the plasma membrane changed when macrophages assumed a multinucleated state and adhered to the CaP surfaces: non-adherent cells revealed a strong homogeneous CD44 signal throughout the whole circumference of the plasma membrane, whereas in adherent multinucleated cells CD44 expression was limited to the basolateral plasma membrane (Fig. 2.1.6 d). This region represented the non-adherent domain of the cells. It has been suggested that CD44 clustering along the non-adherent domain secures the adherence of macrophages. In detail, this distribution pattern caused the lack of CD44 along the apical membrane, which represented the adherent domain of the cell. Due to the lack of CD44, this adherent region could be occupied by molecules that mediated strong adhesion [45, 46]. Recently, it has been documented that synthesis of osteopontin by macrophages is required for optimal cell surface expression of CD44, and that both osteopontin and CD44 are required for normal chemotaxis of macrophages [47].

Nanoparticular HA Paste

In the case of Ostim, the stoichiometry of the product is of importance. According to hydroxyapatite the calcium phosphate ratio of Ostim is 1.67. Its surface is expanded (100 m^2/g) because of the nano-sized crystals, and comparable to the surface area of bone mineral. The biomaterial Ostim is an injectable paste, which is well tolerated in sheep, minipigs and rabbits. It binds to bone

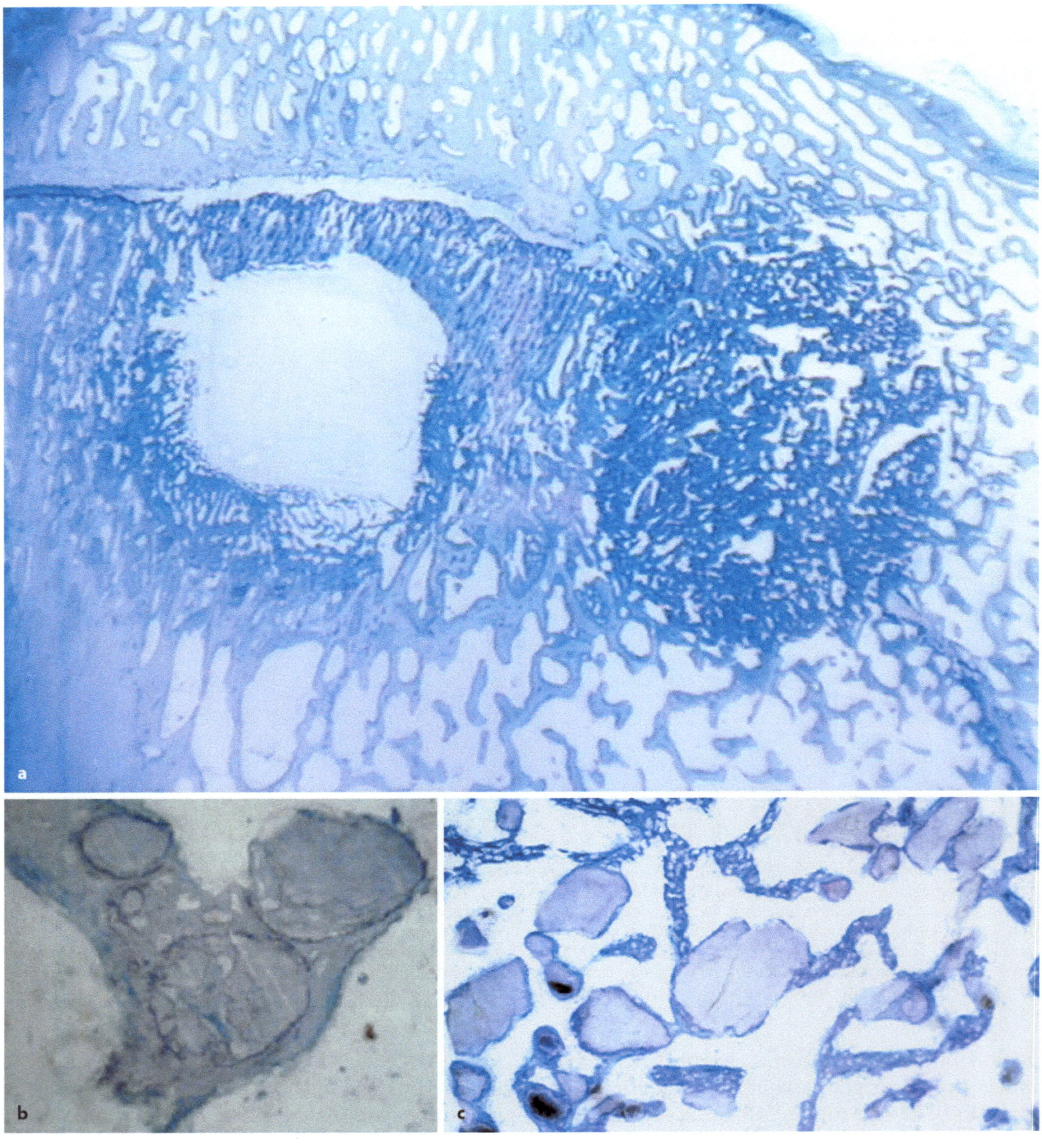

Fig. 2.1.7. a Defect bridging within the tibial head can be seen 60 days after implantation of Ostim in contrast to the empty defect. Histological section, toluidine blue, ×57. b Ostim globules surrounded by newly formed bone. Histological section, toluidine blue, ×250. c Bridging of the critical size defect in the rabbit 4 weeks after implantation of Ostim. Histological section, toluidine blue, ×115

and stimulates bone healing. As the paste does not harden in situ, cell migration into the implantation area coincides with revascularisation. Irrespective of the species used for the experimental procedures, fragmentation of the paste could be observed immediately after implantation. This fragmentation into round particles of different size must be regarded as an essential step toward successful reconstitution of tissue integrity. It enables cellular infiltration of the implantation site and enables osteoblasts to perform bone formation in an osteoconductive manner. After implantation of Ostim into tibial head defects of sheep, the defects were completely filled with new bone even after 60 days (Fig. 2.1.7 a). According to their role as guiding structures for bone formation, the implant particles were covered by newly formed bone (Fig. 2.1.7b). Due to proceeding bone healing, ramifications of trabecular bone could be seen between the implant particles (Fig. 2.1.7c). This spatial ingrowth pattern, taken together with the stimulation of osteoblast activity, supports complete reconstitution (e.g. bridging) of critical size defects of rabbits, sheep, and minipigs within 4 weeks.

Conclusion and Outlook

Autogenous bone grafting used to fill volumetric defects of bone is associated with the risk of morbidity of the patients, while the use of bone graft substitutes fills bony voids and reduces morbidity. Moreover, in contrast to allograft bone, these materials bear no risk of disease transmission. Depending upon the defect location and a determinate capacity of bone formation, the appropriate material must be selected from a number of commercially available bone substitutes. Therefore, knowledge of the characteristic features of bone substitutes is essential. Comparative animal studies are helpful in this field, but the validation of bone graft substitutes in the scope of clinical use provides essential data for approaches to the operative treatment of large bone defects.

Current strategies for bone tissue regeneration focus on rapid cell growth rates and high cell differentiation for the development of implantable matrices that mimic biological tissues [48]. One important approach to bone healing and bone ingrowth is the use of growth factors. Some of these factors, e.g. bone morphogenic proteins [49, 50], TGF-β [51–53], insulin-like growth factor [51, 53], and fibroblast growth factor (FGF) [54–60] act as local regulators of cellular activity and seem to have osteoinductive and angiogenetic potential.

Ikade et al. [61] reported the regeneration of several tissue types after the use of growth factors and different carriers. In a current study [62] bone formation and bone ingrowth in miniature pigs in response to bFGF-coated HA ceramic cylinders have been investigated. The experimental results prove that composite implants provide angiogenesis, bone formation and bone ingrowth that is comparable to the results of autogenous grafts and emphasise the importance of further research in the field of new carrier and release systems for growth factors.

Acknowledgements

We would like to thank Anne Hild, Iris Schütz and Maren Cassens for their excellent technical assistance, and the companies Biomet-Merck and Coripharm for financial support.

References

1. Schnettler R, Dingeldein D, Tausch W, Ritter B. Untersuchungen zur knöchernen Intergration einer Hydroxylapatit-Keramik und bFGF im Vergleich zu autogenen Spongiosazylindern. Osteo Int 1994; 2: 118–126.
2. Tay BK, Patel VV, Bradford DS. Calcium sulfate- and calcium phosphate-based bone substitutes. Mimicry of the mineral phase of bone. Orthop Clin North Am 1999; 30: 615–623.
3. Burstein FD. Bone substitutes. Cleft Palate Craniofac J 2000; 37: 1–4.
4. Collier TO, Anderson JM. Protein and surface effects on monocyte and macrophage adhesion, maturation, and survival. J Biomed Mater Res 2002; 60: 487–496.
5. Collier TO, Anderson JM, Brodbeck WG, Barber T, Healy KE. Inhibition of macrophage development and foreign body giant cell formation by hydrophilic interpenetrating polymer network. J Biomed Mater Res 2004; 69A: 644–650.
6. Matheson LA, Santerre JP, Labow RS. Changes in macrophage function and morphology due to biomedical polyurethane surfaces undergoing biodegradation. J Cell Physiol 2004; 199: 8–19.
7. Zhao Q, Topham NS, Anderson JM, Lodoen GA, Payet CR. Foreign-body giant cells and polyurethrane biostability: in vivo correlation of cell adhesion and surface cracking. J Biomed Mater Res 1991; 25: 177–183.
8. Wada T, Hara K, Quian HY, Wang F, Rosenzweig SA. Ultrastructural and histochemical study of β-tricalcium phosphate resorbing cells in periodontium of dog. J Period Res 1989; 24: 391–401.
9. Dersot JM, Colombier ML, Lafont J, Baroukh B, Septier D, Saffar JL. Multinucleated giant cells elicited around hydroxyapatite particles implanted in craniotomy defects are not osteoclasts. Anat Rec 1995; 242: 166–176.
10. Willert HG, Bertram HB, Buchhorn GH. Osteolysis in alloarthroplasty of the hip: the role of ultra-high molecule weight polyethylene wear particles. Clin Orthop 1990; 258: 95–107.
11. Anderson JM. Multinucleated giant cells. Curr Opin Hematol 2000; 7 (1): 40–47.
12. LeGeros RZ, Daculsi G. In vivo transformation of biphasic calcium phosphate ceramics: ultrastructural and physicochemical characterizations. In: Yamauro, Hench L, Wilson-Hench J, eds. Handbook of bioactive ceramics, Vol II. Florida: CRC Press Boca Raton, 1990; 17–28.
13. LeGeros RZ, LeGeros JP. Bone substitute materials and their properties. In: Schnettler R, Markgraf E, eds. Knochenersatzmaterialien und Wachstumsfaktoren. Stuttgart, New York: Thieme Verlag, 1997; 12–18.
14. De Bruijn JD, Klein CPAT, De Groot K, Van Blitterswijk I. The ultrastructure of the bone-hydroxyapatite interface in vitro. J Biomed Mater Res 1992; 26: 1365–1382.
15. Revell PA, Hing KA, Tanner KE, Best SM, Bonfield W. Osseointegration of porous hydroxyapatite. In: Schnettler R, Markgraf E, eds. Knochenersatzmaterialien und Wachstumsfaktoren. Stuttgart, New York: Thieme Verlag, 1997; 28–30.
16. Hende LL. Bioceramics and the origin of life. J Biomed Mater Res 1989; 23: 685–703.

17. Denissen HW, Van Dijk HJA, De Groot K, Klopper PJ, Vermiden JPW, Gehring AP. In: Hastings GW, Williams DF, eds. Mechanical properties of biomaterials. Wiley & Sons, 1980.
18. Eggli PS, Muller W, Schenk RK. Porous hydroxyapatite and tricalcium phosphate cylinders with two different pore size ranges implanted in the cancellous bone of rabbits. A comparative histomorphometric and histologic study of bony ingrowth and implant substitution. Clin Orthop 1988; 232: 127–138.
19. Bauer HJ, Bauer M, Dingeldein E. Zusammensetzung und Aufbau einer porösen Hydroxylapatitkeramik biologischer Herkunft. Osteo Int 1994; 2: 106–110.
20. Daculsi G, LeGeros RZ, Mitre D. Crystal dissolution of biological and ceramic apatites. Calcif Tiss Int 1989; 45: 95–103.
21. Nordström EG, Hero H, Jorgensen RB. Mechanical properties of hydroxyapatite/mica composite. Biomed Mater Eng 1994; 4: 309–315.
22. Nordström DG, Karson KH. Carbonate-doped hydroxyapatite. J Mater Sci Mater Med 1990; 1: 182–184.
23. Daculsi G, Bouler JM. Bone bioactive ceramic interface: a dynamic process. In: Schnettler R, Markgraf E, eds. Knochenersatzmaterialien und Wachstumsfaktoren. Stuttgart, New York: Thieme Verlag, 1997; 23–27.
24. Daculsi G, Dard M. Bone calcium-phosphate ceramic interface. Osteo Int 1994; 2: 153–156.
25. Knaack D, Goad MEP, Aiolova M, Rey C, Tofighi A, Chakravarthy P, Duke Lee D. Resorbable calcium phosphate bone substitute. J Biomed Mater Res 1998; 43: 399–409.
26. Knaack D, Aiolova M, Tofighi A, Catalano A, Duke Lee D. A fully resorbable calcium phosphate bone substitute. In: Vincenzini P, ed. Materials in clinical applications. Techna Srl 1999; 55–75.
27. Donath K, Breuner G. A method for the study of undecalcified bones and teeth with attached soft tissue. J Oral Path 1982; 11: 318–326.
28. Baslé MF, Chappard D, Grizon F, Filmon R, Delecrin J, Daculsi G, Rebel A. Osteoclastic resorption of Ca-P biomaterials implanted in rabbit bone. Calcif Tissue Int 1993; 53: 348–356.
29. Yamada S, Heymann DM, Bouler JM, Daculsi G. Osteoclastic resorption of biphasic calcium phosphate ceramic *in vitro*. J Biomed Mat Res 1997; 37: 346–352.
30. Yamada S, Heymann D, Bouler JM, Daculsi G. Osteoclastic resorption of calcium phosphate ceramics with different hydroxyapatite/β-tricalcium phosphate ratios. Biomaterials 1997; 18: 1037–1041.
31. Heymann D, Guicheux J, Rouselle AV. Ultrastructural evidence *in vitro* of osteoclastic-induced degradation of calcium phosphate ceramic by simultaneous resorption and phagocytosis mechanisms. Histol Histopathol 2001; 16: 37–44.
32. Wang W, Ferguson DPJ, Quinn JMW, Simpson AHRW, Athanasou NA. Osteoclasts are capable of particle phagocytosis and bone resorption. J Pathol 1997; 182: 92–98.
33. Wang W, Ferguson DPJ, Quinn JMW, Simpson AHRW, Athanasou NA. Biomaterial particle phagocytosis by bone-resorbing osteoclasts. J Bone Joint Surg 1997; 79-B: 849–856.
34. Wenisch S, Stahl JP, Horas U, Heiss C, Kilian O, Trinkaus K, Hild A, Schnettler R. In vivo mechanisms of hydroxyapatite ceramic degradation by osteoclasts: fine structural microscopy. J Biomed Mater Res 2003, 67A (3): 713–718.
35. Kieswetter K, Schwartz Z, Dean DD, Boyan BD. The role of implant surface characteristics in the healing of bone. Crit Rev Oral Biol Med 1996, 7 (4): 329–345.
36. Müller-Mai CM, Voigt C, Gross U. Incorporation and degradation of hydroxyapatite implants of different surface roughness and surface structure in bone. Scanning Microsc 1991; 4: 501–511.
37. Gomi K, Lowenberg B, Shapiro G, Davies JE. Resorption of synthetic hydroxyapatite by osteoclasts *in vitro*. Biomaterials 1993; 14: 91–96.
38. Doi Y, Iwanaga H, Shibutani T, Moriwaki Y, Iwayama Y. Osteoclastic responses to various calcium phosphates in cultures. J Biomed Mater Res 1999, 47: 424–433.
39. Brodbeck WG, Shive MS, Colton E, Nakayama Y, Matsuda T, Anderson JM. Influence of biomaterials surface chemistry on the apoptosis of adherent cells. J Biomed Mater Res 2001; 55: 661–668.
40. Braddock M. The transcription factor Egr-1: a potential drug in wound healing and tissue repair. Ann Med 2001; 33 (5): 313–318.
41. Wahl SM, Hunt DA, Wakefield LM, McCartney-Francis N, Wahl LM, Roberts AB, Spon MB. Transforming growth factor beta induces monocyte chemotaxis and growth factor production. Proc Natl Acad Sci USA 1987; 84 (16): 5788–5792.
42. Cannon GJ, Swanson JA. The macrophage capacity for phagocytosis. J Cell Sci 1992; 101: 907–913.
43. Anderson JM. Implant retrieval and evaluation in biomaterials science: an introduction to materials in medicine. In: Ratner BD, Hoffmann AS, Schoen FJ, Lemons JE, eds. New York: Academic Press, 1996; 451–455.
44. Brodbeck WG, Patel J, Voskerican G, Christenson E, Shive MS, Nakayama Y, Matsuda T, Ziats N, Anderson JM. Biomaterial adherent macrophage apoptosis is increased by hydrophilic and anionic substrates in vivo. PNAS 2002; 99 (16): 10287–10292.
45. Vignery A. Osteoclasts and giant cells: macrophage-macrophage fusion mechanism. Int J Exp Pathol 2000; 81: 291–304.
46. Sterling H, Saginario C, Vignery A. CD44 occupancy prevents macrophage multinucleation. J Cell Biol 1998; 143 (3): 837–847.
47. Zhu B, Suzuki K, Goldberg HA, Rittling SR, Denhardt DT, McCulloch CAG, Sodek J. Osteopontin modulated CD44-dependent chemotaxis of peritoneal macrophages through G-protein coupled receptors: evidence of a role for an intracellular form of osteopontin. J Cell Physiol 2004; 198: 155–167.
48. Liebmann-Vinson A, Hemperly JJ, Guarino RD, Spargo CA, Heidaran MA. Bioactive extracellular matrices: biological and biochemical evaluation. In: Lewandrowski KU, Wise DL, Trantolo DJ, Gresser JD, Yaszemski MJ, Altobelli DE, eds. Tissue engineering and biodegradable equivalents. Scientific and clinical applications. New York: Basel, 2002; 709–764.
49. Urist MR. Bone: formation by autoinduction. Science 1965; 150: 853–899.
50. Urist MR, Lietze A, Dawsen E. Tricalcium phosphate delivery system for bone morphogenetic protein. Clin Orthop 1984; 187: 277–284.
51. Schmidmaier G, Wildemann B, Heeger J, Gabelein T, Flyvbjerg A, Bail HJ, Raschke M. Improvement of fracture healing by systemic administration of growth hormone and local application of insulin-like growth factor-1 and transforming growth factor-beta1. Bone 2002; 31: 165–172.
52. Yu Y, Yang JL, Chapman-Sheath PJ, Walsh WR. TGF-beta, BMPS, and their signal transducing mediators, Smads, in rat fracture healing. J Biomed Mater Res 2002; 60: 392–397.
53. Blumenfeld I, Srouji S, Lanir Y, Laufer D, Livne E. Enhancement of bone defect healing in old rats by TGF-beta and IGF-1. Exp Gerontol 2002; 37: 553–565.
54. Tabata Y, Ikada Y. Vascularization effect of basic fibroblast growth factor released from gelatin hydrogels with different biodegradabilities. Biomaterials 1999; 20: 2169–2175.
55. Rifkin DB, Moscatelli D. Structural characterization and biological functions of basic fibroblast factor. J Cell Biol 1989; 109: 1–6.

56. Abraham JA, Wlang JL, Tunolo A, Mergin A, Friedmann J. Human basic fibroblast growth factor: nucleotide sequence and genomic organization. EMBO J 1986; 5: 2523–2528.
57. Aspenberg P, Wans JS. Basic fibroblast growth factor. Dose- and time dependance in rats. Trans Orthop Res Soc 1994; 19: 18111.
58. Globus RK, Petterson-Bückendahl P, Gospodarowicz D. Regulation of bovine bone cell proliferation by fibroblast growth factor and transforming growth factors. Endocrinology 1988; 123: 98–105.
59. Gospodarowicz D, Ferrara N, Schweigerer G, Neufeld G. Structural characterization and biological functions of fibroblast growth factor. Endocrinol Rev 1987; 8: 95–114.
60. Jingnski S, Hedemann A, Kana SK, Mecey LR, Bolander ME. Acid fibroblast growth factor injection stimulates cartilage enlargement and inhibits cartilage gene expressions in rat fracture. J Orthop Res 1990; 8: 364–371.
61. Ikade Y, Tabata Y, Lewandrowski KU, Wise DL, Tumolo DJ, Gresser JD, Yaszenaski AJ, Altobellio DE. Tissue engineering and biodegradable equivalents. Scientific and clinical applications. New York: Basel, 2002; 145–163.
62. Schnettler R, Alt V, Dingeldein E, Pfefferle HJ, Kilian O, Meyer C, Heiss C, Wenisch S. Bone ingrowth in bFGF coated hydroxyapatite ceramic implants. Biomaterials 2003; 24 (25): 4603–4608.

Osteoinduction: Basic Principles and Developments

R. Capanna, P. De Biase

Introduction

The term osteoinduction applies to the process by which osteogenesis is aroused. The process itself is a complex mechanism that induces, stimulates and regulates the production of calcified bone matrix. This phenomenon regularly takes place in any type of bone healing process. Osteoinduction provides the recruitment of immature cells and the stimulation of the mesenchymal stem cells along an osteoblastic pathway and leads these cells in the formation and apposition of new bone until healing. In the normal healing process osteoinduction plays perhaps the most critical role in effecting bone repair.

Osteoinduction and the intrinsic osteoinductive properties of native bone were emphasized by the historical works of Marshall Urist in 1965. He demonstrated that demineralized bone matrix (DBM) may induce a local inflammatory response, which leads to formation of bone matrix in the muscle pouch of rats. From these experiments the concept of osteoinduction has grown and has been refined over the years to understand the different steps and the different actors playing their roles. Urist [1] defined this discovery of the bone induction principle few years later and he and his co-workers continued the studies until this capacity was attributed to some polypeptides named bone morphogenetic proteins (BMPs). Only 20 years later the genetic sequences of the BMPs were identified and classified with the identification of a number of different BMPs whose precise role in the osteoinduction process is still extensively studied and not well defined. But experimental and preclinical studies have shown also that the BMPs are not playing alone on this stage. Many proteins secreted by the cells are implied in the process of healing and new bone formation; to these factors has been generically assigned the term "growth factors" and an increasing number of these have been identified and used in experimental studies. The more debated are the transforming growth factor-β (TGF-β), the fibroblast growth factor (FGF), the insulin-like growth factor (IGF) and the platelet-derived growth factors (PDGF). Obviously these are only some of the variety of factors that participate in a normal healing process, but are those that seem more implied with bone apposition. More recently osteoinduction has seen the proposal of gene therapy for curing bone diseases such as osteogenesis imperfecta and osteopetrosis, but these experiments are still on the starting blocks and will only be presented here.

Basic Science and Clinical Applications

The repair of bone is a very complex mechanism regulated by numerous factors. All the proteins recognized to be involved in the process have been grouped by the scientific literature under the term "growth factors". Generally growth factors are proteins secreted by the cells or contained in the extracellular matrix that can act on appropriate target cells to initiate or amplify a specific action. They are considered signaling agents for cells and play an important role in bone and cartilage formation and repair. Their signal may be formulated in several ways: autocrine, paracrine or endocrine. The autocrine signal is produced by a cell to influence a cell of the same origin or a cell identical to the signaling cell in phenotype; paracrine signal is produced by a cell that induces a cell of a different phenotype but located close to the first cell; finally, the endocrine signal is intended to induce or influence a cell of a different phenotype and located in a remote site. Growth factors may have all these capacities together and produce a local and distant response with the same mechanism. The protein that constitutes the signal binds to a ligand expressed on the cell membrane, which is a target receptor that activates an intracellular transduction signal; this reaches the nucleus and produces the designated response. This coupling is termed ligand–receptor interaction and may be a very selective process

Table 2.2.1. Summary of growth factor characteristics

Growth factor	Location	Membrane receptor	Proved function
Transforming growth factor beta (TGF-β)	Platelets, bone extracellular matrix, cartilage matrix	Serine threonine sulfate	Pleiotropic growth factor stimulates undifferentiated mesenchymal cell proliferation
Bone morphogenetic protein (BMP)	Osteoprogenitor cells, osteoblasts, bone extracellular matrix	Serine threonine sulfate	Promotes differentiation of mesenchymal cells into chondrocytes and osteoblasts, promotes differentiation of osteoprogenitors into osteoblasts, influences skeletal pattern formation
Fibroblast growth factors (FGF)	Macrophages, mesenchymal cells, chondrocytes, osteoblasts	Tyrosine kinase	Mitogenic for mesenchymal cells, chondrocytes, and osteoblasts
Insulin-like growth factors (IGF)	Bone matrix, osteoblasts, chondrocytes	Tyrosine kinase	Promotes proliferation and differentiation of osteoprogenitor cells
Platelet-derived growth factor (PDGF)	Platelets, osteoblasts	Tyrosine kinase	Mitogen for mesenchymal cells and osteoblasts; macrophage chemotaxis

with only one growth factor coupling with a single type of ligand, or the same protein may bind to several ligands, which in turn may be activated by different growth factors. The final result of the coupling of the growth factor with the membrane receptor is, however, a common pathway descending from the activation of an intracellular transducer. The transmembrane transmission of signal is common to numerous membrane receptors and is based on a conformational change in the transmembrane receptor. The receptors of different growth factors have been identified and studied. In the chain to the nucleus and activation of a specific gene or gene sequence, common to all is a transcription factor that is able to enter the nucleus and activate the message intended by the original ligand bound at the receptor. The receptors for BMP and TGF-β are, not surprisingly, very similar and both proceed by an intracellular signaling process requiring a SMAD protein [2]. The two factors, however, differ because the SMAD activated is different between TGF-β and BMP and also the final effect is different. Also other transmembrane receptors have been identified, like those for FGF and PDGF, which have a tyrosine kinase activity. These latter growth factors show some overlap in the downstream pathways. Growth factors with known activities are summarized in Table 2.2.1. We will now describe in detail the basic science experiments for each growth factor and its relevance in clinical use.

Transforming Growth Factor-β

Transforming growth factor-β is not really a single protein but is the term often used to identify a group of proteins that belong to the so-called TGF-β superfamily. These proteins are related in structure and location and can be found in many tissues around the body, but are more pronounced in bone, cartilage and platelets. The BMPs are also part of this superfamily, as well as some growth differentiation factors. The TGF-β proteins are related to cell proliferation, differentiation and matrix synthesis. In animal experiments (rabbits), when TGF-β was looked for in critical size bone defects, it was found by immunohistochemical staining to be present a few days after the defect was created [3]. It was expressed by endosteal cells, medullary mesenchymal cells and after several more days by osteoblasts and osteocytes. Its appearance was preceded by the presence of basic FGF that was already stained in the inflammatory cells.

In Vitro Results

The effects of TGF-β may also be modulated and enhanced by the presence of other growth factors: TGF-β has been proven in an in vitro model to be capable of stimulating the proliferation and differentiation to chondrogenesis of cells cultured from periosteal explants, i.e. undifferentiated mesenchymal stem cells (MSC). Other growth factors such as IGF-I, when used in combination with TGF-β, enhance the effects on proliferation and cartilage formation, proved by immunohistochemical staining and histomorphometry [4].

The capacity of TGF-β to induce a chondrogenic pathway in MSC in vitro has also been evaluated by another recent study [5]: rat bone marrow cells were cultured and exposed to recombinant TGF-β for 16 days with the addition in the last 2 days of dexamethasone to promote osteogenesis. The culture obtained was transposed in an animal model (rat) and implanted subdermally in a diffusion chamber. The cultures produced cartilage or osteoid matrix depending on the type of TGF-β used, but real bone formation was noted only in another culture where a recombinant bone morphogenetic protein-2 (rhBMP-2) was present. This study therefore supports the most recent hypothesis of the importance of TGF-β as an inducer of replication of osteoblastic progenitors, but its insufficiency in promoting differentiation of these progenitor cells along the osteoblastic lineage. However, the same study demonstrated that the environment does make a difference. When the rat bone marrow cells were cultured in a DBM scaffold, every growth factor was capable of producing all the different phases of bone formation, for the inductive capacities of the DBM were sufficient to fill the gap within the different phases promoted by the independent growth factors. Previous studies in animal models demonstrated the importance of TGF-β to promote recruitment and proliferation of osteoblastic cells in artificially created defects.

In Vivo Results

Beck [6] showed that skull defects of rabbits healed in the presence of locally delivered TGF-β, while the control defects failed to heal without growth factors. However, the preclinical studies facing the fracture-healing model reported some very interesting and contrasting data. Lind [7] studied the effect of TGF-β delivered by injection with a miniosmotic pump in the osteotomy site of adult rabbit tibiae, which were stabilized with plate and screws. TGF-β at doses of 1 or 10 µg per day were administered in two groups for 6 weeks. The control group was treated only with standard plating. At the end of the study period the animals were killed and bone mineral content, the amount of callus formation, and mechanical properties of the callus were evaluated. The results showed no differences among the three groups with respect to bone mineral content or cortical thickness, but a definite, significant increase in callus formation in groups treated with TGF-β compared with the control group ($p=0.01$). The bending strength measured with the use of three-point bending demonstrated a significant increase in normal bending strength only between the group treated with the lower dosage of TGF-β and the control group ($p=0.03$). The author concluded that the mechanical strength was not significantly different due to immature formation of callus, but that TGF-β was efficient in increasing callus size.

One year later, Nielsen [8] evaluated the efficacy of two doses of TGF-β (4 or 40 ng) injected along the line of a rat tibial fracture, every other day for 40 days. Several mechanical tests were performed on the rat tibiae, but the only significant difference was the ultimate load to failure, which was higher in the group that had received the 40-ng dose compared with the group that had received the 4-ng dose and the control group (which had received no growth factor) ($p<0.01$). No difference with respect to stiffness or energy to failure between either of the two experimental groups and the control group was demonstrated. The conclusion of the authors was that the TGF-β induced a dose-dependent increase in the cross-sectional area of the callus and bone at the fracture line.

A final study reported quite different conclusions. Critchlow [9] evaluated the effect of exogenous TGF-β2 on the healing of 25 rabbit tibial fractures. The two groups differed in the mechanical synthesis of the fracture. In the first group the tibiae were fractured and then treated with a dynamic compression plate to achieve a stable mechanical system. In the second group the tibiae were stabilized with a plastic plate designed intentionally to leave a 0.5-mm gap to obtain an unstable mechanical system. The animals in both groups were treated with either 60 or 600 ng of TGF-β2 in a single dose administered after the fracture. The animals were killed at 5, 7, 10, and 14 days and no mechanical testing of the fracture site was performed. Using a point-counting method the authors determined the amount of bone, cartilage and fibrous tissue in the calluses. The animals treated with stable plating showed a callus composed almost entirely of bone, with no effect from the 60-ng injection and abundant callus formation in the animals treated with the 600-ng injections but with no increases in bone content. In contrast, animals with an unstable mechanical construct had minimal bone and cartilage formation after treatment with either 60 or 600 ng of TGF-β2. The author's conclusions were that in the initial healing phase TGF-β is not effective in promoting callus and bone formation.

The conclusion that can be drawn after the presentation of these studies and especially the latter one demonstrates the difficulties that are encountered in translating the results obtained from experimental and preclinical studies in the clinical setting, with several factors that can alter the normal healing process. What seems predictable from these data is that the osteoinductive properties of TGF-β are scarce and to obtain a valuable effect very high doses of this protein are required, which are probably not practical in a clinical setting.

Fibroblast Growth Factor

Fibroblast growth factors are a family of nine structurally related polypeptides that are characterized by their affinity for the glycosaminoglycan heparin-binding sites on cells. The most abundant FGFs in normal adult tissue are acidic fibroblast growth factor (FGF-1 or α-FGF) and basic fibroblast growth factor (FGF-2 or β-FGF). Both these FGFs promote growth and differentiation of a variety of cells, including epithelial cells, myocytes, osteoblasts, and chondrocytes. The FGF family of peptides transduces signals via a group of four receptors that contain distinct membrane-spanning tyrosine kinases. Mutations in FGF receptors have been associated with abnormalities in skeletal development. Mutations in fibroblast growth factor receptor-3 have been linked to several skeletal dysplasias, including achondroplasia, thanatophoric dysplasia (lethal neonatal dysplasia), and hypochondroplasia (a mild form of achondroplasia).

In Vivo Results

On the other hand, Mayahara and coauthors [10] reported data after intravenous administration of human basic FGF: 2 weeks after administration, basic FGF stimulated osteoblast proliferation and new bone formation in various skeletal bones in young and aged rats at dosage levels of 0.1 mg/kg per day and greater. Morphometry of the soft X-ray radiograms of cross-sections of the tibia indicated about a 20% increase in the calcified bone area of the diaphysis at 0.1 mg/kg per day. The Ca and hydroxyproline contents showed statistically significant increases at this dosage. The new bone formation was found only on the endosteal side, and no periosteal bone formation was found. Similar systemic osteogenic potential was seen after intravenous administration of other growth factors of the FGF family, human acidic FGF and human heparin-binding secretory transforming protein-1. However, even if definite activity of FGFs upon the skeleton development and the process of bone formation by the previous and several other studies has been demonstrated, its effect on fracture healing still remains unclear and debated.

Recently Zellin and coauthors [11] studied the activity of recombinant human fibroblast growth factor-2 (rhFGF-2) on the incorporation of autoclaved bone. Twenty-eight adult rats were subjected to bilateral parietal cranioplasties (4×6 mm), and 75% of the grafts were subjected to autoclaving and subsequently treated randomly according to one of the following strategies: no further treatment, or supplementation with bone marrow or rhFGF-2. The remaining 25% of the grafts were replanted as fresh autografts. The results were evaluated after 4 and 12 weeks by radiologic, histologic, and histomorphometric analyses. After 4 weeks, no major differences were observed between treatments. At 12 weeks, however, no distinction in graft revitalization between autografts and autoclaved grafts supplemented with rhFGF-2 was observed, whereas autoclaved grafts with or without bone marrow displayed significantly less revitalization compared with autografts. The authors concluded that the remodeling of autoclaved bone can be increased significantly by simultaneous supplementation with rhFGF-2.

Kato et al. [12] evaluated the effect of a single local injection of rhFGF-2 on the healing of segmental tibial defects in rabbits. In the tibiae of rabbits a 3-mm defect was created and fixed with an external device. Local injections of rhFGF-2 were used with increasing dosages (0, 50, 100, 200, and 400 μg). Healing was assessed with plain radiographs, histological analysis, and an evaluation of bone mineral content with use of dual-energy X-ray absorptiometry. Injection of the growth factor increased the volume and mineral content of newly made bone at the defect in a dose-dependent manner, with significant effects at concentrations of 100 μg or greater. These significant effects were observed at 5 weeks and later. One hundred micrograms of the growth factor increased the volume and mineral content of newly made bone by 95 and 36%, respectively, at 5 weeks.

Nakamura et al. [13] investigated the effect of recombinant human basic FGF on fracture healing using a tibial fracture in beagle dogs. Transverse fractures in the middle of the diaphyses were created in the right tibiae and basic FGF was injected into the fracture sites at a single dose of 200 μg. The fractures were stabilized by intramedullary nails. The time course of changes in callus volume and morphology of the fracture sites was evaluated at weeks 2, 4, 8, 16, and 32 after treatment, and the fracture strength was analyzed at weeks 16 and 32. At week 2, a radiogram of the fracture site showed obvious membranous ossification in the group injected with basic FGF. Basic FGF extended the callus area at week 4 and increased the bone mineral content in the callus at week 8. Basic FGF also increased the osteoclast number in the periosteal callus at weeks 2 and 4. In addition, intramembranous ossification was more pronounced in the rhFGF-2 group. In the basic FGF group, a maximal increase in the osteoclast index was found at week 4, and an identical increase was recognized in the control group at weeks 8 and 16. These findings strongly suggested that basic FGF stimulated not only callus formation but osteoclastic callus resorption. Bone mineral content in the basic FGF group was followed by a rapid decrease from week 8, while that in the control group was identical from week 4. Fracture strength of the basic FGF group showed significant recovery by week 16, and recovery was still evident by week 32. In contrast, callus volume in the control group did not change significantly from 8 to 16 weeks and fracture strength was low at 16 weeks. Mechanical properties of callus (maximum load, bending stress, and energy absorption) were significantly greater in the rhFGF-2 group than in the control group at both 16 ($p<0.05$) and 32 weeks ($p<0.05$), even after the fracture healed in both groups. These results suggest that rhFGF-2 accelerates bone repair and also stimulates remodeling of the callus, a process that restores the biomechanical properties to the bone.

The efficacy of basic FGF to accelerate fracture healing and callus formation was confirmed by Radomsky et al. [14] in a nonhuman primate fracture model. Fibroblast growth factor-2 or basic fibroblast growth factor (4 mg/ml), and hyaluronan, were combined into a viscous gel formulation intended for direct, percutaneous injection into fresh fractures. A bilateral 1-mm noncritical-sized osteotomy defect was surgically created in the fibulae of baboons. One side was injected with the preparation while the contralateral fibula was left untreated to serve as a negative control. Intact fibulae were harvested from an additional group of animals to provide a positive control. The osteotomy sites were treated with three different doses of rhFGF-2. A single direct administration of this hyaluronan/FGF-2 formulation to the defect site significantly promoted local fracture healing, as evidenced by increased callus formation and mechanical strength. Radiographic analysis showed that the callus area was statistically significantly larger at the treated sites than at the untreated sites. There were significant differences between energy to failure ($p\leq0.01$) and load at failure ($p\leq0.05$) between the treated and untreated osteotomy sites, but no differences in torsional stiffness were observed when treated animals were compared with untreated controls. Specimens treated with 0.1, 0.25, and 0.75 ml hyaluronan/FGF-2 demonstrated a 48, 50, and 34% greater average load at failure and an 82, 104, and 66% greater energy to failure than the untreated controls, respectively, without correlation between the dose and the response observed. The histologic analysis showed that the callus size, periosteal reaction, vascularity, and cellularity were consistently more pronounced in the treated osteotomies than in the untreated controls. The conclusion that can be drawn are that FGF-2 is very active in increasing callus formation, especially when combined with an appropriate scaffold, but the dose is not related strictly to the response.

The importance of an adequate scaffold for local delivery of growth factors was confirmed by Schnettler [15]. A cylindrical bone defect was created in both femur condyles of 24 miniature pigs using a saline-coated trephine. Sixteen of the 48 defects were filled with hydroxyapatite (HA) ceramic cylinders coated with 50 µg recombinant human basic FGF, uncoated HA cylinders, and with autogenous transplants, respectively. Fluorochrome-labeled histological analysis, histomorphometry, and scanning electron microscopy were performed. Complete bone ingrowth into basic FGF-coated HA implants and autografts was seen after 34 days compared to 80 days in the uncoated HA group. Also studies using other evaluation methods revealed comparable results of basic FGF-coated HA implants and autogenous grafts regarding angiogenesis, bone synthesis and bone ingrowth.

In a previously published study, data on the influence of FGF on fracture healing were not so successful. Bland and coauthors [16] studied the effect of both FGF-1 (acidic FGF) and -2 (basic FGF) on rabbit tibial fracture healing under stable and unstable mechanical conditions. The mechanical conditions were created by doing an osteotomy in the medial cortex of rabbit tibias and then fracturing them with three-point bending. The fractures were stabilized with two different osteosynthesis devices: a stainless steel dynamic compression plate or a plastic plate. At the fracture line a 0.5-mm gap was left to create instability of the fracture. On day 4 after fracture, 3 µg of either FGF-1 or FGF-2 was injected around the rabbit tibia. The animals were monitored radiographically and weight bearing was unrestricted. At 10 days the fracture site was removed and analyzed. Neither growth factor had a significant effect on either the size of, or the amounts of bone and cartilage in, the 10-day callus irrespective of the mechanical conditions under which the fracture was healing. The 10-day FGF-2-treated calluses were, however, more mature than the FGF-1-treated calluses because the cartilage was separated from the periosteum by bone and endochondral ossification had progressed further. The conclusion drawn from the authors was that the application of FGF-1 or FGF-2 to normally healing fractures of the rabbit tibia does not have a significant effect on the rate of healing.

The differences in the data reported by these studies are probably related to the method used to deliver the FGF at the fracture site and the importance of local release for several days. The sodium hyaluronate appears to be a valid scaffold for this growth factor and other scaffolds are probably also valuable in clinical use. However, it must be said that the data reported from basic science and clinical studies support the potential of FGFs in bone formation and healing but simultaneously underscore its capacity to act as a single regulator of this mechanism in the absence of other growth factors or supportive matrix.

Growth Hormone and Insulin-Like Growth Factor-I

Growth hormone (GH) and IGF-I play critical roles in skeletal growth and development, while their role in bone healing is not certain. Growth hormone is currently used clinically to treat patients with short stature. In addition, because of its systemic effects there is interest in its use to treat osteoporosis and to enhance fracture healing. Back in 1980, Northmore-Ball and coauthors [17] studied the effect of GH on fracture healing experimentally, but they did not find a stimulatory response on bone formation, while previous studies had reported data supporting this hypothesis. What we certainly know is that GH is released by the anterior lobe of the pituitary gland in response to stimulation by growth hormone-releasing hormone, a hormone secreted by the hypothalamus, with an endocrine stimulus. The GH travels through the circulation to the growth plate and the liver, where target cells are stimulated to release IGF. Two IGFs have been identified: IGF-I and IGF-II. Although IGF-II is the type most abundant in bone, IGF-I has been found to be more potent and has been localized in healing fractures in rats and humans. Therefore, experimental studies focused attention on both growth factors for their strict connection in inducing the final effects on skeletal growth and bone formation.

In Vivo Results

Bak et al. [18] reported data on the effect of four doses of biosynthetic human GH (0.08, 0.4, 2.0, and 10.0 mg/kg per day) on fracture healing in rats. Animals received either no injection or twice-daily injections of GH or saline solution (control group), beginning 7 days before the fracture and continuing until the animals were killed, 40 days after the fracture. A positive effect on the mechanical properties of the healed fracture was reported only with the higher doses (2.0 and 10.0 mg) of human GH, with increased ultimate load to failure, stiffness, and energy absorption. Moreover, the increase in the ultimate stress to failure was only seen in association with the 10.0-mg dose.

Carpenter et al. [19] evaluated the effect of intramuscular injection of recombinant human GH versus saline solution in a rabbit fracture model. He produced in the left tibias of 27 rabbits an osteotomy stabilizing the site with an external fixator, and using the contralateral side as control. The GH injections were administered five times a week. The rabbits were killed at 4, 6 and 8 weeks and a four-point mechanical testing was performed. The authors failed to demonstrate any significant difference in the measurements. Also radiological measurements performed weekly for both tibias in each group did not show differences. Also serum levels of IGF-I were monitored to evaluate a systemic response to administration of GH. There was an increase of 33% in the GH-treated group compared to 10% in the control group. No correlation could be done between the serum levels of IGF-I and biomechanical properties of the fracture.

The role of IGF-I in stimulating intramembranous bone formation was studied in a calvarial defect model in rats by Thaller [20]. Animals were subjected to continuous systemic administration of IGF-I for 14 days via a subcutaneous osmotic pump, whereas control animals were treated with saline solution alone. The calvarial defects that had been treated with 2 mg of IGF-I for 2 weeks healed via intramembranous ossification. The results of that study suggest that IGF-I may have a role in enhancing bone formation in defects that heal via intramembranous ossification.

In a more recent study, Bhandari [21] reported data on the indirect importance of IGF-I and -II in the healing process of bone. He treated 24 mice with intramedullary nailing and subsequent femoral fracture, dividing the two groups into reamed and unreamed nail insertion. The mice were killed at 1 week postoperatively and the bone marrow was centrifuged and tested for bone nodule formation. The positive effect reported on the bone marrow from the reamed group was completely inhibited by adding to the culture antibodies to IGF-I or -II. Therefore the study demonstrated ultimately the importance played by IGFs in fracture healing.

The importance of IGF in healing bone defects has also been reported by Meinel et al. [22]. To prolong IGF-I delivery, the authors entrapped 100 μg of IGF-I into biodegradable poly(lactide-co-glycolide) microspheres and evaluated the potential of this system in two defect models of ovine long bones, an 8-mm metaphyseal drill hole and a 10-mm segmental tibia defect. The data showed new bone formation within 3 weeks in the drill hole and bridging of the segmental defect within 8 weeks. The observed increase of 12% newly formed bone in the drill hole defect after 3 weeks was substantial, compared to the measured morphometric bone-to-total area ratio of 31% bone in normal cancellous bone. Administration of the IGF-I delivery system downregulated inflammatory marker gene expression at the site of bone injury, induced new bone formation and reduced bone resorption, and resulted in bridging of 10-mm segmental tibial defects within 8 weeks.

Kandziora and coauthors [23] reported the result of a sheep cervical spine interbody fusion model used to determine the effect of combined IGF-I and transforming growth factor-β1 (TGF-β1) applied by a poly-(D,L-lactide) (PDLLA)-coated cage. Both the carrier properties and the inductive properties of the two growth factors were the object of the study. Thirty-two sheep underwent C3-C4 discectomy and fusion with different devices: autologous tricortical iliac crest bone graft, titanium cage, titanium cage coated with a PDLLA carrier and titanium cage coated with a PDLLA carrier including IGF-I (5% w/w) and TGF-β1 (1% w/w). Blood samples, body weight, and body temperature were recorded, while radiographic scans were performed before and after surgery, then at 1, 2, 4, 8, and 12 weeks, respectively. After 12 weeks, the animals were killed and fusion sites were evaluated using functional radiographic views of the animals in flexion and extension. Quantitative computed tomographic (CT) scans were performed to assess bone mineral density, bone mineral content, and bony callus volume, and biomechanical testing of the motion segment C3-C4 was performed. Also histomorphologic and histomorphometric analyses were performed, and polychrome sequential labeling was used to determine the time frame of new bone formation. No differences between the groups in terms of blood counts, body weight, or temperature were found. After the 12-week period, the groups treated with titanium cage plus PDLLA-coated cages with IGF-I and TGF-β showed significantly lower residual flexion–extension movement and significantly higher values for bone mineral density, bone mineral content, and bony callus volume. The average stiffness in rotation and bending was significantly higher, and the range of motion, neutral zone, and elastic zone in rotation were significantly lower than any other group. However, only one animal demonstrated solid fusion after 12 weeks, although histomorphometric evaluation showed a more progressed bone matrix formation in the group that had PDLLA-coated cages with IGF-I and TGF-β1 than in any other group. The polychrome sequential labeling showed accelerated intervertebral bone matrix formation in this group. The data from the study demonstrated that PDLLA coating of cervical spine interbody fusion cages as a delivery system for growth factors was effective and IGF-I and TGF-β1 application significantly increased the results of interbody bone matrix formation. The authors concluded that longer-term studies were needed to determine whether combined IGF-I and TGF-β1 application leads to a successful spinal fusion.

One year later, Kandziora [24] refined his study, publishing data on the dose-dependent effect of combined IGF-I and TGF-β1 application on intervertebral bone matrix formation in the same sheep cervical spine fusion model. Thirty-two sheep underwent C3-C4 discectomy and fusion. Stabilization was performed using a titanium cage coated with a PDLLA carrier including no growth factors in group 1 and rising doses of IGF-I (75–300 μg) plus gTGF-β1 (15–60 μg). The same method of blood samples, radiographic examinations, quantitative CT scans and biochemical testing was fulfilled. The medium- and high-dose growth factor groups (groups 3 and 4) demonstrated a significantly higher bony callus volume on CT scans, a higher biomechanical stability, an advanced interbody bone matrix formation in histomorphometric analysis, and an earlier bone matrix formation on fluorochrome sequence labeling. No significant difference could be determined between the medium- and the high-dose growth factor groups. The data supported the influence of IGF-I and TGF-β1 in interbody bone matrix formation in a dose-dependent manner, with a plateau reached with the higher doses tested. With an increasing dose of these growth factors, no further stimulation of bone matrix formation was observed. The successful results, however, introduce safety issues because of the high doses necessary to obtain these results.

In conclusion, the results of the studies that evaluated the role of IGF-I as an agent to enhance fracture healing are contrasting: they have been performed in different animal models with the use of different doses and methods of administration to assess the influences of GH and IGF on skeletal repair. Data are not conclusive and therefore even if the importance of GH and IGFs is acknowledged, it is difficult to categorize their role in the enhancement of fracture healing at physiological doses.

Platelet-Derived Growth Factor

Platelet-derived growth factor is secreted by platelets during the early phases of fracture healing and has been identified at fracture sites in both animals and humans. It is not the only growth factor secreted by platelets and therefore its influence on bone formation is often studied together with TGF-β and IGF, which are both present in platelet products. In vitro studies have demonstrated that PDGF provides a mitogenic stimulus for osteoblastic progenitors.

In Vitro Results

Lucarelli et al. [25] studied the effect of platelet-rich plasma (PRP) released by platelet gel on staminal stem cell (SSC) proliferation and differentiation. The results showed that PRP induced SSC proliferation and the effect was dose dependent: 10% PRP is sufficient to induce a marked cell proliferation. Upon treatment with 10% PRP, cells entered logarithmic growth, which was reversed by removal of PRP. SSCs were also evaluated for their ability to differentiate along the chondrogenic and osteogenic lineage. After five passages with PRP, at passage six PRP was washed away and plated cells were treated with dexamethasone. Dexamethasone induced a threefold increase in the number of alkaline phosphatase-positive cells and induced mineralization that is consistent with the differentiation of osteochondroprogenitor cells. In conclusion, 10% PRP promotes SSC proliferation and cells expanded with 10% PRP can mineralize the extracellular matrix once PRP is withdrawn.

Gruber et al. [26] showed that addition of platelets, platelet-released supernatants, platelet membranes, and microparticles to bovine periosteum-derived cells resulted in an increase in ^{3}H-thymidine incorporation and platelet-released supernatants retained their activity after incubation at 56 °C. Of the factors released from activated platelets, basic FGF and PDGF increased ^{3}H-thymidine incorporation; on the contrary the mitogenic activity of platelet-released supernatants was decreased by anti-PDGF, and anti-basic FGF antibodies.

Platelet-released supernatants also resulted in a stimulation of cell proliferation in periosteal explants.

In Vivo Results

Although the role of PDGF in SSC proliferation is defined, its role in fracture healing and bone repair is still unclear. Nash et al. [27] evaluated the efficacy of PDGF in the healing of unilateral tibial osteotomies in 14 rabbits. Three animals died before the experiment was completed, and only six animals with osteotomies and five controls were evaluated. Each osteotomy site was treated with either 80 µg of PDGF in a collagen sponge or with a collagen sponge alone. The animals were killed after 28 days. Radiographic analysis at 2 and 4 weeks demonstrated an increase in callus density and volume in the animals that had been treated with PDGF compared with the controls. Histological analysis demonstrated a more advanced state of osteogenic differentiation both endosteally and periosteally in the animals that had been treated with PDGF than in the controls. A three-point bending test revealed no differences in strength between the tibiae that had been treated with PDGF and the intact, contralateral tibiae, but in the control group the osteotomies were statistically weaker than their nonoperated (contralateral) bones. Although the histological findings suggested that PDGF has a beneficial effect on fracture healing, the principal drawback was that only a small number of animals were analyzed and the mechanical testing data were not significant.

More recently other experimental studies reported data on the role of PRP in healing segmental defects. Zhang et al. [28] created in 24 rabbits a segmental bone defect of 1 cm in the radial bone bilaterally. One side was randomly chosen as the experimental side and filled with artificial bone augmented with PRP. The other side was filled only with artificial bone. Radiological, histological and computer analysis were performed after 2, 4, 8 and 12 weeks of implantation. Two weeks after operation, new bone and fibrous tissue formation in both the experimental and the control sides were observed at the defect ends, but there was much more new tissue in the experimental side. In the 4th and 8th weeks, the surface of the artificial bone was covered with a large amount of new bone trabeculae and in the experimental side it bridged the defect with callus. At 12 weeks after surgery, bone defects were healed in the experimental side, while the control side did not show continuous bone callus.

The positive effect of PRP added to a bony scaffold was not replicated by another study from Denmark by Li and coauthors [29], who investigated whether the combination of β-tricalcium phosphate (β-TCP) and PRP may enhance fusion in 10 pigs used as a spinal fusion model. Three-level anterior lumbar interbody fusion was performed with carbon fiber cages and staples on each pig. Autogenous bone graft, β-TCP, and β-TCP loaded with PRP were randomly assigned to each level and pigs were killed at the end of the third month. Radiographs, CT scanning, and histomorphometric analysis were performed. Platelet concentration used was 4.4-fold after the processing technique. Radiograph examination showed 70% (7/10) fusion rate in the autograft level and all the levels with β-TCP+PRP showed partial fusion, while β-TCP-alone levels had six partial fusions and four nonfusions ($p = 0.08$). CT evaluation of fusion rate demonstrated fusion in 50% (5/10) of the autograft levels while only partial fusion was seen at β-TCP levels and β-CP+PRP levels. Histomorphometric evaluation found no difference between β-TCP and β-TCP+PRP levels. The conclusion drawn was the insufficiency of the PRP at the concentration used in improving the bone-forming capacity of β-TCP biomaterial in anterior spine fusion, with poorer radiological and histological outcomes than autografts after 3 months follow-up.

The poor results of PRP added to artificial bone substitute were also confirmed by Wiltfang et al. [30] in an experimental study on the regeneration of bony defects of pigs. The addition of PRP to bone substitutes hardly influenced bone regeneration or cytokine expression; on the contrary PRP added to autologous bone enhanced bone healing significantly ($p = 0.028$). After 4 weeks, however, no differences were created in bone healing from added PRP in the autogenous group, and at 12 weeks the level of reossification had reached similar values in all groups.

In maxillofacial and oral surgery studies the preliminary results of this technique in humans have been reported. Danesh-Meyer et al. [31] evaluated the potential of PRP to enhance bone formation following sinus augmentation with different bone derivative/substitute materials (DFDBA, FDBA, Xenograft, Bioactive Glass). The subjects of the study were five clinical cases in which sinus augmentation was performed with PRP combined with bone derivatives/substitutes. Histological evaluation of trephine-obtained core samples consistently revealed the presence of residual graft particles surrounded by loose connective tissue, with a limited amount of newly formed bone. The findings suggest that the addition of PRP to bone derivative/substitute materials may not significantly enhance bone formation and confirmed the relative ineffectiveness of adding PRP to bone substitutes. At the present time, the therapeutic role of PDGF in fracture healing remains unclear. The early stages of bone regeneration are associated with a high mitogenic activity of periosteal cells and PRP and PDGF are very effective in both in vitro and in vivo studies in enhancing periosteal cell replication and early differentiation. However, their role in callus formation and new bone apposition is not well defined and accepted. In evaluating the results of the known studies, it should be kept in mind that the potential effects

Table 2.2.2. Effect of growth factors on bone regeneration and healing

Author	Growth factor	Material	Results
Nielsen [8]	TGF-β	Rat tibial fracture, two doses (4 or 40 ng of TGF-β)	TGF-β induces a dose-dependent effect in callus and bone formation at fracture line
Nakamura [13]	FGF-2	Tibial fracture in beagle dogs stabilized with intramedullary nails; bFGF injection vs control	bFGF accelerates bone repair and callus remodeling
Radomsky [14]	FGF-2 + hyaluronan	Fibular defects in baboons; three doses of FGF-2 vs control (contralateral side)	FGF-2 increases callus formation; no correlation dose-response observed, importance of carrier emphasized
Meinel [22]	IGF-I + poly(lactide-co-glycolide) microspheres	Ovine long bone defects Drill holes and segmental defects	Positive effect both in new bone formation and bridging of the defect
Zhang [28]	PRP + artificial bone	Radial defect in rabbits	Healing at 12 weeks in the PRP side, while incomplete callus formation in control side

of PDGF are often evaluated together with other mitogenic polypeptides such as TGF-β and IGF-I, which are all present in the products of platelet degranulation and in PRP, and the final effects of single growth factors are very difficult to identify and are probably questionable separately.

Several studies demonstrating the effects of different growth factors are presented in Table 2.2.2.

Bone Morphogenetic Proteins

Bone morphogenetic proteins are probably the most important and critical growth factors in bone formation and healing. The BMPs are members of the TGF-β superfamily, and 15 individual molecules have been identified, but the different capabilities and targets of these proteins are still lacking. A recent study conducted by Cheng and coauthors [32] found a hierarchy in which BMP-2, -6 and -9 may induce osteoblast differentiation from mesenchymal stem cells, while the other BMPs seem able to stimulate osteogenesis in mature osteoblasts (Fig. 2.2.1). The concept that there is a substance in bone that can induce new bone formation was recognized by Urist in 1965 when he observed that new bone had formed after the implantation of demineralized bone matrix in rat muscle pouch [33]. This phenomenon was called the bone induction principle; later, the protein responsible for this effect was identified by chromatography and further studies led Urist [34] to bovine BMP isolation. Boden [35] studied the efficacy of bovine-derived BMP in inducing spinal fusion in rabbit and primate models and found that high doses of the protein were necessary to obtain healing, but also demonstrated a definite osteoinductive capacity of these proteins.

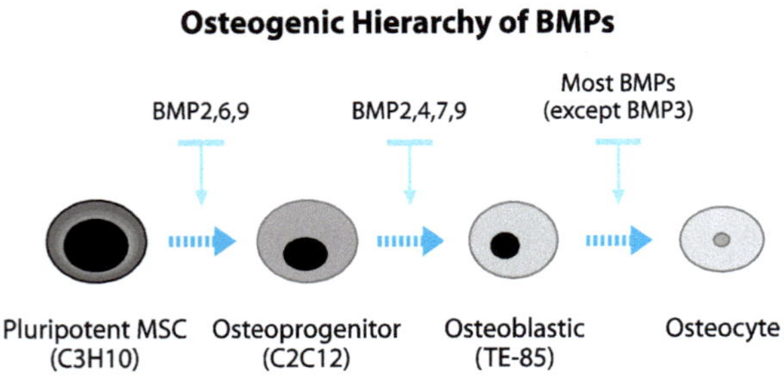

Fig. 2.2.1. Representative illustration of distinct osteogenic activity of human BMPs along the osteoblastic lineage. BMP-2, -6, and -9 may be the most potent agents to induce differentiation of mesenchymal progenitor cells, while most BMPs can effectively promote the terminal differentiation of committed osteoblastic precursors and osteoblasts. (From Cheng et al. [32]. Reprinted with permission from the Journal of Bone and Joint Surgery, Inc.)

Twenty years after Urist's original observation, Wozney et al. [36] identified the genetic sequence of BMP and its various isoforms. The acknowledgement of these data and the use of recombinant gene technology have made it possible to produce recombinant human BMPs (rhBMPs) and a great number of studies have been performed both in vitro and in vivo in preclinical models and clinical trials.

In Vitro Results

Anderson et al. [37] studied two human osteosarcoma cell lineages and their capacity to induce heterotopical bone formation in nude mice. One lineage of the osteosarcoma cells was capable of inducing bone formation in back muscle of rat and of healing surgically created defects in the rat femur. The cells capable of bone induction secreted BMP-1, -2, -3, -4, -6 and TGF-β, while the other cells expressed BMP-2, -3, -4, -5 and -7. The authors concluded that probably the first cell lineage produced an optimal concentration of growth factors that were capable of inducing bone formation. The authors also observed that heterotopic bone formation has a relatively short half-life, while orthotopically induced bone was self-sustaining.

Andrades [38] reported the effect of BMP-7 (also called osteogenic protein-1, OP-1) on selection and amplification of a bone marrow cell population and its induction to an osteogenic lineage. Rat marrow bone cells were cultured in the presence of 40 ng/ml of OP-1 for 16 days and dexamethasone was added to the culture in the last 2 days to promote mineralization. To evaluate in vitro chondro-osteogenic differentiation, expression of alkaline phosphatase, production of osteocalcin and formation of mineralized matrix were assessed. After the in vitro culture, cells were placed inside inactivated DBM cylinders or inside diffusion chambers and implanted in the back of old rats. Cartilage and osteoid tissue was produced in diffusion chambers and bone was observed in DBM cylinders. The author concluded that OP-1 was able to select and induce proliferation of osteoblastic cells both in vitro and in vivo.

A similar experiment was repeated by Chaudhary [39] with normal human bone marrow stromal cells. Cells were treated with BMP-7, PDGF and FGF-2. The sole agent capable of differentiating stromal cells to bone-forming osteoblasts was BMP-7; cultures treated with this factor showed increased alkaline phosphatase activity, bone sialoprotein gene expression and HA crystal deposition. The other growth factors failed to produce the same differentiation and FGF-2 inhibited the effects of BMP-7 on alkaline phosphatase activity and HA formation.

The osteoinductive properties of rhBMP-2 in the muscles of primates was investigated by Kusumoto et al. [40], who evaluated the heterotopic osteoinduction of rhBMP-2 mixed with a collagenous carrier at different doses. Three groups with different concentrations of rhBMP-2 were used and a rat model served as positive control. Four weeks after implanting into the calf muscle pouch, the implant was examined radiographically and histologically. In one specimen of three in the group with higher doses, marked radio-opaque shadow, massive chondrogenesis and partial osteogenesis were observed. In the other two specimens, only microscopic calcification signs were recognized. In the other groups, no findings of heterotopic osteoinduction were observed radiographically. The author concluded that osteoinductive properties of rhBMP-2 were dose dependent and that the heterotopic ossification was less pronounced in primates than in rats.

In vitro assessment of BMP activity has not been the exclusive study method; a number of preclinical studies have also assessed the efficacy of rhBMPs in the healing of critical-sized bone defects, spinal fusion and acceleration of fracture healing and more recently the effects of rhBMP-7 and -2 in inducing bone formation in a hip replacement animal model were also reported.

Bone Morphogenetic Protein-7

In Vivo Results: Critical Defect

Cook et al. [41] evaluated the use of rhBMP-7 in restoration of large segmental ulnar defects in rabbits. A 1.5-cm defect was created in both ulnae. The defect was filled with rabbit bone matrix and variable doses of rhBMP-7 (from 3.13 to 400 μg), while the contralateral side was packed with the matrix alone. The animals were killed at 8 and 12 weeks postoperatively and both histologic examinations and mechanical testing were performed. All implants with rhBMP-7 showed solid union except for those treated with the lowest dosage. Mechanical properties were comparable to the contralateral site. The control lesions showed no bridging of the defects. The same study was repeated by the author on the healing of ulnar and tibial segmental bone defects created in 28 primates (African green monkeys) [42]. The ulnar defects, 2.0 cm long, were treated with 1000 μg of OP-1 in 400 mg of bovine bone-collagen carrier. Control ulnar defects were treated with autogenous bone graft and bovine collagen carrier or with bovine collagen carrier alone. The tibial defects, – 2.0 cm long, – were treated with 250, 500, 1000, or 2000 μg of OP-1 in 400 mg of collagen carrier. Control tibial defects were treated with autogenous bone graft and bovine collagen carrier or with bovine collagen carrier alone. In two animals, the tibial defect was left untreated. At the end of the study after 20 weeks healing of the defects was evaluated radiographically, histologically, and biomechanically. Five of the six ulnae and four of the five tibiae that had been treated with OP-1 healed by 6–8 weeks. None of the six ulnae that had been treated with autogenous bone graft healed, but five of the six tibiae that had been treated with autogenous bone graft healed. None of the defects that had been treated with carrier alone or that had been left untreated demonstrated any signs of healing. Defects treated with OP-1 revealed the presence of normal bone, composed by new cortices, woven and lamellar bone, and normal-appearing marrow elements. The average torsional strength to failure of the ulnae and tibiae treated with OP-1 was 92% and 69% of the contralateral intact ulnae and tibiae, respectively. In contrast, the average torsional strength to failure of the tibiae that had been treated with autogenous bone graft was only 23% of that of the contralateral tibiae, and the ulnae treated with autogenous bone demonstrated sufficient healing to undergo mechanical testing. Similar findings have been reported by the same senior author in healing of critical-sized defects in a canine model [41].

More recently, den Boer et al. [43] evaluated the healing of a segmental bone defect with granular porous HA augmented with OP-1 or autologous bone marrow. A 3-cm segmental bone defect was created in the tibiae of sheep and subsequently fixed with an interlocking intramedullary nail. Five study groups were identified: no implant, autograft, HA alone, HA plus OP-1 and HA plus bone marrow. The results were evaluated at 12 weeks by radiographic and histological examination and mechanical testing. The torsional strength and stiffness of the tibiae were similar in the groups treated with autograft, HA plus OP-1 and HA plus autologous bone marrow. The authors concluded that adding OP-1 to a synthetic scaffold can achieve results similar to those of autografts in bridging segmental defects.

In Vivo Results: Distraction Osteogenesis

Also the timing of application of OP-1 may have importance in inducing osteogenesis. Hamdy and coauthors [44] studied the effect of locally applied OP-1 on distraction osteogenesis in rabbits. Seven days after tibial osteotomy, distraction was started at a rate of 0.25 mm/12 h for 3 weeks. At the end of the distraction period, OP-1 was injected at the site of osteotomy. Four different dosages were tested (0, 80, 800, or 2000 μg; eight rabbits per dose group). Rabbits were killed 3 weeks later, and histologic, densitometric, and biomechanical parameters were assessed. No significant differences were found between groups for any parameter. To explain why this approach was only modestly successful, the expression of BMP receptor protein in the newly formed tissue was analyzed by immunohistochemistry. Strong expression of BMP receptor IA, IB, and II was found during the early distraction phase, but not during later stages of the process. Thus, it appears that the lack of receptor protein in the target tissue impairs the effect of OP-1 given at the end of the distraction period and OP-1 could be more useful when applied early in the distraction phase. Mizumoto et al. [45] applied the conclusions of the previous study and demonstrated the efficacy of OP-1 in distraction osteogenesis. Two groups of seven rats were created and OP-1 versus placebo was tested. An external fixator was applied to the left femur, and a transverse osteotomy was performed. One group was treated with rhBMP-7 in an aqueous solvent, and the other group received the solvent alone and served as the control. Distraction was started 7 days after surgery at a rate of 0.25 mm every 12 h till 10 mm of lengthening.

Radiographs showed accelerated regenerate ossification in the BMP-7 group, with a larger amount of new bone compared with the control group (Fig. 2.2.2). The bone-mineral-density values were dramatically enhanced on day 20 in the BMP-7 group (103.6 ± 12.6 mg/cm^2) compared with the control group (26.2 ± 15.1 mg/cm^2). These differences continued to be greater at 2 and 4 weeks after the cessation of distraction.

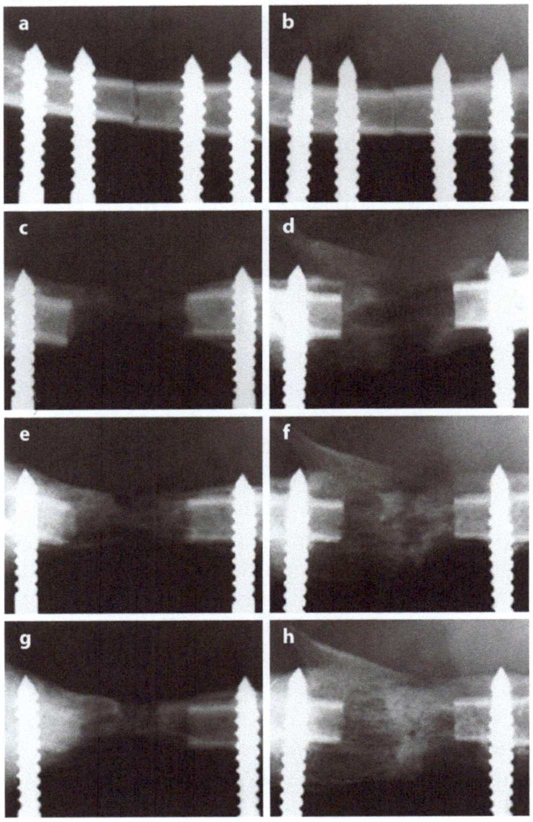

Fig. 2.2.2. The X-rays on the left are representative of the control group at different times; the X-rays on the right are representative of the group treated with osteogenic protein-1 at the corresponding times of treatment. (From Mizumoto et al. [45]. Reprinted with permission from the Journal of Bone and Joint Surgery, Inc.)

In Vivo Results: Fracture Healing

Den Boer [46] evaluated the ability of OP-1 to accelerate normal physiologic fracture healing. In 40 adult female goats a closed tibial fracture was created, stabilized with an external fixator, and treated as follows: (1) no injection; (2) injection of 1 mg OP-1 dissolved in aqueous buffer; (3) injection of collagen matrix; and (4) injection of 1 mg OP-1 bound to collagen matrix. The substances were injected in the fracture under fluoroscopic control. At 2 and 4 weeks, fracture healing was evaluated with radiographs, CT, dual-energy X-ray absorptiometry, biomechanical tests, and histology. At 2 weeks callus diameter, callus volume, and bone mineral content at the fracture site were significantly increased in both OP-1 groups compared to the no-injection group. Bending and torsional stiffness were higher and bony bridging of the fracture gap was observed more often in the group with OP-1 dissolved in aqueous buffer than in uninjected fractures. Treatment with OP-1 plus collagen matrix did not result in improved biomechanical properties or bony bridging of the fracture gap at 2 weeks. At 4 weeks there were no differences between groups, except for a larger callus volume in the OP-1 plus collagen matrix group compared with the control groups. All fractures showed an advanced stage of healing at 4 weeks. In conclusion, the healing of a closed fracture in a goat model can be accelerated by a single local administration of OP-1 and the use of a carrier material does not seem to be crucial.

In Vivo Results: Spinal Fusion

Finally, the OP-1 induction properties have been investigated in spinal fusion in both animal models and pilot clinical human studies [47, 48].

In consequence of animal studies that demonstrated high fusion rates of osteoinductive proteins in noninstrumented posterolateral fusions, Johnsson et al. [47] randomized 20 patients to fusion with either OP-1 implant or autograft bone from the iliac crest, with 10 in each group. The patients were instructed to keep the trunk straight for 5 months after surgery with the aid of a soft lumbar brace. At surgery 0.8-mm metallic markers were positioned in L5 and the sacrum, enabling radiostereometric follow-up analysis during 1 year. The three-dimensional vertebral movements were calculated with an accuracy of 0.5–0.7 mm and 0.5–2.0°. The study failed to show significant differences between the OP-1 implant and fusion with autograft bone. A significant relation between reduced vertebral movements and better bone formation was demonstrated. No adverse effects of the OP-1 implant occurred, while persistent minor pain at the iliac crest was noticed in one patient in the autograft group. In conclusion, there was no significant difference between the two fusion versions. The same outcome of comparable results with OP-1 added to autograft bone was reported also by Vaccaro et al. [48], who showed a successful result of slightly more than 50% in a pilot clinical trial (with no significant difference to the historical results of autograft alone of about 45%).

Clinical Results: Tibial Non-Unions

In another pilot clinical study, Friedlander [49] enrolled 122 patients (124 tibial nonunions) in a controlled, prospective, randomized, partially blinded, multi-center clinical trial and followed them at frequent intervals over 24 months. Each patient was treated by insertion of an intramedullary rod, accompanied by OP-1 in a type I collagen carrier or by fresh bone autograft. Assessment criteria included the severity of pain at the fracture site, the ability to walk with full weight-bearing, the need for surgical re-treatment of the nonunion during the course of this study, plain radiographic evaluation of healing, and physician satisfaction with the clinical course. In addition, adverse events were recorded, and patients were screened for antibodies to OP-1 and type-I collagen at each outpatient visit. At 9 months following the operative procedures, 81% of the OP-1-treated nonunions ($n=63$) and 85% of those receiving autogenous bone ($n=61$) were judged by clinical criteria to have been treated successfully ($p=0.524$). By radiographic criteria, at this same time point, 75% of those in the OP-1-treated group and 84% of the autograft-treated patients had healed fractures ($p=0.218$). These clinical results continued at similar levels of success throughout 2 years of observation, and there was no statistically significant difference in outcome between the two groups of patients at this point ($p=0.939$). More than 20% of patients treated with autografts had chronic donor site pain following the procedure. The authors concluded that OP-1. Implanted with a type I collagen carrier was a safe and effective treatment for tibial nonunions. This molecule provided clinical and radiographic results comparable with those achieved with bone autograft, without donor site morbidity.

The BMP-7 studies are summarized in Table 2.2.3.

Table 2.2.3. Effect of BMP-7 (OP-1) on bone regeneration and healing

Author	Material	Results
Cook [41]	Rabbit ulnar defect, BMP-7 at different doses	Healing of treated defect except for lowest dosage; mechanical testing similar to intact side, no healing in control group
den Boer [46]	Fracture healing in goats	Faster healing with OP-1 independent from collagenous carrier
Mizumoto [45]	Distraction osteogenesis in rats	Accelerated osteogenesis in OP-1 group, with more bone formation also after treatment
Johnsson [47]	Lumbar fusion in humans	No differences between OP-1 and autograft
Friedlander [49]	Tibial nonunions in humans	No differences between OP-1 and autograft

Bone Morphogenetic Protein-2

In Vitro Results

Recombinant human BMP-2 seems to play an important role in the early phases of osteoinduction. Cheng et al. [32] demonstrated the importance of BMP-2 in the early differentiation phases of staminal cells along the osteoblastic lineage. These data indicate that BMP-2 plays an important role in osteoinduction, especially at the early stage, but its osteoinductive properties have also been demonstrated in vivo in the healing of critical-sized defects in rat, rabbit, sheep, and dog models.

In Vivo Results: Critical Defect

Sciadini and Johnson [50] evaluated the efficacy of rhBMP-2 in the healing of a critical-sized radial defect in a dog model. Twenty-seven dogs underwent bilateral radial osteotomy with the creation of a 2.5-cm diaphyseal defect stabilized with an external fixator. All dogs were treated with either autogenous bone graft or a collagen implant containing 0, 150, 600, or 2400 µg of rhBMP-2. The dogs were killed at 12 or 24 weeks after the operative procedure, and a complete analysis was performed. All defects that had been treated with either autogenous bone graft or with the various doses of rhBMP-2 showed union radiographically and histologically. None of the eight defects that had been treated with a collagen carrier alone healed. The biomechanical performance of the defects that had been treated with all three doses of rhBMP-2 was comparable with that of the defects that had been treated with autogenous bone graft and was significantly better than that of the defects that had been treated with the placebo ($p<0.0005$). However, the biomechanical performance of the defects that had been treated with the lowest dose of rhBMP (150 µg) was superior to that of the defects that had been treated with the higher doses: this finding was attributed to the lack of cyst-like voids. The specific mechanism by which these voids developed could not be determined, but the data suggest that the dose of rhBMP-2 protein may have to be adjusted for different clinical applications.

In Vivo Results: Fracture Healing

Bostrom and Camacho [51] evaluated the influence of rhBMP-2 on the healing of fresh fractures in a rabbit ulnar osteotomy model. The authors applied 200 mg of rhBMP-2 in a type-I collagen sponge to 20 ulnar fractures. Limbs that were treated with carrier alone or that were left untreated served as controls. Radiographic evaluation and biomechanical testing were done at 2, 3, 4, and 6 weeks after the operative procedure. BMP-2 accelerated the healing at the osteotomy site as assessed both radiographically and biomechanically. Between 3 and 4 weeks after the procedure, the limbs that had been treated with BMP-2 showed increased stiffness and strength compared with the untreated, intact ulnae. The untreated and collagen-carrier groups attained comparable values.

As for BMP-7, rhBMP-2 was investigated for its effect in healing of fresh fractures. Einhorn et al. [52] tested the hypothesis that a local injection of BMP-2 could accelerate fracture healing. In 278 rats a closed mid-diaphyseal fracture was created and injected after 6 h with buffer, buffer plus rhBMP-2 or received no injection. The animals were killed at different follow-ups and the femurs were tested biomechanically and histologically. From 14 days after the fracture a significant increase in mechanical properties of femur treated with BMP-2 was noted. Histologically examination showed relative maturation of osteochondrogenic cells by day 7 and bridging callus formed earlier in the treated group. The authors concluded that in BMP-2-treated fractures the healing process followed a normal pathway, but at an increased rate.

In Vivo Results: Spinal Fusion

There has also been considerable interest in the use of an osteoinductive agent such as BMP to enhance active spinal fusion in order to avoid the operative morbidity associated with the harvesting of autogenous bone graft. The potential efficacy of rhBMP-2 in the treatment of intertransverse process and posterior segmental spinal fusion has been evaluated in a variety of animal models. In those studies, rhBMP-2 was used in association with a variety of carriers, including collagen, polylactic acid, and copolymers (polylactic acid–polyglycolic acid). All of those investigations demonstrated successful fusion of the spine and, in most instances, the fusion mass at sites that had been treated with rhBMP-2 was greater than that at sites that had been treated with autogenous bone. However, the presence of voids in the fusion mass was noted in two studies in which either an open-cell polylactic acid polymer or a polylactic–polyglycolic acid carrier was used. These voids did not impair the mechanical integrity of the fusion mass as demonstrated by biomechanical testing, but further study of the potential influence of the protein dose and a specific carrier on the formation of these voids is necessary.

Recombinant BMPs have also been used in association with metallic cages to induce lumbar and cervical spinal fusions. Boden et al. [53] reported successful laparoscopic anterior spinal arthrodesis in five adult rhesus monkeys that had been treated with rhBMP-2 in a titanium interbody threaded cage. A solid fusion of the lumbar spine was achieved in association with the recombinant protein independently from doses used. In contrast, a solid fusion was not achieved in two animals that had been treated with a collagen sponge only. Although the results of these preclinical studies have been promising, the relatively high doses of rhBMP required to induce adequate bone formation suggest that large amounts of recombinant protein may be required to produce a clinically important effect.

Clinical Results: Spinal Fusion

Recombinant human BMP-2 has also been tested in controlled clinical human trials regarding spinal fusion and treatment of open fractures. Boden et al. [54] reported the results of lumbar interbody arthrodesis for 14 patients with a single-level lumbar degenerative disc disease. Patients were treated with tapered cylindrical threaded fusion cages filled with rhBMP-2/collagen sponge or autogenous iliac crest bone. They were evaluated with radiographs, CT, and Short-Form 36 and Oswestry outcome questionnaires. All 11 patients who received rhBMP-2 were judged by three independent radiologists to have solid fusions from 6 months postoperatively, whereas only two of the three control patients were deemed to be fused. The Oswestry Disability Questionnaire scores of the rhBMP-2 group improved sooner (after 3 months) than those of the autograft group, with both groups demonstrating similar improvement at 6 months. Short-Form 36 scores continued to improve up to 24 months. In conclusion, the arthrodesis occurred more reliably in patients treated with rhBMP-2-filled fusion cages than in controls with autogenous bone graft. There were no adverse events related to the rhBMP-2 treatment, but we should note that the sample size of this study was limited.

A larger number of patients were evaluated by Burkus et al. [55]. In a prospective randomized study he investigated 42 patients who underwent a single-level anterior lumbar interbody fusion using cylindrical interbody fusion cages. There were two groups: one underwent interbody fusion using two tapered cylindrical fusion cages and rhBMP-2 on an absorbable collagen sponge, and a control group with the cages and autogenous iliac crest bone graft. Plain radiographs and CT scans were used to evaluate the pattern of osteoinduction in the interbody space and the progression of fusion 6, 12, and 24 months after surgery. All the patients who received rhBMP-2 showed radiographic evidence of osteoinduction in the interbody cages 6 months after surgery. New bone formation occurred in the disc space outside the cages by 6 months in 18 of the patients in the investigational group (18/22; 82%). By 24 months, all the investigational patients showed new bone formation outside the cages. In the autograft control group, 10 patients (10/20; 50%) showed evidence of bone formation outside the cages. Therefore definite evidence of osteoinductive properties of rhBMP-2 was supported by these data, which showed in a clinical setting accelerated spinal fusion and new bone apposition under the influence of the morphogenetic protein.

Clinical Results: Open Tibia Fractures

Govender and coauthors [56] presented the data resulting from a prospective, randomized, controlled, single-blind study on 450 patients. Patients with an open tibial fracture were randomized to receive either intramedullary nail fixation and routine soft-tissue management, or the same treatment plus an implant containing either 0.75 mg/ml of rhBMP-2 (total dose of 6 mg), or 1.50 mg/ml of rhBMP-2 (total dose of 12 mg). The rhBMP-2 implant (rhBMP-2 applied to an absorbable collagen sponge) was placed over the fracture at the time of definitive wound closure. At 12 months follow-up, 421 (94%) of the patients were controlled. The 1.50 mg/ml rhBMP-2 group had significantly faster fracture healing ($p=0.0022$) (Fig. 2.2.3) than the control patients and significantly more patients treated with 1.50 mg/ml of rhBMP-2 had healing of the fracture at the postoperative visits from 10 weeks through 12 months ($p=0.0008$). Patients treated with 1.50 mg/ml of rhBMP-2 also had significantly fewer infections and faster wound healing. The authors concluded that the rhBMP-2 implant was safe and, when 1.50 mg/ml was used, significantly superior to the standard of care in reducing the frequency of secondary interventions and the overall invasiveness of the procedures, accelerating fracture and

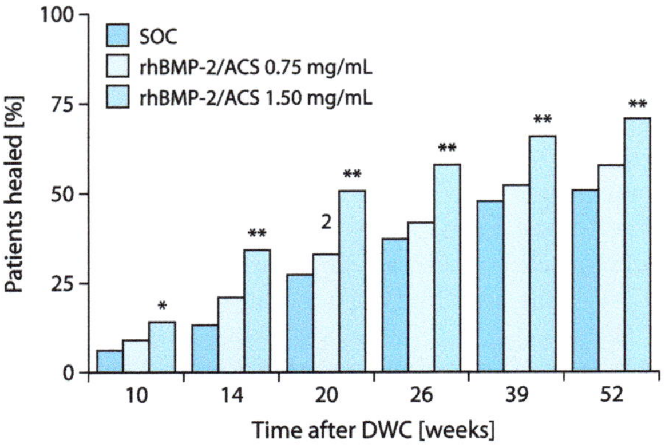

Fig. 2.2.3. Rate of fracture healing according to the treatment group and visit. The determination of fracture healing was based on the treating surgeons' clinical and radiographic assessment. *SOC* standard-of-care (control) group, *rhBMP-2/ACS* groups treated with recombinant human bone morphogenetic protein-2 in an absorbable collagen sponge implant, *DWC* definitive wound closure. $*p<0.05$, $**p<0.01$. (From Govender et al. [56]. Reprinted with permission from the Journal of Bone and Joint Surgery, Inc.)

wound healing, and reducing infection rates after open tibia fractures.

The BMP-2 studies are summarized in Table 2.2.4.

Conclusion

However, the satisfactory results obtained by the use of rhBMPs in clinical settings do not address completely the concerns regarding safety and cost. BMP-7 has been shown to elicit a subclinical immune response in one-third of the patients. BMP-2 does not seem to produce an immune response, but its utility in the healing process has been limited by experimental studies only to the initial phases. What still seems challenging is the difference between the experimental in vitro studies and the preclinical and clinical data. The results of the studies are often contradictory and too many variables are present that can influence the end result of the BMP: the matrix or carrier used, the delivery method and timing of adding the BMPs and the contamination of naturally delivered growth factors in animal and human trials. Delivery methods of BMP or other growth factors are currently under investigation. Recent studies by Wildemann [57] have tested the possibility of coating osteosynthesis devices with growth factors and showed the efficacy of this technique, introducing new concepts of growth factor delivery in addition to established fixation devices. This concept could lead to the development of specialized fixation devices for nonunion, which already deliver in a controlled way the necessary growth factor creating true bioactive plating or nailing.

However, there are also other areas that cause great interest for the future applications of growth factors to enhance bone healing: acceleration of fracture healing (particularly in patients who are at high risk for nonunion) and treatment of established nonunions by injectable preparations of BMPs; enhancement of primary spinal fusion and treatment of established pseudarthrosis of the spine; enhancement of prostheses fixation to bone and gap filler in revision arthroplasty. Growth factors are not the only strategy affordable by the orthopedist to enhance bone repair in the future: mesenchymal stem cell research and gene therapy are already at the preclinical stage.

Gene Therapy

Some very interesting experimental and preclinical studies on the delivery of growth factors via genetic therapy have been published in the past few years. Gene therapy involves the transfer of genetic information to cells. When the gene is transferred to a target cell, the protein encoded by that gene is synthesized. The duration of the effect is determined by the transfer procedure chosen. A long-term effect is desired in a chronic disease, like rheumatoid arthritis, while a short-term

Table 2.2.4. Effect of BMP-2 on bone regeneration and healing

Author	Material	Results
Sciadini [50]	Dog radial defect; external fixator and different doses of BMP-2	Healing of defects treated with BMP-2, no healing of untreated controls. Better mechanical performance of lower dosage of BMP-2
Bostrom [51]	Fracture healing of rabbit ulnae	Accelerated healing of BMP-2-treated fractures compared to controls
Burkus [55]	Single-level lumbar fusion in humans; BMP-2 + cages vs autograft	Accelerated spinal fusion and increased bone formation inside and outside the cages in BMP-2-treated group
Govender [56]	Healing of open fractures in 450 patients	The BMP-2-treated group showed faster bone and wound healing, less need for reoperation, lower infection rate

effect is probably necessary to obtain segmental bone repair. Gene therapy can be also defined by the use of systemic or regional techniques. Moreover the DNA sequence may be implanted in the patient (in vivo technique) or specific target cells can be harvested, manipulated and infected with the genetic sequence and reimplanted in the patient (ex vivo technique; Fig. 2.2.4). Every technique has advantages and disadvantages. Systemic gene therapy should probably be used to treat disorders resulting from a gene mutation with a long-term action. Local disease such as nonunion of a fracture is probably best treated with regional therapy. The in vivo technique is technically simple and low cost, but the efficacy is reduced. The ex vivo technique requires a longer time, but it affords the possibility to select the target cells, adding to the growth factor properties also the cells participating in the process and provides a safer profile, for no viral particles or DNA sequences are introduced into the patient. As for BMPs and other growth factors, the carrier used for local delivery plays a critical role; in gene therapy the vector of genes must be well selected. Viruses are efficient vectors because the delivery and expression of DNA is a critical aspect of their normal life cycle. When a virus is used, essential

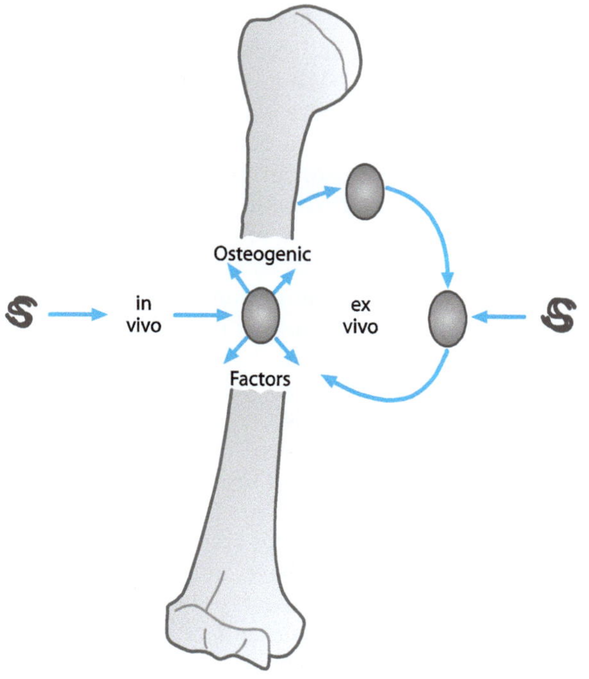

Fig. 2.2.4. In the ex-vivo approach (*right-hand side*) cells are removed from the individual, genetically modified outside the body and introduced into the fracture site. In the in vivo approach (*left-hand side*), vectors are introduced directly into the fracture site. (From Niyibizi et al. [64]. Reprinted with permission from Clin Orthop Rel Res)

portions of its genome must be deleted to render it replication deficient and to create space in its genome for the insertion of the therapeutic DNA. This process is known as homologous recombination. The process that involves the transfer of functional genetic information from the recombinant vector (virus) into the target cell is known as transduction. The DNA brought by the virus enters the nucleus of the cell, where it may become integrated into the host genome or may remain extrachromosomal. A major concern related to the use of viral vectors is the possibility of the defective virus to regain viral sequences present in the host, resulting in the generation of replication-competent viruses with the ability to multiply in the patient. In addition, cells infected with certain viruses (e.g., adenoviruses) produce not only the transgene product but also other viral proteins that may elicit an immune response, which in turn can limit the duration of protein expression by the transduced cells.

Both viral and nonviral vectors have been used to heal critical-sized defects and to induce fusion in the spine in both rabbits and rats. Lee et al. [58], using ex vivo gene transfer methods, genetically engineered freshly isolated human skeletal muscle cells with adenovirus and retrovirus to express human BMP-2. These cells were then implanted into nonhealing bone defects (skull defects) in severe combined immune deficiency mice. Mice that received BMP-2-producing human muscle-derived cells experienced a full closure of the defect by 4–8 weeks post-transplantation. Remodeling of the newly formed bone was evident histologically during the 4- to 8-week period. A small fraction of the transplanted human muscle-derived cells was found within the newly formed bone, where osteocytes normally reside. These results indicate that genetically engineered human muscle-derived cells enhance bone healing primarily by delivering BMP-2, while a small fraction of the cells seems to differentiate into osteogenic cells. Dumont et al. [59], using ex vivo gene therapy with the use of hMSCs and the BMP-9 gene, evaluated the efficacy in promoting spinal fusion in the rat. Sixteen athymic nude rats were treated with hMSCs transduced with adenovirus containing either the BMP-9 (Ad-BMP-9) or the β-galactosidase (Ad-ß-gal) gene, which served as the control. Each animal received a percutaneous, paraspinal injection of 10(6) hMSCs transduced, with Ad-BMP-9 on the left and Ad-β-gal on the right. At 8 weeks post injection, CT scans of the lumbosacral spine were obtained, and the lumbosacral spine specimens were examined histologically. CT scans and histological analysis clearly demonstrated large volumes of ectopic bone at the Ad-BMP-9-transduced hMSC injection sites, resulting in successful spinal fusion and no evidence of nerve root compression or local or systemic toxicity. The contralateral regions showed no evidence of osteogenesis.

Rose et al. [60] tried to improve the healing of bone lesions with severe soft tissue damage. An animal model with a femoral osteotomy lesion associated with soft tissue damage was developed in rats and muscle-derived cells, genetically engineered to express BMP-4, were inserted within the osteotomy gap. The groups were subdivided with regard to the fixation method: stable and unstable fixation. The rats were killed at 3 and 6 weeks post surgery. No callus formation was found in the control group at any time point, whereas sufficient callus formation appeared in the treatment group after 6 weeks. A bridging callus with woven bone and hypertrophic chondrocytes was achieved in the treatment group when a stable fixation was used, but failed to appear in unstable fixation, as a demonstration that mechanical issues are still a concern in treating fractures.

Rundle [61] used in vivo gene therapy to accelerate the repair of bone fractures. A murine leukemia virus-based retroviral vector has been transduced with a hybrid gene that consists of a BMP-4 transgene with the BMP-2 secretory signal to enhance the secretion of mature BMP-4. The vector was administered at the lateral side of the fracture periosteum at 1 day after fracture in the rat femoral fracture model. X-ray examination by radiograph and peripheral quantitative CT at 7, 14, and 28 days after fracture revealed a highly significant enhancement of fracture tissue size in the MLV-BMP-2/4-treated fractures compared to the control fractures. The newly formed bone exhibited normal bone histology. There was no evidence of viral vector infection of extraskeletal tissues, suggesting that this in vivo gene therapy for fracture repair is safe. The authors succeeded in demonstrating for the first time that a MLV-based retroviral vector is a safe and effective means of introducing a transgene to a fracture site and that this procedure caused an enormous augmentation of fracture bone formation.

Wang et al. [62] used ex vivo adenoviral gene transfer to create BMP-2-producing bone marrow cells, and used these autologous cells to induce a posterolateral fusion of the spine in syngenic rats. Ten groups were created. Each specimen underwent plain radiography, manual palpation, and histological analysis. All spines in groups I and II (BMP-2-producing bone marrow cells) and all spines in groups III and IV (BMP locally administered) were fused at 4 weeks postoperatively, whereas none of the spines in the other groups had fused at a minimum of 8 weeks after implantation. Histological analysis of the specimens revealed that the spines that had received BMP-2-producing bone marrow cells (groups I and II) were filled with coarse trabecular bone postoperatively, whereas those that had received rhBMP-2 (groups III and IV) were filled with thin, lace-like trabecular bone. All of the other spines, including those that had been treated with autogenous iliac crest bone grafting (group V), produced little or no new bone. The conclusion was that gene therapy was successful in producing spinal fusion.

Southwood et al. [63] recently evaluated the use of adenoviral transfer of the BMP-2 gene (Ad-BMP-2) for enhancing healing in an infected defect fracture model. A femoral defect stabilized with plates and screws was created in 64 rabbits. Four experimental groups were identified: (1) noninfected Ad-luciferase (Ad-LUC, NONLUC), (2) noninfected Ad-BMP-2 (NONBMP), (3) infected Ad-LUC (INFLUC), and (4) infected Ad-BMP-2 (INFBMP). A sclerosing agent facilitated osteomyelitis. Rabbits in the noninfected and infected groups that were treated with Ad-BMP-2 had earlier initial healing and bridging-callus formation, and a higher overall external callus grade compared to rabbits in the Ad-LUC groups. These data suggest that Ad-BMP-2 enhances the early stages of healing in an infected defect fracture.

A few years ago, BMP for clinical use and gene therapy for bone disease was still a fantasy. Now there is experimental and clinical evidence of new possibilities offered to orthopedic surgeons in treating challenging situations or in facilitating and accelerating the normal process of bone formation, healing of fractures, bone ingrowth to prosthesis and treatment of nonunions. The recent advances in gene therapy will eventually lead to the treatment of systemic bone diseases such as osteogenesis imperfecta and osteoporosis and will bring new powerful tools into clinical practice. At the time of writing, two rhBMPs have been cleared for clinical use in Europe and in the USA: OP-1 and BMP-2. Both have strict indications and bring the negative aspect of a very high cost. The clinical trials till now have not shown an outstanding superiority of these proteins when compared to well-known, safe and relatively low-cost autogenous bone, but their use will give more evidence of their safety and usefulness and will definitively confirm their safety and efficacy.

References

1. Urist MR, Silverman BF, Buring K, Dubuc FL, Rosenberg JM. The bone induction principle. Clin Orthop & RR 53: 243–283, 1967.
2. Lieberman JR, Daluiski A, Einhorn TA. The role of growth factors in the repair of bone. JBIS 84A, 6: 1032–1044, 2002.
3. Massague 1996
4. Fukumoto T, Sperling JW, Sanyal A, Fitzsimmons JS, Reinholz GG, Conover CA, O'Driscoll SW. Combined effects of insulin-like growth factor-1 and TGF-beta1 on periosteal mesenchymal cells during chondrogenesis in vitro. Osteoarthritis Cartilage 2003; 11(1): 55–64.
5. Andrades JA, Han B, Nimni ME, Ertl DC, Simpkins RJ, Arrabal MP, Becerra J. A modified rhTGF-beta1 and rhBMP-2 are effective in initiating a chondro-osseous differentiation pathway in bone marrow cells cultured in vitro. Connect Tissue Res 2003; 44(3–4): 188–197.
6. Beck LS, Amento EP, Xu Y, Deguzman L, Lee WP, Nguyen T, Gillett NA. TGF-beta 1 induces bone closure of skull defects: temporal dynamics of bone formation in defects exposed to rhTGF-beta 1. J Bone Miner Res 1993; 8(6): 753–761.
7. Lind M, Schumacker B, Soballe K, Keller J, Melsen F, Bunger C. Transforming growth factor-beta enhances fracture healing in rabbit tibiae. Acta Orthop Scand 1993; 64: 553–556.
8. Nielsen HM, Andreassen TT, Ledet T, Oxlund H. Local injection of TGF-beta increases the strength of tibial fractures in the rat. Acta Orthop Scand 1994; 65: 37–41.
9. Critchlow MA, Bland YS, Ashhurst DE. The effect of exogenous transforming growth factor-beta 2 on healing fractures in the rabbit. Bone 1995; 16: 521–527.
10. Mayahara H, Ito T, Nagai H, Miyajima H, Tsukuda R, Taketomi S, Mizoguchi J, Kato K. In vivo stimulation of endosteal bone formation by basic fibroblast growth factor in rats. Growth Factors 1993; 9(1): 73–80.
11. Zellin G, Alberius P, Linde A. Autoclaved Bone for Craniofacial Reconstruction: Effects of Supplementation with Bone Marrow or Recombinant Human Fibroblast Growth Factor-2. Plastic & Reconstructive Surgery 102(3): 792–800, September 1998.
12. Kato T, Kawaguchi H, Hanada K, Aoyama L, Hiyama Y, Nakamura T, Kuzutani K, Tamura M, Kurokawa T, Nakamura K. Single local injection of recombinant fibroblast growth factor-2 stimulates healing of segmental bone defects in rabbits. J Orthop Res 1998; 16: 654–659.
13. Nakamura T, Hara Y, Tagawa M, Tamura M, Yuge T, Fukuda H, Nigi H. Recombinant human basic fibroblast growth factor accelerates fracture healing by enhancing callus remodelling in experimental dog tibial fracture. J Bone Miner Res 1998; 13: 942–949.
14. Radomsky ML, Aufdemorte TB, Swain LD, Fox WC, Spiro RC, Poser JW. Novel formulation of fibroblast growth factor-2 in a hyaluronan gel accelerates fracture healing in nonhuman primates. J Orthop Res 1999; 17: 607–614.
15. Schnettler R, Alt V, Dingeldein E, Pfefferle HJ, Kilian O, Meyer C, Heiss C, Wenisch S. Bone ingrowth in bFGF-coated hydroxyapatite ceramic implants. Biomaterials 2003; 24(25): 4603–4608.
16. Bland YS, Critchlow MA, Ashhurst DE. Exogenous fibroblast growth factors-1 and -2 do not accelerate fracture healing in the rabbit. Acta Orthop Scand 1995; 66(6): 543–548.
17. Northmore-Ball 1980
18. Bak B, Jorgensen PH, Andreassen TT. Dose response of growth hormone on fracture healing in the rat. Acta Orthop Scand 1990; 61: 54–57.
19. Carpenter JE, Hipp JA, Gerhart TN, Rudman CG, Hayes WC, Trippel SB. Failure of growth hormone to alter the biomechanics of fracture-healing in a rabbit model. J Bone Joint Surg Am 1992; 74: 359–367.
20. Thaller SR, Dart A, Tesluk H. The effects of insulin-like growth factor-1 on critical-size calvarial defects in Sprague-Dawley rats. Ann Plast Surg 1993; 31: 429–433.
21. Bhandari M, Schemitsch EH. Bone formation following intramedullary femoral reaming is decreased by indomethacin and antibodies to insulin-like growth factors. J Orthop Trauma 2002; 16(10): 717–722.
22. Meinel L, Zoidis E, Zapf J, Hassa P, Hottiger MO, Auer JA, Schneider R, Gander B, Luginbuehl V, Bettschart-Wolfisberger R, Illi OE, Merkle HP, von Rechenberg B. Localized insulin-like growth factor I delivery to enhance new bone formation. Bone 2003; 33(4): 660–672.
23. Kandziora F, Schmidmaier G, Schollmeier G, Bail H, Pflugmacher R, Gorke T, Wagner M, Raschke M, Mittlmeier T, Haas NP. IGF-I and TGF-beta1 application by a poly-(D,L-lactide)-coated cage promotes intervertebral bone matrix formation in the sheep cervical spine. Spine 2002; 27(16): 1710–1723.
24. Kandziora F, Pflugmacher R, Scholz M, Schafer J, Schollmeier G, Schmidmaier G, Duda G, Raschke M, Haas NP. Dose-dependent effects of combined IGF-I and TGF-beta1 application in a sheep cervical spine fusion model. Eur Spine J 2003; 12(5): 464–473.
25. Lucarelli E, Beccheroni A, Donati D, Sangiorgi L, Cenacchi A, Del Vento AM, Meotti C, Bertoja AZ, Giardino R, Fornasari PM, Mercuri M, Picci P. Platelet-derived growth factors enhance proliferation of human stromal stem cells. Biomaterials 2003; 24(18): 3095–3100.
26. Gruber R, Karreth F, Frommlet F, Fischer MB, Watzek G. Platelets are mitogenic for periosteum-derived cells. J Orthop Res 2003; 21(5): 941–948.
27. Nash TJ, Howlett CR, Martin C, Steele J, Johnson KA, Hicklin DJ. Effect of platelet-derived growth factor on tibial osteotomies in rabbits. Bone 1994; 5: 203–208.
28. Zhang CQ, Yuan T, Zeng BF. Experimental study on effect of platelet-rich plasma in repair of bone defect. Zhongguo Xiu Fu Chong Jian Wai Ke Za Zhi 2003; 17(5): 355–358.
29. Li H, Zou X, Xue Q, Egund N, Lind M, Bunger C. Anterior lumbar interbody fusion with carbon fiber cage loaded with bioceramics and platelet-rich plasma. An experimental study on pigs. Eur Spine J 2004; Jan 17.
30. Wiltfang J, Kloss FR, Kessler P, Nkenke E, Schultze-Mosgau S, Zimmermann R, Schlegel KA. Effects of platelet-rich plasma on bone healing in combination with autogenous bone and bone substitutes in critical-size defects. An animal experiment. Clin Oral Implants Res 2004; 15(2): 187–193.
31. Danesh-Meyer MJ, Filstein MR, Shanaman R. Histological evaluation of sinus augmentation using platelet rich plasma (PRP): a case series. J Int Acad Periodontol 2001; 3(2): 48–56.
32. Cheng H, Jiang W, Phillips FM, Haydon RC, Peng Y, Zhou L, Luu HH, An N, Breyer B, Vanichakarn P, Szatkowski JP, Park JY, He TC. Osteogenic activity of the fourteen types of human bone morphogenetic proteins (BMPs). J Bone Joint Surg Am 2003; 85-A(8): 1544–1552.
33. Urist MR. Bone formation by autoinduction. Science 1965; 50: 893–899.
34. Urist MR, Huo YK, Brownell AG, Hohl WM, Buyske J, Lietze A, Tempst P, Hunkapiller M, DeLange RJ. Purification of bovine bone morphogenetic protein by hydroxyapatite chromatography. Proc Natl Acad Sci USA 1984; 81(2): 371–375.
35. Boden SD, Moskovitz PA, Morone MA, Toribitake Y. Video-assisted lateral intertransverse process arthrodesis. Validation of a new minimally invasive lumbar spinal fusion technique in the rabbit and nonhuman primate (rhesus) models. Spine 1996; 21(22): 2689–2697.

36. Wozney JM, Rosen V, Celeste AJ, Mitsock LM, Whitters MJ, Kriz RW, Hewick RM, Wang EA. Novel regulators of bone formation: molecular clones and activities. Science 1988; 242: 1528–1534.
37. Anderson HC, Hsu HH, Raval P, Hunt TR, Schwappach JR, Morris DC, Schneider DJ. The mechanism of bone induction and bone healing by human osteosarcoma cell extracts. Clin Orthop 1995; 313: 129–134.
38. Andrades JA, Santamaria JA, Nimni ME, Becerra J. Selection and amplification of a bone marrow cell population and its induction to the chondro-osteogenic lineage by rhOP-1: an in vitro and in vivo study. Int J Dev Biol 2001; 45(4): 689–693.
39. Chaudhary LR, Hofmeister AM, Hruska KA. Differential growth factor control of bone formation through osteoprogenitor differentiation. Bone 2004; 34(3): 402–411.
40. Kusumoto K, Bessho K, Fujimura K, Akioka J, Okubo Y, Wang Y, Iizuka T, Ogawa Y. Osteoinduction by recombinant human bone morphogenetic protein-2 in muscles of nonhuman primates. J Int Med Res 2002; 30(3): 251–259.
41. Cook SD, Baffes GC, Wolfe MW, Sampath TK, Rueger DC. Recombinant human bone morphogenetic protein-7 induces healing in a canine long-bone segmental defect model. Clin Orthop 1994; 301: 302–312.
42. Cook SD, Wolfe MW, Salkeld SL, Rueger DC. Effect of recombinant human osteogenic protein-1 on healing of segmental defects in non-human primates. J Bone Joint Surg Am 1995; 77: 734–750.
43. den Boer FC, Wippermann BW, Blokhuis TJ, Patka P, Bakker FC, Haarman HJ. Healing of segmental bone defects with granular porous hydroxyapatite augmented with recombinant human osteogenic protein-1 or autologous bone marrow. J Orthop Res 2003; 21(3): 521–528.
44. Hamdy RC, Amako M, Beckman L, Kawaguchi M, Rauch F, Lauzier D, Steffen T. Effects of osteogenic protein-1 on distraction osteogenesis in rabbits. Bone 2003; 33(2): 248–255.
45. Mizumoto Y, Moseley T, Drews M, Cooper VN 3rd, Reddi AH. Acceleration of regenerate ossification during distraction osteogenesis with recombinant human bone morphogenetic protein-7. J Bone Joint Surg Am 2003; 85-A Suppl 3: 124–130.
46. den Boer FC, Bramer JA, Blokhuis TJ, Van Soest EJ, Jenner JM, Patka P, Bakker FC, Burger EH, Haarman HJ. Effect of recombinant human osteogenic protein-1 on the healing of a freshly closed diaphyseal fracture. Bone 2002; 31(1): 158–164.
47. Johnsson R, Stromqvist B, Aspenberg P. Randomized radiostereometric study comparing osteogenic protein-1 (BMP-7) and autograft bone in human noninstrumented posterolateral lumbar fusion: 2002 Volvo Award in clinical studies. Spine 2002; 27(23): 2654–2661.
48. Vaccaro AR, Patel T, Fischgrund J, Anderson DG, Truumees E, Herkowitz H, Phillips F, Hilibrand A, Albert TJ. A pilot safety and efficacy study of OP-1 putty (rhBMP-7) as an adjunct to iliac crest autograft in posterolateral lumbar fusions. Eur Spine J 2003; 12(5): 495–500. Epub 2003 Aug 08.
49. Friedlaender GE, Perry CR, Cole JD, Cook SD, Cierny G, Muschler GF, Zych GA, Calhoun JH, LaForte AJ, Yin S. Osteogenic protein-1 (bone morphogenetic protein-7) in the treatment of tibial nonunions. J Bone Joint Surg Am 2001; 83 Suppl 1: S151–158.
50. Sciadini MF, Johnson KD. Evaluation of recombinant human bone morphogenetic protein-2 as a bone-graft substitute in a canine segmental defect model. J Orthop Res 2000; 18: 289–302.
51. Bostrom MP, Camacho NP. Potential role of bone morphogenetic proteins in fracture healing. Clin Orthop 1998; 355 Suppl: S274–282.
52. Einhorn TA, Trippel SB. Growth factor treatment of fractures. Instr Course Lect 1997; 46: 483–486.
53. Boden SD, Martin GJ Jr, Horton WC, Truss TL, Sandhu HS. Laparoscopic anterior spinal arthrodesis with rhBMP-2 in a titanium interbody threaded cage. J Spinal Disord 1998; 11: 95–101.
54. Boden SD, Zdeblick TA, Sandhu HS, Heim SE. The use of rhBMP-2 in interbody fusion cages. Definitive evidence of osteoinduction in humans: a preliminary report. Spine 2000; 25: 376–381.
55. Burkus JK, Dorchak JD, Sanders DL. Radiographic assessment of interbody fusion using recombinant human bone morphogenetic protein type 2. Spine 2003; 28(4): 372–377.
56. Govender S, Csimma C, Genant HK, Valentin-Opran A, Amit Y, Arbel R, et al. Recombinant human bone morphogenetic protein-2 for treatment of open tibial fractures: a prospective, controlled, randomized study of four hundred and fifty patients. J Bone Joint Surg Am 2002; 84-A(12): 2123–2134.
57. Wildemann B, Bamdad P, Holmer Ch, Haas NP, Raschke M, Schmidmaier G. Local delivery of growth factors from coated titanium plates increases osteotomy healing in rats. Bone 2004; 34(5): 862–868.
58. Lee JY, Peng H, Usas A, Musgrave D, Cummins J, Pelinkovic D, Jankowski R, Ziran B, Robbins P, Huard J. Enhancement of bone healing based on ex vivo gene therapy using human muscle-derived cells expressing bone morphogenetic protein 2. Hum Gene Ther 2002; 13(10): 1201–1211.
59. Dumont RJ, Dayoub H, Li JZ, Dumont AS, Kallmes DF, Hankins GR, Helm GA. Ex vivo bone morphogenetic protein-9 gene therapy using human mesenchymal stem cells induces spinal fusion in rodents. Neurosurgery 2002; 51(5): 1239–1244.
60. Rose T, Peng H, Usas A, Kuroda R, Lill H, Fu FH, Huard J. Gene therapy to improve osteogenesis in bone lesions with severe soft tissue damage. Langenbecks Arch Surg 2003; 388(5): 356–365.
61. Rundle CH, Miyakoshi N, Kasukawa Y, Chen ST, Sheng MH, Wergedal JE, Lau KH, Baylink DJ. In vivo bone formation in fracture repair induced by direct retroviral-based gene therapy with bone morphogenetic protein-4. Bone 2003; 32(6): 591–601.
62. Wang JC, Kanim LE, Yoo S, Campbell PA, Berk AJ, Lieberman JR. Effect of regional gene therapy with bone morphogenetic protein-2-producing bone marrow cells on spinal fusion in rats. J Bone Joint Surg Am 2003; 85-A(5): 905–911.
63. Southwood LL, Frisbie DD, Kawcak CE, Ghivizzani SC, Evans CH, McIlwraith CW. Evaluation of Ad-BMP-2 for enhancing fracture healing in an infected defect fracture rabbit model. J Orthop Res 2004; 22(1): 66–72.
64. Niyibizi, C et al. Potential role for gene therapy in the enhancement of fracture healing. Clin Orthop Rel Res 1998; 335S: 148–153.

Intramedullary Reaming of Long Bones

J.P. Frölke

Introduction

In Küntscher's original design he inserted a cloverleaf-shaped nail in the medullary cavity to achieve fixation in the isthmus through the elastic expansion of the nail [1]. It was a dynamic compression nail that guaranteed rotational stability providing a three-point contact between nail and bone (Fig. 2.3.1). Essential in this technique was a good match between the nail and medullary canal. A snug fit between nail and medullary canal controls rotational deformity at the fracture site. If the nail is too large to fit the isthmus, it impedes the insertion and results in either jamming of the nail or iatrogenic fracture [2].

In order to avoid these problems, Küntscher proposed reaming of the medullary cavity [1, 3]. After preparing and exposing the right point of entry in the bone, the awl is used to open the medullary cavity. Sometimes in young bone, an extra small hand reamer is necessary to pass through the cortical defect into the medullary canal. After removal of the hand reamer, an olive-tipped guide wire is passed down the medullary canal as far as the fracture site and after closed reduction into the distal fragment. The olive-tipped guide wire should be passed into the center of the distal fragment. The reamers and the nail will always follow the guide wire and therefore an eccentrically located guide wire will result in a malpositioned nail. It should be placed firmly into the metaphyseal bone of the distal fragment to minimize the risk of it backing out later. The reamers are introduced over the olive-tipped guide wire.

Depending on the reamer design, it has an end-cutting or a side-cutting reamer head. The initial reamer is always end-cutting and enlarges the track to allow the reamers to expand the track in 0.5-mm increments. Reaming should always be carried out so that the resultant track in the medullary cavity is at least 1 mm wider than the intramedullary nail that is proposed to be used [4].

Reaming increases the inner diameter of the medullary canal by removing the inner cortical bone and a larger diameter nail can be used. This provides better stability by increasing the interference and thus the mechanical properties of the nail [2, 5]. The indication for this nail was limited to midshaft transverse or oblique fractures.

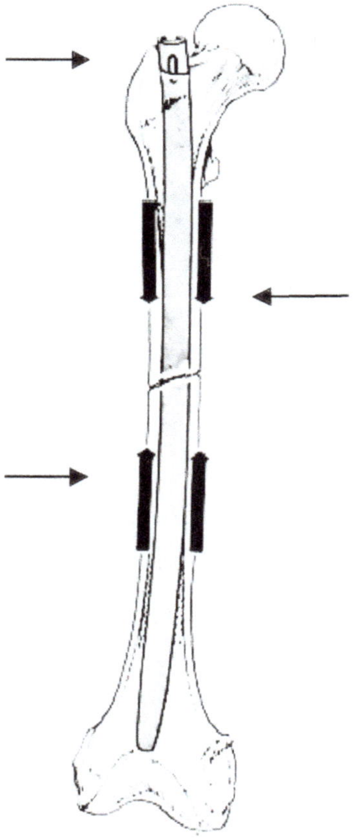

Fig. 2.3.1. Küntscher's design of intramedullary nail with three-point fixation (*small arrows*) and dynamic compression (*large arrows*) in a fractured femur

Since Küntscher's first design, the evolution of the reamed nail has followed two main paths. First the femoral nail shape was altered to correspond with the natural anterior bow of the femur, although the overall shape of the tibial nail remained essentially unchanged. The second modification involved perforation of the nail to allow

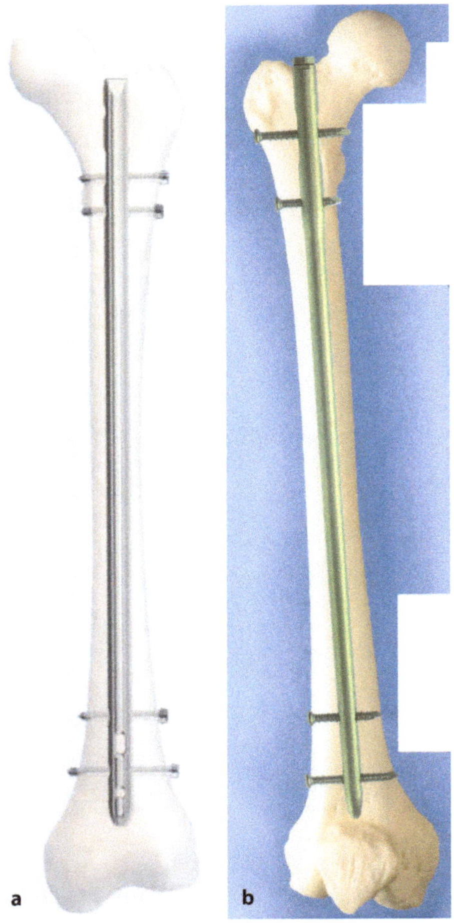

Fig. 2.3.2 a, b. Examples of interlocking femoral nails with a a large, reamed nail and b a small, unreamed nail

the introduction of cross-bolts capable of transfixing both bone and nail. This type of "locking" or "interlocking" nail was initially introduced by Küntscher, but the design was modified several times later on [3, 6–8].

The development of the interlocking nail permitted intramedullary nailing with smaller nails with subsequent less extensive or no reaming [9, 10]. The indications for intramedullary nailing were extended to long, oblique, spiral, comminuted and open fractures in the whole diaphysis of the bone (Fig. 2.3.2) [6, 11, 12].

Most reamed and unreamed locked nails can be inserted in dynamic or static modes. Dynamic locking refers to the practice of placing cross-bolts at one end of the nail only, while in the static mode there are cross-bolts at both ends. Dynamic locking can be distal for more proximally located fractures and proximal for more distally located fractures. Some nails have a special longitudinal cross-bolt perforation to provide rotational stability in an axially dynamic mode. The theoretical advantage of dynamic locking is that it permits axial movement and thus compression at the fracture site during weight bearing. This mode is used when there is a fracture above or below the isthmus of a type that is stable after nailing. If there is any comminution, or if the fracture is segmental, a static lock should be used. This gives stability to the fracture, allowing for the maintenance of length and correct alignment. However, axial loading of the fracture is minimized. Dynamization is the practice of converting the static mode to either a proximal or distal dynamic mode. This is usually carried out between 6 and 8 weeks after fracture treatment [4].

A small-diameter nail makes the insertion easy and the operation time shorter, but the stiffness of the nail is decreased, resulting in nail bending, breakage and migration postoperatively [13]. It provides a weaker fixation and a higher rate of implant complications compared to larger nails like nonunion or malunion and nail or interlocking bolt breakage [14–16]. This phenomenon, however, has predominantly been described for tibial nailing and not so much for femoral nailing [17–19].

Systemic Effects of Reaming

Fat Embolism Syndrome

During the 1990s, a new generation of intramedullary locking nails was designed, which did not need previous reaming of the intramedullary cavity. This was the result of a discussion about the relationship of the reaming procedure with systemic adverse effects such as fat embolism (Table 2.3.1) and subsequent acute respiratory distress

Table 2.3.1. Diagnostic criteria for fat embolism syndrome. One major and three minor criteria or two major and two minor criteria are considered to show an established fat embolism syndrome [30]

Major criteria
Petechial rash
Respiratory symptoms plus bilateral signs with positive radiographic changes
Cerebral signs unrelated to head injury or any other condition
Minor criteria
Tachycardia
Pyrexia
Retinal changes (fat or petechiae)
Urinary changes (anuria, oliguria, fat globules)
Sudden drop in hemoglobin level
Sudden thrombocytopenia
High erythrocyte sedimentation rate
Fat globules in the sputum

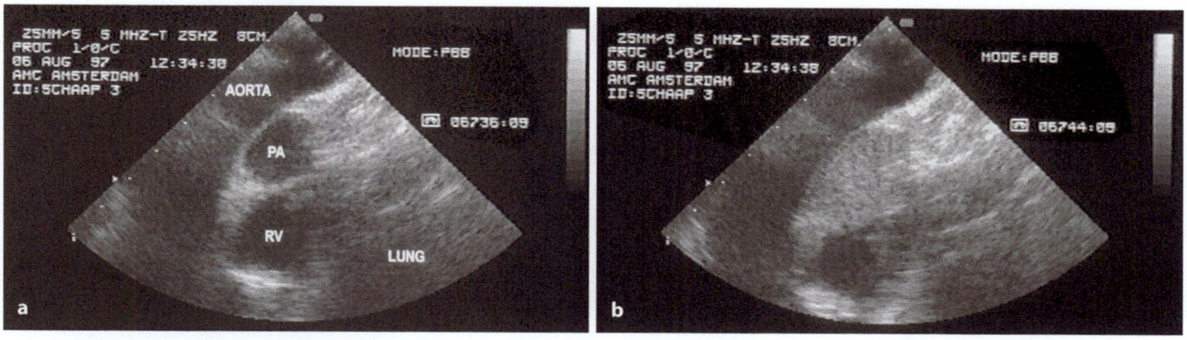

Fig. 2.3.3 a, b. Example of transesophageal echocardiography of a a preoperative sheep and b after reaming the femoral medullary cavity with a storm of fat embolisms in the pulmonary artery. *PA* pulmonary artery, *RV* right ventricle

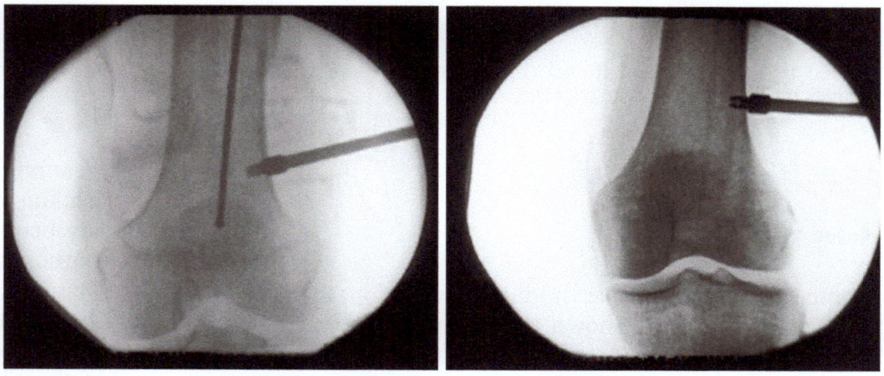

Fig. 2.3.4. Anteroposterior roentgenograms of pressure sensor position at the supracondylar region

syndrome (ARDS), especially in cases of multitraumatized patients [20–28]. However, these adverse effects were predominantly observed in animal studies (Fig. 2.3.3) and case reports [29].

In primary conventional reamed intramedullary nailing, the combination of thoracic trauma with a femoral shaft fracture may lead to postoperative pulmonary complications. Patients with multiple injuries and lung contusions have their compensatory mechanism fully stressed. In these circumstances, an additional stress factor, such as intramedullary nailing, may trigger the development of ARDS. Direct blockade of the pulmonary vascular system by embolized bone marrow fat particles associated with an acute rise in pulmonary artery pressure may lead to this decompensation after reaming the femoral canal [21, 22].

Another cause for this decompensation may be the agglutination of activated platelets and leukocytes in the pulmonary vascular system, resulting in endothelial damage by releasing proteolytic enzymes and other cytotoxic mediators [31–34]. These factors, however, could also be activated by the operative trauma itself [35, 36].

During the reaming procedure, the intramedullary pressure (Fig. 2.3.4) increases in a certain manner [37–39], and various studies have reported a positive correlation between intramedullary pressure and the amount of bone marrow fat embolized to the intravascular compartment [10, 40, 41].

Efforts to minimize intramedullary hypertension resulted in the development of different reamer head designs (Fig. 2.3.5) [42–45], venting during nailing [46], an irrigation-suction technique [37, 39] and unreamed nailing techniques [21, 47].

To decide if one or the other nailing modality would be of any benefit to prevent these systemic complications, reamed or unreamed nailing has been an important subject of research during the last decade. Large prospective randomized clinical studies have been performed to compare these two treatment modalities [9, 48–50]. A meta-analysis of 676 studies showed no difference of systemic complications in reamed versus unreamed nailing of femoral or tibial fractures [51].

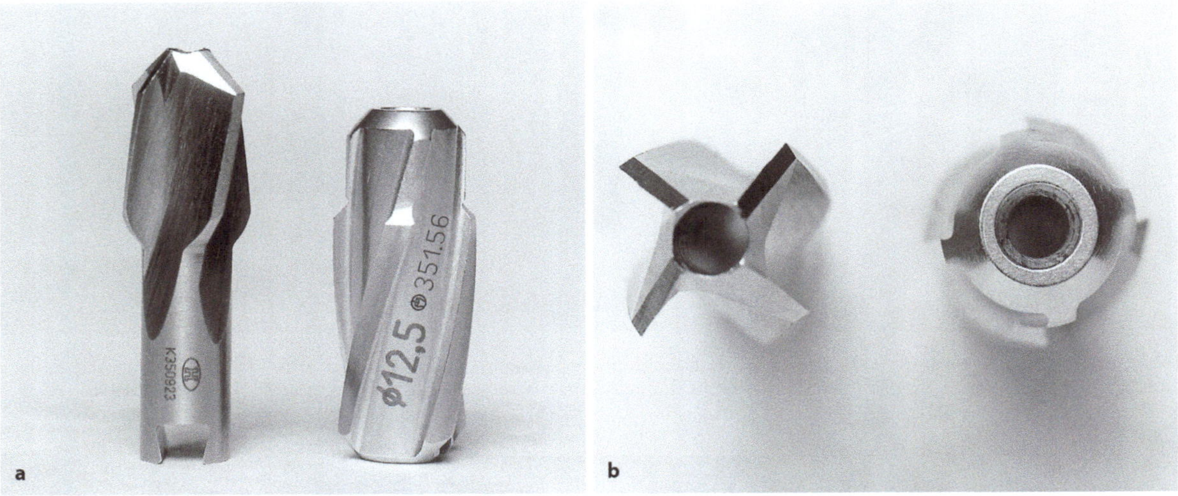

Fig. 2.3.5 a, b. Side (a) and frontal (b) view of 12.5-mm large fluted reamer head with small core (*left*) and small fluted reamer head with large core (*right*)

Local Effects of Reaming

Autografting

Comparative prospective studies focused on the time of healing have shown that fractures treated with reamed nailing have a significantly shorter healing time [50–52].

A number of surgeons suggest that the reamings from the endosteal surface of the cortex have a bone graft effect and thereby enhance bone union [4, 53]. This so-called "bone autograft theory" assumes a local release of reaming debris in the fracture gap when reaming the medullary cavity.

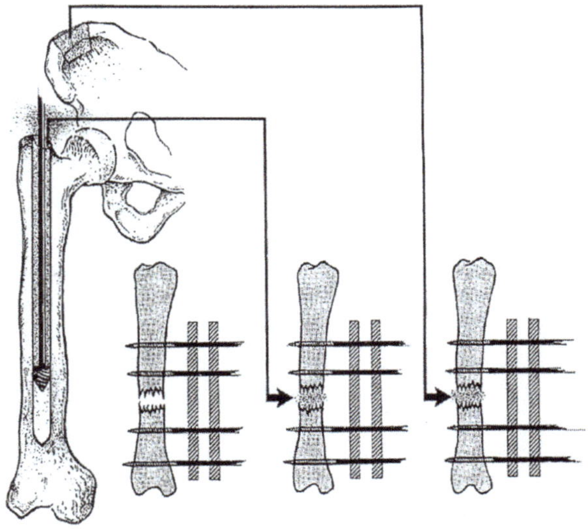

Fig. 2.3.6. Animal model to evaluate the osteoinductive effect of isolated reaming debris

The use of reaming debris as a free graft to stimulate the healing of a bone defect or non-union has already been applied clinically even before the exact pathophysiological mechanism was revealed [54]. The effect of isolated reaming debris on fracture healing therefore was studied in an animal model [45]. Thirty sheep were treated with an osteotomy of the tibia with 5-mm distraction. In one group, the osteotomy gap was left empty. In the second group, the gap was packed with reaming debris from the ipsilateral femur, and in the third group, the gap was packed with cancellous bone from the iliac crest (Fig. 2.3.6). At follow-up, callus volume was measured on standard X-rays. After 3 weeks, callus volume from the reamings group as well as the iliac crest group had increased significantly compared to the empty group (Fig. 2.3.7). The conclusion of this study was that isolated reaming debris supports callus

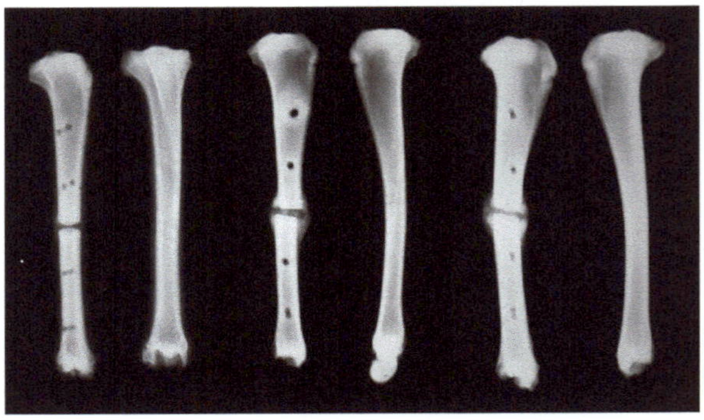

Fig. 2.3.7. Lateral roentgenograms of the left tibia of three sheep at 3 weeks follow-up. From left to right: empty gap, reaming debris grafting and iliac crest grafting

formation as much as conventional autologous bone grafting.

Exchange nailing – from unreamed to reamed – is a useful method to promote union of fractures when slow consolidation occurs after initial treatment with an unreamed nail [4, 55]. The exact cause of fracture healing by this exchange of nail is not yet clear, but it is assumed that the combination of providing more stability together with the collection of reaming debris at the fracture site could have local effects on fracture healing [56–59].

Distribution of Cortical Reamings

It is indeed likely that reamings, which are moved up and down with the reamer under a certain pressure during reaming of the medullary cavity, collect at the place of least resistance. This can be at the opening in the proximal cortex, made to insert the reaming tool, or at the fracture site. The first step in understanding the influence of autografting on fracture healing is how much reamings actually settle in the fracture gap during reaming of the medullary cavity.

A sheep cadaver model was used to measure the distribution of cortical reamings in 10 sheep femurs during reaming of the medullary cavity with 0.5-mm increments and with moderate speed and pressure (Fig. 2.3.8). Twenty-four per cent of the total amount of reamings at the gap was found (Fig. 2.3.9), but depending on the size and location of the fracture cleft and the amount of distraction in a real fracture situation, the amount of reaming debris may vary [60].

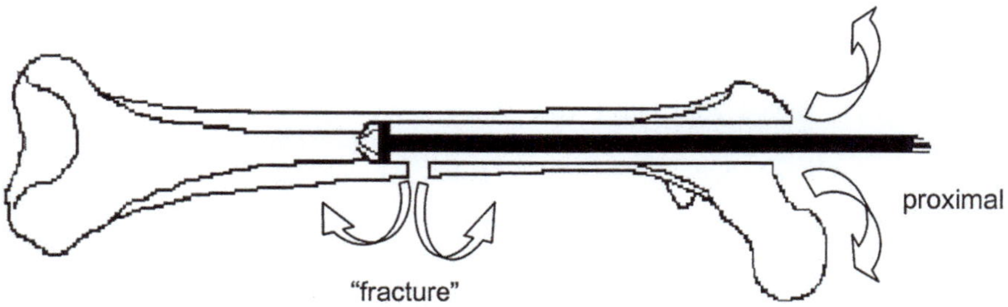

Fig. 2.3.8. Sheep cadaver model: *arrows* with "*fracture*" indicate the place where reaming debris collects at the fracture site, whereas *arrows* with "*proximal*" indicate the place where reaming debris escapes through the working channel of the reaming tool

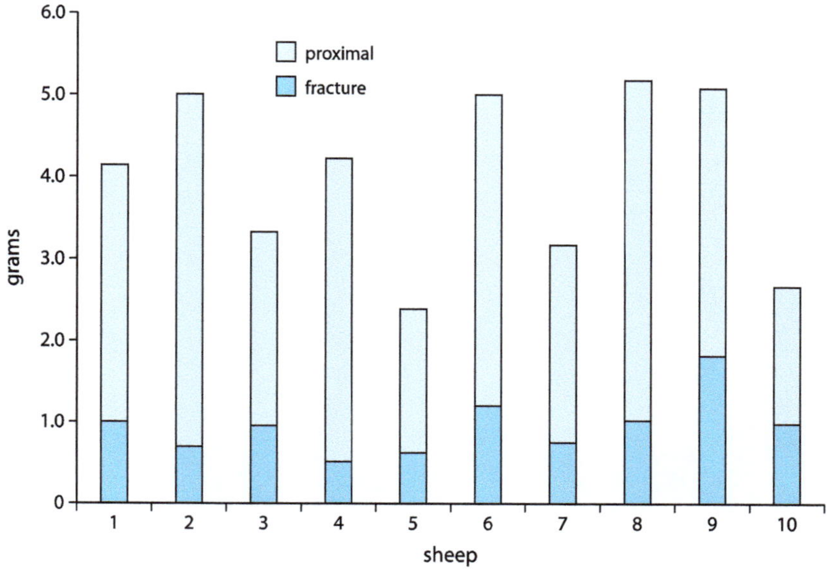

Fig. 2.3.9. Amounts of reaming debris in grams per sheep femur, weighed separately from the artificial fracture gap ("*fracture*") and from the proximal opening in the medullary cavity ("*proximal*")

Viable Osteoblastic Potential of Cortical Reamings

Reaming debris seems to have excellent properties for bone healing. All three components of reaming debris may be of certain value to stimulate fracture healing: bone marrow, blood and bone scrapings. Bone marrow and blood have been proven to have osteogenic properties [61, 62]. Bone scrapings can provide a scaffold in a passive way similar to iliac crest grafting, but it is not yet clarified how and whether bone cells actively contribute to fracture healing [63]. In a small series of patients, intramedullary reamings seem vital and retain their viability for at least 7 days. The osteoinductive potential of intramedullary reamings in the treatment of bone loss was equal and possibly better than the currently utilized iliac crest graft [56].

The viability of bone cells in reaming debris has also been assessed for continued calcification by placing human reamings in muscle tissue of living rats [64], and the incidence of heterotopic ossification in reamed nailing has been related to the generation of osteogenic reaming debris [59].

To further reveal a possible role of bone cells in the biology of fracture repair in reamed nailing, the reaming debris of 10 sheep femora was cultivated in a standard manner, and compared with cultivated cancellous bone fragments from the iliac crest of 10 other sheep [65]. The aim of this study was to test whether viable cells are present and if so, to test the cells for osteoblastic characteristics and assess to what level cells from reaming debris resemble cells from iliac crest bone. The question to be answered in this study was whether cells from reaming debris respond similarly to 1,25-dihydroxyvitamin D3 (vitD) by enhanced alkaline phosphatase activity as bone cells derived from the iliac crest bone [66].

In all cases, cells started to grow from the reaming debris or the iliac crest fragments within 2–5 days. They proliferated rapidly and covered the entire culture flask within 9–13 days. Cells from reaming debris and iliac crest fragments had a similar osteoblastic appearance, with a spindle-shaped, somewhat cuboidal form (Fig. 2.3.10).

All cultures derived from sheep reaming debris responded to vitD with enhanced alkaline phosphatase activity in a manner that is largely similar to the response of bone cells obtained from the iliac crest [66]. VitD reduced the protein content of both the reaming debris cultures and the iliac crest cultures in a similar manner, indicating that in both cases vitD inhibited cell proliferation, a response that is typical of osteoblasts (Fig. 2.3.11). This is the first study to show these osteoblastic characteristics in reaming debris, which means that reaming debris is as vital as iliac crest bone and may act similarly to an osteoinductive autograft.

Compartment Syndrome

Due to the effect of the reamer like a piston in a syringe, the intramedullary pressure increases when moving the reamer along the medullary cavity [67]. The muscle compartment pressures may rise as well during that phase of the reaming procedure because the fracture is continuous with most of these compartments. Comparable to the piston effect in the syringe, the pressure is decreased and eventually a suction effect is caused by removal of the reamer [9].

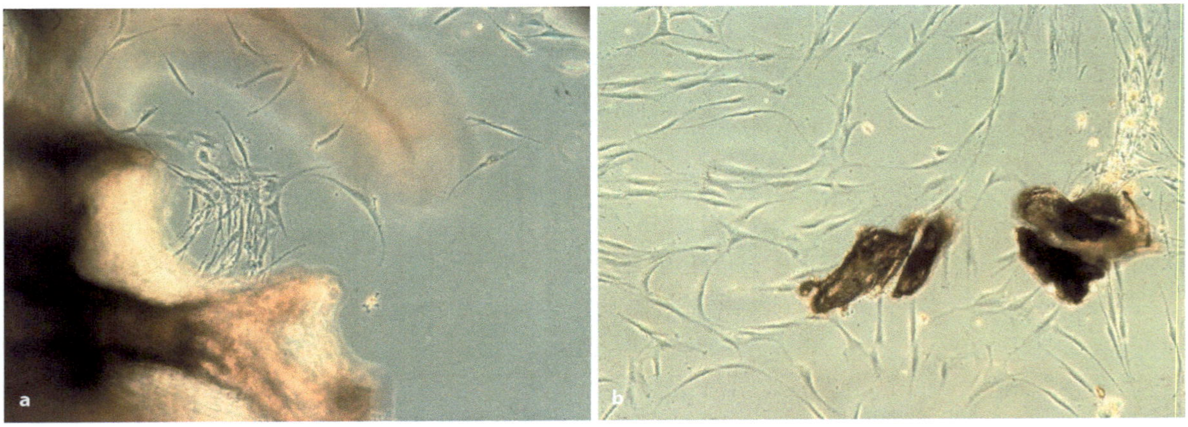

Fig. 2.3.10 a, b. Spindle-shaped and somewhat cuboidal cells from the iliac crest (a) and from reaming debris (b) after 1 week of cultivation (magnification 10×). Cells from reaming debris and iliac crest show a similar morphology

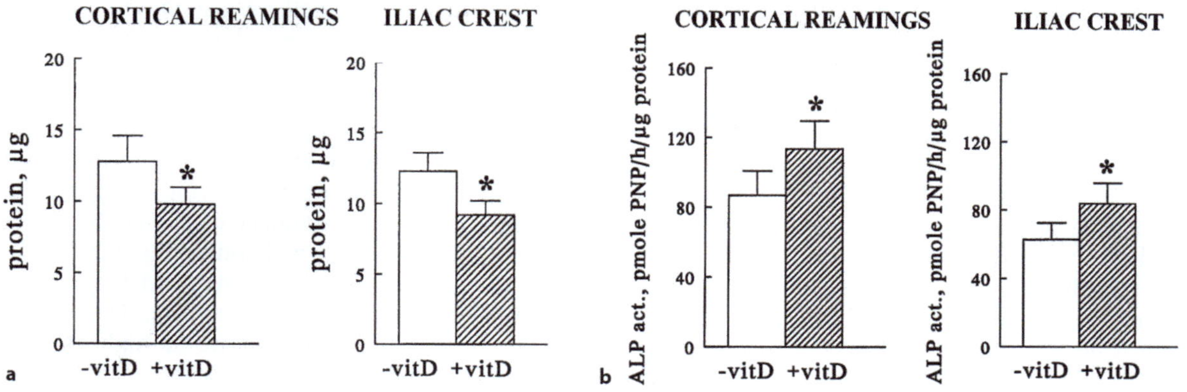

Fig. 2.3.11 a, b. The effect of 1,25-dihydroxyvitamin D3 on the protein content of the cell layer (a) and alkaline phosphatase activity (b) in bone cell cultures from reaming debris and from iliac crest bone biopsies. Values are means ± SEM of triplicate cultures of reaming debris or iliac crest bone biopsies from 10 sheep each. *Significant effect of vitD, $p < 0.05$

Animal studies have shown an increased compartment pressure during reaming [68, 69], but no clinical data exist supporting the hypothesis that the reaming procedure can cause a compartment syndrome. A large meta-analysis could not confirm a higher incidence of the compartment syndrome in reamed nailing [51].

Cortical Circulation

Fracture healing cannot occur without an adequate blood supply. The diaphysis of long bones receives its blood supply predominantly from the nutrient artery and its endosteal tributaries. The periosteal vessels that are fed from the surrounding muscular envelope and the vessels of the metaphysis anastomose with the endosteal vessels of the nutrient artery (Fig. 2.3.12). In the mid-diaphysis, the inner two-thirds of the cortex receives its blood supply from endosteal vessels and only 10–30% of the outer cortex receives its blood supply from extramedullary vessels [70, 71].

Reaming and intramedullary nailing have dramatic acute effects on the diaphyseal blood flow. Reaming removes the marrow contents, endosteum and inner cortical bone and destroys the medullary blood vessels. This surgical intervention alters the blood flow from centrifugal to centripetal, resulting in an initial decreased blood flow in the remaining cortex and may lead to cortical bone necrosis in the inner half of the cortex [72–74]. Animal studies have shown that, as long as space remains within the intramedullary canal after insertion of the nail, the bone is revascularized through centripetal blood flow within 6 weeks [75].

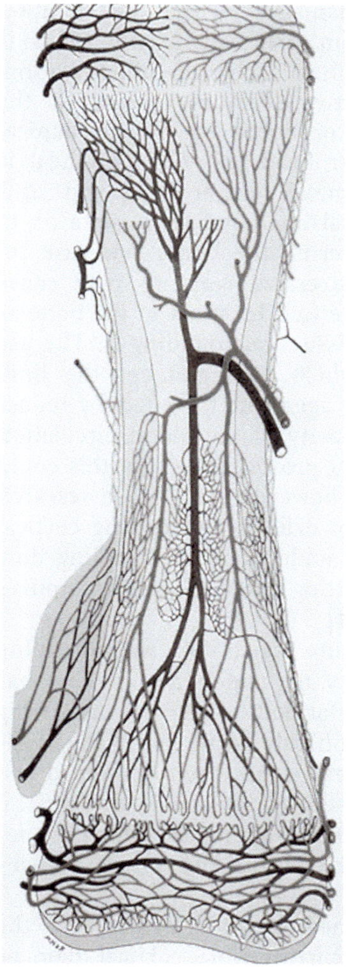

Fig. 2.3.12. Schematic frontal section of vascularization of long bone in a child. *Light gray vessels* arterial pole, *dark gray vessels* venous pole

After reamed intramedullary nailing, the fracture-healing process is dependent on the revascularization response from the periosteum and surrounding soft tissues. Also the circulation of the overlying muscles and skin increases by reaming and may have a stimulatory effect on fracture healing [76, 77]. Interruption of the periosteal and surrounding soft tissue vascular supply to the cortex, either by excessive surgical exposure during open intramedullary nailing or by traumatic loss in open fractures, would be expected to have a deleterious effect on revascularization of the cortex and fracture healing [78]. This is the rationale for surgeons to use unreamed nailing techniques in fractures with severe loss of soft tissue coverage.

Heat Necrosis

Bone cells can be damaged by the lack of blood supply but also from heat denaturation. This is more a theoretical than a clinical differentiation. An important negative effect of reaming is the generation of heat produced by the mechanical power of the reamer head [42, 79]. This heat is generated by the metal reamer head and conducted to the cortical bone and from there on to the soft tissues covering the bone. Few case reports show that excessive reaming may cause thermal injury to the full thickness of the bone as well as to the soft tissues surrounding it. The use of a tourniquet, which exsanguinates the limb during surgery, may aggravate the effect by reducing the cooling capacity of the blood circulation [80, 81]. In a clinical prospective study this could not be confirmed, however [82]. Most research has been focused on drilling and cutting cortical bone and it is well understood that cooling during drilling and cutting cortical bone minimizes heat necrosis [83, 84].

Cortical temperature registration when reaming the medullary cavity of long bones in vivo has not often been performed [82]. The measuring method remains a difficult point. No reliable, validated measuring method has been developed yet, because the attachment of sensors in the cortical wall requires a surgical approach, which is not desired in closed reduction and intramedullary nailing techniques.

Using different methods of determination, the threshold value for irreversible cortical damage varies and depends on the exposed temperature and the time of exposure. Bone necrosis becomes morphologically visible at 47 °C when using a direct microscopic method with an exposure time of 1 min [85].

Histochemical as well as histological methods underestimate the thermal damage. Despite that, reaming is a procedure that can easily be performed in less than 1 min under normal conditions, Lundskog has shown that heat necrosis can also occur in a much shorter exposure time [86]. Assuming that the time of inserting and removing a reamer from the medullary canal should not go beyond 40 s under normal conditions, the time of true contact between the reamer and inner cortical wall may be even less than 15 s. Therefore it is safe to assume a temperature as high as 77 °C for any amount of time to cause irreversible thermal injury to the bone [87].

Thermal complications of reaming in bone have been described [80, 81], but no method of measuring shows that the temperature indeed reaches the threshold level of osteonecrosis. The introduction of new, sharp reamers, designed to minimize the development of cortical heat necrosis, therefore cannot be evaluated. The danger of this phenomenon is that the evaluation of different reamers with the existing measuring method can lead to false conclusions [42].

An experimental study was performed to compare different in vitro methods of measuring the cortical temperature when reaming the medullary cavity [88]. This was done to validate an approved mathematical model, which can be used to determine the temperature gradient in the cortical bone in the presence or absence of sensors (Fig. 2.3.13). Artificial bone was used with an intramedullary heat source instead of a reamer. Temperatures were measured with thermocouples placed radially and axially in the cortical wall (Fig. 2.3.14). These two measurement positions were compared and used to validate an approved mathematical model in order to determine the temperature gradient in cortical bone in the absence of sensors.

It appeared that the measurement of the cortical temperature with the thermocouples in a radial position only reflects maximally 14% of the temperature of the reamer (calculated 55%). The measurement with the thermocouples in the axial position reflects 65% (calculated 70%) of the reamer temperature at most, which is similar to undisturbed bone (Fig. 2.3.15). The measuring method with the thermocouples in a radial position therefore could not be recommended [89].

The limitations of this study seem obvious: a theoretical model with artificial bone and a controlled heat source instead of a true reamer. An environment with a constant temperature of 37 °C is necessary to compare measurements and calculations in this study but the cooling effect of soft

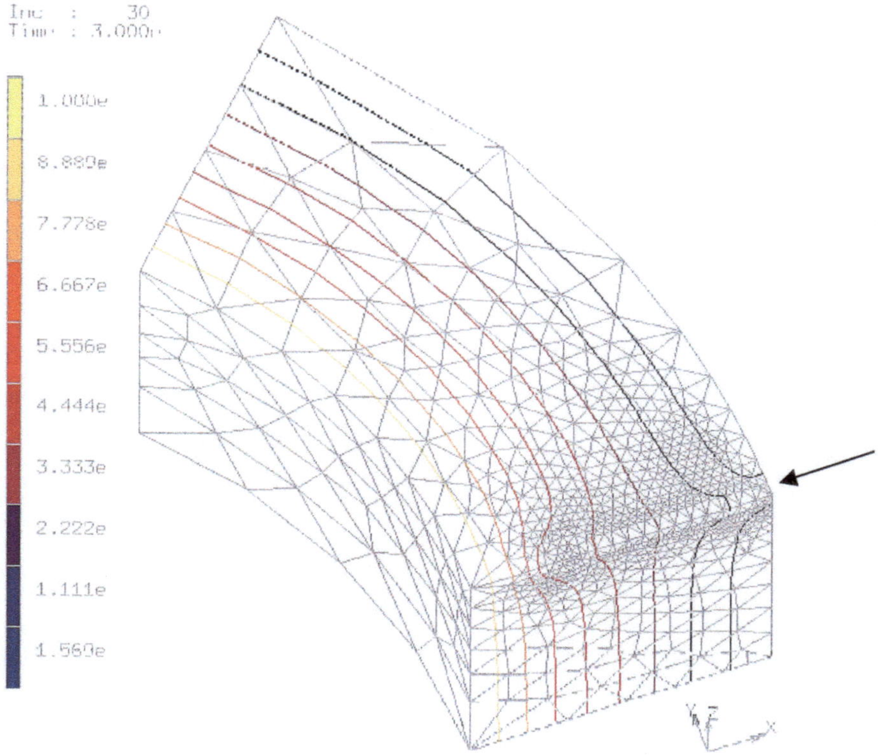

Fig. 2.3.13. Finite element model of bone segment with radial sensor position showing disturbance of heat conduction. *Colored lines* indicate 1 °C, *arrow* indicates virtual sensor position

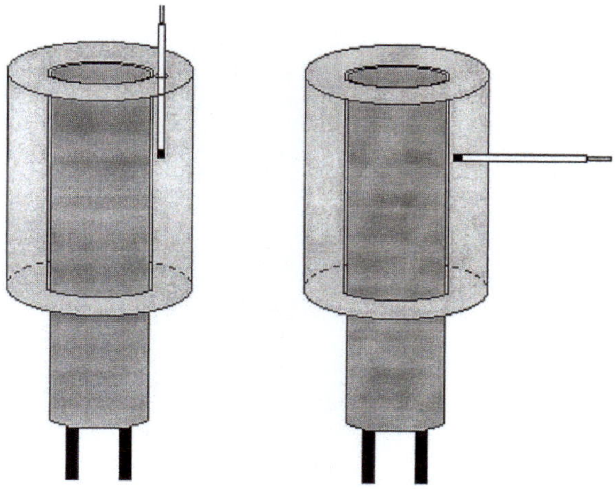

Fig. 2.3.14. Longitudinal cross-section of long bone with sensor positioning in this study. *T* (in °C) is the difference between source temperature and temperature of the environment

tissue coverage and blood circulation never reaches this level or the clinical picture of heat blisters on the skin would not appear.

To gather information about the generated temperature it is important that measurements take place on the nearest point where the temperature is generated, which is the reamer head. Thermocouples have been mounted on the tip of Kirschner wires [90], but to our knowledge no experiments have yet been performed with a measuring device on the reamer head. These data combined with the mathematical method shown in this study would make a clinical application possible. Comparison of different reamer head designs can be performed and guidelines for reaming techniques could be defined. Technically this is all possible but the lack of clinical importance has meant that research teams have not yet pursued those developments.

It is likely that a much higher temperature is generated and conducted through reaming than has been presumed until now. There is no clinical importance of these observations in normal circumstances but it might play a role when the reamer becomes obstructed in a narrow or scarred medullary cavity. Therefore several guidelines have to be emphasized, which have been postulated before [91, 92]. Be sure about the geometry of the medullary canal. Any narrowing, scarring or obstruction should be anticipated. Pay attention to the quality of the reamer heads. The use of a tourniquet should not be stimulated because it exsanguinates the limb and may prevent the circulating blood from cooling. Moderate

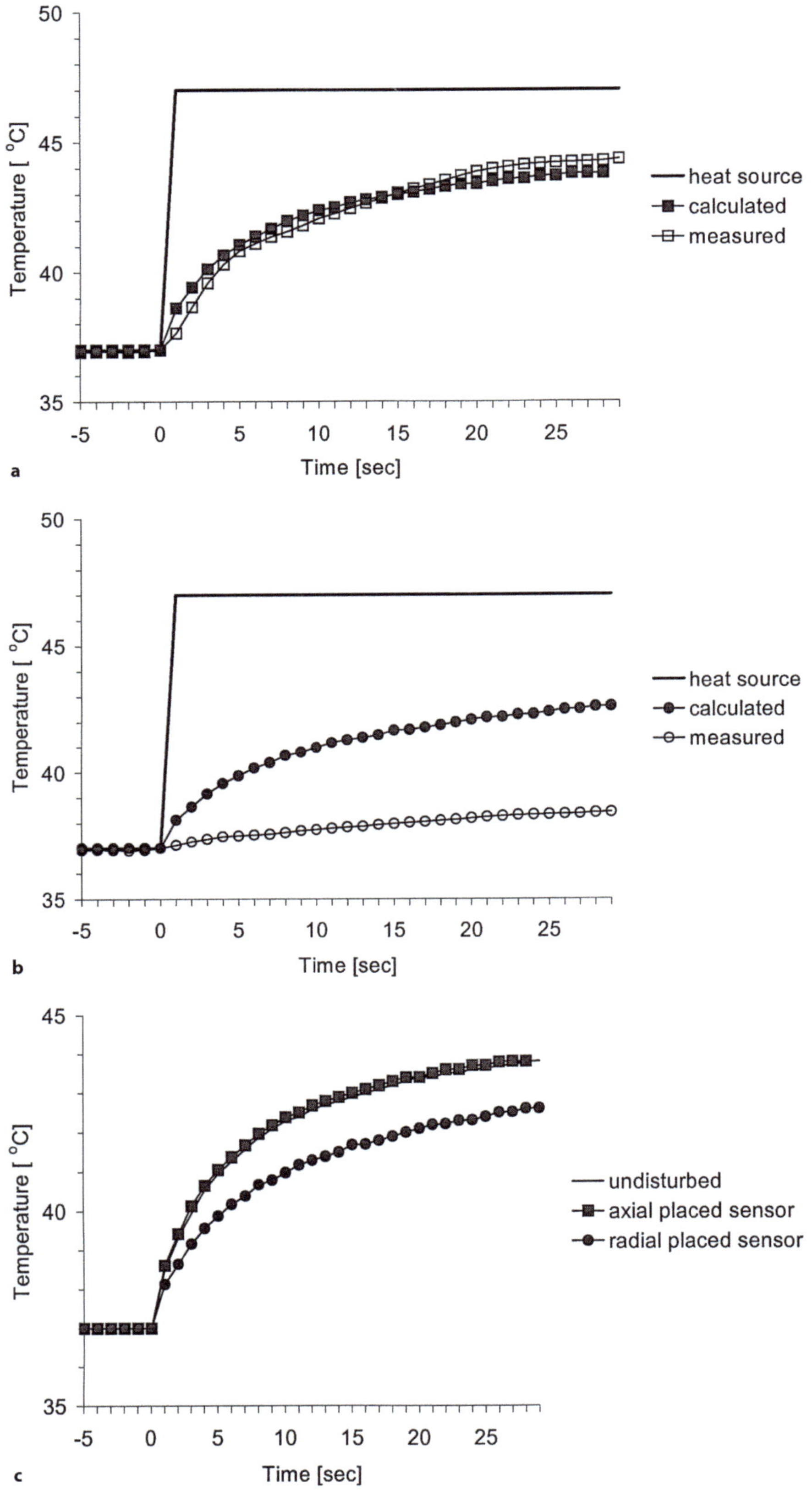

Fig. 2.3.15 a–c. Calculated and measured temperature assessment during "reaming" with the sensor in the radial position

power and speed with every insertion of the reamer promotes a smooth procedure and steps of more than 0.5 mm, especially in young patients, are to be avoided. Drilling with a blunt reamer for too long in the same position may stimulate heat production and a step back to a smaller and sharper reamer should overcome this problem.

Conclusions

1. In vivo as well as ex vivo studies provide more proof for the "autograft theory" assuming that a considerable amount of debris that is produced during reaming of the medullary cavity releases at the fracture site and stimulates callus formation by adding vital bone cells to the fracture.
2. The potential detrimental effect of heat, which is generated and conducted by the reamer, does not seem to play an important role in physiologic reaming conditions. However, the current methods of measuring this temperature underestimate the temperature in the cortical wall during reaming. It is likely that a much higher temperature is generated and conducted through reaming than has been presumed until now. Again, there is no clinical importance of these observations in normal circumstances but it might play a role when the reamer becomes obstructed in a narrow or scarred medullary cavity, especially in the tibia because of its marginal soft tissue coverage.
3. The increase of intramedullary pressure can be measured in patients with femoral shaft fractures. A significant difference can be demonstrated between standard reamers and the new-generation reamers, which are especially designed to depressurize the medullary cavity. However, no difference in clinical symptoms of a fat embolism syndrome was noted, but study groups are small and do not include polytraumatized patients. In patients with multiple injuries, priority should be given to survival rather than fracture healing and intramedullary reaming should be avoided. If necessary, however, this could be an ultimate indication to use the new-generation reamers, which may cause less collection of reaming debris at the fracture site but also less intramedullary hypertension.
4. Comparing reamed and unreamed nailing with respect to the time to healing can only be judged in high quality prospective studies with more than 1000 patients enrolled, which are not available at this time. A limited number of smaller prospectively designed studies published so far show a reduction of healing time and less nonunions in fractures treated with reamed nailing. Lack of consensus in the assessment of fracture healing by surgeons is a confounder. Reaming takes time, so it is not surprising that the operation time was significantly shorter in the unreamed group in every citation. Therefore unreamed nailing may be a better choice in order to gain time, particularly in severely injured patients with cerebral and pulmonary contusion.

Recommendations

Primary Reaming

Reaming is beneficial for any fresh long bone fracture, thus the question should rather be: is there any strong indication not to ream? In a polytraumatized patient with cerebral and pulmonary contusion, unreamed nailing may be a better choice for the benefit of gaining time and avoiding complications. Fractures combined with severe soft tissue injury can be a relative contraindication for reamed nailing.

Secondary Reaming

Exchange nailing, or the substitution of one intramedullary nail for a larger second nail, is usually performed because of actual or incipient nonunion in a previously nailed fracture. Especially high-energy femoral and tibial type C fractures are at high risk for nonunion, regardless of their method of treatment. The conversion to a reamed nail may enhance healing in several ways. Reaming ameliorates the cortical vascularization by providing a condition to stimulate vascular ingrowth from the periosteal side of the cortex and together with the osteogenic effect of reaming debris this enhances atrophic nonunions to heal. The insertion of a larger nail increases the mechanical stability, allowing weight-bearing and physiological loading of the fracture site, enhancing a hypertrophic nonunion to heal.

Reaming for Infection

Intramedullary reaming to debride the medullary cavity after removing or during replacement of an infected nail can be a useful treatment. This technique has to be considered when local measures have failed to control chronic osteomyelitis of long bones and must be supported by local and systemic antibiotic treatment. Reaming debrides the medullary cavity with removal of sequesters and other sources of infection as a mechanical cleaning device. Reaming relieves intramedullary pressure and restores the continuity of the medullary cavity and the amelioration of cortical vascularization by providing a condition to stimulate vascular ingrowth from the periosteal side of the cortex. The access that is created this way can also be utilized for treatment with local antibiotics.

Technique of Reaming

The geometry of the medullary canal has to be studied preoperatively. Any narrowing, scarring or obstruction should be anticipated. The reamer set with small-diameter reamers has to be complete. Attention should be paid to the quality and sharpness of the reamer heads. Always check the connection of the reamer head with the flexible drive. Make sure you do not lose the head or guiding rod in the medullary cavity and use a rod with sufficient length. The setup of the operation is standard with maximum antiseptic precautions. A tourniquet should be avoided. The guide rod is inserted preferentially as central in the medullary cavity as possible. The tissue protector should be fixed not with tape but with a clamp to prevent loose tape remnants in the medullary cavity. Moderate power and speed should be used with every insertion of the reamer and steps of more than 0.5 mm should be avoided, especially in young patients. Never drill too long on the same position to prevent overheating. If the reamer does get stuck inside the medullary canal, gentle use of the drill may free the reamer and a smaller-diameter reamer should be used. The flexible drive of the reamer can also be reversed; however, when the flexible reamer is made of coiled steel, reversal of the reamer may cause it to uncoil. A slotted hammer can be positioned over the reamer against the drill attachments and the assembly tapped out. If these maneuvers are unsuccessful, open operative removal will be necessary but fortunately this is rarely required.

References

1. Küntscher G: The Küntscher method of intramedullary fixation. J Bone Joint Surg 1958; 40A:17–26
2. Fairbank AC, Thomas D, Cunningham B, Curtis M, Jinnah RH: Stability of reamed and unreamed intramedullary tibial nails: a biomechanical study. Injury 1995; 26:483–485
3. Küntscher G: Intramedullary surgical technique and its place in orthopaedic surgery. My present concept. J Bone Joint Surg 1964; 47A:809–818
4. Court-Brown CM. An atlas of closed nailing of the tibia and femur. Springer, Berlin Heidelberg New York 1991
5. Bucholz RW: Fatigue fractures of the interlocking nail for the femur. J Bone Joint Surg 1987; 69A:1391–1399
6. Kempf I, Grosse A, Beck G: Closed intramedullary nailing: its application to comminuted fractures of the femur. J Bone Joint Surg 1985; 67A:709–720
7. Huckstep RL: The Huckstep intramedullary compression nail. Clin Orthop 1986; 212:48–61
8. Klemm KW, Borner M: Interlocking nailing of complex fractures of the femur and tibia. Clin Orthop 1986; 212:89–100
9. Court-Brown CM, Christie J, McQueen MM: Closed intramedullary tibial nailing. Its use in closed and type I open fractures. J Bone Joint Surg 1990; 72B:605–611
10. Kröpfl A, Berger U, Neureiter H, Hertz H, Schlag G: Intramedullary pressure and bone marrow fat intravasation in unreamed femoral nailing. J Trauma 1997; 42:946–954
11. Kyle RF, Schaffhausen JM, Bechtold JE. Biomechanical characteristics of interlocking femoral nails in the treatment of complex femoral fractures. Clin Orthop 1991; 267:169–173
12. O'Brien PJ, Meek RN, Powell JN, Blachut PA: Primary intramedullary nailing of open femoral shaft fractures. J Trauma 1991; 31:113–116
13. Watson Jones R, Coltart WD: The classic. Slow union of fractures with a study of 804 fractures of the shafts of the tibia and femur. Clin Orthop 1982; 168:2–16
14. Weckbach A, Blattert TR, Kunz E: Differentialindikation zur Marknagelung der Tibia in aufgebohrter und nicht aufgebohrter Technik. Zentralbl Chir 1994; 119:556–563
15. Hutson JJ, Zych GA, Cole JD, Johnson KD, Ostermann P, Milne EL, Latta L: Mechanical failures of intramedullary tibial nails applied without reaming. Clin Orthop 1995; 315:129–137
16. Whittle AP, Wester W, Russell TA: Fatigue failure in small diameter tibial nails. Clin Orthop 1995; 315:119–128
17. Boenisch UW, de Boer PG, Journeaux SF: Unreamed intramedullary tibial nailing – fatigue of locking bolts. Injury 1996; 27:265–270
18. Boyer MI, Ribeiro E, Hu R, Powell JN: Small versus large diameter closed-section femoral nails for the treatment of femoral shaft fractures; is there a difference? J Trauma 1996; 41:279–282
19. Reynders PA, Broos PLO: Healing of closed femoral shaft fractures treated with the AO unreamed femoral nail. A comparative study with the AO reamed femoral nail. Injury 2000; 31:367–371
20. Fabian TC. Unraveling the fat embolism syndrome. N Engl J Med 1993; 329:961–963
21. Pape HC, Dwenger A, Regel G, Krettek C, Mehler D, Sturm JA, Tscherne H: Pulmonary damage after intramedullary femoral nailing in traumatized sheep – is there an effect from different nailing methods? J Trauma 1992; 33:574–581
22. Pape HC, Giannoudis PV, Grimme K, van Griensven M, Krettek C. Effects of intramedullary femoral fracture fixation: what is the impact of experimental studies in regards to the clinical knowledge? Shock 2002; 18:291–300

23. Pell ACH, Christie J, Keating JF, Sutherland GR: The detection of fat embolism by transoesophageal echocardiography during reamed intramedullary nailing. J Bone Joint Surg 1993; 75B:921–925
24. Heim D, Regazzoni P, Tsakiris DA, Aebi T, Schlegel U, Marbet GA, Perren SM: Intramedullary nailing and pulmonary embolism: does unreamed nailing prevent embolization? An in vivo study in rabbits. J Trauma 1995; 38:899–905
25. Made WJ van der, Smit EJM, van Luyt PA, van Vugt AB: Intramedullary femoral osteosynthesis: an additional cause of ARDS in multiple injured patients? Injury 1996; 27:391–393
26. Bosse MJ, MacKenzie EJ, Riemer BL, Brumback RJ, McCarthy ML, Burgess AR, Gens DR, Yasui Y: Adult respiratory distress syndrome, pneumonia and mortality following thoracic injury and a femoral fracture treated either with intramedullary nailing with reaming or a plate. J Bone Joint Surg 1997; 79A:799–809
27. Bulger EM, Smith DG, Maier RV, Jurkovich GJ: Fat embolism syndrome. A 10-year review. Arch Surg 1997; 132:435–439
28. Schemitsch EH, Jain R, Turchin DC, Mullen JB, Byrick RJ, Anderson G, Richards RR: Pulmonary effects of fixation of a fracture with a plate compared with intramedullary nailing. J Bone Joint Surg 1997; 79A:984–996
29. Duwelius PJ, Huckfeldt R, Mullins RJ, Shioto T, Woll TS, Lindsey KH, Wheeler D: The effects of femoral intramedullary reaming on pulmonary function in a sheep lung model. J Bone Joint Surg 1997; 79A:194–202
30. Gurd A: Fat embolism: an aid to diagnosis. J Bone Joint Surg 1970; 52B:732–737
31. Barie PS, Malik AB: Role of intravascular coagulation and granulocytes in lung vascular injury after bone marrow embolism. Circ Res 1982; 50:830–838
32. Schnaid E, Lamprey JM, Viljoen MJ, Joffe BI, Seftel HC: The early biochemical and hormonal profile of patients with long bone fractures at risk for fat embolism syndrome. J Trauma 1987; 27:309–311
33. Strecker W, Gonschorek O, Fleischmann W, Brückner, Beyer M, Kinzl L: Thromboxane-cofactor of pulmonary disturbances in intramedullary nailing. Injury 1993; 24(Suppl):S68–S72
34. Jones JP: Fat embolism, intravascular coagulation and osteonecrosis. Clin Orthop 1993; 292:294–308
35. Cinat M, Waxman K, Vaziri ND, Daughters K, Yousefi S, Scannell G, Tominaga GT: Soluble cytokine receptors and receptor antagonists are sequentially released after trauma. J Trauma 1995; 39:112–118
36. Keel M, Ecknauer E, Stocker R, Ungethüm U, Steckholzer U, Kenney J, Gallati H, Trentz O, Ertel W: Different pattern of local and systemic release of proinflammatory, anti-inflammatory mediators in severely injured patients with chest trauma. J Trauma 1996; 40:907–914
37. Stürmer KM: Measurement of intramedullary pressure in an animal experiment and propositions to reduce the pressure increase. Injury 1993; 24(Suppl):S7–S21
38. Frölke JPM, Bakker FC, Patka P, Haarman HJThM: Intramedullary pressure in reamed femoral nailing with two different reamer designs. Eur J Trauma 2001; 27:235–241
39. Müller CA, Rahn BA. Intramedullary pressure increase and increase in cortical temperature during reaming of the femoral medullary cavity: the effect of draining the medullary contents before reaming. J Trauma 2003; 55:495–503
40. Wozasek GE, Simon P, Redl H, Schlag G: Intramedullary pressure changes and fat intravasation during intramedullary nailing: an experimental study in sheep. J Trauma 1994; 36:202–207
41. Christie J, Robinson, Pell ACH, McBirnie J, Burnett R: Transcardiac echocardiography during invasive intramedullary procedures. J Bone Joint Surg 1995; 77B:450–455
42. Müller Chr, Rahn BA, Pfister U, Weller S: Intramedullary pressure, strain on the diaphysis and increase in cortical temperature when reaming the femoral cavity – a comparison of blunt and sharp reamers. Injury 1993; 24(Suppl):S22–S30
43. Peter RE, Selz T, Koestli A: Influence of the reamer shape on intraosseus pressure during closed intramedullary nailing of the unbroken femur. A preliminary report. Injury 1993; 24(Suppl):S48–S55
44. Pape HC, Dwenger A, Grotz M, Kaever V, Negatsch R, Kleemann W, Regel G, Sturm JA, Tscherne H: Does the reamer type influence the degree of lung dysfunction after femoral nailing following severe trauma? An animal study. J Orthop Trauma 1994; 8:300–309
45. Frölke JPM, Bakker FC, Patka P, Haarman HJThM: Reaming debris in osteotomized sheep tibiae. J Trauma 2001; 50:65–69
46. Martin R, Leighton RK, Petrie D, Ikejiani C, Smyth B: Effect of proximal and distal venting during intramedullary nailing. Clin Orthop 1996; 332:80–89
47. Cole AS, Hill GA, Theologis TN, Gibbons CLMH, Willett K: Femoral nailing for metastatic disease of the femur: a comparison of reamed and unreamed femoral nailing. Injury 2000; 31:25–31
48. Blachut PA, O'Brien PJ, Meek RN, Broekhuyse HM: Interlocking intramedullary nailing with and without reaming for the treatment of closed fractures of the tibial shaft. A prospective, randomized study. J Bone Joint Surg 1997; 79A:640–646
49. Keating JF, O'Brien PI, Blachut PA, Meek RN, Broekhuyse HM: Reamed interlocking intramedullary nailing of open fractures of the tibia. Clin Orthop 1997; 338: 182–191
50. Tornetta P, Tiburzi D: Reamed versus unreamed anterograde femoral nailing. J Orthop Trauma 2000; 14:15–19
51. Bhandari M, Guyatt GH, Tong D, Adili A, Shaughnessy SG: Reamed versus nonreamed intramedullary nailing of lower extremity long bone fractures: a systematic overview and meta-analysis. J Orthop Trauma 2000; 14:2–9
52. Court-Brown CM, Will E, Christie J, McQueen MM: Reamed or unreamed nailing for closed tibial fractures. A prospective study in Tscherne C1 fractures. J Bone Joint Surg 1996; 78B:580–583
53. Stedtfeld HW: Verriegelungsnagelung – unaufgebohrt, gebohrt? Unfallchirurg 1998; 101:500–505
54. Chapman MW: Closed intramedullary bone-grafting and nailing of segmental defects of the femur. J Bone Joint Surg 1980; 62A:1004–1008
55. Templeman D, Thomas M, Varecka T, Kyle R: Exchange reamed intramedullary nail for delayed union and non union of the tibia. Clin Orthop 1995; 315:169–175
56. Tydings JD, Martino LJ, Kircher M, Alfred R, Lozman J: The osteoinductive potential of intramedullary canal bone reamings. Curr Surg 1986; 43:121–124
57. Kreusch-Brinker R, Schwetlick G: Korrekturosteotomien an Femur- und Tibiaschaft mit dem Verriegelungsnagel. Unfallchirurgie 1990; 16:236–243
58. Cornell CN, Lane JM: Newest factors in fracture healing. Clin Orthop 1992; 277:297–311
59. Furlong AJ, Giannoudis PV, Smith RM: Heterotopic ossification: a comparison between reamed and unreamed femoral nailing. Injury 1997; 28:9–14
60. Frölke JPM, Krol E van de, Bakker FC, Patka P, Haarman HJThM: Destination of reaming debris during intramedullary reaming. Acta Orthop Belg 2000; 66:337–340
61. Sakata H, Takagi K: Effect of bone marrow mononuclear phagocytes on the bone matrix-induced bone formation in rats. Clin Orthop 1987; 220:253–258
62. Connolly J, Guse R, Lippiello L, Dehne R: Development of an osteogenic bone-marrow preparation. J Bone Joint Surg 1989; 71A:684–691

63. Colterjohn NR, Bednar DA: Procurement of bone graft from the iliac crest. J Bone Joint Surg 1997; 79A:756–759
64. Tydings JD, Martino LJ, Kircher M, Alfred RH, Lozman J: Viability of intramedullary canal bone reamings for continued calcification. Am J Surg 1987; 15:306–309
65. Frölke JP, Klein Nulend J, Semeins CM, Bakker FC, Patka P, Haarman HJThM. Viable osteoblastic potential of cortical reamings from intramedullary nailing. J Orthop Res 2004; 22:1271–1275
66. Sterck JGH, Klein-Nulend J, Lips P, Burger EH. Response of normal and osteoporotic human bone cells to mechanical stress in vitro. Am J Physiol 1998; 274: E1113–1120
67. Tischenko GJ, Goodman SB: Compartment syndrome after intramedullary nailing of the tibia. J Bone Joint Surg 1990; 72A:41–44
68. Moed BR, Strom DE: Compartment syndrome after closed intramedullary nailing of the tibia: a canine model and report of two cases. J Orthop Trauma 1991; 5:71–77
69. Hupel TM, Aksenov SA, Schemitsch EH: Muscle perfusion after intramedullary nailing of the canine tibia. J Trauma 1998; 48:256–260
70. Rhinelander FW, Baragry RA: Microangiography in bone healing. J Bone Joint Surg 1962; 44A:1273–1298
71. Lopez-Curto JA, Bassingthwaighte JB, Kelly P: Anatomy of the microvasculature of the tibial diaphysis of the adult dog. J Bone Joint Surg 1980; 62A:1362–1369
72. Danckwardt-Lillieström G, Lorenzi L, Olerud S: Intracortical circulation after intramedullary reaming with reduction of pressure in the medullary cavity. A microangiographic study on the rat tibia. J Bone Joint Surg 1970; 52A:1390–1394
73. Schemitsch EH, Kowalski MJ, Swiontkowski MF, Senft D: Cortical bone blood flow in reamed and unreamed locked intramedullary nailing: a fractured tibia model in sheep. J Orthop Res 1994; 8:373–382
74. Nakamura T, Itoman M, Yokoyama K: Cortical revascularization after reamed and unreamed intramedullary nailing in the rabbit femur: a microangiographic histometric analysis. J Trauma 1999; 47:744–751
75. Rhinelander FW: Effects of medullary nailing on the normal blood supply of the diaphyseal cortex. Instr Course Lect 1973; 22:161–187
76. Lindstrom T, Gullichsen E, Lertola K, Niinikoski J: Leg tissue perfusion in simple shaft fractures treated with unreamed and reamed nailing. J Trauma 1997; 43:636–639
77. Hupel TM, Aksenov SA, Schemitsch EH: Effect of limited and standard reaming on cortical bone blood flow and early strength of union following segmental fracture. J Orthop Trauma 1998; 12:400–406
78. Chapman MW: The effect of reamed and nonreamed intramedullary nailing on fracture healing. Clin Orthop Rel Res 1998; 355(Suppl):S230–S238
79. Henry SL, Adcock RA, von Fraunhofer JA, Selgson D: Heat of intramedullary reaming. South Med J 1987; 80:173–176
80. Leunig M, Hertel R: Thermal necrosis after tibial reaming for intramedullary nail fixation. A report of three cases. J Bone Joint Surg 1996; 78B:584–587
81. Ochsner PE, Baumgart F, Kohler G: Heat-induced segmental necrosis after reaming of one humeral and two tibial fractures with a narrow medullary canal. Injury 1998; 29(Suppl):S1–S10
82. Giannoudis PV, Snowden S, Matthews SJ, Smye SW, Smith RM. Friction burns within the tibia during reaming. Are they affected by the use of a tourniquet? J Bone Joint Surg Br 2002; 84:492–496
83. Matthews LS, Hirsch C: Temperatures measured in human cortical bone when drilling. J Bone Joint Surg 1972; 54A:297–308
84. Toksvig-Larsen S, Ryd L, Lindstrand A: Temperature influence in different orthopaedic saw blades. J Arthropl 1992; 7:21–24
85. Eriksson RA, Albrektsson T: Temperature threshold levels for heat-induced bone tissue injury: A vital microscopy study in the rabbit. Journal of Prosthetic Dentistry 1983; 50:101–107
86. Lundskog J: Heat and bone tissue. Scand J Plast Reconstr Surg 1972; Suppl 9
87. Fuchsberger A: Die schädigende Temperature bei der spanenden Knochenbearbeitung. Unfallchirurgie 1988; 14:173–183
88. Frölke JPM, Peters R, Boshuizen K, Patka P, Bakker FC, Haarman HJThM: The use of thermocouples in the assessment of cortical heat during intramedullary reaming of long bones. Injury 2001; 32:683–688
89. Frölke JP, Reeling Brouwer GC. Friction burns within the tibia during reaming. J Bone Joint Surg Br 2004; 86:149
90. Egmond van DB, Hovius SER, van der Meulen JC, den Ouden A: Heat recordings at tips of Kirschner wires during drilling through human phalanges. J Hand Surg 1994; 19A:648–652
91. Mousavi M, David R, Ehteshami J, Pajenda G, Vécsei V: Pressure changes during reaming with different parameters and reamer designs. Clin Orthop 2000; 373:295–303
92. Baumgart F, Kohler G, Ochsner PE: The physics of heat generation during reaming of the medullary cavity. Injury 1998; 29(Suppl):S11–25

Differentiation Capacity and Characterisation of Cells Growing Out of Human Reaming Debris

K. Trinkaus, S. Wenisch, C. Siemers, R. Schnettler

Introduction

In about 10% of all reconstructive operations caused by traumatic, resectional or congenital defects, bone grafts or bone substitutes are necessary. In the course of reconstructive surgery reaming debris has not been mentioned yet, because it was designated as a necrotic material, which does not contain vital cells.

Autogenic bone grafting is still regarded as the golden standard to treat large bone defects. However, collection of the autogenic material from the iliac crest requires a second site of surgery, which can be associated with complications such as pain, infections and haematoma [1, 2].

Bone substitutes comprise a wide range of materials. Based upon their chemical and physical features, these materials closely mimic the mineral phase of natural bone. These biomimetic properties promote the process of bone healing. However, in contrast to the natural bone, anorganic bone substitutes reveal no signs of biological activity due to the lack of growth or differentiation factors and cells, whose participation in the process of bone healing is of great functional importance [3–5].

Therefore, new strategies have been developed to treat large bone defects. These innovations of tissue engineering are based upon the knowledge about complex interactions between osteoinductive factors and cells in vivo. Consequently, bone healing is improved by using implants in combination with autogenic or recombinant growth factors and/or cells [6].

The clinical use of autogenic cells requires their collection prior to their expansion in vitro before growth on a suitable matrix can be carried out [6]. Cancellous bone [6–8] and bone marrow [9] represent sources of osteoblastic cells and multipotential mesenchymal stem cells (MSCs) [10–14]. Because of their differentiation capacity, MSCs have a therapeutic potential that is already used regarding the composition of newly developed bone graft substitutes [10].

Up to now, discussion of osteoregenerative effects of reaming debris has been controversial. It has been assumed that the cells undergo necrosis during the reaming procedure due to temperature elevations [15] and the influence of mechanical forces [15–19]. In contrast, experimental studies in the sheep and a few clinical studies in humans refer to the osteoinductive potential of reaming debris in vivo. Additionally, in vitro culturing of ovine reaming debris [19] has proven the vitality of the cells and has confirmed their osteoblast-like properties. In accordance with these findings, clinical studies have documented that fractures of long bones showed distinctly shorter times of healing when treated with reamed nails, than fractures treated with non-reamed nails [20–25]. Although the cause of this phenomenon has still to be clarified, it has been assumed that reaming creates a high potential of regeneration caused by the osteoinductive effects of blood and bone marrow, whereas dispersed bone fragments promote healing in an osteoconductive manner [26]. However, it has been taken into consideration that reaming of bones bears the risk of fat embolism or it can cause the adult respiratory distress syndrome.

Although there is no final scientific evidence for the assumption that reaming debris has stimulatory effects on bone healing, it might represent an autogenous source of vital cells, which could be used in the scope of bone tissue grafting. With special regard to this potential clinical significance, cells of human reaming debris have been investigated in the present in vitro study. The purpose was to prove vitality of the cells by means of cell culturing and by transmission electron microscopy and – if so – to characterise the viable cells phenotypically by means of morphology, antigenic properties and their capacity to differentiate in multiple cell lineages.

Materials and Methods

Reaming debris ($n = 13$) was collected from the reamer head and was immediately transferred into F12K medium. In the laboratory each specimen was divided into four parts. The first part was used for transmission electron microscopic examination (Zeiss EM 109). These specimens – weighing 1–1.5 g – were embedded in Epon (Serva, Heidelberg).

The second part was placed directly into the culture dish. The standard medium contained F12K medium, 20% fetal calf serum (FCS), 0.05 U/ml penicillin and 0.05 µg/ml streptomycin. The third part was washed in Hank's balanced salt solution until the components of blood and fat were macroscopically removed. The fourth part of each specimen was treated with collagenase for 2 h at 37 °C before it was placed in the culture dish. The cells were placed in the standard medium until they were grown to confluence. The medium was replaced every week. Then the cells were transferred into 24-well dishes.

In order to elucidate their differentiation repertoire, cells were incubated in osteogenic medium (DMEM low glucose with L-glutamine, 10% FCS, 0.1 µM dexamethasone, 0.05 mM ascorbic acid-2-phosphate, 10 mM β-glycerolphosphate, 0.05 U/ml penicillin and 0.05 µg/ml streptomycin) and in adipogenic induction medium (DMEM high glucose with L-glutamine, 1 µM dexamethasone, 0.2 mM indomethacin, 0.01 mg/ml insulin, 0.5 mM 3-isobutyl-1-methyl-xanthine, 10% FCS, 0.05 U/ml penicillin and 0.05 µg/ml streptomycin). After 3–4 days the adipogenic induction medium was substituted by adipogenic culture medium (DMEM high glucose with L-glutamine, 0.01 mg/ml insulin, 10% FCS, 0.05 U/ml penicillin and 0.05 µg/ml streptomycin), in which the cells were incubated for 1 week. For chondrogenic differentiation, cell pellets were created by centrifugation and were incubated in chondrogenic medium (Cambrex, Apen) for 28 days.

After 3 weeks of incubation within the osteogenic medium, the cells were stained with Von Kossa and alizarin Red S. Osteocalcin expression was investigated immunohistochemically (Chemicon, Hampshire, UK). Additionally, cells induced to the osteoblastic phenotype were embedded in Epon for transmission electron microscopy.

The cells incubated within the adipogenic medium were stained with Oil Red O.

Cell pellets of the chondrogenic medium were embedded in paraffin and the expression of collagen II (Cambrex, Apen, anti-collagen type II, human) was investigated immunohistochemically.

Fluorescence-activated cell sorter (FACS) analysis was performed to determine the antigenic properties of the cells incubated within the standard medium. In accordance with the investigations of Deans and Moseley [27], Pittenger et al. [13] and Hung et al. [28], the following surface markers were selected out of a long list of antibodies that are suitable to characterise MSCs: CD29, CD44, CD90, CD105, CD106, CD71, CD34, and CD45.

For FACS analysis, the cells were harvested from the standard medium, washed in phosphate-buffered saline (PBS) and incubated on ice for 30 min with fluorescein isothiocyanate or phycoerythrin-conjugated primary antibodies. Then they were resuspended in PBS and examined by FACS analysis.

Results

Transmission electron microscopy of reaming debris demonstrated that few free cells survived the reaming procedure (Fig. 2.4.1). These cells did not exhibit signs of degeneration or necrosis. However, cells with distinct morphological alterations such as condensation of the nuclear chromatin and the cytoplasm and disintegration of their membranes could also be detected.

By means of cell culturing, cell outgrowth became evident in all specimens ($n = 13$). However, the time of appearance of the cells was dependent on the treatment of the reaming debris prior to the incubation within the standard medium. Those parts of the specimens that were transferred directly into the medium showed cell outgrowth after 4–5 days. The cells revealed a large, flattened morphology.

In specimens treated with Hank's balanced salt solution, small spindle-shaped cells started to grow out of the bone fragments after 7 days, whereas in collagenase-treated samples outgrowth of cells could be seen for the first time after 2 weeks.

All in all, within all samples investigated, cell outgrowth started from the bone fragments (Fig. 2.4.2). Interestingly, even bone fragments from reaming debris that had been kept in culture for 6 months were still a source of outgrowing cells.

As shown in Fig. 2.4.3, cells could be also detected in regions of the culture dish where bone fragments were lacking, particularly in specimens that had not been treated with Hank's balanced salt solution. This is in accordance with the electron microscopic investigation, which revealed free and intact cells in human reaming debris. It

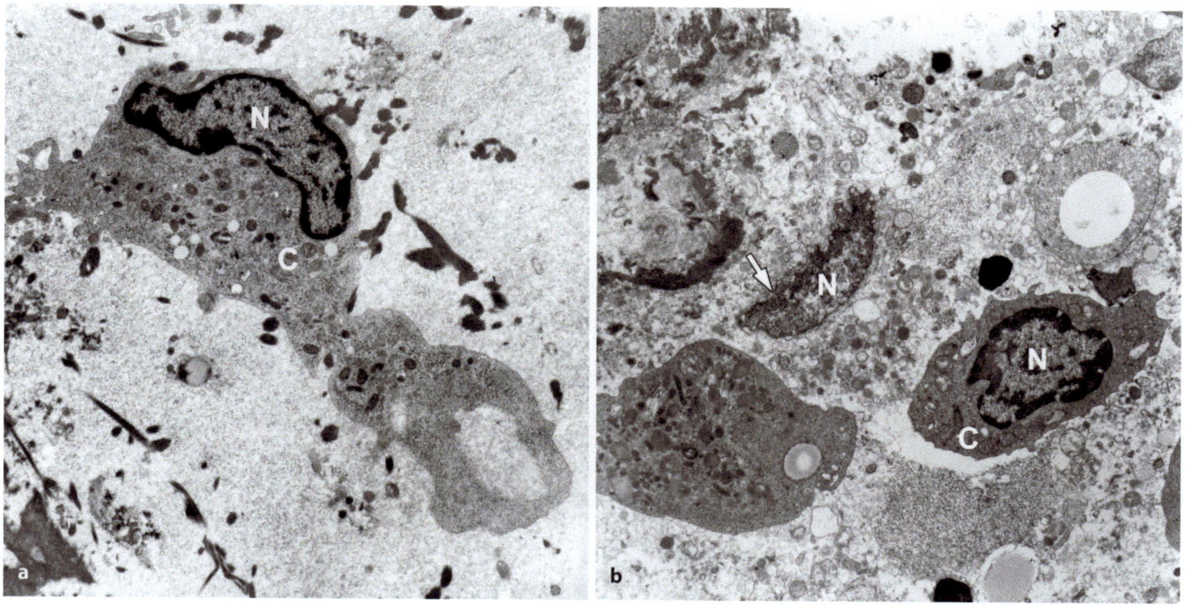

Fig. 2.4.1. Reaming debris examined by transmission electron microscope. a Free and intact cells. b Cells with signs of degeneration such as disintegration of chromatin, cytoplasm and membranes (*arrow*). *N* nucleus, *C* cytoplasm

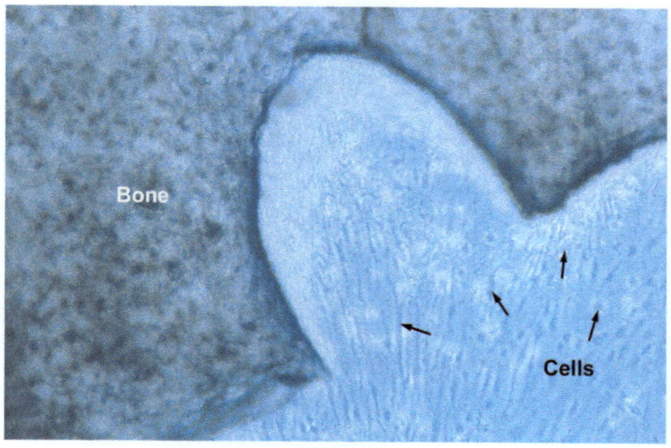

Fig. 2.4.2. Cells (*arrows*) are growing out of the small bone fragments of reaming debris

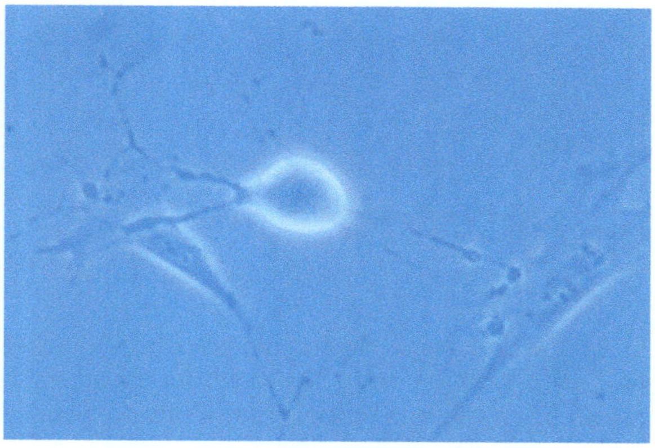

Fig. 2.4.4. Rapidly self-renewing cell (RS cell)

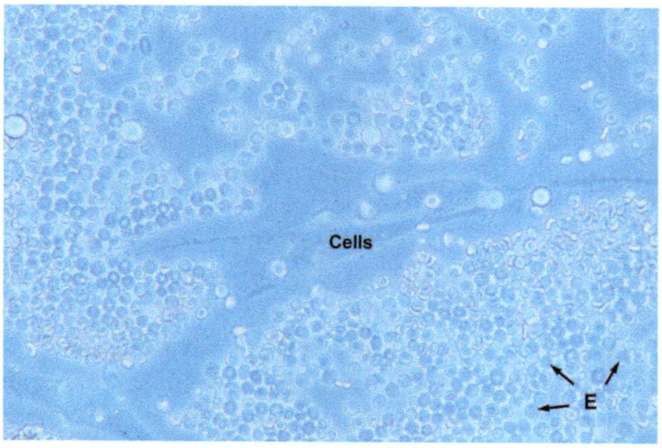

Fig. 2.4.3. Cells also appear between erythrocytes (*E*) in regions of the culture dish without bone fragments. Presumably those are the free cells that have survived the reaming procedure as shown in Fig. 2.4.1a

should be mentioned that non-adherent components such as erythrocytes and bone fragments were removed subsequently due to the exchange of the medium.

Irrespective of the different treatment procedures prior to the incubation in the standard medium, three types of cells could be seen in all culture dishes. The first were small cells revealing polygonal to round shapes (Fig. 2.4.4) adhered to the culture dish; they could also be seen as free-floating cells within the medium. The second, spindle-shaped cell type was larger in size (Fig. 2.4.5), while the third type was extremely large, of flattened morphology, often binucleate and intensively granulated (Fig. 2.4.6).

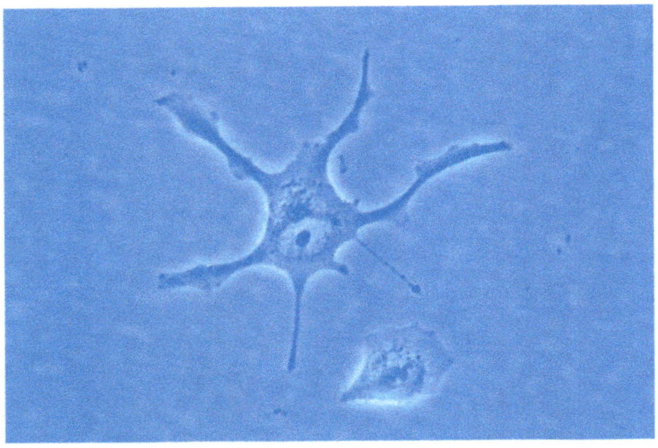

Fig. 2.4.5. Spindle-shaped cell

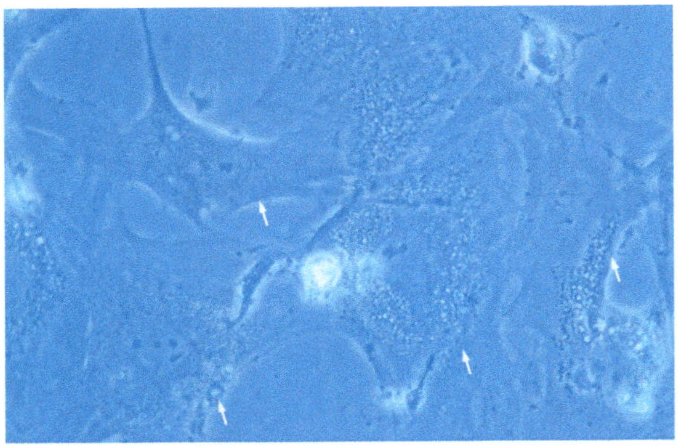

Fig. 2.4.6. Mature mesenchymal stem cells (*arrows*)

As the small cell type could also be identified as a non-adherent cell, the medium was centrifuged. Then the remaining pellet was resuspended and placed back in the culture dish. After incubation for a few days, all three cell types could be seen again within the expanding cell culture. When the small cells were seeded in numbers less than five per cm^2 they did not adhere or propagate.

Cells of different passages were transferred into the differentiation media in order to elucidate the differentiation capacity. The results have shown that the expansion through sequential passages did not influence their differentiation repertoire. However, the cells did not differentiate adequately when plated at high densities.

After 1 week of incubation in the osteogenic medium, the majority of cells flattened and assumed a cubic shape. During the second week, the onset of extracellular matrix production became visible (Fig. 2.4.7), and intensive staining by means of Von Kossa, alizarin Red and osteocalcin could be seen after 4 weeks.

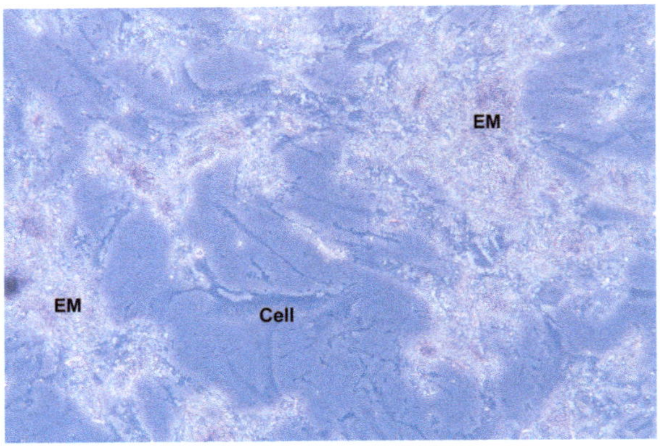

Fig. 2.4.7. Cells from human reaming debris that have been incubated in osteogenic medium for 3 weeks. The cells grow adherently and the extracellular matrix (*EM*) lays above the cells

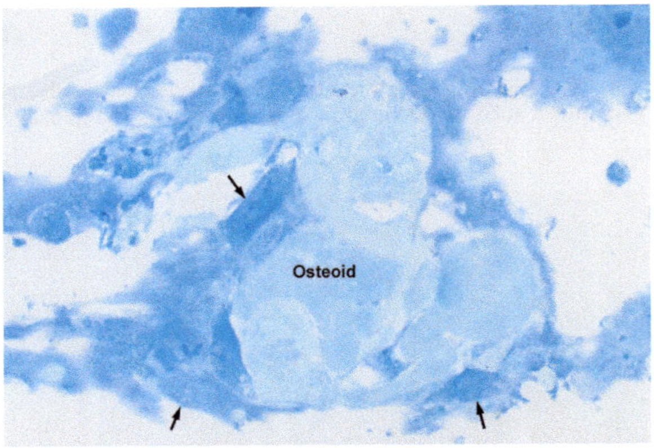

Fig. 2.4.8. Semithin section of MSCs after incubation in osteogenic medium, stained with toluidine blue. The cells (*arrows*) produce osteoid matrix

Moreover, it could be shown ultrastructurally that the cells induced to the osteoblastic phenotype (Fig. 2.4.10) produced a matrix composed of collagen fibres, and mineral (Figs. 2.4.8 and 2.4.9).

After 6 days of incubation within the adipogenic medium, the cells assumed morphological features of adipocytes and were stained positively with Oil Red O.

The cell pellets incubated within the chondrogenic medium revealed strong expression of collagen II (Fig. 2.4.11), and in a few regions the formation of chondrons could be observed.

The data of FACS analysis showed corresponding results even when the cells were harvested from different passages. However, the expression pattern of some surface markers (CD29, CD105, CD106) was obviously dependent upon the cell type (Table 2.4.1).

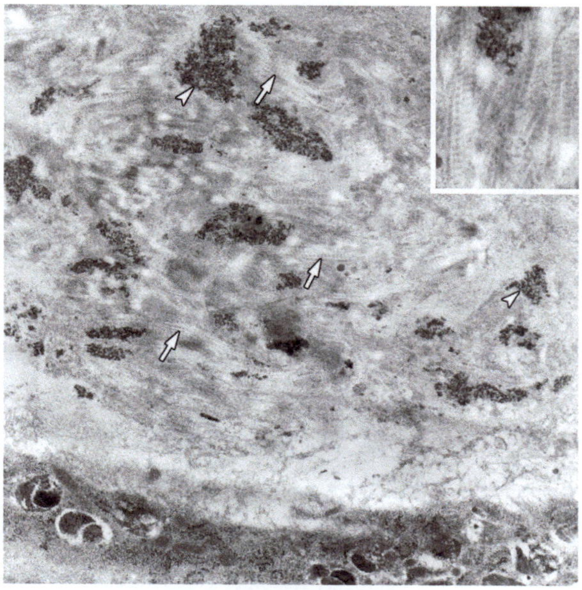

Fig. 2.4.9. Ultrastructural view of the osteoid matrix shown in Fig. 2.4.8. Collagen fibres (*arrows*) and deposits of mineral (*arrowheads*) can be detected. *Inset*: typical banded collagen fibres

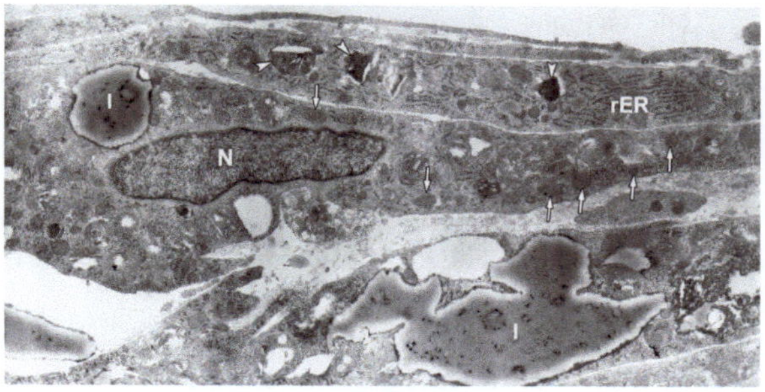

Fig. 2.4.10. Ultrastructure of osteoblast-like cells of the osteogenic medium. The cells have abundant rough ER (*rER*) and show many mitochondria (*arrows*) and lipofuscin granules (*arrowheads*). Inclusion bodies (*I*) of unknown origin could be detected. *N* Nucleus

Discussion

In accordance with the results of Frölke [19], the present investigation has demonstrated that cells have survived the harsh reaming procedure. Moreover, the cells have been characterised as MSCs due to their morphological and antigenic features and due to their differentiation capacity.

This result favours the idea of using human reaming debris as a tissue graft. Simple culture conditions enable the expansion of MSC in vitro: after washing, the reaming debris can be natively transferred into the culture dish instead of isolating the cells by density gradient centrifugation, as is commonly done in the case of bone marrow-derived MSC [13]. It has been shown that cell outgrowth is delayed but not altered when the washing procedure is performed prior to the incubation. Therefore, it might be assumed that rinsing of the samples removes not only non-adherent cells but also growth-promoting factors.

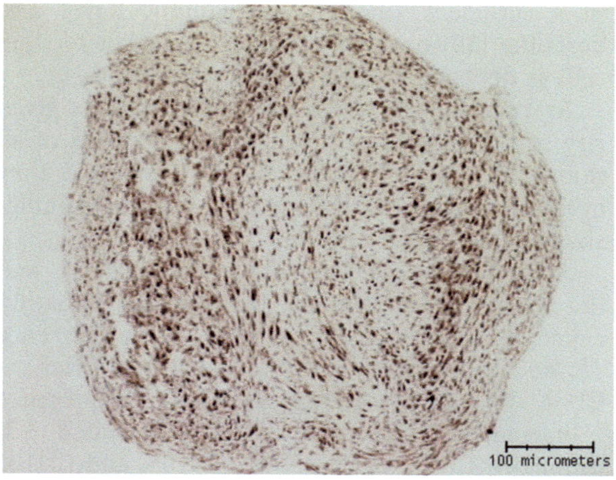

Fig. 2.4.11. Section of a cell pellet after 3 weeks of incubation in chondrogenic medium. The collagen II is stained immunohistochemically, and is visualised by the brown-coloured reaction product

Table 2.4.1. Surface marker profile: FACS analysis

Antibody	Spindle-shaped cells	Large flat cells
CD29	Negative	Positive
CD34	Negative	Negative
CD44	Positive	Positive
CD45	Negative	Negative
CD71	Negative	Negative
CD90	Positive	Positive
CD105	Negative	Positive
CD106	Negative	Positive

In all samples of reaming debris, cell outgrowth started from the bone fragments. This finding is in accordance with the assumption that reaming promotes bone healing in both an osteoinductive and an osteoconductive pattern [19].

Three kinds of morphologically distinct cells could be seen after culturing. Based upon the results of Colter et al. [29], these cells are termed rapidly self-renewing (RS) cells, spindle-shaped cells and mature mesenchymal stem cells (mMSCs).

RS cells are characterised by their small size (in the present investigation approximately 7 μm), their high nucleus/cytoplasm ratio, and their round to polygonal shape. They adhere to the culture dish, but were also found in suspension [28].

These small RS cells were capable of establishing a new population of stem cells when seeded in a sufficient amount. Accordingly, Reyes and Verfaillie [30] have shown that expansion of stem cells is dependent upon critical cell densities.

As culturing of resuspended RS cells has given rise to a population of stem cells composed of all three cell types, it might be assumed that they bear the capacity to differentiate into the spindle-shaped cells and the mMSC.

According to the morphological criteria and the results concerning the cellular differentiation capacity, FACS analysis has revealed the presence of MSCs in human reaming debris. In brief, as CD34 and CD45 were not expressed, the presence of haematopoietic stem cells can be excluded. Additionally, CD29, CD44, CD90, CD105, and CD106 – commonly used as stem cell markers [13, 27, 28] – were detectable at the surfaces of MSCs. According to the lack of CD71 expression found presently, CD71 is known to be expressed by cells of the chondrogenic lineage, but not from those of the osteogenic lineage [31].

All in all, the present investigation has shown that human reaming debris is a source of vital cells that are capable of differentiating under appropriate culture conditions into osteoblasts, adipocytes and chondrocytes. This finding supports the observations made by most surgeons that fractures treated with reamed nails have a shorter healing time than those treated with unreamed nails [20–25]. To our knowledge this is the first report giving a detailed characterisation of human reaming debris-derived cells. However, the clinical and therapeutic benefit of reaming debris used as a bone graft instead of – or in combination with – commercially available bone substitutes remains to be elucidated.

References

1. Arrington ED, Smith WJ, Chambers HG, Bucknell, Davino NA (1996) Complications of iliac crest bone graft harvesting. Clin Orthop Rel Res 329: 300–309
2. Dütting A, Thomas W, Lorenz H, Holst A (1988) Komplikationen nach autologer Knochentransplantation am Entnahmeort. Z Orthp 126: 44–47
3. Einhorn L (1998) Fracture repair. Clin Orthop 355: 353–360
4. Probst S (1997) Cellular mechanisms of bone repair. J Invest Surg 10: 77–86
5. Zellin G (1998) Growth factors and bone regeneration. Implications of barrier membranes. Swed Dent J Suppl 129: 7–65
6. Behrens P, Wolf E, Bruns J (2000) In-vitro-Anzüchtung humaner autogener osteoblastärer Zellen auf natürlichem Knochenmaterial. Orthopäde 29: 129–134
7. Nolan PC, Nicolas RM, Mulholland BJ, Mollan RAB, Wilson DJ (1992) Culture of human osteoblasts on demineralised human bone. Possible means of graft enhancement. J Bone Joint Surg Br 74: 284–286
8. Schneider U (1998) Die autogene Knochenzelltransplantation. Orthopäde 27: 143–146
9. Louisia S, Stromboni M, Meunier A, Sedel L, Petite H (1999) Human osteoblastic cells: a potential tool to assess the etiology of pathologic bone formation. J Bone Mineral Res 9: 1847–1850
10. Alison MR, Poulson R, Forbes R, Wright NA (2002) An introduction to stem cells. J Pathol 197: 419–423
11. Jiang Y, Jahagirdar BN, Reinhardt RL, Schwartz RE, Keene CD, Ortiz-Gonzales XR, et al. (2002) Pluripotency of mesenchymal stem cells derived from adult marrow. Nature 418: 41–49
12. Lodie TA, Blickarz CE, Devarakonda TJ, He C, Dash AB, Clarke J, Gleneck K, Shihabuddin L, Tubo Ross (2002) Systematic analysis of reportedly distinct populations of multipotent bone marrow-derived stem cells reveals a lack of distinction. Tissue Engineering 8: 739–751.
13. Pittenger MF, Mackay AM, Beck SC, Jaiswal RK, Douglas R, Mosca JD, Moorman MA, Simonett DW, Craig S, Marshak DR (1999) Multilineage potential of adult human mesenchymal stem cells. Science 284: 143–147
14. Shur I, Marom R, Lokiec F, Socher R, Benayahu D (2002) Identification of cultured progenitor cells from human marrow stroma. J Cell Biochem 87: 51–57
15. Ochsner PE, Baumgart F, Kohler G (1998) Heat-induced segmental necrosis after reaming of one humeral and two tibial fractures with a narrow medullary canal. Injury 29 (Suppl): 1–10
16. Henry SL, Adcock RA, von Fraunhofer JA, Selgson D (1987) Heat of intramedullary reaming. South Med J 80: 173–176
17. Brisman DL (1996) The effect of speed, pressure, and time on bone temperature during the drilling of implant sites. Int J Oral Maxillofac Implants 11(1): 35–37
18. Leunig M, Hertel R (1996) Thermal necrosis after tibial reaming for intramedullary nail fixation. A report of three cases. J Bone Joint Surg 78B: 584–587
19. Frölke JP (2001) Intramedullary reaming of long bones. Ponsen and Looijen, Wageningen
20. Anglen JO, Blue JM (1995) A comparison of reamed and unreamed nailing of the tibia. J Trauma 39: 351–355
21. Court-Brown CM, Will E, Christie J, McQueen MM (1996) Reamed or unreamed nailing for closed tibial fractures. A prospective study in Tscherne C1 fractures. J Bone Surg 78B: 580–583
22. Giannoudis PV, Furlong AJ, Macdonald DA, Smith RM (1997) Reamed against unreamed nailing of the femoral diaphysis: a retrospective study of healing time. Injury 28 (1): 15–18
23. Clatworthy MG, Clark DI, Gray DH, Hardy AE (1998) Reamed versus unreamed femoral nails. A randomized prospective trial. J Bone Joint Surg 80B: 485–489
24. Finkemeier CG, Schmidt AH, Kyle RF, Templeman DC, Varecka TF (2000) A prospective, randomized study of intramedullary nails inserted with and without reaming for the treatment of open and closed fractures of the tibial shaft. J Orthop Trauma 14:187–193
25. Tornetta P 3rd, Tiburzi D (2000) Reamed versus nonreamed anterograde femoral nailing. J Orthop Trauma 14(1): 15–19
26. Furlong AJ, Giannoudis PV, Smith RM (1997) Heterotopic ossification: a comparison between reamed and unreamed femoral nailing. Injury 28: 9–14
27. Deans RJ, Moseley AB (2000) Mesenchymal stem cells: biology and potential clinical uses. Experimental Hematology 28: 875–884
28. Hung SC, Chen NJ, Hsieh SL, Li H, Ma HL, Lo WH (2002) Isolation and characterisation of size sieved stem cells from human bone marrow. Stem Cells 20: 249–258
29. Colter DC, Sekiya I, Prockop DJ (2001) Identification of a subpopulation of rapidly self-renewing and multipo-

tential adult stem cells in colonies of human marrow stromal cells. Proc Natl Acad Sci USA 98(14): 7841–7845

30. Reyes M, Verfaillie CM (2001) Characterisation of multipotent adult progenitor cells, a subpopulation of mesenchymal stem cells. Ann NY Acad Sci 938: 231–235
31. Haynesworth SE, Baber MA, Caplan AI (1992) Cell surface antigens on human marrow-derived mesenchymal cells are detected by monoclonal antibodies. Bone 13: 69–80

Section 3 Materials Used for Intramedullary Devices

Implant Alloys and Interfacial Engineering

P. Procter, G. von Oldenburg, H. von Wieding, A. Speitling

Introduction

This chapter surveys the different aspects of "state-of-the-art" implant material performance. Today implant failure is less common than bone failure and implant design now focuses upon modifying the interface properties between implant and bone. The text discusses femoral implant design in particular but the principles apply equally to all long bone fracture fixation devices.

The Nature of In Vivo Loading

While there have been many attempts to estimate the nature of loading on human long bones [1], there have been few direct measurements made with which to validate such models. There have been many attempts to measure directly the effects of loading on the long bones but only a few have succeeded in providing any data of value to the implant designer.

Bergmann et al. [2] made an elegant series of measurements on patients in whom an instrumented prosthesis was implanted. The implant (Fig. 3.1.1 a) was calibrated to measure three components of hip force (Fig. 3.1.1 b), and patients then undertook a series of locomotion activities. External force actions and gait kinematics were also measured. The key aspects of the hip joint force components are significant magnitude and variation in direction. The vertical force component is typically 300% of body weight. The anterior–posterior component is significant and in each step taken by a subject alternates between posterior and anterior directions. Reversed torsional loading plays an important role in the mechanical failure of implants. Surgeons have intuitively recognised this, which has led to the addition of cross-locking screws proximally and distally in all intramedullary rod designs. There have been only a few studies in which implants that were indicated for trauma have been instrumented and implanted. Brown et al. [3] developed an instrumented hip nail that revealed for the first time that the "horizontal" component of movement was significant and should be taken into account in the design of devices used for fixation of the hip (Fig. 3.1.2).

The development of instrumented hip nails has continued and fully implantable implant/sensor/telemetry devices have now been developed after Burny et al. [4] (Fig. 3.1.3). Finally, Schneider et al. [5] developed an intramedullary nail (Fig. 3.1.4 a), which was implanted in a patient who had experienced a femoral fracture. The nail loads were transduced as strains and sent via telemetry to a receiver where the force actions were then decoded as shown in Fig. 3.1.4 b. This was a closed-section clover profile nail of 16 mm diameter. While the data are interesting as the only such measurement on record, they do not follow the expected pattern of reducing with time as the fracture heals and the bone takes over the task of load-bearing.

To summarise, the key aspects of loading in the lower limb are that the forces are large, dynamic, and three dimensional in nature, and the design of implants has to take into account the in vivo force environment specific to each implant in its indication range.

General Requirements of Implant Materials

In addition to recognising in vivo loading duty that the implant has to perform, there are other aspects that have to be considered in every implant material:

- Biocompatibility. This is the biological tolerance of the body to an implanted material. At one time it was considered that the ideal material would have no biological impact and result in no adverse body reactions. Now devices are being designed that are intended by surface treatment or some other modification to impact on the local biological environment. Examples are: the addition of hydroxyapatite

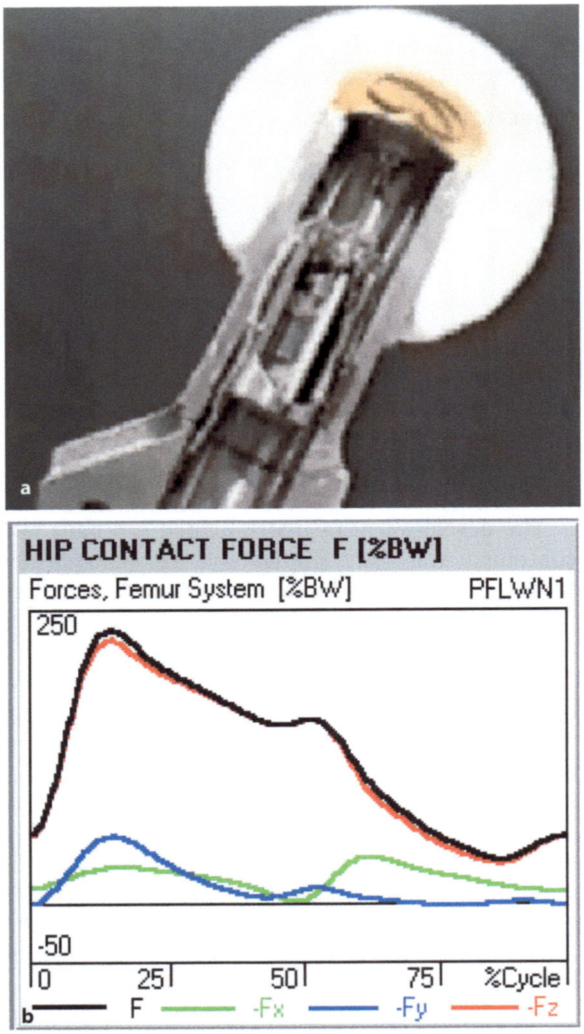

Fig. 3.1.1. a Instrumented hip prosthesis [2]. b Hip force components and resultant force [2]

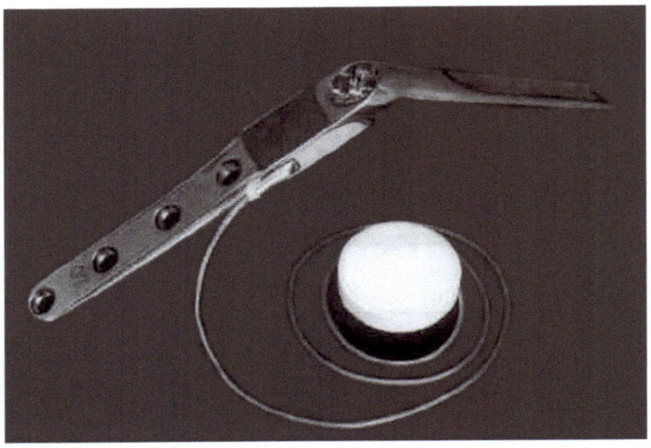

Fig. 3.1.3. Implantable hip nail (after Burney et al. [4])

coatings designed to promote bony ingrowth; anodisation type II designed to protect titanium implant surfaces and modify the interface between bone and implant. Interfacial bioengineering implants have now become a significant aspect of implant design and will become increasingly important in the future.

- Biomechanical equivalence. An ideal implant should restore physiological loading and result in strains and stresses that are compatible with the requirements of the adjacent bony and soft tissue structures.
- Clinical compliance. The implant should allow all imaging modes, e.g. magnetic resonance imaging (MRI), computed tomography (CT) and ultrasound, with minimum distortion and induction of artefacts.
- Implantation and explantation. The safe and easy implantation and removal of the device must be assured. In general, trauma implants are designed to minimise bony ingrowth to

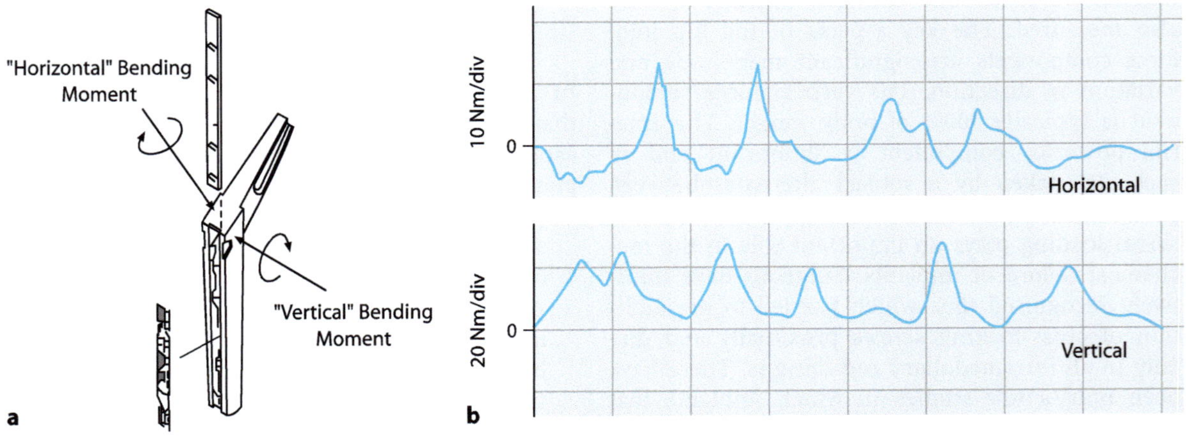

Fig. 3.1.2. a Instrumented hip nail (after Brown et al. [3]). b Horizontal and vertical moments (after Brown et al. [3])

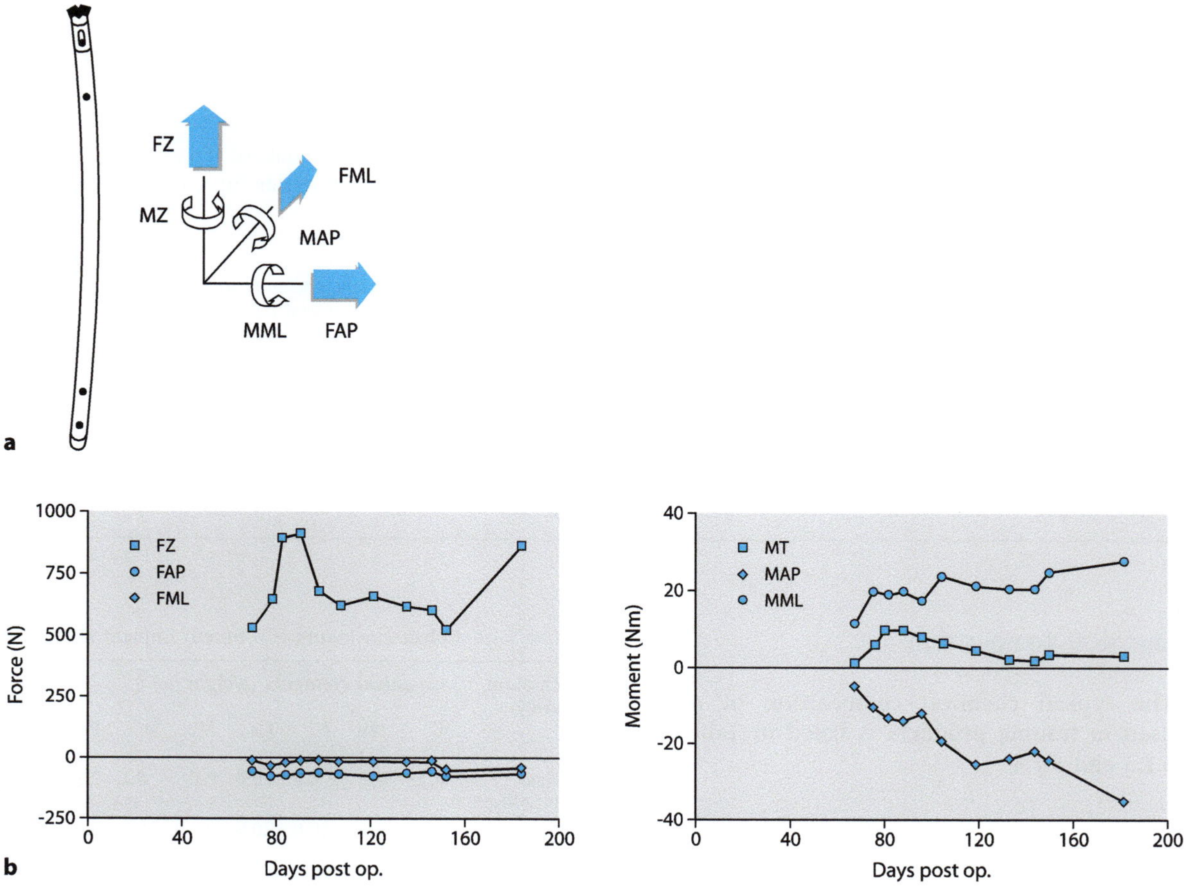

Fig. 3.1.4. a Instrumented intramedullary nail (Schneider et al. [5]). b Forces and moments measured directly from an implanted intramedullary nail (Schneider et al. [5])

ease explantation, and the use of non-standard screws and coupling devices should be avoided.

- Manufacturing considerations. To meet the demands for cost-effective implant and instrumentation systems, the material availability, material price and manufacturing cost of implants must be in an acceptable economical range.

Implant Materials

The most widely used materials within the trauma implant manufacturing industry are the stainless steel 316 LVM, Orthinox and 22-13-5 grades of stainless steel. More recently titanium alloys have been increasingly favoured. Of the dozen or so titanium alloys, Ti-6Al-4V and TAV are most often used. To characterise these alloys: TAV provides a slightly higher strength than 316 LVM in cold working (CW) conditions. Due to the absence of chromium (Cr) and Nickel (Ni), TAV is recommended for patients with Ni/Cr allergy. The steels Orthinox and 22-13-5 are further developments of 316 LVM with higher strength and higher corrosion resistance. 22-13-5 and Orthinox are parallel developments of two different steel manufacturers. Since Orthinox is standardised by an ASTM as well as an ISO standard, it is more established and is preferred to 22-13-5, which is only standardised by an ASTM standard. Where a stainless steel of high strength is indicated, Orthinox, a high nitrogen grade of stainless steel, combines the highest strength together with excellent corrosion resistance. Its superior properties come at a higher manufacturing cost, so Orthinox is usually targeted at applications that require superior mechanical strength. The titanium alloy Ti-6Al-7Nb (TAN) is less frequently used and was developed to eliminate the vanadium used in other grades of titanium. While the strength and corrosion resistance of cobalt-based alloys like Vitallium are on a par with implant steels, they are suitable for casting and wrought conditions, the advantages of casting are, in general, not significant for trauma implants (Table 3.1.1).

Table 3.1.1. List of implant materials used within trauma and their common applications

Material/ref. standard	Alloy	Typical applications
Orthinox/ASTM F 1586/ISO 5832-9	Austenitic stainless steel	Proximal femoral nails
22-13-5/ASTM F 1314	Austenitic stainless steel	Compression hip screws, cannulated screws
316 LVM/ASTM F 138 ISO 5832-1	Austenitic stainless steel	IM nails, ex fix pins, compression hip screws, cannulated screws
CP Ti/ASTM F 67 ISO 5832-2	Commercial pure titanium	Craniomaxillofacial plating
Ti 6Al 4V/ASTM F 136 ISO 5832-3	Titanium alloy	Plating systems, IM nails, compression hip screws, cannulated screws, proximal femoral nails
TMZF/ASTM F 1813	Titanium alloy	IM nail cross-locking screws, high strength
Ti 6Al 7Nb/ASTM F 1295 ISO 5832-11	Titanium alloy	Plating systems
Wrought vitallium/ ASTM F 90 ISO 5832-5	Cobalt chromium alloy	Staples
Cast vitallium/ASTM F 75 ISO 5832-4	Cobalt chromium alloy	Staples

Chemical Composition

The typical chemical composition of materials used in trauma products is listed in Tables 3.1.2, 3.1.3 and 3.1.4.

Implant Steels

These are based on Iron (Fe). The main alloy components are chromium (Cr), nickel (Ni), molybdenum (Mo) and manganese (Mn). To increase strength and corrosion resistance, the steels Orthinox and 22-13-5 are alloyed with nitrogen (N) and niobium (Nb) and have higher chromium and manganese content.

Table 3.1.2. Stainless-steel (Fe-based) implant alloys

Implant alloy	Chemical elements (weight %)							
	C	Mn	Ni	Cr	Mo	N	Nb	Fe
Orthinox	0.03	4.0	9.0	20.5	2.2	0.4	0.3	Bal.
22-13-5	0.02	5.0	12.7	21.4	2.3	0.3	0.2	Bal.
316 LVM	0.02	1.2	13.5	18.0	2.8	–	–	Bal.

Table 3.1.3. Titanium (Ti-based) implant alloys

Implant alloy	Chemical elements (weight %)					
	C	O	Fe	Al	Other	Ti
CP titanium grade 4	0.01	0.37	0.26	–	–	Bal.
Ti 6Al 4V	0.03	0.12	0.14	6.0	V 4.0	Bal.
Ti 6Al 7Nb	0.08	0.20	0.25	6.0	Nb 7.0	Bal.

Table 3.1.4. Cobalt-chromium (Co-based) implant alloys

Implant alloy	Chemical elements (weight %)							
	C	Mn	Ni	Cr	Mo	W	Fe	Co
Cast vitallium	0.22	0.7	0.2	28.0	6.0	0.1	0.3	Bal.
Wrought vitallium	0.1	1.5	10.0	20.0	–	15.0	0.2	Bal.

Titanium and Its Alloys

Commercially pure titanium is available in four grades designated 1, 2, 3 and 4. As the grade number increases, the chemical composition is slightly modified to improve the strength while maintaining the percentage of titanium above 99%. To increase strength and/or increase elasticity, Ti is alloyed with other elements. In general the names of Ti alloys indicate the main alloy components by weight percentage, e.g. Ti-6Al-4V refers to 6% weight of aluminium (Al) and 4% weight of vanadium (V).

Cobalt–Chromium Alloys

These are not commonly used today and are mentioned for completeness. Vitallium is a brand name and is available in both cast and wrought forms. The main components of cast Vitallium are cobalt, chromium and molybdenum with minimal nickel. In wrought Vitallium, cobalt is alloyed with chromium, nickel and tungsten.

Mechanical Characteristics of Implant Materials

As demonstrated earlier, the loads imposed on implants are both large and either static or dynamic depending upon the joint and the activity undertaken.

The term "static load" describes a constant load during certain actions, for example standing on one leg, or lifting a weight to a fixed position. Static overload leads to plastic deformation of the implant (Fig. 3.1.5). Plastic deformation occurs when a material is deformed beyond the elastic limit and means that the material is permanently deformed.

The term "dynamic load" means that the loads vary, usually in both directions and magnitude. This is typical of in vivo cyclic loading and unloading of an implant during walking. Dynamic loads that are sufficiently large and frequent may result in a fatigue fracture (Fig. 3.1.6). The lack of bony support in this instance resulted in the implant taking continued dynamic loading and this loading was magnified by the stress-concentrating effect of the reduced cross-section in the region of the lower lag screw. An example of how this can be overcome will be described later.

Mechanical Behaviour Under Static Load

The static material property tensile strength is determined by a tensile test (Fig. 3.1.7). In this test a material specimen of standardised size is loaded in tension in a tensile test machine (Figs. 3.1.8 and 3.1.9) until fracture.

During the test a stress vs. strain diagram is recorded from which the material properties such as yield strength, ultimate tensile strength, plastic deformation at fracture and modulus of elasticity are derived (Fig. 3.1.9). Stress represents the intensity of force applied to a given cross-section. Stress is calculated by dividing the applied force by the area of that cross-section and is given in the unit newtons per millimetre squared (N/mm^2) or megapascals (MPa). Strain is a measure of change in length. Strain is calculated by dividing the change in length of the specimen by its original length and is given in %.

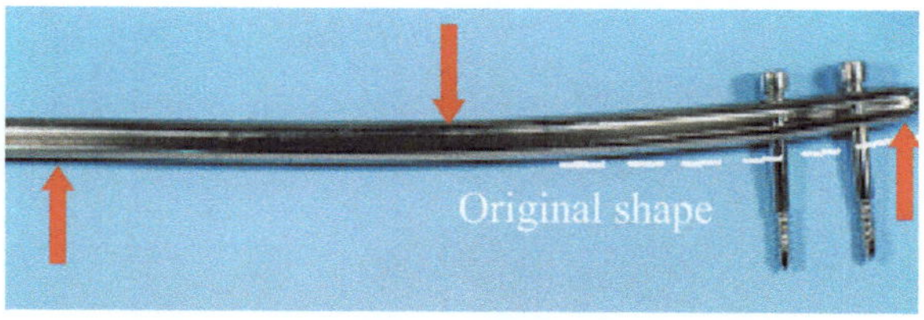

Fig. 3.1.5. Plastic deformation of intramedullary nail due to static overload

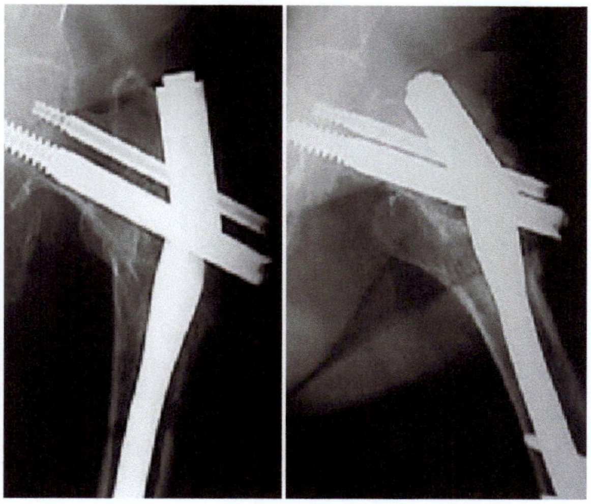

Fig. 3.1.6. Dynamic fracture of a proximal femoral nail

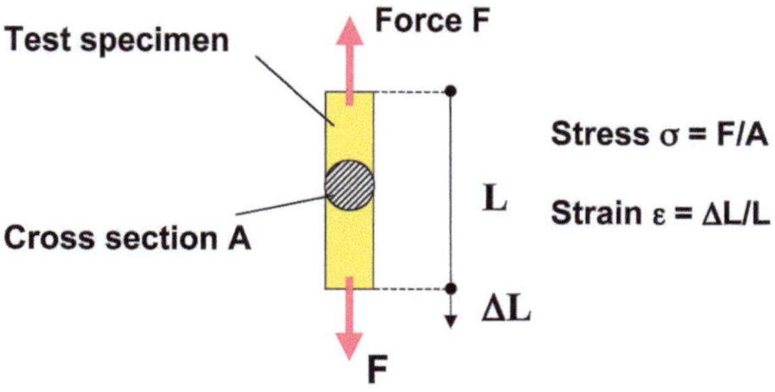

Fig. 3.1.7. Tensile test, principle

Definitions of Standard Terms

Elasticity is defined as the ability of a material to undergo non-permanent (elastic) deformation in response to an applied stress. The elasticity is expressed as elastic modulus or Young's modulus, after the 18th-century English physician and physicist Thomas Young. It is the ratio of stress unit per strain unit in the linear part of the stress–strain curve and represents the slope of the curve (Fig. 3.1.9). Materials with a low modulus of elasticity such as polymers are more flexible than those with a higher modulus such as metals.

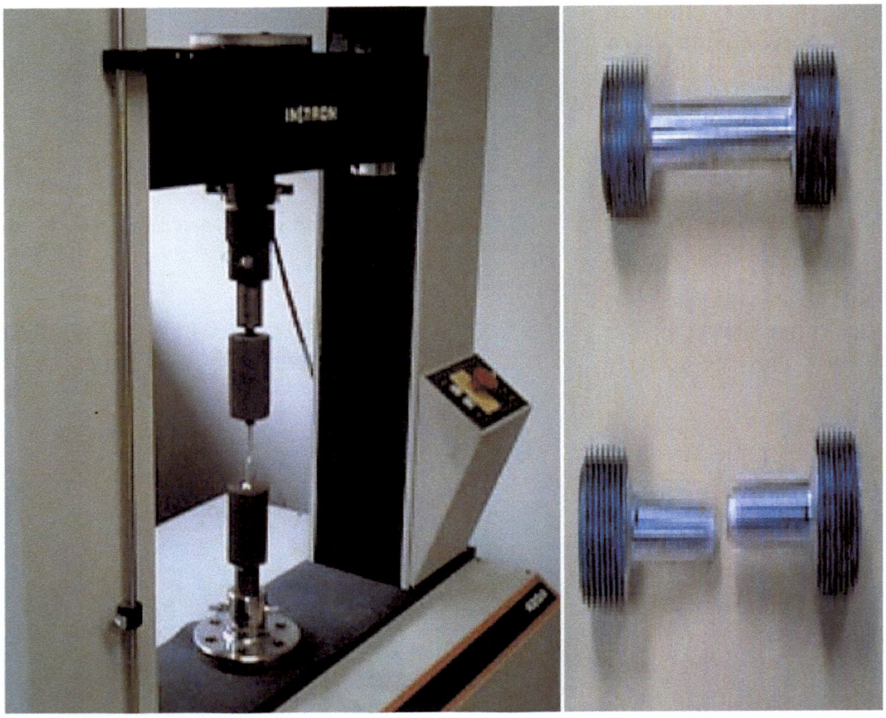

Fig. 3.1.8. Tensile test machine and tensile test pieces (pictures courtesy of Instron Corporation)

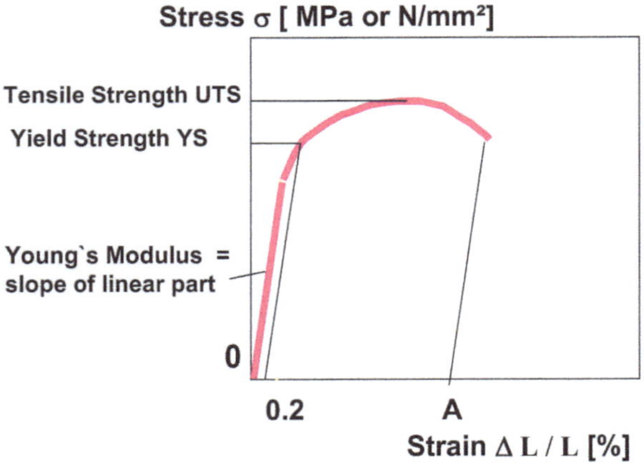

Fig. 3.1.9. Stress–strain curve derived from tensile test

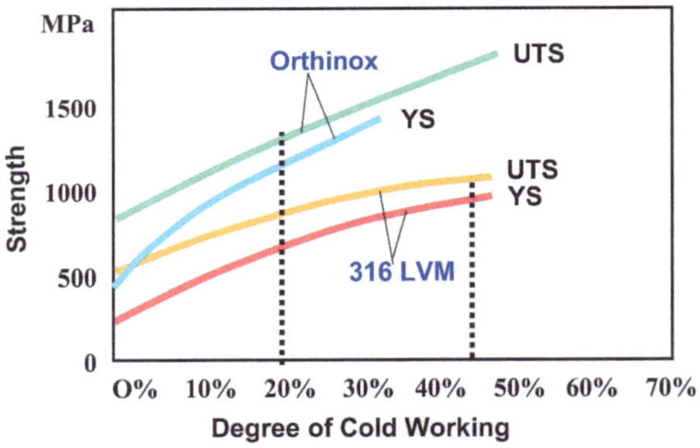

Fig. 3.1.10. Strength resulting from degree of cold working

Yield tensile strength is the stress required to cause a permanent deformation (strain) of 0.2%.

Ultimate tensile strength (UTS) is the stress required to cause a material to fracture.

Elongation at fracture (A) is the maximum plastic deformation (strain) before fracture occurs. Elongation at fracture will be determined by comparing the length of the broken specimen with its original length.

Material Properties

The implant steels can be used in annealed and CW conditions. Annealed steel provides low strength and very high potential for plastic deformation. By CW/cold deformation during or prior to manufacturing, the material strength can be increased (Fig. 3.1.10).

For steel implants, which might have to be contoured during surgery, for example some bone plates, annealed steel is used. For all other steel implants, CW material is usually preferred. The

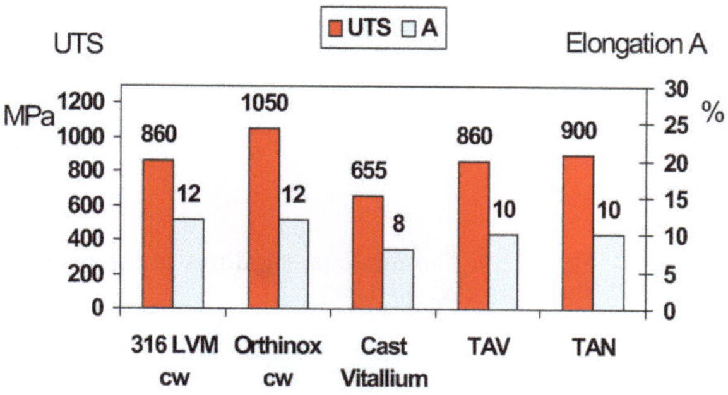

Fig. 3.1.11. Comparison of tensile strength and elongation at fracture

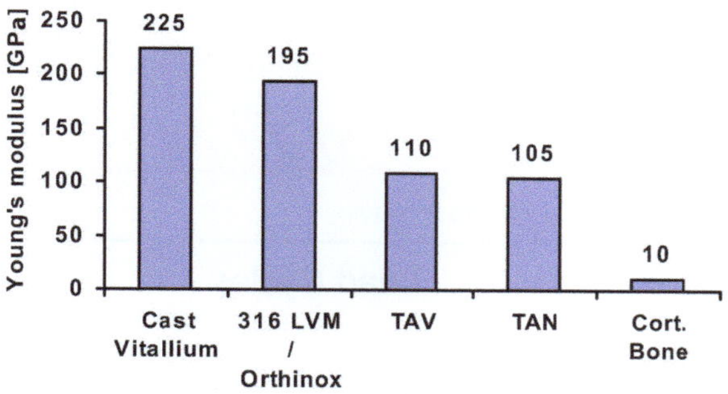

Fig. 3.1.12. Young's modulus for different materials

Orthinox material is used in 20% CW conditions and 316 LVM in 40–50% CW conditions. In Fig. 3.1.11 a comparison of the minimum requirements on tensile strength and elongation is shown according to the standards for the different materials. While the elongation values of the titanium and stainless-steel alloys are in the same range, the strength of CW Orthinox is significantly higher.

Young's modulus for the different materials is given in Fig. 3.1.12. Cortical bone has the lowest Young's modulus and therefore has the highest elasticity. Young's modulus of TAN and TAV is approximately ten times higher than that of cortical bone. For Vitallium, 316 LVM and Orthinox it is approximately 20 times higher. That means titanium is ten times as rigid as cortical bone and Vitallium, 316 LVM and Orthinox 20 times as rigid as cortical bone.

Implant Properties

While implant properties are very important, they are just one part of the behaviour of a final design. Historically, when titanium was first introduced it was assumed that it was a better material choice because it had a modulus of elasticity closer to that of bone. In practice, titanium nails often had a thicker wall to compensate strength, while they might have the same outside diameter. Some intramedullary nail cross-sections are shown in Fig. 3.1.13a and it can be seen that the four 12-mm designs have completely different cross-sectional shapes. When these are tested, the bending rigidities adapted from Eveleigh [6] (Fig. 3.1.13b) show that the ACE titanium 12-mm design is as rigid as the 12-mm RT stainless-steel design. So Young's modulus alone should not be used to judge the behaviour of implants.

Similarly in torsion (Fig. 3.1.14), the results show that the effect of a slot in the cross-section is to greatly reduce the torsional rigidity compared with closed-section or solid-section nails. In the slotted designs, the 10-mm ACE titanium nail is stiffer than the 12-mm AO Universal design in stainless steel. Once again, the design of the nail cross-section is more significant in determining performance than material alone.

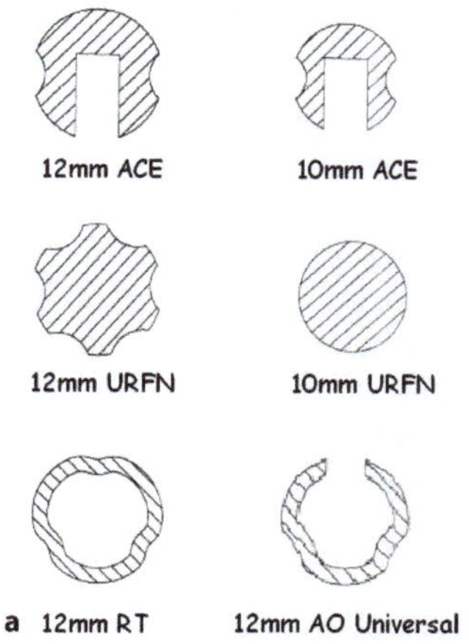

b

NAIL DESIGNS	Average Bending Rigidity Nmm^2	Material
10mm ACE	35	Titanium
10mm AO URFN	48	Titanium
12mm AO universal	59	Stainless Steel
12mm AO URFN	67	Titanium
12mm ACE	77	Titanium
12mm RT	79	Stainless Steel

Fig. 3.1.13. a Intramedullary nail cross-sections. b The bending rigidities of the nails shown in a

NAIL DESIGNS	Average Torsional Rigidity Nm per degree	Material
10mm ACE	3	Titanium
10mm AO URFN	25	Titanium
12mm AO universal	2	Stainless Steel
12mm AO URFN	27	Titanium
12mm ACE	8	Titanium
12mm RT	69	Stainless Steel

Fig. 3.1.14. The torsional rigidities of the nails shown in Fig. 3.1.13 a

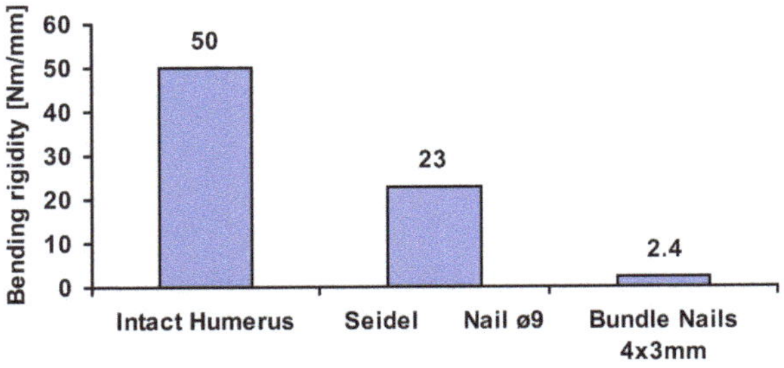

Fig. 3.1.15. Structural rigidity determined according to ASTM F 383, bending test

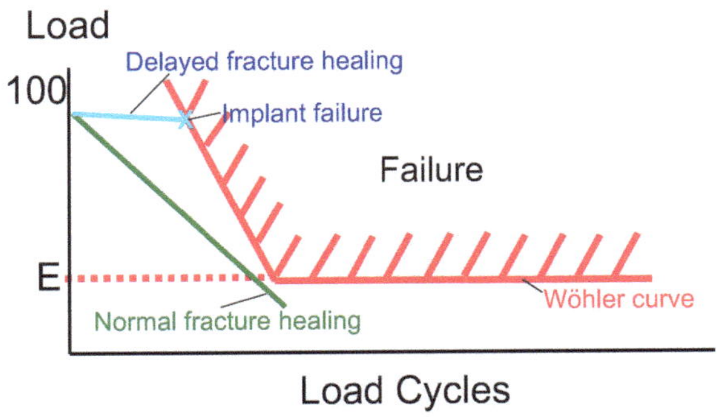

Fig. 3.1.16. Wöhler curve

A comparison of the structural rigidity between an intact humeral bone and different implants is given in Fig. 3.1.15. The rigidity of the intact bone is twice as high as for a stainless-steel Seidel humeral nail ∅ 9 mm. Therefore, it is important to discuss implant rigidity in terms of implant design and Young's modulus. It is equally important to discuss bone rigidity in the same terms.

Mechanical Behaviour Under Dynamic Load

Fatigue is the most common cause of implant failure (>99%). The material's behaviour under dynamic load can be described by the Wöhler curve (Fig. 3.1.16). When a material is cyclically loaded by a load lower than the load E, the material can withstand an infinite number of load cycles without failure; this is termed the "endurance limit". When the repetitive load is higher than E, material failure will occur after a certain number of load cycles. The higher the load, the smaller the number of load cycles the specimen can bear before failure. Implants for fracture fixation are designed for initial weight-bearing and if normal fracture healing occurs, the load on the implant will decrease as the bone heals and takes more and more load (Fig. 3.1.16, green line). Implant failure may occur when fracture healing is delayed or fails (non-union) and the implant is continuously loaded at a high load level (Fig. 3.1.16, blue line).

Test Method: The material data are determined by dynamic tensile or bending tests. Specimens of standard size are loaded dynamically with predefined load amplitude until fracture. The result from the failure of each specimen is one point on the Wöhler curve. The test is continued with a new specimen at lower load amplitude and so on until a load is reached at which a specimen survives up to a defined number of load cycles (e.g. 10 million cycles) without failure.

Characteristic Values: Fatigue strength is defined as the maximum load level below which all tested specimens reach 10^7 cycles without failure.

Materials Data: In Fig. 3.1.17 the fatigue strength is given for different materials. The values were determined for smooth surface test specimen. Orthinox in CW conditions provides the highest fatigue strength compared to all other generally used trauma implant materials. When the material surface is notched, caused by a thread or a scratch, the fatigue strength will be reduced depending on the notch geometry, as shown in Fig. 3.1.25.

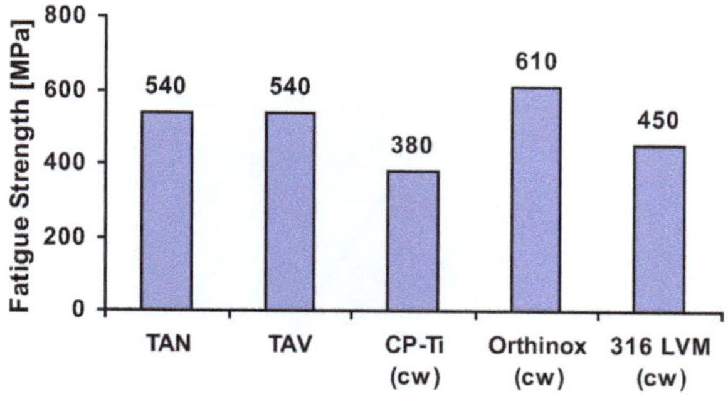

Fig. 3.1.17. Fatigue strength of different materials

Corrosion

Corrosion is electrolytic material dissolution caused by a corrosive solution. There is a cathodic solution reaction with a parallel anodic material dissolution (Fig. 3.1.18). Usually all implant materials will spontaneously form a passive surface oxide layer (e.g. CrO_2, TiO_2, etc.) in the presence of oxygen. To inhibit further corrosion of implants, manufacturers have developed processes that grow an enhanced protective oxide film through a process of surface oxidation or passivation. This is usually the last step in the implant manufacturing process. Corrosion of metallic implants embedded in the human body may occur by the mechanism of passive layer breakdown. Pitting corrosion, crevice corrosion and fretting corrosion are the most important forms of corrosion of implants.

Pitting Corrosion: Pitting occurs when the ratio of the anode to the cathode area on the metal surface is very small. This drives intense corrosion at the anodic site and leads to the formation of pits. With increasing depth of pit, the oxygen supply to the bottom of the pit becomes very limited. This lowers the local pH value and prevents repassivation and accelerates the pitting corrosion.

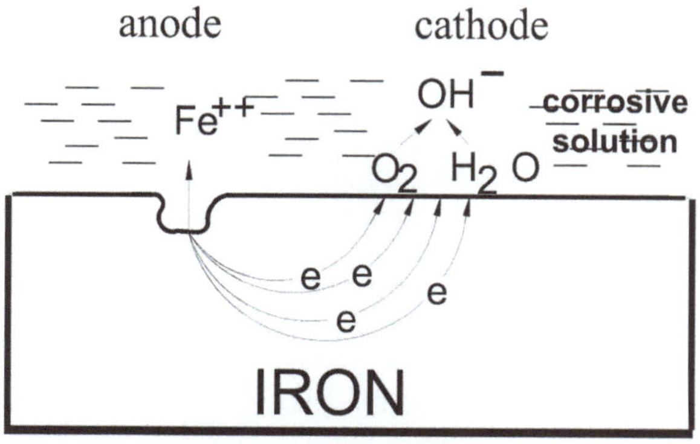

Fig. 3.1.18. Corrosion of metals, principle

It is very important to avoid scratching the surface of an implant as any small scratch may act as an anodic point and initiate corrosion.

Crevice Corrosion: Gaps or cracks between parts of multicomponent implants provide sites for crevice corrosion to take place. When crevice corrosion commences, there is a depletion of local oxygen, which further accelerates the corrosion process as described for pitting corrosion.

Fretting Corrosion: Fretting occurs when two components of a device are subjected to relative oscillatory movement. If the amplitude of oscillation is small, a fretting situation exists, but at larger amplitudes this becomes a wear phenomenon. The presence of a corrosive environment accelerates fretting and the existence of crevice conditions may intensify the corrosion conditions. By adding certain surface coatings, it is possible to enhance the resistance to fretting. Titanium, which is more susceptible to fretting than stainless steels, can be protected from fretting corrosion by a process known as anodisation type II. This will be described in more detail below.

Test Method: Corrosion resistance is determined by electrochemical measurements, where a material specimen is immersed in Ringer's solution and subjected to defined electric voltages leading to corrosion. The voltage at which corrosion starts is determined for the different forms of corrosion.

Pitting Potential Data: Corrosion data for pitting potential are listed in Fig. 3.1.19. The higher the pitting potential, the higher the corrosion resistance. The physiological corrosion potential in biosystems is about 200 mV_{SCE}. All implant materials provide corrosion resistance above this level. There are some very demanding implant applications, e.g. unstable hip fractures, in which implants are subjected to a combination of crevice

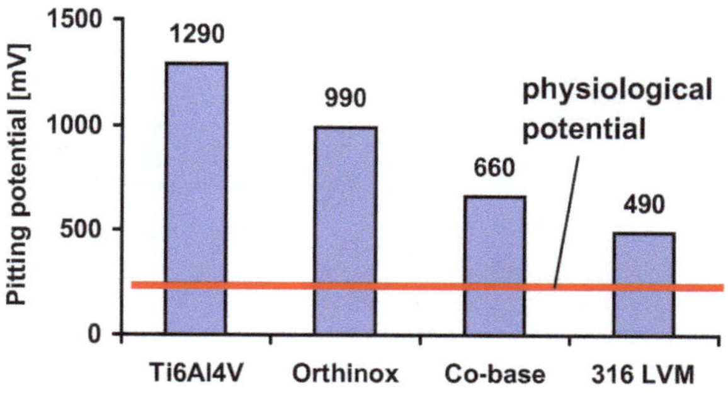

Fig. 3.1.19. Pitting potential of implant materials

and fretting corrosion and high mechanical load. The Gamma locking nail, Orthinox, or anodisation type II protected titanium alloys are ideal for such implants.

Titanium Surface Modifications

An untreated titanium surface shows strong wear and friction when sliding against all kinds of surfaces. This produces wear particles, tissues may blacken, and it may ultimately lead to failure of the implant. Titanium surfaces are susceptible to bony ingrowth and while this may be desirable in a cementless hip stem, it is less desirable in a trauma implant that may have to be removed. To improve both friction and wear behaviour of titanium, anodisation can be very effective. Anodisation modifies a titanium or titanium alloy surface by oxidisation in an electrolyte bath. Depending on electrolytic conditions and surface finishing after the electrolytic process, either anodisation type II or anodisation type III occurs.

Non-Anodised Titanium Surface

A non-anodised surface structure is shown in Fig. 3.1.20. The material surface is covered by a thin, porous layer of titanium oxide (TiO_2). Titanium is highly reactive in air and rapidly forms the passive oxide layer that confers good corrosion resistance.

Anodisation Type II

The first stage in the anodisation type II process is an electrolytic treatment in an alkaline bath. A voltage is applied between material and bath. The procedure removes the original oxide layer and causes oxygen and silicon diffusion into the material surface. In addition a new porous oxide layer grows on the surface. In the second stage this porous oxide layer is removed by blasting with glass beads. The resultant surface structure is shown in Fig. 3.1.21.

The diffused oxygen is partly forming oxides, which are very hard. Oxygen and oxides are embedded in material interstitially; they are an integral part of the material. The area of diffusion is called the conversion layer.

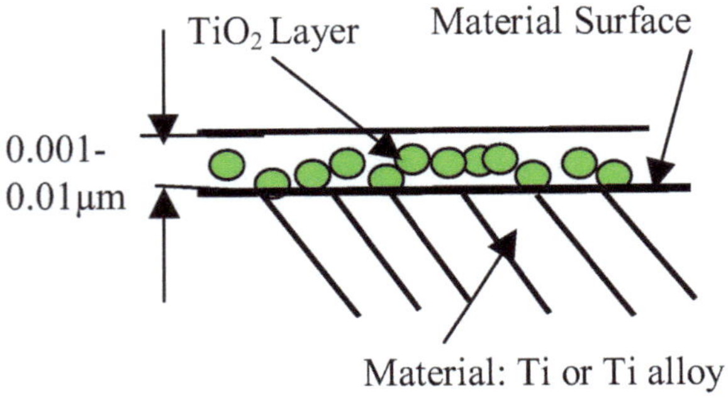

Fig. 3.1.20. Structure of non-anodised surface

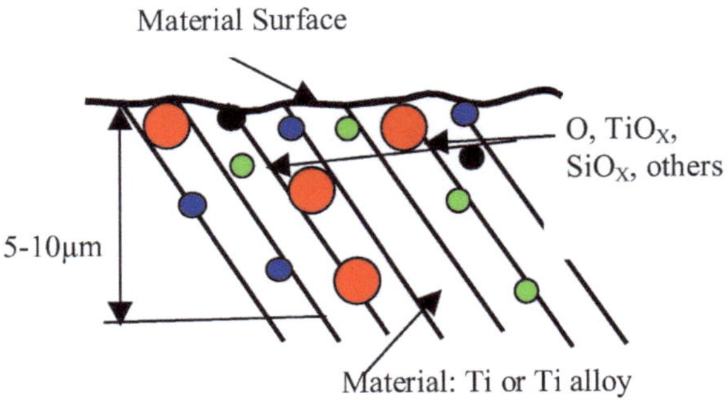

Fig. 3.1.21. Resultant structure of anodised type II surface

Anodisation Type III

Anodisation type III is a completely different process to type II and is used by some manufacturers to add colour to titanium implants. At the first stage the original oxide layer is removed in an acid bath. The second stage is an electrolytic process in which a voltage is applied between material and acid bath. The voltage is used to control the thickness of a new TiO_2 oxide layer on the surface. The resultant surface structure is shown in Fig. 3.1.22.

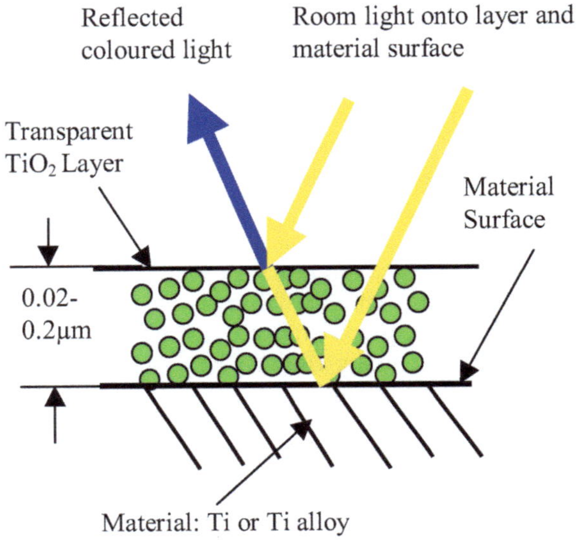

Fig. 3.1.22. Resultant structure of anodised type III surface

The anodised type III surface shows a similar structure to the non-anodised surface. The main difference is the thickness of layer, which is increased by more than one order of magnitude and it has a specific colour. The colour is generated by interference of light, partly reflected from the layer surface, partly reflected from the bulk material surface. The colour depends on the thickness of the layer and this can be precisely controlled during the anodisation process.

Properties of Different Anodised Surfaces

Anodisation modifies the interface properties of an implant. The following section quantifies this influence.

Metal-to-Metal Friction: Titanium components exhibit high friction when sliding against a surface of equal kind. In vivo, this may cause malfunction at sliding connections, e.g. between lag screw and nail. The friction coefficient μ represents the characteristic value for sliding resistance. Low friction coefficient means low friction. Values for different materials are listed in Fig. 3.1.23.

The results in Fig. 3.1.23 show that anodisation type II and III reduces the friction coefficient to one-quarter of non-anodised titanium. Anodised titanium surface friction is even slightly lower than that determined for Orthinox stainless steel.

Metal-to-Metal Wear: Ti shows excessive wear. It is affected by abrasion of hard surface oxides, which do not show sufficient adhesion to the base material. The abrasion process is followed by material microwelding and surface reoxidisation, then abrasion again, and so on. The removed oxides are seen as black particles. Non-anodised as well as type III anodised surfaces show similar surface structure. For both, the hard oxide layers are located on the material surface and are easily removed during friction. The easy removal will result in excessive wear. For anodisation type II the hard oxides are integrated in the material and thus are not removed as easily during friction. Therefore anodisation type II will show considerably lower wear rates.

Metal-to-Bone Wear: Ti also shows excessive wear when sliding against bone. The wear products are responsible for the black debris found around implants. They may affect bone resorption. Pin-on-disc tests show the influence of anodisation on wear against bone. The mass loss Δm is the characteristic value for wear rate. Results are shown in Fig. 3.1.24. In this test pins manufactured from bone cement were used to simulate cortical bone.

The results show anodisation type II to reduce wear rate to 1/500th of non-anodised control. Anodisation type III blue colour reduces wear to one-seventh of non-anodised control. Type II wear rate is in the same range as for steel Orthinox. In contrast to non-anodised control, surface type II did not generate black debris. Wear products consist mainly of oxidised titanium. Therefore the wear rate gives an indication of the release rate of metal ions.

Effect of Anodisation Type II on Fatigue Strength: In vivo implants may fail by fatigue fracture due to dynamic loading. Results from dynamic nail-bending tests simulating in vivo loading of the locking hole area are shown in Fig. 3.1.25.

Results demonstrate that anodisation type II increases the fatigue strength of nail shafts by 15% compared to non-anodised control.

Bony Ingrowth: In vivo, bony ingrowth into trauma implants can lead to complications during ex-

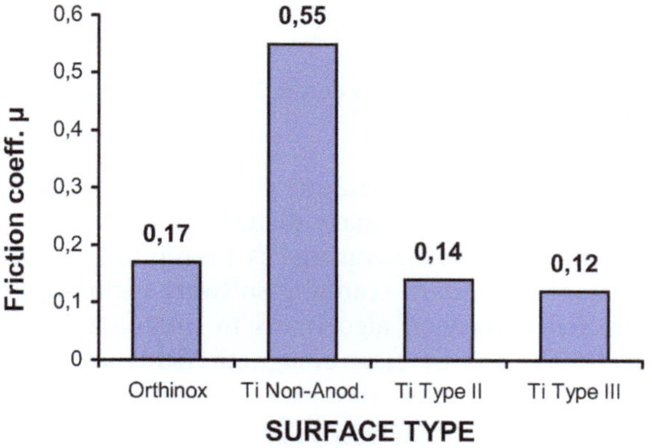

Fig. 3.1.23. Friction coefficients μ for movement between equal surface types

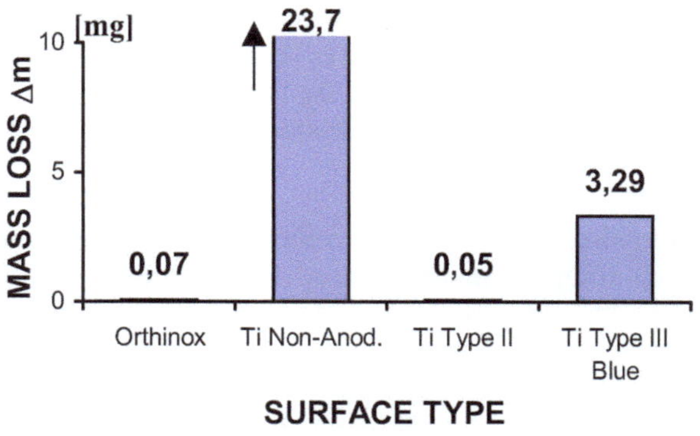

Fig. 3.1.24. Wear rate of metal in contact with bone cement

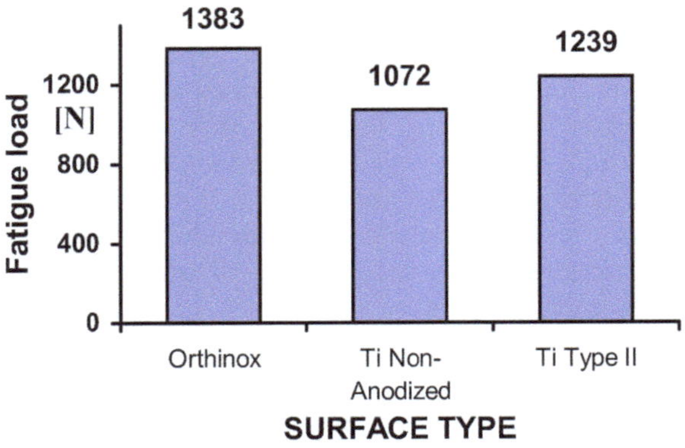

Fig. 3.1.25. Fatigue failure load determined for drilled nail shafts in bending

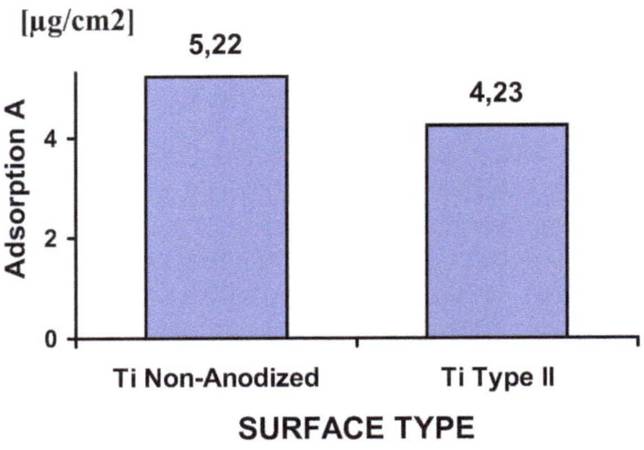

Fig. 3.1.27. Protein adsorption determined in immersion tests

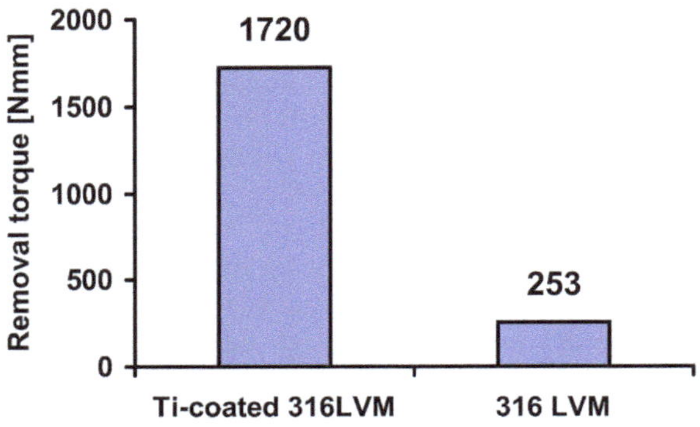

Fig. 3.1.26. Pin removal torque after 6 weeks implantation in sheep (tibia)

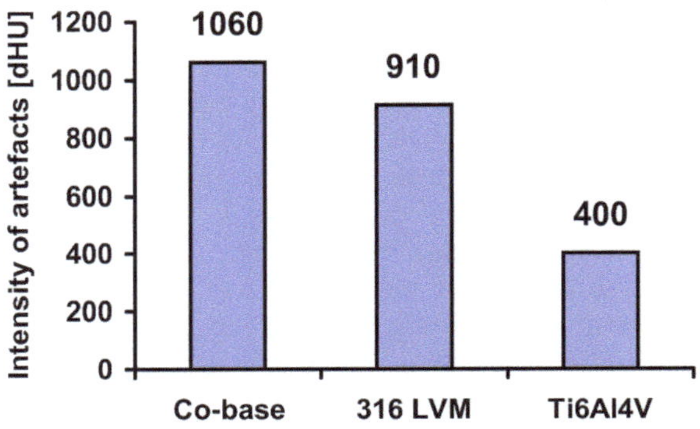

Fig. 3.1.28. Intensity of artefacts during CT scanning

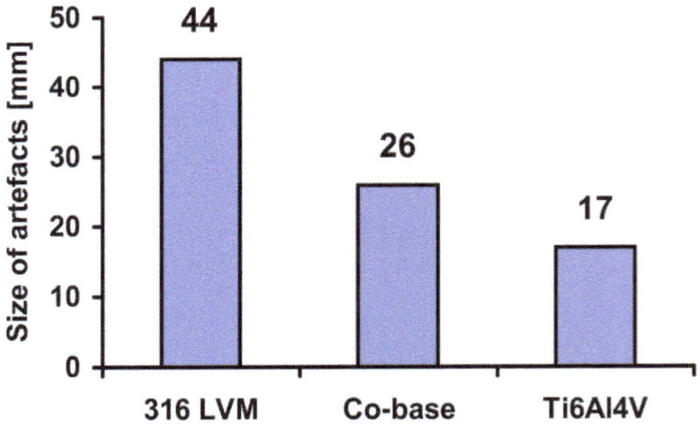

Fig. 3.1.29. Size of artefacts during MRI scanning

plantation, e.g. bone refractures. Ingrowth testing of titanium-coated and uncoated 316 LVM pins in sheep (tibia) showed a higher removal torque for titanium-coated pins than for the uncoated 316 LVM pins (Fig. 3.1.26).

Further tests were performed to determine the influence of anodisation on bony ingrowth. This was done by measuring protein adsorption on different surfaces, since protein adsorption is the first stage in bony ingrowth.

Results demonstrate that anodisation type II reduces protein adsorption by approximately 20% compared to non-anodised control (Fig. 3.1.27). The reduction is effected by the dense silicon surface layer that reduces interaction between material and tissue.

Response to Imaging Procedures: MRI and CT are well-accepted methods used for diagnostic imaging. The effectiveness of these technologies is influenced by implant material, imaging system, scan protocol and configuration of implant. While all commonly used implant materials cause image artefacts during CT and MRI, as shown in Figs. 3.1.28 and 3.1.29, titanium is often preferred because it causes less image disturbance.

This perceived advantage is becoming less important as modern scanning software includes optimised correction algorithms to minimised artefacts. The intense electromagnetic fields used during MRI scanning may also cause movement or heating of an implant and this has led to the concept of MRI safe devices in which these effects are below defined values.

A Practical Example

A practical example will serve to show how some of the concepts introduced above are used in implant design to make state-of-the art implants.

The trochanteric Gamma nail (TGN), in both regular and long version, is accepted as a standard treatment in traumatology, particularly in unstable fractures of the femur. The TGN was made from Orthinox in order to meet the high loading typical of these fractures. Surgeons also wished to have a titanium proximal femoral nail that would perform at least as well clinically as the TGN and better where possible. This led to the Gamma3 design and some of the key elements of this design are described below (Fig. 3.1.30).

Surface Treatment

Gamma3 components are protected by anodisation type II. This is particularly important in any proximal femoral nail with a lag screw as the region between the lag screw and the nail is dynamically loaded with significant alternating loads. The gap between screw and nail also might act as a crevice and there is sliding between both components.

Strength Enhancements

One of the clinical goals was to reduce the proximal diameter of the nail while at the same time maintaining strength. To maintain nail strength with a reduced proximal diameter implied a reduction in lag-screw diameter. The challenge was to maintain high lag-screw cut-out performance with a reduced lag-screw diameter. This was achieved by adding a patented strength improvement groove feature to the lateral margin of the nail in the region of the lag-screw hole, as shown in Fig. 3.1.31.

Paradoxically this removal of material results in an increase in strength as it reduces the local stress concentration in the highly loaded rim of the lag-screw hole. This is illustrated in Fig. 3.1.32 from the results of finite element models showing that, by reducing the nail diameter and moving from stainless steel to titanium material, the stress in the region of the lag-screw hole increases by 24%. By adding the stress improvement groove, the stress is reduced and becomes equivalent to that in the TGN under the same boundary conditions. (Note that red denotes higher stress and blue lower stress.)

Fatigue Strength of Screws

To minimise the distal diameter of the nail, the distal locking screws were reduced in size from 6.28 mm (TGN) to 5.00 mm (Gamma3). The design challenge of doing this while maintaining strength is significant. Many of the screw features were modified (thread profile, thread depth, core diameter, etc.) to increase strength as much as possible. As shown in Fig. 3.1.33, these measures

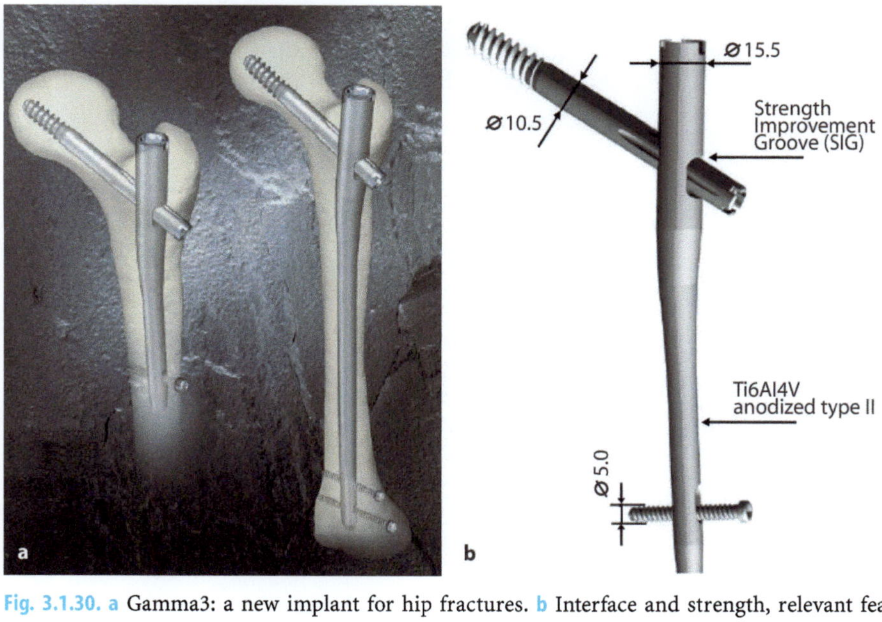

Fig. 3.1.30. a Gamma3: a new implant for hip fractures. b Interface and strength, relevant features

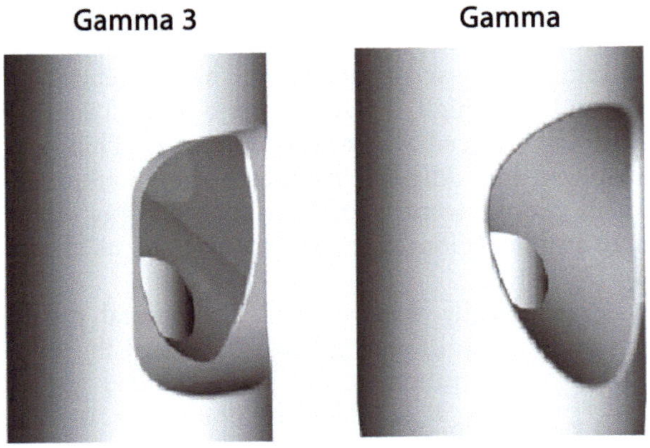

Fig. 3.1.31. Strength improvement groove feature in the Gamma3 nail

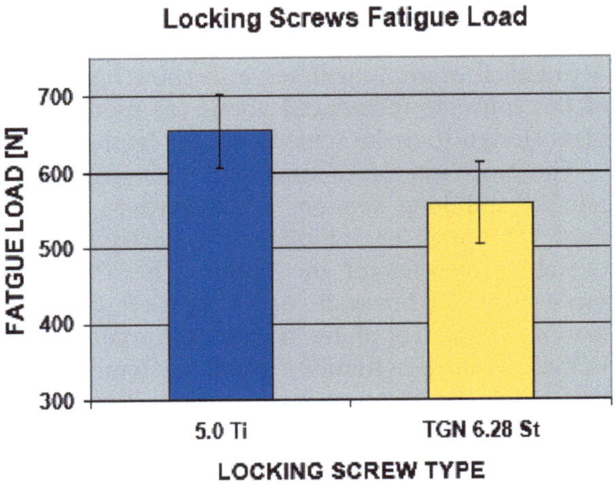

Fig. 3.1.33. The fatigue strength of distal screws

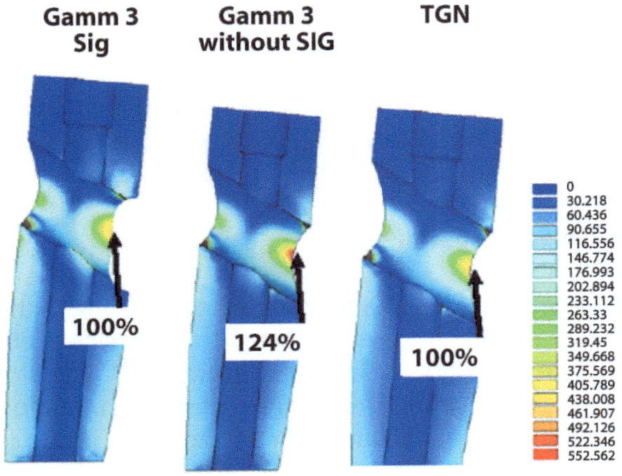

Fig. 3.1.32. Effect of the strength improvement groove on stress

were effective and resulted in an increase in strength while at the same time reaching the clinical goal of reducing screw diameter.

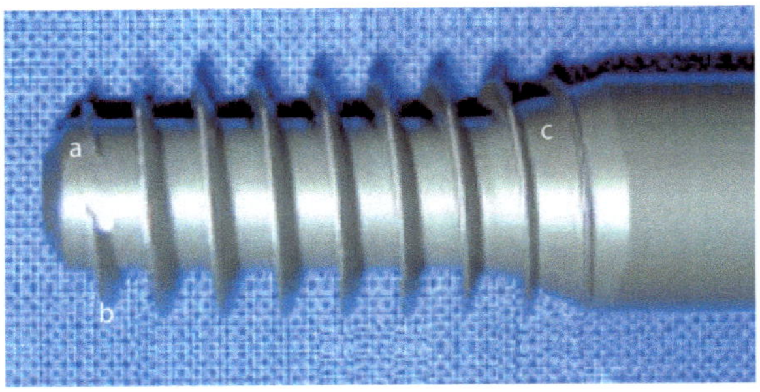

Fig. 3.1.34. Gamma3 lag screw

Lag Screw to Bone Interface Design

The reduction in lag-screw diameter necessitated a reduction in the diameter of the threaded portion of the lag screw. The screw (Fig. 3.1.34) was re-engineered to make it as bone friendly as possible, reducing the risk of cut-out, while at the same time making it both easy to insert and for the surgeon

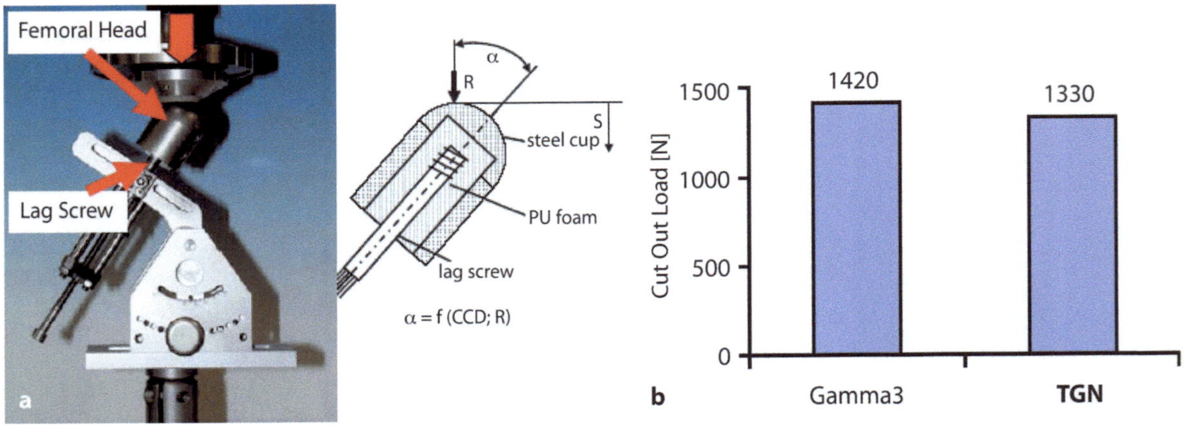

Fig. 3.1.35. a Cut-out test rig. b Cut-out test results

to feel when it was properly tightened even in osteoporotic bone. The cutting flutes (a) were modified to reduce cancellous bone damage. A negative flank and thinner thread flanks (b) were added. The core diameter was tapered up to the screw major diameter and the thread run out continuously (c).

While these changes might seem small, their effect of performance was dramatic and the best test to demonstrate this is the dynamic cut-out test (depicted in Fig. 3.1.35 a) in which the cut-out load is determined as the load level at which significant screw migration in a bone simulation material starts. The higher the cut-out load, the higher the cut-out resistance. The results of this test (Fig. 3.1.35 b) show that in spite of having a smaller diameter (10.5 mm) than the TGN (12 mm), the Gamma3 lag screw demonstrated a higher resistance to cut-out.

Conclusion

In the manufacturing of implants there are many aspects to be considered in selection of materials, their treatment and design features, all of which have to be assessed against the demands of a specific application. The advances in clinical experience combine with advances in biomechanical knowledge and new technologies to enable significant improvements to be made in implants designed for fracture fixation.

Note: All test data shown in this chapter are data on file, Stryker Trauma GmbH.

References

1. Paul JP, 1966-67. Forces transmitted by the joints in the human body. Proc Inst Mech Eng 181 (3J), 8–15.
2. Bergmann G, Graichen F, Rohlmann A, 1993. Hip joint loading during walking and running measured in two patients. J Biomech 26(8), 969–990.
3. Brown RH, Burstein AH, Frankel VH, 1982. Telemetering in-vivo loads from nail implants. J Biomech 15 (11), 815–823.
4. Burny F, Donkerwolke M, Moulart F, Bourgeois R, Puers R, Van Schuylenbergh K, Barbosa M, Paiva O, Rodes F, Bégueret JB, Lawes P, 2000. Concept, design and fabrication of smart orthopedic implants. Med Eng & Physics (22), 469–479.
5. Schneider E, Michel MC, Genge M, Perren SM, 1990. Loads acting on an intramedullary femoral nail. In: Implantable telemetry in orthopaedics, Bergmann, Graichen and Rohlmann, eds. Forschungsvermittlung der FU, Berlin, 221–227.
6. Eveleigh RJ, 1997. A biomechanical evaluation of intramedullary nails during simulated fracture healing. PhD Thesis, University of Bath, England.

Section 4 New Designs of Intramedullary Nails

A New Titanium Nail for the Femur: Concept and Design

T. Mückley, V. Bühren

Introduction

Intramedullary nailing of the femur is an established and widely used technique in traumatologic and orthopedic surgery, with a broad spectrum of indications. It has become the preferred treatment for diaphyseal fractures due to good alignment at the fracture site, preservation of the periosteal blood supply and soft tissue, and the early restoration of function. Kuentscher's basic principles of mechanical and biological fracture healing with closed reduction, preservation of the fracture hematoma, and fixation with an intramedullary nail according to the fracture pattern, is still valid today [37].

Fixation of the original intramedullary Kuentscher nail is based on the cylindrical reaming principle and transversal spring locking of the cloverleaf nail profile. The original idea, to obtain stability with a larger intramedullary blocked nail, was abandoned with the development of locking nails. With this remarkable development, the spectrum of indications expanded widely. However, to achieve axial and rotational stability, the new generation of intramedullary nails has to be interlocked proximally and distally [2, 9, 16, 34]. Using these technical principles, it has been demonstrated by numerous authors that intramedullary fixation of diaphyseal long bone fractures is more effective and mechanically superior to plate fixation [2, 20, 34, 52]. Conventionally, locked intramedullary nailing requires pre-reaming of the medullary canal for insertion of a larger diameter nail. Nevertheless, there are experimental and clinical data indicating that reaming may have adverse consequences of systemic embolization [55], pulmonary damage [45], hemostatic activation [27], reduction of bone strength [46] and destruction of the endosteal blood supply [50, 51]. Accordingly, the trend in nailing shaft fractures led to unreamed and limited-reamed techniques and the use of small-diameter nails. However, a high incidence of complications including implant failure, delayed unions, nonunions and malunions has been reported with the use of small-diameter nails and unreamed techniques [1, 5, 17, 26, 30, 53]. Many of the complications mentioned above are due to the poor primary stability of the osteosyntheses. Another disadvantage of unreamed nailing is the occasional appearance of distraction at the fracture site, due to endosteal resistance during the insertion process. The resulting fracture diastasis is a well-known cause of prolonged bone healing and nonunion.

Clear improvement concerning the aforementioned issues has been achieved with the development of new implant materials and different locking options, as well as the development of an integrated compression mechanism. With the same nail diameter, for the appropriate fracture, better primary stability can be achieved with the compression nail compared to other intramedullary locking nails [6, 7, 21, 39]. In addition, through the compression mechanism, which allows dispensed fragment apposition, a primary fracture diastasis can be avoided [43].

Instruments, Implants and Surgical Technique

The biomechanical concept of compressed or appositioned nailing consists in the use of an intramedullary device that is inserted into the medullary cavity without jamming and that allows, after proximal and distal locking, a relative movement of the fragments against each other. First, the implant is firmly attached to the distal main fragment (or the proximal fragment, if a retrograde technique is being employed), using fully threaded locking screws at the nail tip. Next, the other main fragment, which contains the nail entry portal, is fixed via a partially threaded locking screw (shaft screw) that has been placed in an oblong hole. The compression screw is inserted from the top of the nail, and is pushed against the shaft screw (Fig. 4.1.1), drawing either the distal or the proximal segment toward the fracture site, resulting in apposition or compression of the fracture gap (Fig. 4.1.2).

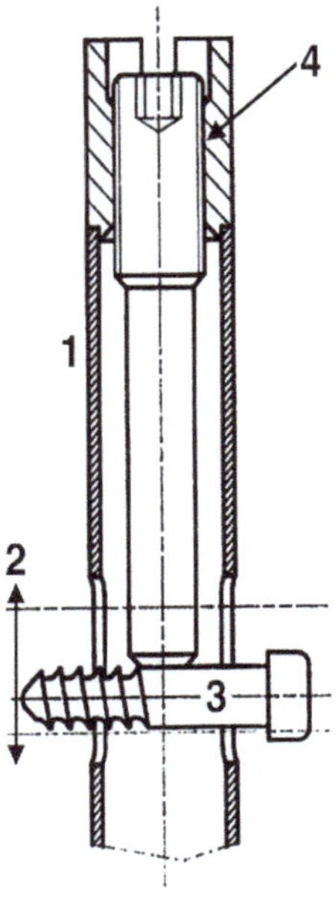

Fig. 4.1.1. Cutaway view of compression mechanism at the proximal nail end (*1*). Compression screw (*4*) is tightened and its reaction against the transverse shaft screw (*3*) in the oblong hole (*2*) causes compression at the fracture/osteotomy site

Therefore, the devices used for compression nailing should be free to slide in the medullary canal, and should be of sufficient size and strength to transmit the forces applied via the compression screw into the bone, without undergoing major deformation. The former condition means that there is no need for a slot along the nail to obtain a tight intramedullary fit. This is also beneficial, since slotting would obviously, and unnecessarily, reduce the stiffness of the implant.

The T2 nails (T2 Nailing System, Stryker Trauma) are cannulated devices, with diameters that allow insertion without reaming or with limited reaming techniques. Typically used femoral nails are 9–13 mm in diameter. These nail diameters allow for the use of 5-mm locking screws, which with a core diameter of >4 mm are strong enough to withstand the compression applied without major bending. With this new generation of compression nails, we have titanium alloy implants (Ti6Al4V, anodization type II), which can be implanted using the ante- or retrograde technique with the same instruments and implants (Fig. 4.1.3) [43]. According to the fracture type, the system offers the option of different locking modes. In addition to static locking, a controlled dynamization with rotational stability is optional. Compression nailing can be performed using two different locking patterns: actively pre-compressed dynamic locking, and actively appositioned/pre-compressed static locking. The actively pre-com-

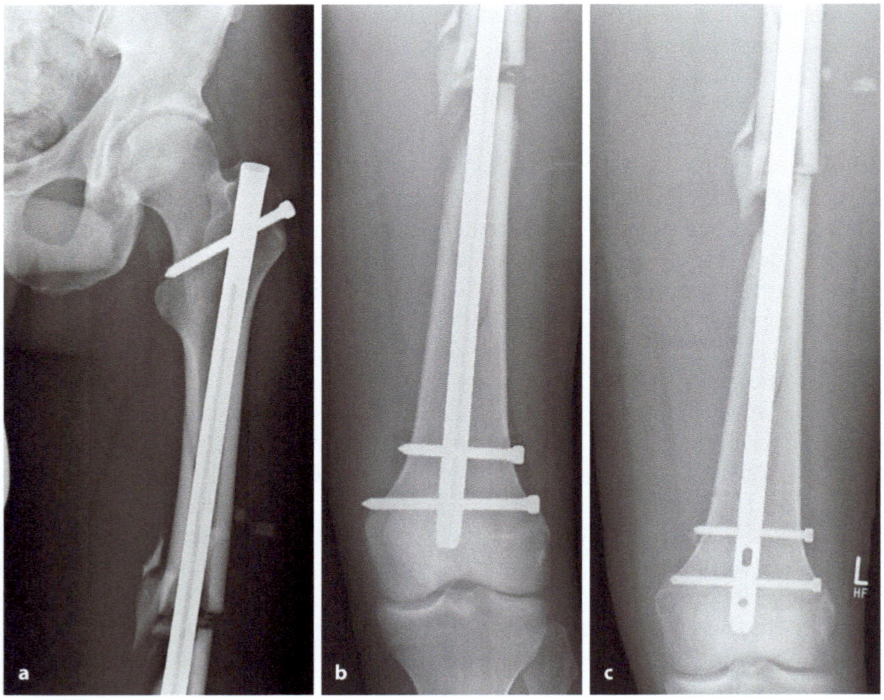

Fig. 4.1.2. a Persisting fracture gap of 5–7 mm after nailing with a locked GK-nail. b, c After nail exchange, sound apposition and compression is performed with the axially inserted compression screw

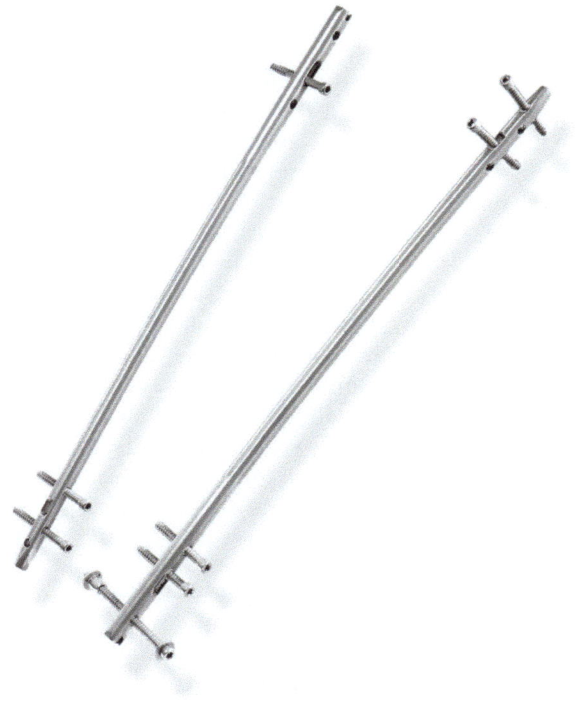

Fig. 4.1.3. The T2 femur nail can be used in antegrade or retrograde fashion in combination with multiple locking modes

pressed dynamic mode involves compression of transverse (AO type 32-A3.2) or short oblique (AO type 32-A2.2) fractures and hypertrophic nonunions via the compression screw, which the surgeon tightens by hand "with feeling" and monitoring on the image intensifier. The force used should not exceed that normally used to seat a cortical screw. Once a torque of 2–3 Nm has been reached, and the shaft screw starts bending, tightening must be stopped. In this way, the remaining distance of the shaft screw in the oblong hole constitutes a means of dynamization of the fracture in the further course of treatment.

When the nail is being used in the actively appositioned/pre-compressed static mode, apposition or active compression is applied to AO type 32-A1.2 or AO B-type fractures as described above but with less torque and under online image intensifier control. After apposition or pre-compression a second proximal locking screw is applied, to occupy a round hole. This will ensure the static locking of the bone fragments. This special locking mode is called "advanced locking mode" (Fig. 4.1.4). Locking in the static mode has the disadvantage of not allowing the shaft screw to displace distally in the oblong hole for fracture dynamization. On the other hand, this locking mode has the advantage of enhancing the stability

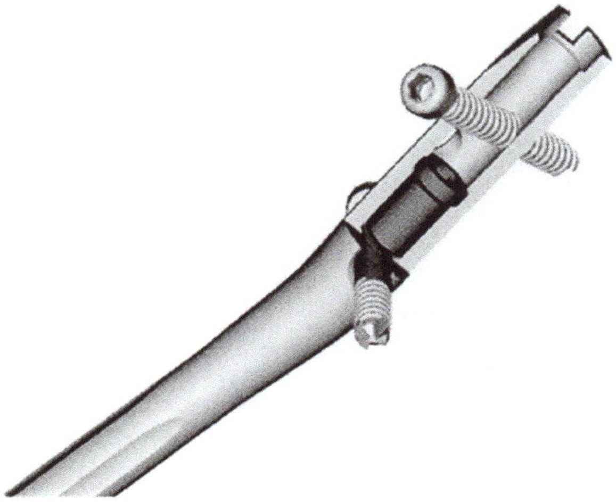

Fig. 4.1.4. With short compression screws, more unstable fracture patterns can be stabilized after apposition with additional static locking screws located close to the nail end. This type of locking is called "advanced locking mode"

of the bone fragments, since the locking screw in the round hole will provide markedly better fixation of the fragment. This is particularly beneficial when the fracture pattern involves a short proximal or distal fragment, with little intramedullary guidance of the nail. Static locking may also be used if apposition or pre-compression is desired, but there are concerns about the axial stability at the fracture site.

Evolution of the Compression Concept

From the very beginning, the AO has considered interfragmentary compression as a main issue in their search for stable osteosyntheses. The idea of compressing a fracture or osteotomy site via an internal fixation device was realized early on, in plate and screw fixation techniques, with the use of lag screws, plate-tensioning devices, and the provision of specially shaped holes in plates to allow dynamic compression.

The first attempts to apply this concept to intramedullary nails were made by Olerud [44] and Kaessmann [32, 33] in the late 1950s. The special interest in compression nailing started in the late 1960s as a reaction to the then innovative method of compression plating. As a result of the first experiments, a tie rod was placed within a Kuentscher nail and anchored to the distal fragment by cross-pinning. An external system provided the application of compression, which was maintained on the proximal end of the nail by a collar locker with a set screw [32]. A few results regarding this system were published in the

1970s, but no regular clinical use ever took place [31]. The main problem in those early days was the transmission of the interfragmentary compressive forces into the bone [8, 18, 31, 33]. It was found that implants fixed mainly in the cancellous bone of the metaphysis were incapable of withstanding controlled compression for longer periods of time. According to the studies of Ritter, the bone surface that supports a sustained compression force must be 100 times bigger in cancellous bone compared to cortical bone [49].

Later on, additional compression nail designs were introduced proposing external compression devices and static fixation. While the main advantage described by all authors was the greater stability during the first postoperative weeks with less pain [8, 29], the technique did not become widely used. At the same time, Ritter [48] and Mittelmeier et al. [38] were developing intramedullary compression nails with cortically supported locking screws and an axially inserted compression screw as a simple internal compression device that allowed high compressive forces to be applied. The concept was first employed in antegrade nailing of the femur, and is now an established feature of compression nailing techniques for upper and lower limb long bone fractures.

Biomechanics

The concept of compression nailing relies on the significant increase in the primary stability of the osteosyntheses brought about by the compression of the fracture or osteotomy site [6, 20, 39, 47].

Richardson et al. [47] confirmed this after performing biomechanical tests on different intramedullary femur osteosyntheses. Compared with dynamically and statically interlocked nails, only the compression nail showed any fracture site compression in the unloaded state, and the compressed fracture configuration was also demonstrated to be more stable. Fracture site angulation, shear and distraction were less with the compression nail. For clinical use, this should lead to less macromotion at the fracture site and minor postoperative pain, less bone resorption and faster bone healing.

A higher rotational stability achieved with compressed intramedullary nailing, compared to uncompressed systems, could be proven by Blum et al. [6]. For a statically locked nail with corresponding pre-compression, a clearly higher four-point bending stiffness and a significantly higher strength were demonstrated.

The results of Gonschorek et al. [21] showed that the amount of the resulting compression forces at the osteotomy site is dependent on the quality of the bone stock and can be reduced for example by osteoporosis. With our own specific

Table 4.1.1. Inter-fragmentary compression force (N) versus applied torque (Nm) for femur T2 nails depending on environmental conditions (lubricant/dry)

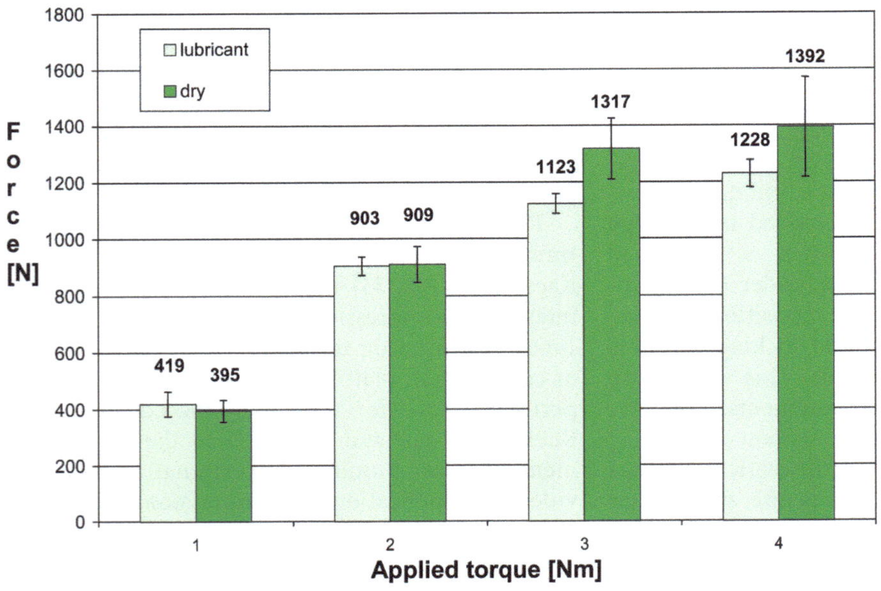

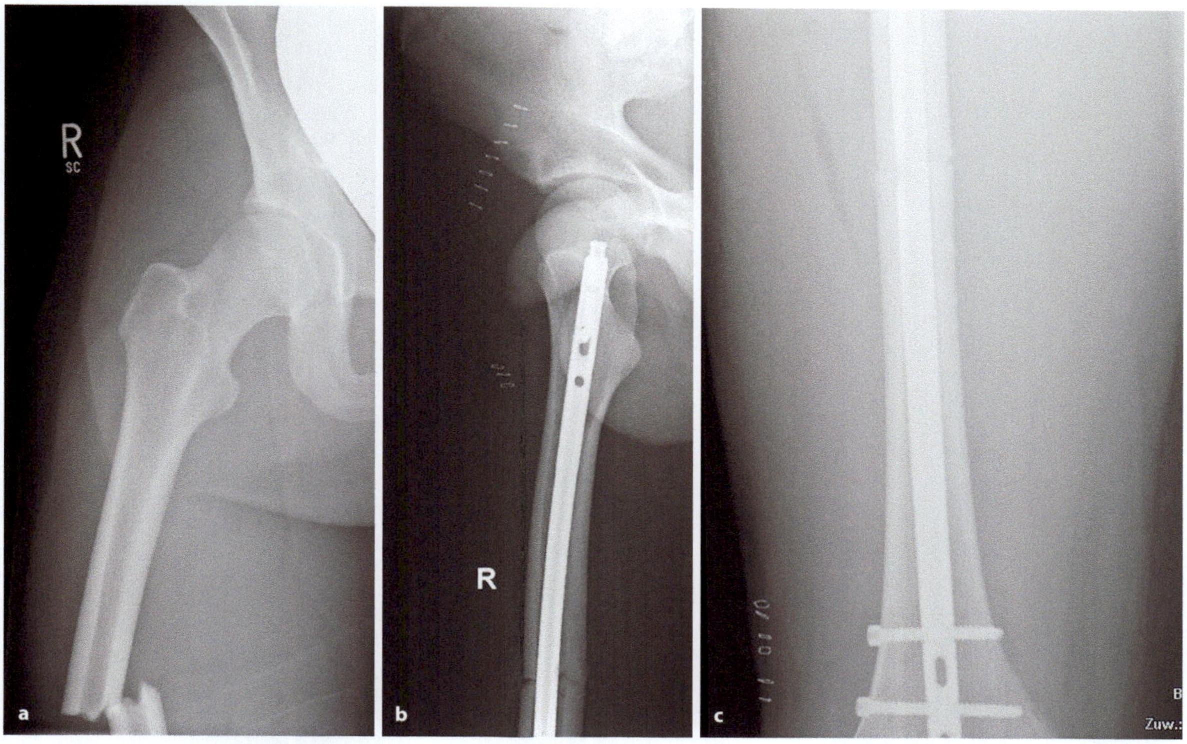

Fig. 4.1.5 a–c. An excellent indication for compression nailing is a noncomminuted transverse fracture at the mid-shaft level with interdigitation of the projecting cortical spikes over a large surface area

tests on the T2 femoral nailing system, we could demonstrate the relation of interfragmentary forces and compression screw torque (Table 4.1.1). Tests showed, in accordance with the clinical experience, that at about 2000 N, which is achievable in theory, deformation of the locking screw and shifting of the screw in the cortex can be seen. Utilizing the appropriate screw driver and a two-finger technique to hold the screw driver, the torque typically applied to the T2 compression screw amounts to 2–3 Nm. The applied torque onto compression screw is transmitted into inter-fragmentary compression force proportionally. For the femur the typical clinical used torque results in a compression force of approximately 900–1400 N.

The extent and duration of the increase in stability will be a function of the quality and vitality of the patient's bone stock, the fracture pattern, the resorption process at the fracture surface, the fatigue of the implants and the autodynamization by weight-bearing [11]. The ideal case for compression nailing is that of a noncomminuted transverse fracture at the mid-shaft level with interdigitation of the projecting cortical spikes over a large surface area (Fig. 4.1.5) [36]. In such a case, the bone will have excellent rotational stability. In the stabilization of transverse osteotomy, the flat mating bone surfaces produced by the surgeon tend to offer less favorable conditions [10–12]. However, several studies have shown the primary resistance to rotational forces achieved with intramedullary compression nailing to be far superior to that which can be obtained with conventionally locked nails [6, 20, 39, 47].

Another aspect of compression nailing is the biomechanical advantage of creating active circumferential compression to the fracture site, transferring axial load to the bone, and reducing the function of the nail as a load-bearing device [47]. This ability to transfer load back to the bone (load sharing) can reduce the incidence of implant failure secondary to fatigue. Typical statically locked unreamed nails with distraction at the fracture site function as load-bearing devices, and failure rates in excess of 20% have been reported (Fig. 4.1.6) [30].

Compression nailing differs from conventional dynamic locking in that it involves actively applied levels of fracture-site compression. With physiological loading, conventional dynamic intramedullary nailing can produce stress reversal at the fracture site, with the load pattern passing through zero: in the loaded state, compressive

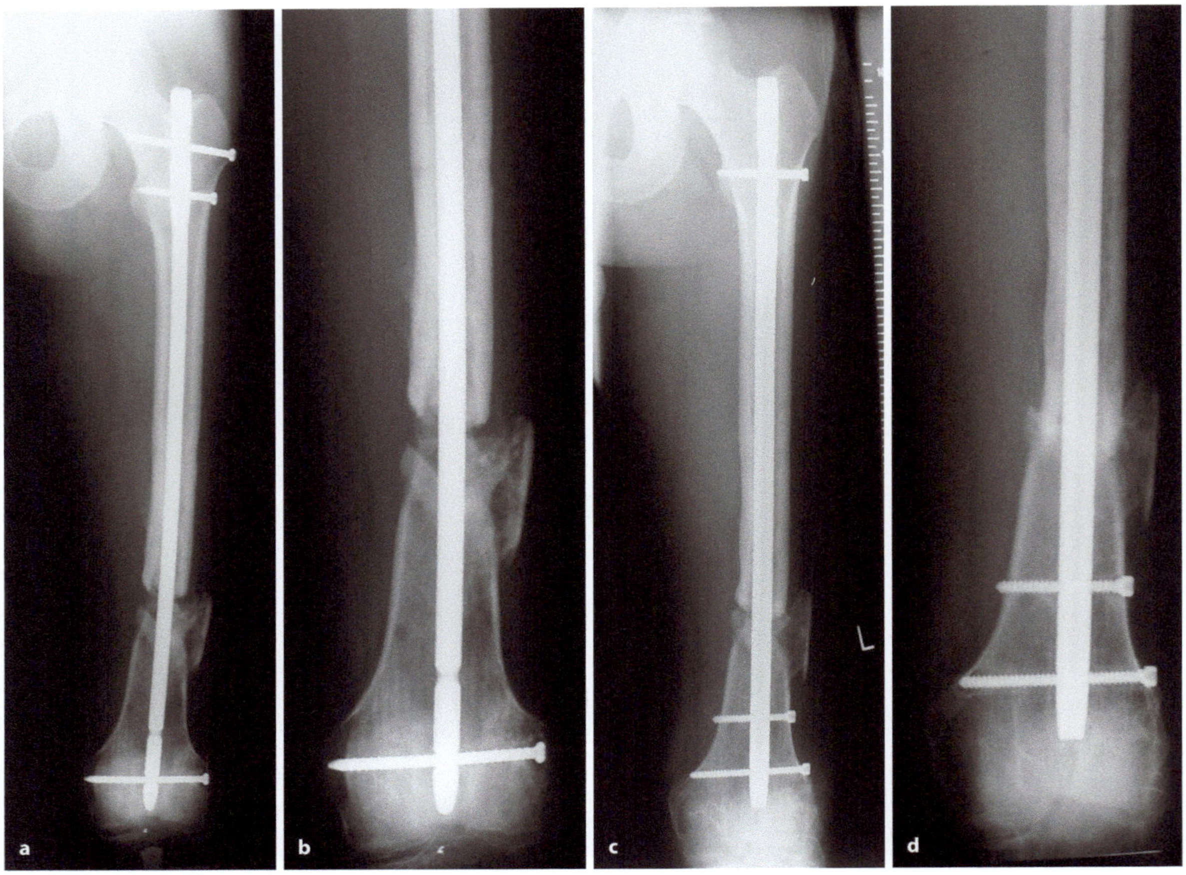

Fig. 4.1.6. a, b Statically locked unreamed femur nail with distraction at the fracture site resulting in nonunion. c Compression nailing after intramedullary reaming with apposition of the bone fragments and d consolidation after 6 months

forces amounting to the subject's body weight are produced; in the unloaded state, the weight of the extremity will cause tensile stresses that may pull the fragments apart. With active compression, the amount of compression applied will be additive to the body weight in the loaded state, while, in the unloaded state, the active compression will counteract distraction. Thus, throughout all phases of physiological movement, there will always be a baseline level of compression at the fracture site and reduced macromotions. The reduction of zero crossing represents reduced mechanical stress of the implants.

While the biomechanical patterns have been reasonably researched and described in cadaver and synthetic bone studies, there is little information on the in vivo postimplantation behavior of actively pre-compressed intramedullary nails in humans. Clinical experiences have indicated that the compression forces or at least a part of the compression forces sustain over a time period of 2–4 weeks. Just in this time period, an increased stability due to the continued compression on the fracture gap, as shown in studies on animal experiments, can have a positive impact on the new vessel formation at the fracture site [54]. For its use in the lower limb, it must be assumed that, with physiological load bearing, the initially applied level of compression will be reduced as a result of micro loosening of the locking screws, and of resorption at the fracture surfaces. However, since the shaft screw could still move distally in the oblong hole, even the total loss of the initially applied compression would leave the bone in the favorable situation of a conventional dynamic locking mode with rotational stability [11].

Indications

The potential indications for intramedullary compression nailing cover axial stable fractures of the shaft region and an important part of reconstructive surgery: pseudarthrosis treatment and osteotomies [11, 13–15, 20]. Compression nailing may be of special value for situations in which load bearing of the affected extremity is not possible [11, 47]. Indications include multiple injuries of the lower limb and polytrauma, which make axial loading of the affected limb impossible [11].

Whether or not compression nailing can be used will depend on the axial stability of the fracture [11, 14, 24, 43]. This means that simple fracture patterns (AO 32-A3.2, AO 32-B2.2 with small bending wedge), nonunions without bone loss (e.g. hypertrophic nonunions) and elective osteotomies are excellent indications [3, 4, 23, 25, 40, 42]. Metaphyseal fractures or osteotomies are inherently unsuitable for management with compression nailing [11]. This is because the metaphysis has a markedly lower proportion of compression-resistant cortical bone. Also, the difference in caliber may lead to the slender, harder shaft being telescoped into the wider, softer metaphysis. Since the fragment that contains the nail entry portal is locked only with one screw, in an oblong hole rather than a round hole, this fragment must provide a reasonably long medullary canal trajectory for the nail. Accordingly compression nailing will need to be confined to the management of diaphyseal fractures. More precisely, the fractures considered for this fixation should be in the central three-fifths of the long bone. Among several hundred patients, comprising both solitary and multiple injuries, almost exactly 40% of femoral fractures were found to be suitable for treatment with compression nailing. In reconstructive surgery for delayed fracture healing, nonunion, the correction of axial or rotational malalignment and the restoration of limb length, 90% of the patients proved suitable [11, 20].

Due to the developments of short compression screws, of additional static locking holes located more at the nail end as well as the option for either the antegrade or retrograde approach, the T2 nailing system extends the spectrum of indications to nearly all diaphyseal fracture types and also to fractures at the metaphyseal region [43]. In these cases we are no longer talking about the classical compression locking mode but the options for the appositioning of the main fragments and the different static locking options. Besides severe soft tissue damage and insufficient intraoperative stabilizing of the fracture, one of the major risks for delayed unions or pseudarthrosis is mainly considered to be the fracture diastasis. Postoperative fracture diastasis could mainly be observed in poorly managed unreamed intramedullary nailing techniques. The difficulties and the absence of a secondary dynamization in such osteosyntheses have been described already [28]. The possibility of a mechanically controlled appositioning of the main fragments with the aid of an integrated "compression mechanism" or "appositioning mechanism" respectively, is not only able to prevent a fracture diastasis effectively but also increases the primary stability of the assembly.

Fractures

In the treatment of femoral shaft fractures, correct length and axial alignment are the principal objectives and have to be assessed radiographically and clinically. We choose the lateral decubitus position on a fracture table for antegrade and the supine position with the knee 40–50° flexed for the retrograde approach.

In nearly all cases of shaft fractures we perform reduction as a closed procedure. After determination of the exact entry point, a guide wire is inserted and placed very carefully in the center of the distal fragment. Provided that the entry portal is also exactly in the line of the intramedullary canal, for simple fracture patterns the insertion of a nail of sufficient size will automatically oppose the cortical surfaces and reduce the main fragments.

In cases of severe soft-tissue injury or high-degree open fractures, we recommend primary external fixation. In severely polytraumatized patients and especially in patients with risk of post-traumatic pulmonary failure, we also recommend primarily external fixation of the long bone fractures. Conversion to an intramedullary fixation should be performed within 1–2 weeks.

Since the femur has a good soft-tissue envelope, femoral shaft fractures are more often closed than open. The treatment by intramedullary nailing is, therefore, more straightforward and less risky than for the tibia. For standard treatment of closed femoral fractures without severe soft-tissue injury, we use limited reaming techniques without cortical reaming. As a matter of principle, we use at least two locking screws in the frontal plane at the nail tip; where the fragment at the nail tip is short (e.g. for antegrade nailing at the junction of the middle and the distal third, or for retrograde nailing at the junction of the middle and the proximal third of the shaft), perpendicular (mediolateral plus anteroposterior) screws will be used (Fig. 4.1.7). For highly unstable fractures there is the option to block axially two locking screws at the driving end of the nail by introducing a compression screw and an end cap (Fig. 4.1.8). This can prevent an early loosening or a screw back out respectively and additionally lead to more stability of the osteosyntheses. Whether

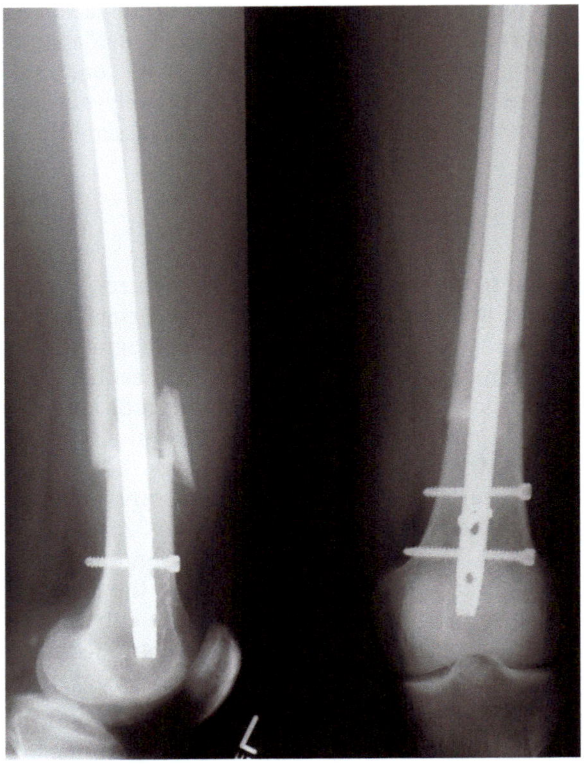

Fig. 4.1.7. Short distal fragments should be stabilized with perpendicular locking screws (mediolateral plus anteroposterior)

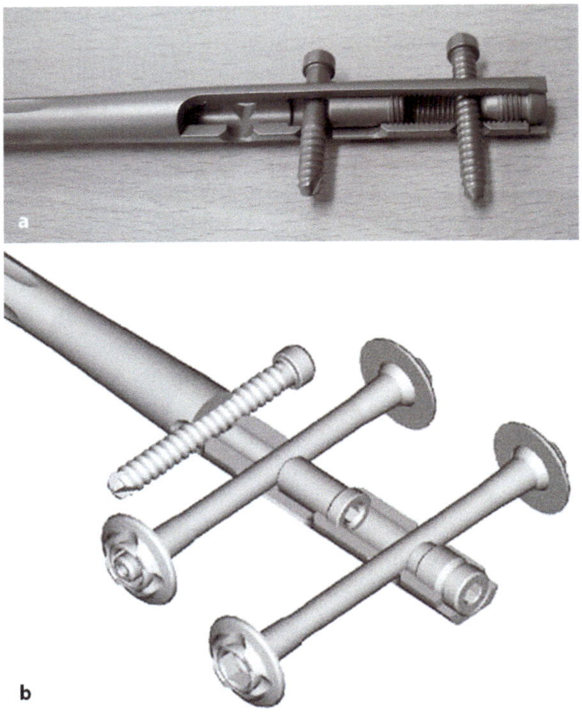

Fig. 4.1.8 a, b. Blocking of two locking screws with the short compression screw and the end cap prevents early loosening and offers higher stability of the osteosyntheses

or not a particular fracture can be compressed will depend upon the cortical contact between the two main fragments [41]. This contact may be reduced if small fragments have split off, as in a butterfly fracture, or if inadequate reduction has been obtained. As a rule of thumb, the main fragments should have good cortical contact over at least half the circumference of the shaft [11, 41]. Compression at the fracture site should always be monitored on the image intensifier. If during compression, incipient telescoping of the fragments is observed, compression must be stopped and static locking mode is adopted. In our experience, equally good compression may be obtained regardless of whether nailing is performed using the anterograde or retrograde technique [11, 41].

If apposition is used for long spiral fractures, it must be done very carefully, since the fragments may slide and rotate, causing bone shortening as well as twisting of the screw in the oblong hole. In these special cases additional static locking should be used (advanced locking mode) [41, 43].

In segmental fracture patterns involving several levels, the locking mode should be chosen to suit the component with the poorest axial stability. In clinical terms, this will virtually always mean static locking of the bone fragments. In a very small number of cases, detailed analysis may show that an intermediate diaphyseal fragment can be picked up with a guide wire and reduced with compression. The more complex patterns will not infrequently be found to be suitable for secondary compression, which may be used after the healing of the metaphyseal component, to speed up the union of the shaft fracture.

Since no controlled comparative studies have been carried out to date, it is impossible to tell whether compression nailing is clinically superior to the established unreamed or limited reamed intramedullary nailing techniques that offer static or dynamic locking but do not provide compression. Also, simple femoral fractures should heal without complications following correct nailing by any of the techniques available. However, a more detailed analysis will show certain trauma patterns that could benefit from intramedullary nailing with active compression.

Due to the increased use of unreamed intramedullary nailing, there has, over the last few years, been a growth in the number of fractures failing to heal because of fragment dehiscence caused by the advancement of the nail [20, 28]. Under these conditions, static locking, without dynamization, may result in nonunion. To prevent this primary dehiscence, it has been suggested that the limb should be axially compressed, either by direct soft-tissue manipulation or by driving the nail back after distal locking [35]. The compression mechanism of the intramedullary nail permits more subtly controlled fragment apposition, which can be set, under image intensification, to within 1 mm. This means that nearly anatomical reduction is achieved even with a closed technique of intramedullary nailing. Obviously, a similar mechanism will be at work in fractures with dynamic locking, as weight-bearing on the affected limb is being increased. However, weight-bearing will not be possible for some patients (in severe trauma cases, same limb injury that cannot be loaded). In such cases, compression will ensure sound apposition of the fracture fragments, even in the unloaded state.

Nonunions

Nonunions can be either hypertrophic or atrophic. Hypertrophic nonunions can be successfully treated by altering the biomechanical environment of the fracture. For femur shaft nonunions, reamed intramedullary nailing is well established. Reaming of the nonunion site should be used to remove the fibrous tissue at the fracture site, which stimulates new bone formation even in cases of poor blood supply. This is due to the flow change between endosteal and periosteal blood supply on the one hand and to the pressing of reamed bone debris in the nonunion area, on the other hand [4].

Except for atrophic or infected nonunions with bone loss, failure of long-bone shaft fractures to unite is the indication par excellence for compression nailing. Hypertrophic nonunions are particularly likely to benefit from the essential features of compression nailing: opening of the medullary canal and freshening of the bone surfaces; fixation with strong compression and sound stability to promote undisturbed bone healing (Fig. 4.1.9) [3, 4, 22, 23].

In such cases, we perform moderate reaming of the medullary canal, of 1–1.5 mm after entering the medullary canal with cortical contact. The chosen nail diameter will be 1 mm less than that of the last reamer used. Compression is applied using 3 Nm torque. Femoral nonunions managed with this technique are inherently suitable for mobilization with full weight-bearing; once the swelling has gone down a few days after surgery, patients tend to cooperate with the early postopera-

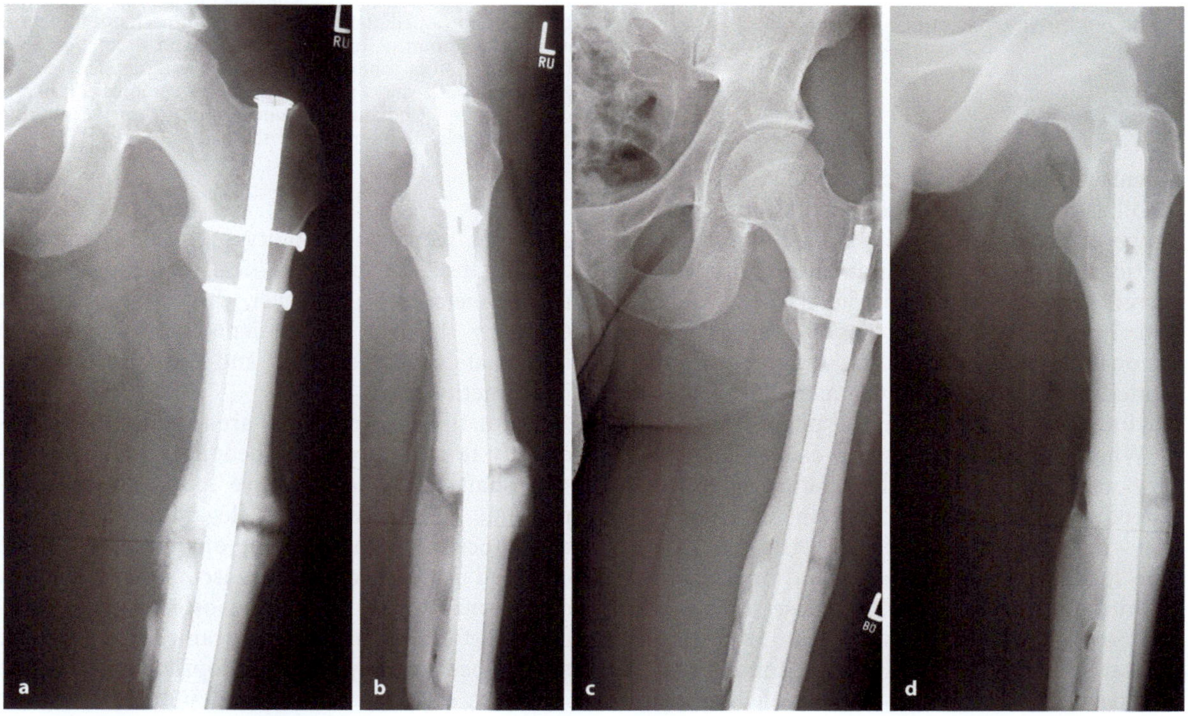

Fig. 4.1.9. a, b Hypertrophic nonunion after intramedullary nailing. **c, d** Reaming and compression nailing offer high stability and promote bone healing

tive weight-bearing regime [11, 23]. In cases of atrophic and infected nonunions, there are some additional points that need to be taken into account. Atrophic nonunions do not generally unite without additional open bone grafting, although reaming debris may act as an internal bone graft. The basic principles in the treatment of infected nonunions are the establishment of adequate bone stability and the eradication of the infection. This is achieved with repetitive surgical debridements and with antibiotic administration. In the initial management of an infected nonunion, external fixation is probably the method of choice for stabilization. After eradication of the infection, conversion to an internal osteosynthesis can be performed, from our point of view preferably compression nailing, and will fasten up the bone healing.

In an earlier study, patients with tibial and femoral nonunions were included and analyzed, over a period of 3.5 years: a total of 112 patients with 56 femoral and 56 tibial nonunions, ranging in age from 18 to 82 years, were referred from other hospitals [20]. In more than one-third of the patients, pretreatment consisted of intramedullary nailing. In 91.1% the nonunions healed using the above outlined concept in time without any further intervention being necessary. Four secondary recompressions and four exchange nailings had to be performed, as well as two septic revisions. Active compression was performed in 86.6% of the patients.

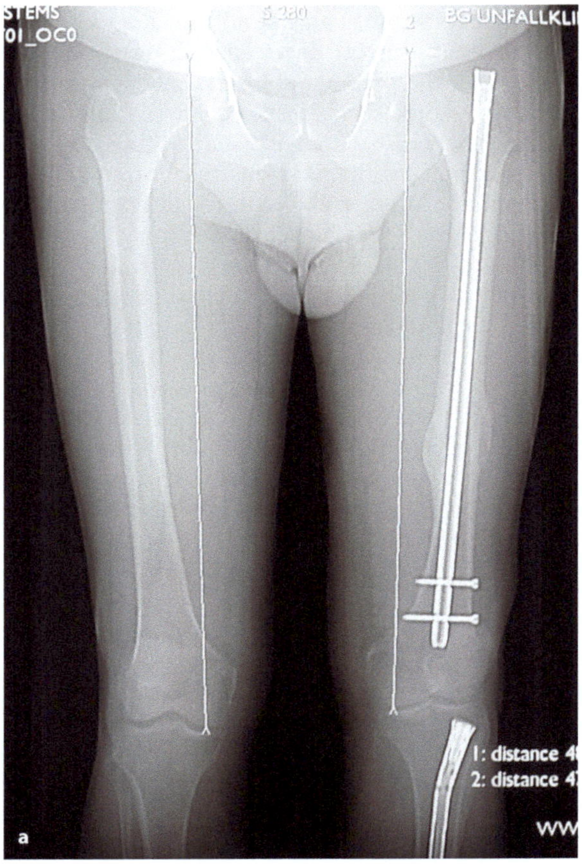

Fig. 4.1.10. a, b A 62-year-old patient with external malrotation of 38° after intramedullary nailing of a femur shaft fracture 2 years before. **c** The osteotomy was performed using an intramedullary saw at the biomechanically most appropriate point. After nail insertion and derotation with the nail in situ, compression locking was applied. **d** The postoperative X-ray confirmed the good compression of the osteotomy. **e, f** Undisturbed bone healing confirmed by the X-ray controls after removal of the nail

Osteotomies

Kuentscher used his intramedullary nail for the stabilization of osteotomies carried out for a wide range of indications, such as axial alignment corrections, derotation and limb shortening. His preferred tool was the intramedullary saw, which optimally preserves the soft-tissue envelope. The rotational stability provided by the jamming of his slotted unlocked nail in the medullary canal was obviously adequate for clinical purposes.

Where contemporary small-caliber intramedullary nails are used for the fixation of transverse osteotomies, dynamic locking in an oblong hole may not produce sufficient rotational stability. The locking bolts have a certain amount of play within their holes, which will cause some instability. Some nail patterns have been found to have almost 20° of play [11]. Hence it follows that if a derotational transverse osteotomy of the diaphysis is to be performed with an small-caliber nail, compression must be used, in order to achieve sufficient rotational stability [12, 19]. Diaphyseal osteotomies take longer to heal than those nearer to the metaphysis; however, this disadvantage is offset by the fact that patients may weight-bear immediately after surgery, and thus are not limited functionally.

Derotational osteotomies are required fairly frequently in the era of intramedullary nailing of femur shaft fractures. We have found closed compression nailing to be an elegant technique for this procedure. The amount of derotation to be obtained is marked with transcutaneous K-wires or external fixator pins. The osteotomy is carefully performed, using an intramedullary saw at the biomechanically most appropriate point in the midshaft, away from the healed site of the former fracture. The K-wires are aligned with the nail in situ, and compression locking is applied (Fig.

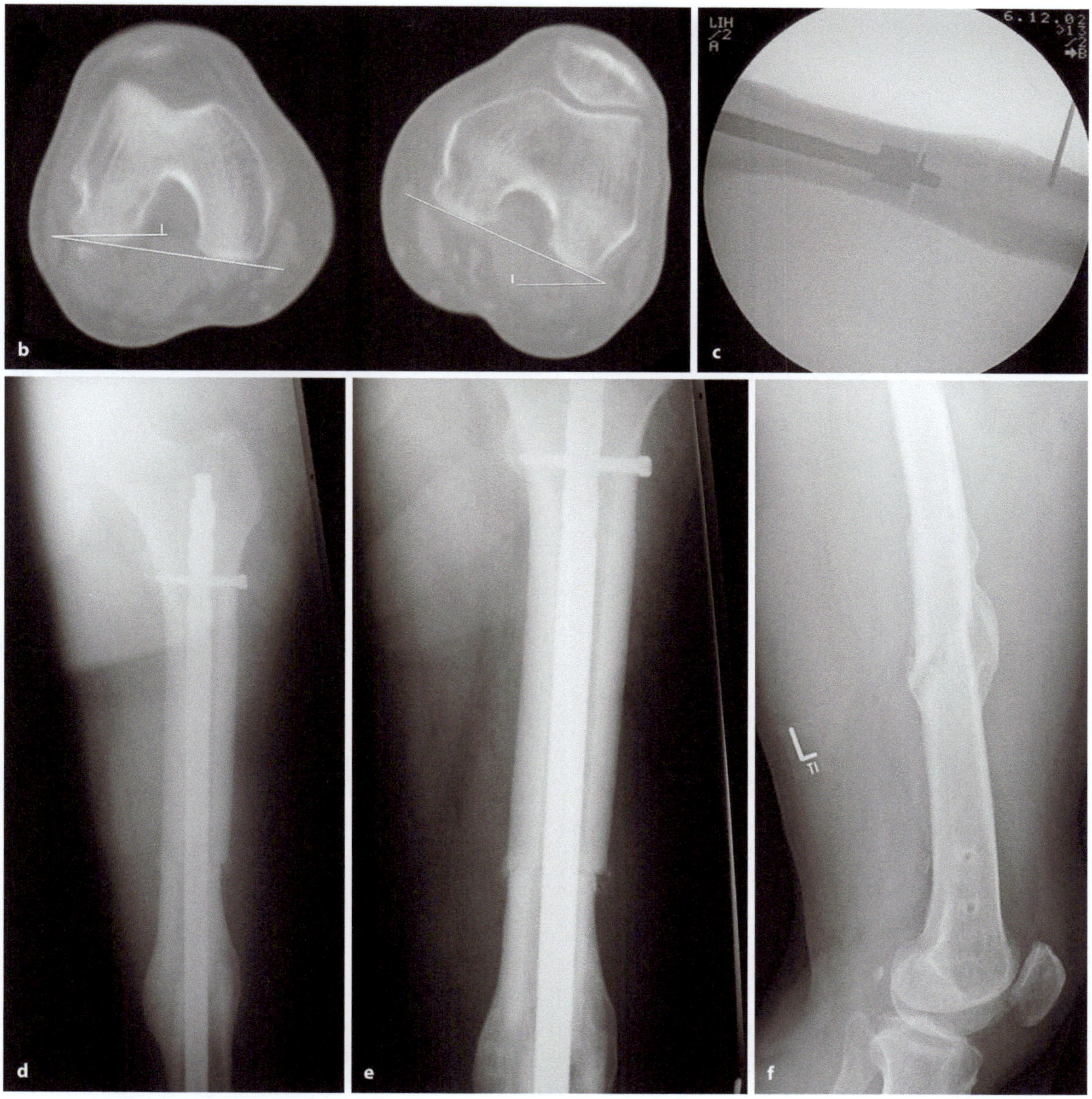

Fig. 4.1.10.

4.1.10). Over a 3-year period, we corrected 41 deformities, of which 19 were rotational deformities of the femur [20]. Patient satisfaction was above average, not least because of the possibility of early weight-bearing and the healing, in normal time, of all the osteotomies in the series. There was only one septic complication in a patient with a femoral valgus correction.

Axial malalignment that is mainly in the diaphysis may also be corrected with intramedullary nailing. After wedge resection or mobilization of a nonunion site, thanks to the stiffness of the implant, the device will hold the osteotomized bone in correct alignment. Additional bone graft may be required. Deformities close to the metaphysis will need to be analyzed very carefully, and are often not suitable for fixation with an intramedullary nail.

Limb lengthening after shaft fractures that have healed with bone shortening may be done in one session, using the nail, providing that the amount of lengthening required does not exceed 2 cm. In such cases, we perform an open transverse osteotomy. A retractor is inserted to create the desired lengthening at the osteotomy site. The space then will be filled with bicortical iliac crest grafts. After moderate apposition is applied the nail will be locked statically, to prevent secondary displacement and crushing of the grafts (Fig. 4.1.11).

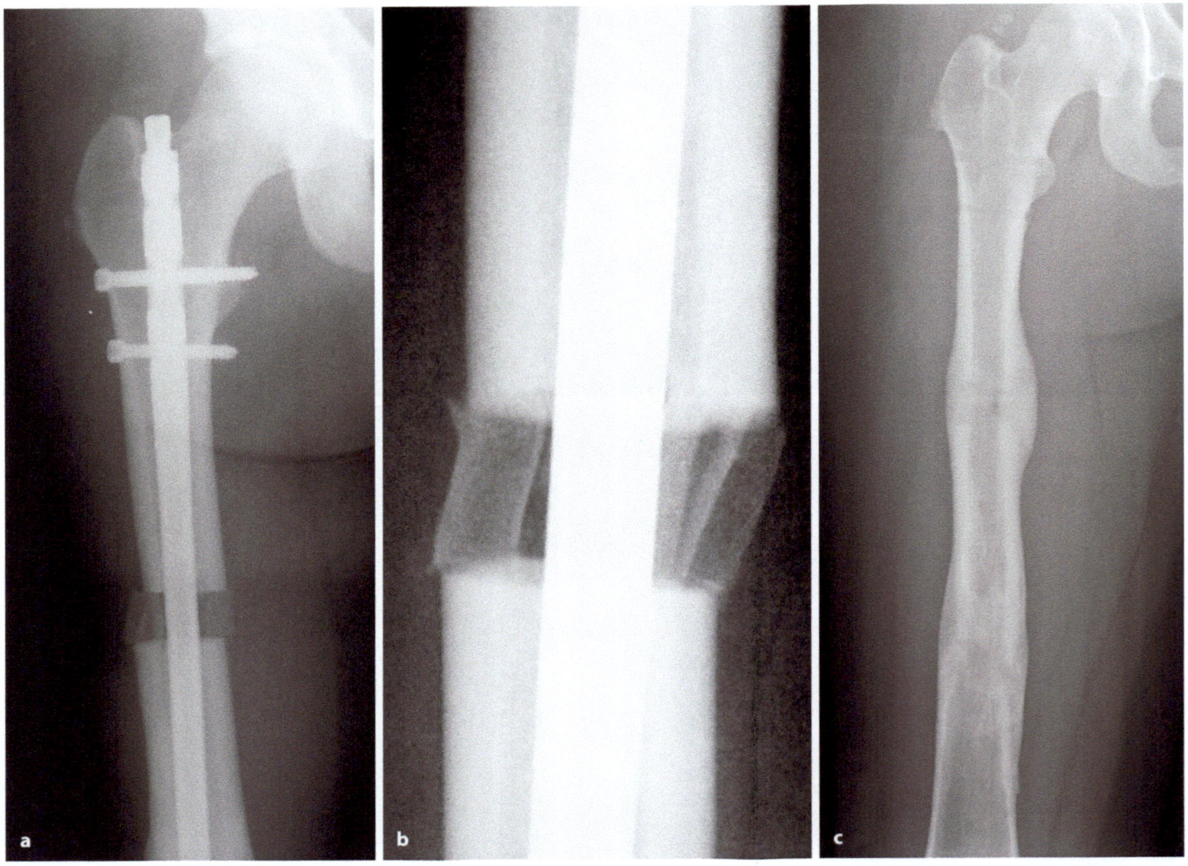

Fig. 4.1.11. a A 28-year-old female with shortening of the right leg after nailing of a comminuted femur shaft fracture. After transverse osteotomy with the intramedullary saw and insertion of a femur nail, lengthening of about 2 cm with interposition of bicortical bone graft was performed. b Moderate compression and supplementary static locking were applied. c Bone healing and removal of the implant after 1.5 years

Conclusion

Intramedullary nailing has been in worldwide use for more than 60 years. However, its innovative potential appears to be far from exhausted [11].

Compression nails must meet certain design requirements, which were listed by Ritter in the early 1990s [49]. The holes for locking screws should not be in the metaphyseal region, which will not support much load bearing, but in the diaphyseal part of the long bone. This requirement conflicts with the present-day trend to have holes arranged extremely at the nail ends, in order to extend the use of the nails to the management of more proximally and distally located fractures. With the T2 nailing system, a compromise could be found using different locking modes, blocking techniques and additional end caps. These nails are suitable for conventional antegrade and for retrograde intramedullary nailing of long bones, as well as for metaphyseal fractures and hold up for controlling the fragments apposition through the integrated compression mechanism.

With the foreseeable growth in long bone fractures and nonunions in elderly people, more use should be made of compression nailing, which offers the benefits of controlled fragment apposition and sound primary stability.

References

1. Anglen JO, Blue JM (1995) A comparison of reamed and unreamed nailing of the tibia. J Trauma 39:351–355
2. Angliss RD, Tran TA, Edwards ER, Doig SG (1996) Unreamed nailing of tibial shaft fractures in multiply injured patients. Injury 27:255–260
3. Baas N, Gonschorek O, Beickert R, Bühren V (1999) Entwicklung eines neuen Marknagels mit internem Kompressionsmechanismus zur Behandlung von Oberarmpseudarthrosen. Hefte Unfallchirurg 275:35
4. Beickert R, Smieja S (2001) Kompressionsmarknagelung bei Pseudarthrosen. Trauma Berufskrankh 3:195–202
5. Blachut PA, O'Brien PJ, Meek RN, Broekhuyse HM (1993) Interlocking intramedullary nailing with and without reaming for the treatment of closed fractures

of the tibial shaft: a prospective, randomized study. J Bone Joint Surg [Am] 75:1583–1584
6. Blum J, Machemer H, Högner M, Baumgart F, Schlegel U, Wahl D, Rommens PM (2000) Biomechanik der Verriegelungsmarknagelung bei Oberarmschaftfrakturen. Unfallchirurg 103:183–190
7. Blum J, Rommens PM (2001) Komprimierte Marknagelung bei Oberarmschaftfrakturen. Trauma Berufskrankh 3:188–194
8. Böstmann O, Vainionpää S, Saikku K (1984) Infra-isthmal longitudinal fractures of the tibial diaphysis: results of treatment using closed intramedullary compression nailing. J Trauma 24:964–969
9. Braten M, Terjesen T, Rossvoll I (1995) Femoral shaft fractures treated by intramedullary nailing. A follow-up focusing on problems related to the method. Injury 26:379–383
10. Brug E (1977) Modell eines intramedullären Kompressionsosteosynthese-Verfahrens für den Oberarm. Fortschr Med 95(4):239–244
11. Bühren V (2000) Kompressionsmarknagelung langer Röhrenknochen. Unfallchirurg 103:708–720
12. Bühren V, Gonschorek O (1998) Indikation, Lokalisation und Technik von Torsionskorrekturen am Femurschaft. Unfallmedizinische Tagungen der Landesverbände der gewerblichen Berufsgenossenschaften 101: 111–118
13. Bühren V, Potulski M, Marzi I (1993) Konzept und Ergebnisse der pirmär komprimierten Verriegelungsnagelung ohne Kortikalisaufbohrung an Femur und Tibia. Langenbecks Arch Chir 378 [Suppl]:937–939
14. Bühren V, Potulski M, Mittelmeier H, Mittelmeier W (1993) Klinische Erfahrungen mit einem neuen Kompressions-Verriegelungsnagel. Orthop Prax 9:588–590
15. Bühren V, Potulski M, Mittelmeier W, Mittelmeier H (1993) Kompressions-Verriegelungs-Nagel zur Frakturbehandlung an Femur und Tibia. Hefte Unfallchirurg 230:799–802
16. Court-Brown CM, Keating JF, Christie J, McQueen MM (1994) Exchange intramedullary nailing: its use in aseptic tibial nonunion. J Bone Joint Surg [Br] 77:407–411
17. Court-Brown CM, Will E, Christie J, McQueen MM (1996) Reamed or unreamed nailing for closed tibial fractures. J Bone Joint Surg [Br] 78:580–583
18. Derweduwen J (1979) A new intramedullary compression device for fractures and pseudarthroses of the long bones. Acta Orthop Belg 45:6–12
19. Gonschorek O, Beickert R, Hofmann GO, Bühren V (1998) Minimalinvasive Technik zur Derotationsosteotomie des Femurs unter Verwendung von Innenraumsäge und Verriegelungs-Kompressionsmarknagelung. Osteosynthese Intern 6 [Suppl 1]:11
20. Gonschorek O, Hofmann GO, Bühren V (1998) Interlocking compression nailing: a report on 402 applications. Arch Orthop Trauma Surg 117:403–437
21. Gonschorek O, Hofmann GO, Bühren V (2001) Kompressionsmarknagelung; Biomechanik und Implantate. Trauma Berufskrankh 3:174–179
22. Gonschorek O, Hofmann GO, Hofmeister M, Bühren V (1997) Der Einsatz der Kompressionsmarknagelung zur Behandlung von Pseudarthrosen an Femur und Tibia. Hefte Unfallchirurg 242:500–502
23. Gonschorek O, Hofmann GO, Hofmeister M, Bühren V (1999) Treatment of femoral pseudarthrosis by using a reamed IM nail with active compression (Interlocking Compression Nail). Osteosynthese Intern 7 [Suppl 1]: 27–30
24. Gonschorek O, Hofmann GO, Kirschner MH, Bühren V (1999) Hochstabile Versorgung von Unterschenkelfrakturen durch Kompressionsmarknagelung. Osteosynthese Intern 7 [Suppl 2]:92–94
25. Gonschorek O, Hofmann GO, Wagner FD, Bühren V (1999) Reamed interlocking compression nailing for the treatment of tibial pseudarthrosis. Osteosynthese Intern 7 [Suppl 1]:142–145
26. Gregory P, Sanders R (1995) The treatment of closed, unstable tibial shaft fractures with unreamed interlocking nails. Clin Orthop 315:48–55
27. Heim D, Regazzoni P, Tsakiris DA, Aebi T, Schlegel U, Marbet GA, Perren SM (1995) Intramedullary nailing and pulmonary embolism: does unreamed nailing prevent embolization? An in vivo study in rabbits. J Trauma 38:899–906
28. Hofmann GO, Gonschorek O, Bühren V (2000) Deficient fracture dynamization employing unreamed nails in tibial fractures. Osteosynthese Intern 8:109–112
29. Huckstep RL (1986) The Huckstep intramedullary compression nail. Indications, technique und results. Clin Orthop 212:48–61
30. Hutson JJ, Zych GA, Cole JD, Johnson KD, Ostermann P, Milne EL, Latta L (1995) Mechanical failures of intramedullary tibial nails applied without reaming. Clin Orthop 315:129–137
31. Hutter CG, Oden R, Kirk R (1977) The intramedullary compression rod. Clin Orthop 122:165–173
32. Kaessmann HJ (1966) Stabile Osteosynthese durch den Kompressionsnagel. Chirurg 37:272–276
33. Kaessmann HJ (1969) Der Kompressionsnagel, eine Modifikation des Marknagels nach Küntscher. Bruns Beitr z Klin Chir 217:315–320
34. Kempf I, Grosse A, Beck G (1985) Closed locked intramedullary nailing: its application to comminuted fractures of the femur. J Bone Joint Surg [Am] 67:709–720
35. Krettek C, Schandelmaier P, Tscherne H (1995) Nonreamed interlocking nailing of closed tibial fractures with severe soft tissue injury. Clin Orthop 315:34–47
36. Kummer FJ, Hickey DG, Maurer SG, Baitner AC, Jazwari LM, Jamal J, Koval KJ (1999) The self-compressing tibial intramedullary nail. Bull Hosp Jt Dis 58(4):181–183
37. Küntscher GBG (1958) The Küntscher method of intramedullary fixation. J Bone Joint Surg [Am] 40:17–26
38. Mittelmeier H, Trennheuser M, Mittelmeier W (1989) Biomechanische Untersuchungen über die interfragmentären Kompressionskräfte mit einem neuen kombinierten Kompressions-Verriegelungsnagel. Hefte Unfallheilkunde 207:305
39. Mittelmeier H, Trennheuser M, Mittelmeier W (1990) Vergleichende biomechanische Messungen der Torsionsstabilität von intramedullären Nagel-Osteosynthesen. Hefte Unfallheilkunde 212:468–471
40. Mückley T, Baas N, Goebel M, Beickert R, Bühren V (2002) Die Kompressionsmarknagelung der Oberarmschaftpseudarthrose. Hefte Unfallchirurg 284:195–196
41. Mückley T, Gonschorek O, Bühren V (2003) Compression nailing of long bones. Eur J Trauma 29:113–128
42. Mückley T, Hofmann GO, Bühren V (2002) Fehlstellungen und Verkürzungen nach Oberschenkelschaftfrakturen. Trauma Berufskrankh 4:242–248
43. Mückley T, Hofmann GO, Bühren V (2002) Weiterentwickelter Kompressions-Verriegelungs-Nagel zur kontrollierten Fragmentapposition. Biomaterialien 3:38–41
44. Olerud S (1970) Intramedullary nailing after reaming. Acta Orthop Scand 134 [Suppl]:1–78
45. Pape HC, Regel G, Dwenger A, Krumm K, Schweitzer G, Krettek C, Sturm JA, Tscherne H (1993) Influences of different methods of intramedullary femoral nailing on lung function in patients with multiple trauma. J Trauma 35:709–716
46. Pratt DJ, Papagiannopoulos G, Rees PH, Quinnell R (1987) The effects of medullary reaming on the torsional strength of the femur. Injury 18:177–179
47. Richardson T, Voor M, Seligson D (1998) Fracture site compression and motion with three types of intramedullary fixation of the femur. Osteosynthese Intern 6:261–264

48. Ritter G (1989) Biomechanische Voraussetzungen für die Kompressionsosteosynthese mit dem neuen AO-Universal-Marknagel. Hefte Unfallheilkunde 207:304
49. Ritter G (1991) Kompressionsosteosynthesen mit dem neuen AO-Universalnagel. Funktionsprinzip und biomechanische Voraussetzungen. Unfallchirurg 94:9–12
50. Schemitsch EH, Kowalski MJ, Swiontkowski MF, Harrington RM (1995) Comparison of the effect of reamed and unreamed locked intramedullary on blood flow in the callus and strength of union following fracture of the sheep tibia. J Orthop Res 13:382–389
51. Schemitsch EH, Kowalski MJ, Swiontkowski MF, Senft D (1994) Cortical bone blood flow in reamed and unreamed locked intramedullary nailing: a fractured tibia model in sheep. J Orthop Trauma 8:373–382
52. Tencer AF, Johnson KD, Johnston DW, Gill K (1984) A biomechanical comparison of various methods of stabilization of subtrochanteric fractures of the femur. J Orthop Res 2:297–305
53. Whittle AP, Wester W, Russell TA (1995) Fatigue failure in small diameter nails. Clin Orthop 315:119–128
54. Wolf JW Jr., White AA, 3rd, Panjabi MM, Southwick WO (1981) Comparison of cyclic loading versus constant compression in the treatment of long-bone fractures in rabbits. J Bone Joint Surg [Am] 63:805–810
55. Wozasek GE, Simon P, Redl H, Schlag G (1994) Intramedullary pressure changes and fat intravasation during intramedullary nailing: an experimental study in sheep. J Trauma 36:202–207

Advances in Tibial Nailing

J.R. Hsu, K.F. Dickson

Closed intramedullary nailing has become the "gold standard" in the treatment of displaced fractures of the tibial shaft [1, 3, 11, 12, 24, 26, 58, 59]. Intramedullary nailing has led to faster healing times and better fracture alignment than nonoperative management [6]. Indications for the use of intramedullary nails have expanded in recent years to include treatment of metaphyseal fractures of the tibia, both proximally and at the extreme distal end [36]. Since very little "nail" effect occurs in the metaphyseal region due to diameter mismatch between the nail and the bone, surgical techniques and surgical implants have been revised to deal with these more troublesome fractures. Newer surgical implants allow for compression of appropriate fractures, which has certain advantages. In addition, some controversy still exists over reaming and nail size.

Reaming and Nail Size

Open and closed tibia fractures seem to benefit from reaming. Faster healing times and fewer hardware failures have been demonstrated in several studies [13, 29, 45, 64]. However, concern should remain when reaming open fractures beyond Gustillo and Anderson grade II, as these high-grade open fractures have higher rates of deep infection after reaming [9, 35]. In rabbit studies, Melcher et al. [46, 47] demonstrated a statistically significant increase in infection rate with bacteria-inoculated tibias when reaming was used.

In addition to allowing the placement of a larger nail, reaming has some biological benefits as well. Both Frolke [16] and Hoegel [25] have demonstrated that viable bone cells can be cultured from intramedullary reamings. Both of the authors also showed that these cells retained the capability for biological activity.

Current trends with reamed nailing involve limited reaming or "ream to fit" techniques. This technique seems to balance the benefits and detriments of reaming. Limited reaming is associated with lower cortical temperatures [18–20, 34] and a higher percentage of viable bone cells in the reamings [37]. Hupel et al. [27, 28] have shown a smaller negative impact on tibia cortical blood flow in limited reaming versus standard ($p=0.009$) as well as lower cortical porosity for the limited reaming in a series of canine tibia studies. The cortical bone density in the limited reaming group was better than both the standard reamed and unreamed groups. This limited reaming technique has shown improved clinical results in open fractures versus unreamed nailing in a recent study by Ziran et al. [64]. No difference in infection was noted between limited reamed nailing and unreamed nailing. Unreamed nailing resulted in a significantly higher number of secondary procedures to achieve bony union.

Muller et al. [48–52] have done multiple experiments to show that reamer design also has a significant impact on intramedullary pressure and temperature. Narrow driving shafts, small reamer heads, and sharp, deep, end-cutting and side-cutting reamers perform best. Currently, irrigation-suction reamer designs are in their early phases. These reaming systems show some promise with regard to improved biology of reaming as well as decreasing intramedullary pressures and fat intravasation [30, 31].

Attention to the detrimental effects of traditional reaming has led surgeons to use smaller-diameter nails either placed without reaming or with limited reaming. Unfortunately, these more biologically friendly small-diameter nails have shown a much higher rate of fatigue failure of the implant, with need for subsequent surgery. Most of the implant failures involved interlocking screw breakage in several series [13, 22, 29, 63]. Thus, small-diameter nails with larger (5.0 mm) interlocking bolts should perform better [17]. A 20% increase in interlocking bolt diameter has been shown to increase fatigue strength by 25–70% [17].

The effect of reaming in the severely injured with lung trauma is still controversial [5, 7, 54,

55]. In patients with poor perfusion and oxygenation from a severe pulmonary injury, an unreamed nail should be considered.

Titanium Versus Stainless Steel

Biocompatibility of titanium alloy implants has been well studied in the laboratory setting [38, 57]. Kraft et al. [38] recently published data from a hamster study comparing the microvascular response to stainless-steel versus titanium bulk implants and debris. Both the stainless-steel bulk implant and the wear debris created a massive inflammatory response with increased endothelial permeability and leakage of activated leukocytes. Extensive edema resulted, creating a compromise of the microcirculation. Titanium bulk and debris only created a transient increase in inflammatory response without macrovascular leakage.

Clinically, there is some evidence of improved performance of titanium alloy nails compared to their stainless-steel predecessors. Titanium tibial intramedullary nails showed a statistically significant lower incidence of implant failure versus stainless steel in a series by Riemer et al. [56]. In 67 fractures there was a 2% versus 25% failure rate for titanium versus stainless-steel nails respectively ($p<0.01$). In a biomechanical study, Gabler et al. showed increased fatigue strength of interlocking bolts made from titanium alloy versus stainless steel ($p<0.001$) [17].

Finally, diaphyseal and metaphyseal fractures around the knee are often associated with intra-articular knee pathology. Magnetic resonance imaging of knees with adjacent titanium intramedullary nails shows less interference than with stainless-steel implants [10]. In an inoculation study of rabbits, titanium seemed to have less infection than stainless steel [2]. In general, titanium seems to have better biocompatibility, modulus of elasticity (closer to bone), fatigue strength, and yield strength. Furthermore, with the availability of cannulated titanium bar stock, the cost difference between titanium and stainless steel should be minimum.

Compression Nailing

An evolution in intramedullary nailing of both the tibia and femur involves the use of compression or apposition mechanisms within the intramedullary device. The concept of compression nailing is not new, but seems to be gaining in popularity due to the benefits of improved stability despite the increasingly popular use of limited reaming and smaller-diameter nails. In addition, compression nailing has a use in nonunion and malunion surgery using intramedullary techniques.

The compression or apposition mechanism can improve the reduction in a fracture that becomes distracted during nail insertion (Fig. 4.2.1). Fracture gap in the tibia has been implicated in the predictable development of a nonunion (relative risk 8.33, 95% CI 3.03–25.0) in a review of 200 tibia fractures treated at two level-one trauma centers [4]. In these fractures the apposition mechanism will decrease the gap between the fracture fragments. Compression of the bony surfaces improves fracture site stability providing a better mechanical environment for fracture healing as well as possibly decreasing patient discomfort and allowing early weight-bearing [21].

Compression nailing is possible for axially stable fracture patterns such as transverse and short oblique fractures. Compressing fractures with limited cortical contact can result in angula-

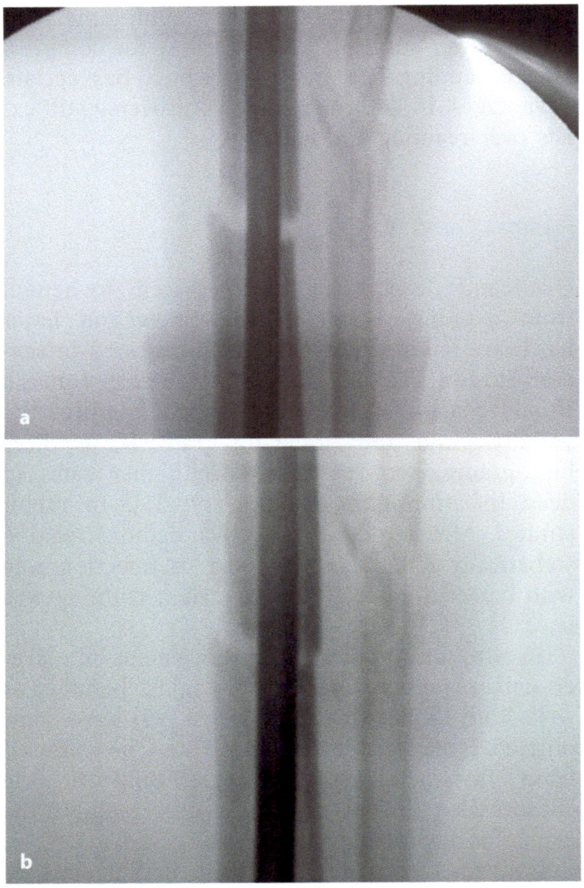

Fig. 4.2.1. a Fracture gap prior to compression. b Fracture gap after compression

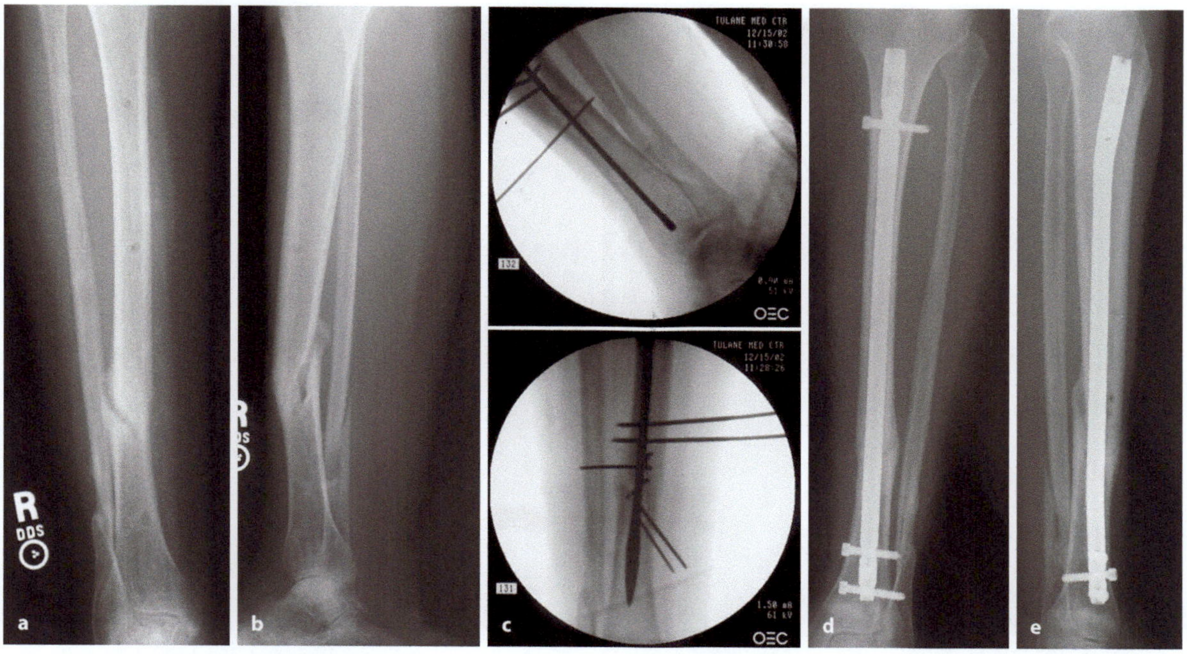

Fig. 4.2.2. a Anteroposterior view of a nonunion of the tibia initially treated with external fixation. b Lateral view of the nonunion of the tibia. c Blocking wires used to guide the guide wire and subsequently the reamers into a good position. d Anteroposterior view after the compression nail with union within 2 months. e Lateral view with the compression nail after healing

tion while compressing comminuted fractures will create unacceptable shortening. Compression nailing is more suited for treatment of diaphyseal fractures. Attempted compression of metaphyseal fractures may result in telescoping with resultant shortening.

In the treatment of axially stable nonunions and malunions, the compression mechanism can create good apposition and stability of the nonunion or osteotomy site (Fig. 4.2.2) [23]. This can be accomplished through "minimally invasive" techniques with surgical access remote from the desired healing bed [21]. In this case blocking wires were used to ensure proper reaming and nailing.

Metaphyseal Fractures

Treatment of proximal one-third and distal one-third tibia fractures with an intramedullary device is an attractive option. It offers the potential for minimally invasive surgery with skin incisions remote from the fracture site. Unfortunately, nailing of metaphyseal fractures has proven to be difficult. It has led to unacceptably high percentages of malalignment due to mismatch between the diameter of the bone and the diameter of the nail [15, 44]. This mismatch prevents intimate contact between the nail and the endosteal surface. Thus the nail does not aid in reduction of the fracture. In fact, the geometry of some nails may contribute to a malreduction.

Proximal one-third tibia fractures have an alarmingly high rate of malalignment [15, 44]. The malalignment is usually valgus and apex anterior angulation. Posterior translation of the tibial diaphysis relative to the proximal fragment can also occur. This displacement is exacerbated in older nail designs with a more distal Herzog bend by creating a wedge effect on the fracture (Fig. 4.2.3). Nail designs employing a more proximal bend like the Herzog bend (10° at 50 mm) result in a shorter overall offset from the anterior-most aspect of the top of the nail to the apex of the bend (Fig. 4.2.4). Such a design may help in reducing the resultant displacement of the fracture site with insertion of the nail.

Freedman and Johnson [15] found a 58% malalignment rate with proximal one-third fractures compared to only 7% of middle one-third and 8% of distal one-third fractures. Lang et al. reported on a series of 32 proximal one-third extra-articular tibia fractures treated with an intramedullary nail. Eighty-four per cent had a 5° or greater magnitude of angulation; 59% had greater than 1 cm of displacement. These authors called into question the further use of intramedullary nails for these fractures [44].

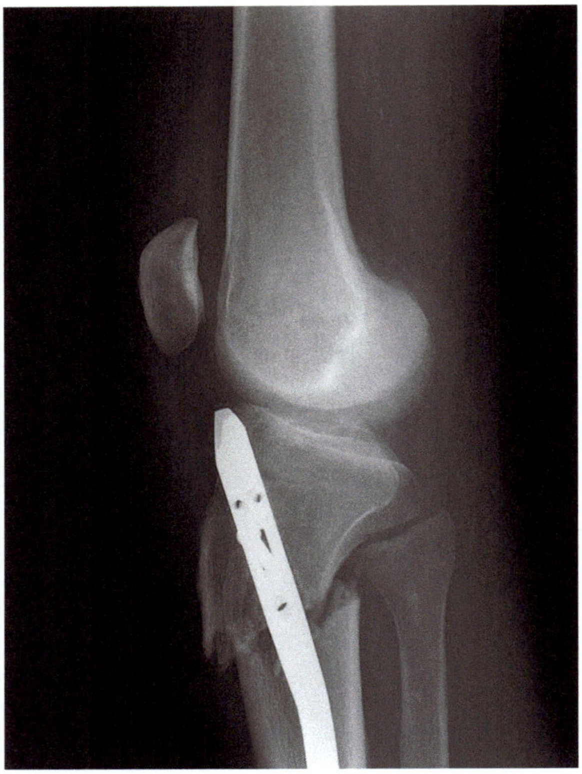

Fig. 4.2.3. Proximal tibia nailed with a nail with a distal bend causing a classic apex anterior deformity

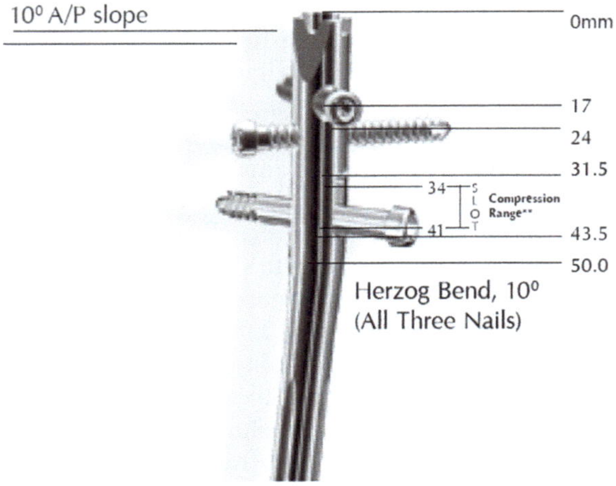

Fig. 4.2.4. Standard T2 tibia nail with oblique screws, a compression slot and a proximal bend

Adaptive techniques to avoid malalignment include the use of an external fixator, a medial unicortical plate, a more proximal and lateral entry point, blocking screws (poller screws) [39–42] and placing proximal interlocking bolts with knee extended [8, 61, 62]. This extended position for proximal interlocking helps to eliminate the negative influence of the extensor mechanism on fracture angulation. Only a few nailing systems have standard proximal targeting guides that allow proximal interlocking with the knee in extension without significant impingement of the patella and patellar tendon. Some tibial nail systems have a dedicated proximal tibial nail as well as a dedicated distal tibial nail (Fig. 4.2.5).

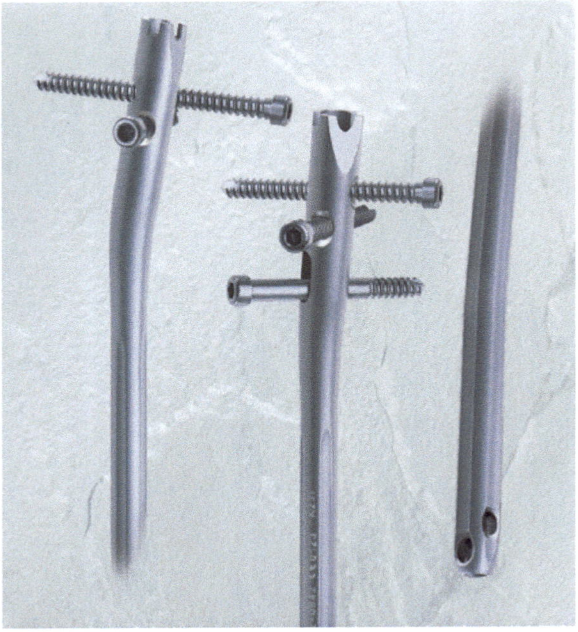

Fig. 4.2.5. Proximal, standard, and distal tibial T2 nails

Newer nail designs with oblique proximal interlocking screws demonstrate improved biomechanical stability over nails with parallel proximal interlocking screws for these proximal one-third tibia fractures [43].

Distal one-third tibia fractures can create similar problems with angulation due to the same type of diameter mismatch [53]. An additional problem with very distal fractures is related to nail designs with multiple different holes. Several nail designs have three or more holes necessitating leaving a hole in the nail open near the fracture site with the nail fixed above and below. A stress riser exists at this empty hole near the fracture site, which may be slow to heal. This is the likely location for a nail fracture [14].

A nail specifically designed for this fracture pattern, with only two very distal holes, avoids this problem. A nail specifically designed for treating extreme distal tibia fracture is ideal for dealing with the difficult problem of a tibial shaft fracture with extension into the tibial plafond (Fig. 4.2.6). This is a truly "minimally invasive" technique with remote surgical access and percutaneous screw placement in the fracture zone (Fig. 4.2.6).

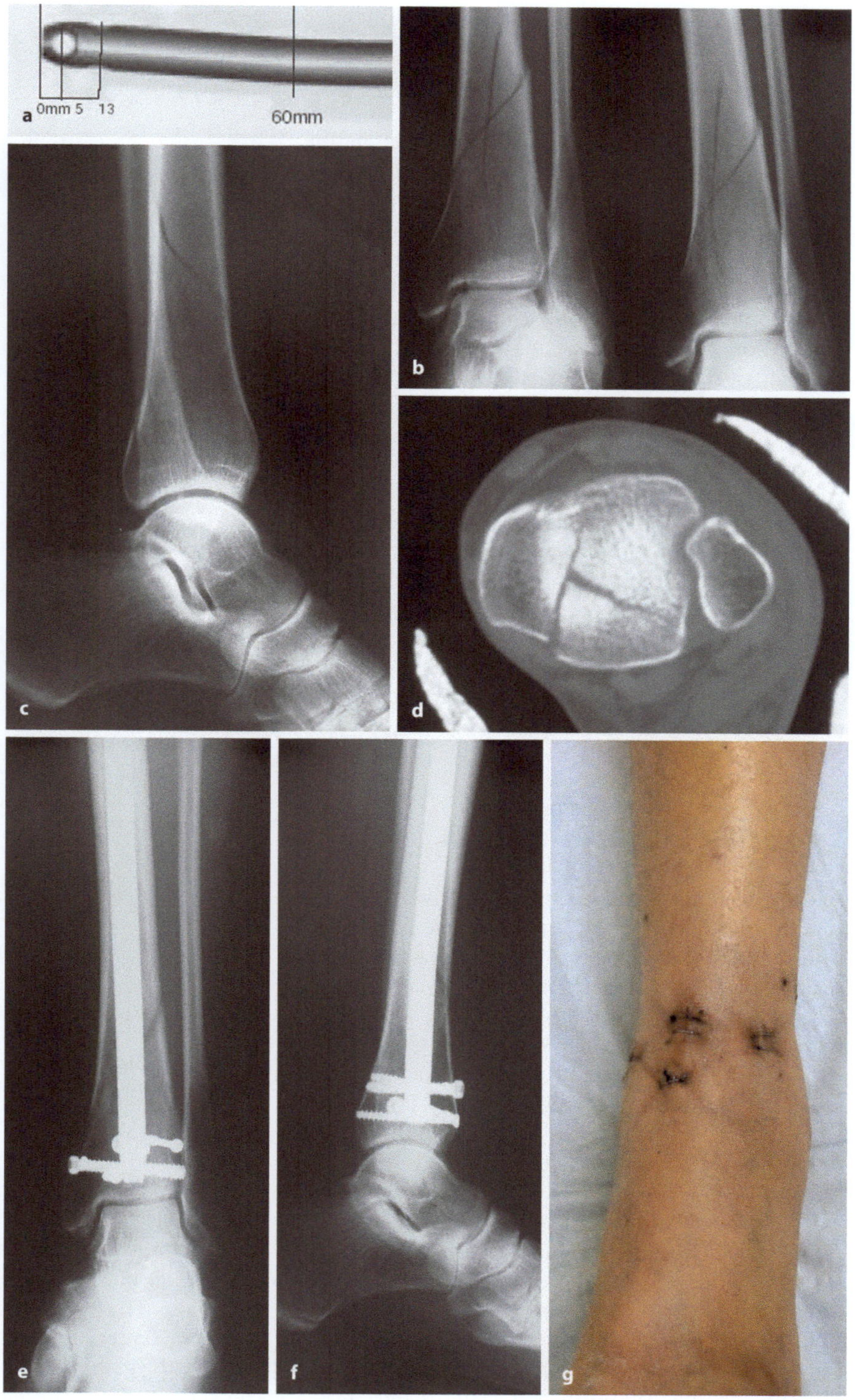

Fig. 4.2.6. a Distal T2 tibial nail with only two holes distally at 90° to each other. b Mortise and anteroposterior view of a distal tibia fracture with extension into the joint. c Lateral view of distal tibia fracture with extension into the joint. d Computed tomography of distal tibial plafond showing joint displacement. e Postoperative mortise view after closed reduction of joint with clamp and lag-screw fixation and a distal tibial nail. f Lateral postoperative view. g Skin incisions used on distal tibial plafond fracture

Fracture-Specific Implants

In order to encompass the wide variety of expanding indications for intramedullary nails in the tibia, a surgeon must have multiple nailing systems available, a modular nail, or a nailing system containing several types of fracture-specific nails. There seem to be clear advantages to the last option, since multiple nailing systems create an inventory and cost issue for the hospital.

Although modular nails seem to be an attractive option, their track record in the past is quite inconclusive [32, 33]. Jones et al. [33] reported on 27 patients with modular stainless-steel nails for diaphyseal femur fractures or nonunions. Retrieved specimens demonstrated fretting corrosion and stainless-steel corrosion at the junctions with a granulomatous reaction in the tissue surrounding the junctions. Twenty-three of 27 patients demonstrated osteolysis, periosteal reaction, and/or cortical thickening at one or both junctions. Eighteen of these patients showed severe bony reactions. When compared to a control group of patients with a one-piece nail, a significant level of thigh pain was demonstrated ($p = 0.03$).

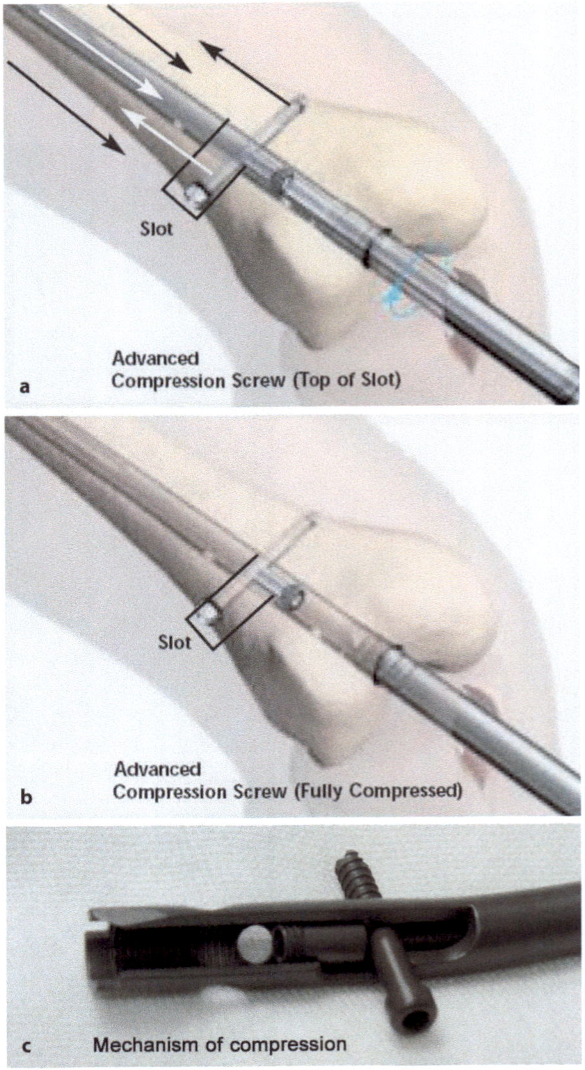

Fig. 4.2.7. a Distal femur prior to compression. b Distal femur after compression. c Cut away of proximal tibial nail showing compression screw

A New Titanium Nail for the Tibia

In response to the aforementioned advances in intramedullary nailing of the tibia, the Stryker T2 tibial nailing system has been developed. The reamer system (Bixcut) is an end-cutting and side-cutting reamer. It has a narrow, short head with deep flutes and a narrow driving shaft.

The nail itself has 5.0-mm interlocking bolts even for the 9-mm diameter nails. This allows smaller, more biologically friendly nailing while retaining the benefit of the larger interlocking bolts.

The nail is constructed of type II anodized titanium alloy (Ti6AL4V). This has improved fatigue strength and decreased wear rate compared to nonanodized or type III anodized titanium alloy. The surface has been treated to prevent bony ingrowth of the titanium that has made extraction difficult in other titanium nail systems [60].

The T2 tibial nailing system is truly a system of nails. It consists of three different nails (Fig. 4.2.5). There is a standard nail to accommodate the majority of fractures. There are also two fracture-specific nails in the system (proximal and distal).

The T2 tibial nail (standard and distal) has a self-contained compression mechanism available. The nail is first fixed into the distal fragment with interlocking bolts. A partially threaded interlocking bolt is placed through the compression slot in the nail. The compression screw is introduced into the center of the nail from the top. As it is tightened against the partially threaded screw in the slot, it draws the nail up through the proximal fragment pulling the distal fragment as it goes (Figure 4.2.7). This creates a tremendous compressive force at the fracture site. Stability can be improved to such an extent that early weight-bearing and improved comfort is possible even with smaller-diameter nails.

The proximal nail is specifically designed to treat those very difficult proximal one-third tibia

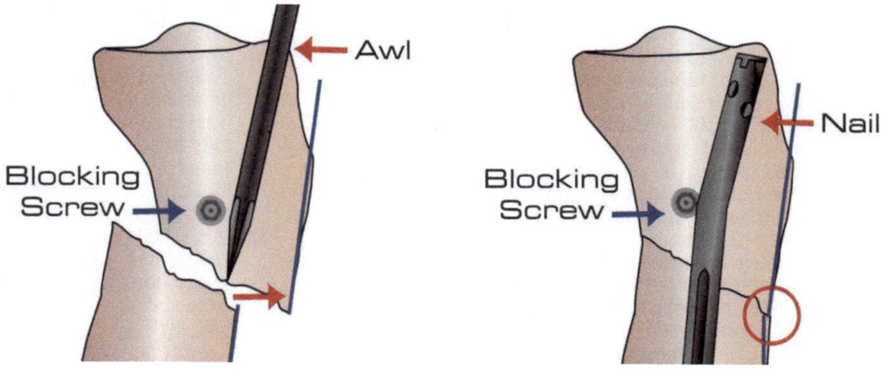

Fig. 4.2.8. Use of blocking screw to guide path of awl and nail to maintain reduction

fractures. For fractures of the proximal quarter of the tibia, the proximal tibial nail offers the benefits of the proximal Herzog bend (10° at 50 mm). Since no nailing effect is expected for a proximal fracture, the proximal interlocking bolts are designed to cross in a static mode to improve the stability of the short metaphyseal fragment over parallel screws. This nail does not include the compression slot to avoid having a large stress riser at the proximal fracture site. Blocking or poller screws are often used to help maintain reduction (Fig. 4.2.8).

At the other end of the tibia, very distal fractures can be treated with the third nail in the system. The distal nail has two very distal, static interlocking bolts. The centers of the holes are 5 mm and 13 mm from the tip of the nail (Fig. 4.2.6 a). The bolts are oriented at 90° to each other to improve stability. Unlike the standard nail, there is no third more proximal hole in the nail. This third hole in other nails often creates a weak point in the nail near the fracture site. Since distal tibia fractures are slow to heal, having a solid tube in this area should decrease the chances of nail fracture.

Summary

A better understanding of the biological consequences and benefits of reamed tibial nailing is leading to incremental changes in our operative technique as well as the design of the intramedullary implants and their reamers. Improved material and implant design may ultimately contribute to a decrease in the number of clinical failures. Furthermore, the addition of compression seems to benefit certain fractures as well as nonunions and malunions undergoing osteotomy. Although closed nailing of tibia fractures is nothing new, the expanding indications for tibial nailing have created problems of their own, specifically with regard to nailing metaphyseal fractures. The solutions to these problems include both refinements of technique as well as improvements in technology.

References

1. Alho A, Benterud JG, Hogevold HE, Ekeland A, Stromsoe K. Comparison of functional bracing and locked intramedullary nailing in the treatment of displaced tibial shaft fractures. Clin Orthop (277): 243–250, 1992.
2. Ahrens S, Schlegel U, Printzen G, Ziegler WJ, Perren SM, Hansis M. Influence of materials for fixation implants on local infection: an experimental study of steel versus titanium DCP in rabbits. J Bone Joint Surg Br 78(4): 647–651, 1996.
3. Bhandari M, Adili A, Leone J, Lachowski RJ, Kwok DC. Early versus delayed operative management of closed tibial fractures. Clin Orthop (368): 230–239, 1999.
4. Bhandari M, Tornetta P, 3rd, Sprague S, Najibi S, Petrisor B, Griffith L, Guyatt GH. Predictors of reoperation following operative management of fractures of the tibial shaft. J Orthop Trauma 17(5): 353–361, 2003.
5. Bone LB, Johnson KD, Weigelt J, et al. Early versus delayed stabilization of femoral fractures: a prospective randomized study. J Bone Joint Surg Am 71: 336–340, 1989.
6. Bone LB, Sucato D, Stegemann PM, Rohrbacher BJ. Displaced isolated fractures of the tibial shaft treated with either a cast or intramedullary nailing. An outcome analysis of matched pairs of patients. J Bone Joint Surg Am 79(9): 1336–1341, 1997.
7. Bosse MJ, MacKenzie EJ, Riemer BL, et al. Adult respiratory distress syndrome, pneumonia, and mortality following thoracic injury and a femoral fracture treated either with intramedullary nailing with reaming or with a plate: a comparative study. J Bone Joint Surg Am 79: 799–809, 1997.
8. Buehler KC, Green J, Woll TS, Duwelius PJ. A technique for intramedullary nailing of proximal third tibia fractures. J Orthop Trauma 11(3): 218–223, 1997.
9. Court-Brown CM, Keating JF, McQueen MM. Infection after intramedullary nailing of the tibia. Incidence and protocol for management. J Bone Joint Surg Br 74(5): 770–774, 1992.
10. Dickson KF, Galland MW, Barrack RL, Neitzschman HR, Harris MB, Myers L, Vrahas MS. Magnetic resonance imaging of the knee after ipsilateral femur fracture. J Orthop Trauma 16(8): 567–571, 2002.
11. Dickson KF, Hoffman WJ, Delgado ED, Contreras DM. Unreamed rod with early wound closure for Grade IIIA

and IIIB open tibial fractures: analysis of 40 consecutive patients. Orthopaedics 21: 531–535, 1998.
12. Dickson KF, Katzman S, Delgado E, Contreras D. Delayed unions and nonunions in open tibia fractures. Clinic Orthop 302: 189–193, 1994.
13. Finkemeier CG, Schmidt AH, Kyle RF, Templeman DC, Varecka TF. A prospective, randomized study of intramedullary nails inserted with and without reaming for the treatment of open and closed fractures of the tibial shaft. J Orthop Trauma 14(3): 187–193, 2000.
14. Franklin JL, Winquist RA, Benirschke SK, Hansen ST, Jr. Broken intramedullary nails. J Bone Joint Surg Am 70(10): 1463–1471, 1988.
15. Freedman EL, Johnson EE. Radiographic analysis of tibial fracture malalignment following intramedullary nailing. Clin Orthop (315): 25–33, 1995.
16. Frolke JP, Nulend JK, Semeins CM, Bakker FC, Patka P, Haarman HJ. Viable osteoblastic potential of cortical reamings from intramedullary nailing. J Orthop Res 22(6): 1271–1275, 2004.
17. Gaebler C, Stanzl-Tschegg S, Heinze G, Holper B, Milne T, Berger G, Vecsei V. Fatigue strength of locking screws and prototypes used in small-diameter tibial nails: a biomechanical study. J Trauma 47(2): 379–384, 1999.
18. Garcia OG, Mombiela FL, De La Fuente CJ, Aranguez MG, Escribano DV, Martin JV. The influence of the size and condition of the reamers on bone temperature during intramedullary reaming. J Bone Joint Surg Am 86-A(5): 994–999, 2004.
19. Giannoudis PV, Snowden S, Matthews SJ, Smye SW, Smith RM. Friction burns within the tibia during reaming. Are they affected by the use of a tourniquet? J Bone Joint Surg Br 84(4): 492–496, 2002.
20. Giannoudis PV, Snowden S, Matthews SJ, Smye SW, Smith RM. Temperature rise during reamed tibial nailing. Clin Orthop (395): 255–261, 2002.
21. Gonschorek O, Hofmann GO, Bühren V. Interlocking compression nailing: a report on 402 applications. Arch Orthop Trauma Surg 117(8): 430–437, 1998.
22. Greitbauer M, Heinz T, Gaebler C, Stoik W, Vecsei V. Unreamed nailing of tibial fractures with the solid tibial nail. Clin Orthop (350): 105–114, 1998.
23. Gupta A. Dynamic compression nail: a preliminary report. BMC Musculoskelet Disord 2(1): 6, 2001.
24. Henley MB, Chapman JR, Agel J, Harvey EJ, Whorton AM, Swiontkowski MF. Treatment of type II, IIIA, and IIIB open fractures of the tibial shaft: a prospective comparison of unreamed interlocking intramedullary nails and half-pin external fixators. J Orthop Trauma 12(1): 1–7, 1998.
25. Hoegel F, Mueller CA, Peter R, Pfister U, Suedkamp NP. Bone debris: dead matter or vital osteoblasts. J Trauma 56(2): 363–367, 2004.
26. Hooper GJ, Keddell RG, Penny ID. Conservative management or closed nailing for tibial shaft fractures. A randomised prospective trial. J Bone Joint Surg Br 73(1): 83–85, 1991.
27. Hupel TM, Aksenov SA, Schemitsch EH. Effect of limited and standard reaming on cortical bone blood flow and early strength of union following segmental fracture. J Orthop Trauma 12(6): 400–406, 1998.
28. Hupel TM, Weinberg JA, Aksenov SA, Schemitsch EH. Effect of unreamed, limited reamed, and standard reamed intramedullary nailing on cortical bone porosity and new bone formation. J Orthop Trauma 15(1): 18–27, 2001.
29. Hutson JJ, Zych GA, Cole JD, Johnson KD, Ostermann P, Milne EL, Latta L. Mechanical failures of intramedullary tibial nails applied without reaming. Clin Orthop (315): 129–137, 1995.
30. Joist A, Schult M, Frerichmann U, Frebel T, Spiegel HU, Koppe M, Joosten U. [A new irrigation-suction boring system facilitates low-pressure intramedullary boring of isolated swine femurs]. Unfallchirurg 106(10): 874–880, 2003.
31. Joist A, Schult M, Ortmann C, Frerichmann U, Frebel T, Spiegel HU, Kropfl A, Redl H. Rinsing-suction reamer attenuates intramedullary pressure increase and fat intravasation in a sheep model. J Trauma 57(1): 146–151, 2004.
32. Jones DM, Marsh JL. Osteolysis of the femur at the junction of a modular intramedullary nail. A case report. Iowa Orthop J 18: 136–141, 1998.
33. Jones DM, Marsh JL, Nepola JV, Jacobs JJ, Skipor AK, Urban RM, Gilbert JL, Buckwalter JA. Focal osteolysis at the junctions of a modular stainless-steel femoral intramedullary nail. J Bone Joint Surg Am 83-A(4): 537–548, 2001.
34. Karunakar MA, Frankenburg EP, Le TT, Hall J. The thermal effects of intramedullary reaming. J Orthop Trauma 18(10): 674–679, 2004.
35. Keating JF, O'Brien PJ, Blachut PA, Meek RN, Broekhuyse HM. Locking intramedullary nailing with and without reaming for open fractures of the tibial shaft. A prospective, randomized study. J Bone Joint Surg Am 79(3): 334–341, 1997.
36. Konrath G, Moed BR, Watson JT, Kaneshiro S, Karges DE, Cramer KE. Intramedullary nailing of unstable diaphyseal fractures of the tibia with distal intraarticular involvement. J Orthop Trauma 11(3): 200–205, 1997.
37. Kouzelis AT, Kourea H, Megas P, Panagiotopoulos E, Marangos M, Lambiris E. Does graded reaming affect the composition of reaming products in intramedullary nailing of long bones? Orthopedics 27(8): 852–856, 2004.
38. Kraft CN, Diedrich O, Burian B, Schmitt O, Wimmer MA. Microvascular response of striated muscle to metal debris. A comparative in vivo study with titanium and stainless steel. J Bone Joint Surg Br 85(1): 133–141, 2003.
39. Krettek C, Miclau T, Schandelmaier P, Stephan C, Mohlmann U, Tscherne H. The mechanical effect of blocking screws ("poller screws") in stabilizing tibia fractures with short proximal or distal fragments after insertion of small-diameter intramedullary nails. J Orthop Trauma 13: 550–553, 1999.
40. Krettek C, Schandelmaier P, Rudolf J, Tscherne H. Aktueller Stand der operativen Technik für die unaufgebohrte Nagelung von Tibiaschaftfrakturen mit dem UTN. Unfallchirurg 97: 575–599, 1994.
41. Krettek C, Schandelmaier P, Tscherne H. Non-reamed interlocking nailing of closed tibial fractures with severe soft tissue injury: indications, technique and clinical results. Clin Orthop 315: 34–47, 1994.
42. Krettek C, Stephan C, Schandelmaier P, Richter M, Pape HC, Miclau T. The use of Poller screws as blocking screws in stabilising tibial fractures treated with small diameter intramedullary nails. J Bone Joint Surg Br 81: 963–968, 1994.
43. Laflamme GY, Heimlich D, Stephen D, Kreder HJ, Whyne CM. Proximal tibial fracture stability with intramedullary nail fixation using oblique interlocking screws. J Orthop Trauma 17(7): 496–502, 2003.
44. Lang GJ, Cohen BE, Bosse MJ, Kellam JF. Proximal third tibial shaft fractures. Should they be nailed? Clin Orthop (315): 64–74, 1995.
45. Larsen LB, Madsen JE, Hoiness PR, Ovre S. Should insertion of intramedullary nails for tibial fractures be with or without reaming? A prospective, randomized study with 3.8 years' follow-up. J Orthop Trauma 18(3): 144–149, 2004.
46. Melcher GA, Hauke C, Metzdorf A, Perren SM, Printzen G, Schlegel U, Ziegler WJ. Infection after intramedullary nailing: an experimental investigation on rabbits. Injury 27 Suppl 3: SC23–26, 1996.
47. Melcher GA, Metzdorf A, Schlegel U, Ziegler WJ, Perren SM, Printzen G. Influence of reaming versus nonream-

ing in intramedullary nailing on local infection rate: experimental investigation in rabbits. J Trauma 39(6): 1123–1128, 1995.
48. Muller C, Frigg R, Pfister U. Effect of flexible drive diameter and reamer design on the increase of pressure in the medullary cavity during reaming. Injury 24 Suppl 3: S40–47, 1993.
49. Muller C, McIff T, Rahn BA, Pfister U, Weller S. Intramedullary pressure, strain on the diaphysis and increase in cortical temperature when reaming the femoral medullary cavity – a comparison of blunt and sharp reamers. Injury 24 Suppl 3: S22–30, 1993.
50. Muller C, Rahn BA, Pfister U, Weller S. Extent of bluntness and damage to reamers from hospitals. Injury 24 Suppl 3: S31–35, 1993.
51. Muller CA, Baumgart F, Wahl D, Perren SM, Pfister U. Technical innovations in medullary reaming: reamer design and intramedullary pressure increase. J Trauma 49(3): 440–445, 2000.
52. Muller CA, Schavan R, Frigg R, Perren SM, Pfister U. Intramedullary pressure increase for different commercial and experimental reaming systems: an experimental investigation. J Orthop Trauma 12(8): 540–546, 1998.
53. Obremskey WT, Medina M. Comparison of intramedullary nailing of distal third tibial shaft fractures: before and after traumatologists. Orthopedics 27(11): 1180–1184, 2004.
54. Pape HC, Auf'm'Kolk M, Paffrath T, et al. Primary intramedullary femur fixation in multiple trauma patients with associated lung contusion: a cause of posttraumatic ARDS? J Trauma 34: 540–548, 1993.
55. Pape HC, Regel G, Dwenger A, et al. Influences of different methods of intramedullary femoral nailing on lung function in patients with multiple trauma. J Trauma 34: 540–548, 1993.
56. Riemer BL, DiChristina DG, Cooper A, Sagiv S, Butterfield SL, Burke CJ, 3rd, Lucke JF, Schlosser JD. Nonreamed nailing of tibial diaphyseal fractures in blunt polytrauma patients. J Orthop Trauma 9(1): 66–75, 1995.
57. Ryhanen J, Kallioinen M, Serlo W, Peramaki P, Junila J, Sandvik P, Niemela E, Tuukkanen J. Bone healing and mineralization, implant corrosion, and trace metals after nickel-titanium shape memory metal intramedullary fixation. J Biomed Mater Res 47(4): 472–480, 1999.
58. Schandelmaier P, Krettek C, Rudolf J, Kohl A, Katz BE, Tscherne H. Superior results of tibial rodding versus external fixation in grade 3B fractures. Clin Orthop (342): 164–172, 1997.
59. Schmidt AH, Finkemeier CG, Tornetta P, 3rd. Treatment of closed tibial fractures. Instr Course Lect 52: 607–622, 2003.
60. Takakuwa M, Funakoshi M, Ishizaki K, Aona T, Hamaguchi H. Fracture of removal of the ace tibial nail. J Bone Joint Surg Br 79(3): 444–445, 1997.
61. Tornetta P, 3rd. Technical considerations in the surgical management of tibial fractures. Instr Course Lect 46: 271–280, 1997.
62. Tornetta P, 3rd, Collins E. Semiextended position of intramedullary nailing of the proximal tibia. Clin Orthop (328): 185–189, 1996.
63. Uhlin B, Hammer R. Attempted unreamed nailing in tibial fractures: a prospective consecutive series of 55 patients. Acta Orthop Scand 69(3): 301–305, 1998.
64. Ziran BH, Darowish M, Klatt BA, Agudelo JF, Smith WR. Intramedullary nailing in open tibia fractures: a comparison of two techniques. Int Orthop 28(4): 235–238, 2004.

The Development of Retrograde Nailing for Distal Femur Fractures

D. Seligson

Introduction

Osteosynthesis of the distal femur has always been problematic. At the turn of the last century, Albin Lambotte of Antwerp fabricated and used a custom implant on the lateral side of the distal femur. The Lambotte plate was broad, had multiple holes for the distal condylar block, and used a row of unicortical screws for the femur shaft [13, 14]. Following the Second World War, mass-produced implants for fracture treatment became available and were increasingly accepted for use for specific fractures. The bent or angled plate for the proximal femur was turned around and applied in the supracondylar area. This technique of angled plate fixation, initially introduced in New York [26], was adapted by the Association for the Study of Internal Fixation, and became a regular part of the education for fracture surgeons [19, 20]. The method was one of the more arcane techniques of the "Swiss school" and not all were convinced either that the operation was straightforward or that it reliably produced good results [23, 24].

At the same time that open methods of fracture care using plates and screws were promoted by the Swiss, medullary nailing came into general use thanks to the work of the Seattle group of Clawson, Smith, Hanson, and Winquist. The American orthopedists researched the work of Gerhard Küntscher, purchased implants and an image intensifier, and systematically proved that closed medullary nailing was a safe and effective method of fracture care. Winquist and Hanson were effective teachers and developed a strong following in the USA. With the advent of interlocking introduced and developed by Klemm and Schellmann in Germany [11], and Grosse and Kempf in France, the indications for intramedullary stabilization of fractures was extended to more comminuted fracture patterns, and, pertinent to supracondylar nailing, to fractures ever more distal in the femur. Ted Hanson, in particular, used to say that the indications for nailing extended from the lesser trochanter to the adductor tubercle of the femur.

Interestingly, Anoch Lewert had performed medullary nailing of supracondylar fractures as early as 1956 [15]. Modny and Bambara [17] had developed an I-beam nail to be inserted in a fracture site. This nail had multiple perforations and could be locked in place with screws placed at different angles. Both Küntscher in Germany and Harris in the USA passed nails from the distal femoral condyles retrograde for the fixation of trochanteric fractures. The Rush group of Meridian Mississippi routinely recommended retrograde flexible pins for the treatment of femur shaft fractures [21], as did Ender of Vienna. Later Brunner and Weber published a case of nailing of a femur shaft from the knee [1]. Prof. Ronald Huckstep of New South Wales, Australia developed a titanium alloy nail for antegrade insertion with multiple holes for interlocking. Huckstep's nail could also be inserted through a fracture site, moved into position and then interlocked. Huckstep's nailing was used for supracondylar fractures. However, traumatologists involved in the development of fracture treatment methods in the last part of the twentieth century observed the advantages of intramedullary stabilization, particularly when the technique was used for closed fracture fixation. In the last decade there has been continuous improvement in the armamentarium for fracture treatment as well as inexorable increases in implant costs and patient expectations.

Development of the Idea

On September 28–30, 1986, Dr. David Seligson and Dr. Stuart Green attended an external fixation symposium – Recent Advances in External Fixation – at Riva del Garda, Italy. The weather was beautiful, and neither having a talk to give, they decided to take a hike up one of the hills alongside the lake. The talk turned to methods for the care of supracondylar fractures and the general difficulty of getting a good result, particularly in the elderly. They decided to solve the problem. They discussed the regimented approach of the "Swiss group" to fracture fixation, pointing particularly to the Swiss-German concept of a right way to do something, and resolved there and then not only to consider new technical options for this fracture but also to find a method that was more orthopedic so that the performance of the operation would allow decision making. They continued the conversation at dinner. Both had experience with Huckstep's nail and also with Zickel's supracondylar nailing. The Zickel nailing used two flat flexible rods that were inserted from the medial and lateral distal femoral condyles and held in place with large condylar anchoring screws [29]. At dinner, Green and Seligson discussed supracondylar nailing again and Dr. Green sketched out their first concepts. Finally the best solution seemed to be to insert the nail through an entrance point in the trochlea right in the central axis of the distal femur. Nailing from a joint had precedence since Küntscher and Maatz nailed the humerus from the shoulder. Although infection and arthrosis were worrisome possibilities, the advantages of the central entrance point in the distal femur seemed considerable. Furthermore, did not a nail in the distal femur with transfixing screws in reality communicate with the joint through the fracture lines in the distal condylar block?

In the coming months Green and Seligson discussed the new nailing. They initially planned to use Huckstep's titanium nail. Green made models and sent slides of his findings to Seligson (Fig. 4.3.1 a, b). Both encountered difficulties with obtaining the Huckstep nail from the distributor. The locking screws of the Huckstep nail fit the nail with little clearance, so open insertion of the screws was usually necessary. Since both Green and Seligson had worked with Smith & Nephew, they decided to ask if a nail and guide system could be fabricated for supracondylar nailing. A young engineer, David Brumfield, with the encouragement of the trauma group led by Frank Navarra, developed a guide based on the Russell-Taylor nailing system for supracondylar nailing. The nails were standard Russell-Taylor closed-section nails, and the screws were the 6.4-mm locking screws from the femur nail. The instrumentation used the same sleeves and drills as the Russell-Taylor nails (Fig. 4.3.2). In accordance with the anatomic studies done by Dr. Green, the nail was designed with a bend to match the axis of the distal femur in the lateral plane. In general the nail was to be inserted with the apex of the angle anterior, but both Green and Seligson agreed that there should be no "right way" to place the implant. The traumatologist should use judgment in placing the implant in the most suitable position for the reduction of the fracture.

The unique features of the intramedullary supracondylar nail as developed by Green and Seligson with the Smith & Nephew group were as follows:

1. Closed-section nail with multiple holes for interlocking: concepts from Modny, Huckstep and Russell-Taylor
2. Nail-mounted guide: concepts of Küntscher, Klemm and Schellmann, Grosse and Kempf
3. Fully cannulated nails for insertion over a guide wire: Küntscher, Russell-Taylor.

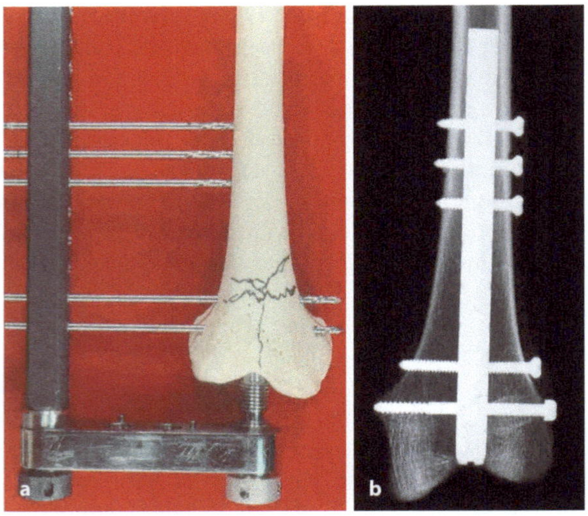

Fig. 4.3.1. a Model of a supracondylar nail prepared by Dr. Stuart A. Green, of Los Alamitos, CA in 1987 using the Huckstep nail. b The X-ray of the model demonstrates the concept of a locked nail placed from the trochlea with screws inserted with a guide

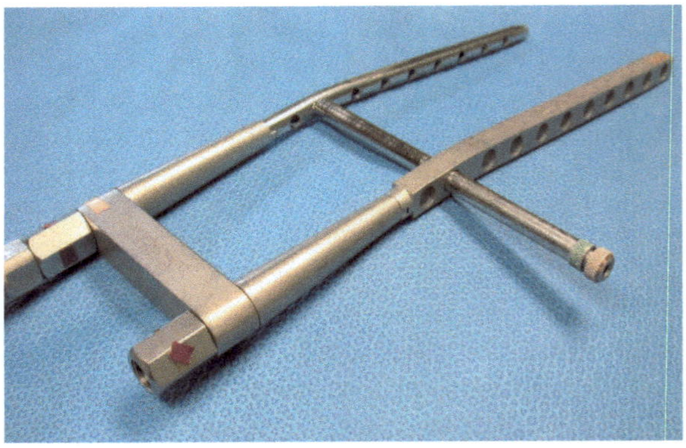

Fig. 4.3.2. The nail and guide as manufactured by Smith & Nephew. Note the first nails had 6.4-mm locking holes along the length of the nail

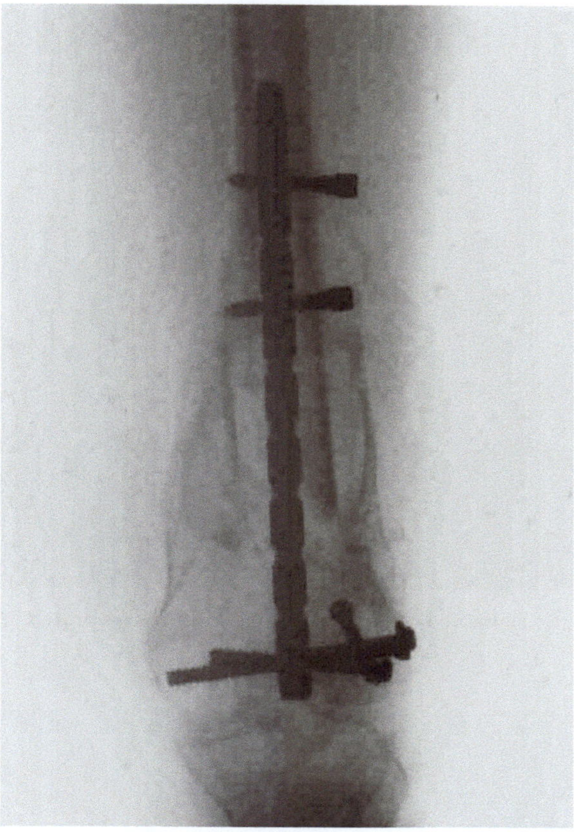

Fig. 4.3.3. An early case of supracondylar nailing. Since the implant is inserted into the medullary canal and the nailing is not rigid, there is abundant callus formation

The new implant was expressly designed for insertion across the knee from a portal in the trochlea. The final prints for the new nail were dated 6 April 1987. Dr. Seligson placed the first of the new nails in Louisville, KY on 29 April 1987. The second and third procedures were done 1 June 1987 and 29 June 1987, also in Louisville (Fig. 4.3.3).

Introduction of the New Implant [25]

The first paper about the new concept was an article by Dr. Green in an issue of Bruce Browner's *Techniques in Orthopedics* on medullary nailing, in 1988 [3].

The nail was shown at Dr. Robert D'Ambrosia's fracture workshop in New Orleans in November 1988. The method of retrograde nailing for supracondylar fractures was then presented at the meeting of the Gerhard Küntscher Society in Vienna on 18 March 1989. Dr. Jörg Böhler of the Böhler Accident Hospital commented that the method was interesting, but he wondered if the authors had "forgotten about gravity."

Drs. Browner and Seligson held a course at the Waldorf in New York on "Problem Fractures and Fracture Problems", 10 November 1989, in which Dr. Steven Henry of Louisville lectured on supracondylar nailing. The nailing was shown in a scientific exhibit at the American Academy of Orthopedic Surgery in New Orleans in February 1990 [4]. By this time Dr. Henry, a young attending in Louisville, began using the nail for younger patients, and the implant came to be known in the USA as the GSH nail (for Green, Seligson, Henry). The nailing was pictured in a 1990 review article on femoral nailing [2]. The method and case results were shown at the 20th Anniversary Symposium on Interlocking Nailing at the BG Unfallklinik Frankfurt am Main, 28–30 September 1990 (Fig. 4.3.4 a–d).

The nails in the original series were 150 or 200 mm in length, 11 mm in diameter with 6.4-mm locking screws. The nails were fabricated in stainless steel and were closed-section tubes with a 2-mm wall thickness. The longitudinal cannulation was gun-drilled and the nail had an 8° bend 38 mm from the driving end. Problems in the early series were few since most of the patients were elderly with low activity demand and the nails were short, which made interlocking relatively easy using the guide. Dr. Henry lectured about the clinical series at the AAOS Anaheim meeting in March 1991 and published a preliminary series [5]. The first combined American case series of 55 cases was presented at the OTA meeting in Seattle in 1991 [6]. Clinical papers also appeared in *Orthopedic Transactions* 1991 [7], *Unfallchirurg* 1993 and *Clinical Orthopedics* 1993 [16].

In Europe, the first case has an interesting story. In 1990, Seligson visited Dr. Dietrich Hempel in Hamburg and brought a nail along in his luggage. Since the implant was marked "sample", Dr. Hempel said "Let's try (sample) it." So the two went to the shop and shooting range of the famous gun maker Hartmann and Weiss, and besides seeing the fabulous underground shooting range and store, had a driver made for the nail. The next day they successfully implanted the "sample" in an elderly patient who healed her fracture uneventfully. Prof. Sáváry of Budapest, who had attended the initial presentations at the Küntscher Society, went on to fabricate and use supracondylar nails in Budapest in 1991 and published several reports [22]. Similarly, the Dutch made a version based on the gamma trochanteric nail [12].

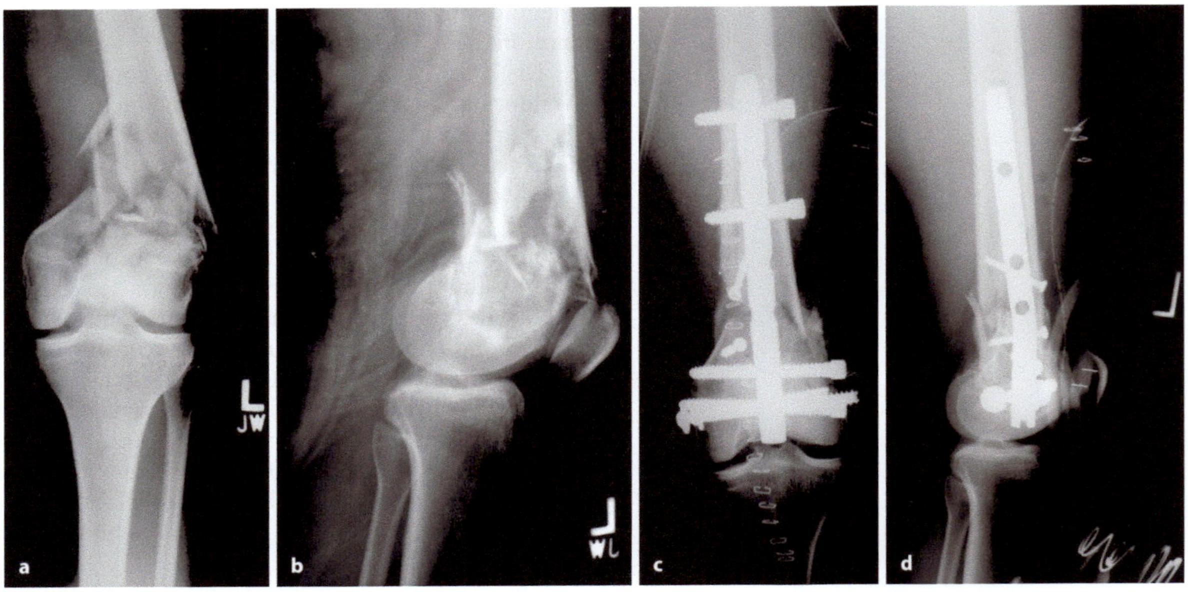

Fig. 4.3.4. a, b Preoperative and c, d postoperative radiographs of a supracondylar nailing done with an open approach. In such cases open bone grafting was usually used

It is difficult to recall the tremendous resistance to the introduction of supracondylar nailing in the early 1990s. "The concept was doomed to failure." The technique was "not approved", "unbiologic". One case report raised the specter of synovial chondromatosis and worse [10]. Subsequent research and clinical experience in many centers answered these criticisms and established the anatomical, mechanical, and clinical basis for the procedure. At grand rounds with the Department of Orthopedics at the University of Vermont after the presentation, Dr. Robert Johnson, a sports medicine doctor with a special interest in the anterior cruciate ligament, finally pronounced that one could "stop worrying, the nail isn't near the cruciates."

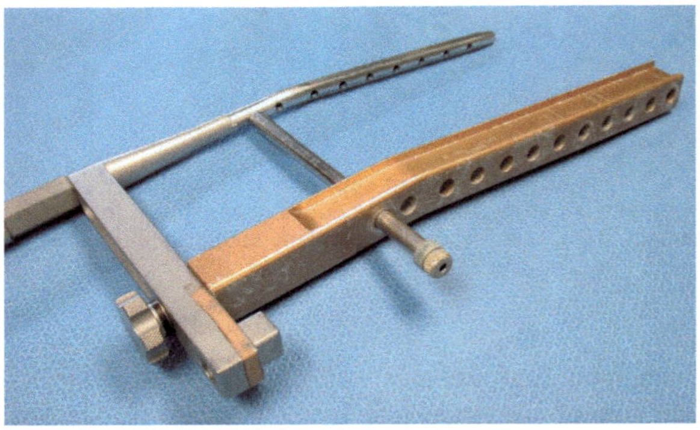

Fig. 4.3.5. Evolution of the nail and guide. In this instrument the position of the guide can be adapted to the width of the thigh. The screw holes are smaller (5 mm) to reduce nail breakage

Development of the Method

In the first series of cases both from Louisville and from Camden, there was a small, but definite incidence of broken nails [9, 16]. As the method of supracondylar nailing became widespread, the manufacturer, Smith & Nephew, first collected information about these cases and then set out to make changes in nail design. This problem emerged as younger patients with higher activity demand and more complex high-energy fractures were treated. As more cases were collected, it was observed that the greatest incidence of nail breakage was at the second hole proximal to the bend (the fourth hole from the driving end). The first solution was to decrease the size of the locking holes in the nail so that they fit 5-mm rather than 6.4-mm screws (Fig. 4.3.5). Although this gave good fixation in the femoral shaft, often the screws in the condyles had little hold. Next the screw holes were cold worked to increase their fatigue resistance.

In 1994, the manufacturer proposed that the nail be manufactured without holes in the middle portion. Working in the Orthopedic Research Laboratory in Louisville, Dr. Michael Voor, the engineer, studied the fatigue properties of nail sections with and without holes and found a marked increase in the endurance limit of the nail when the hole was not present [27]. Several different configurations of "five-hole" nails were pro-

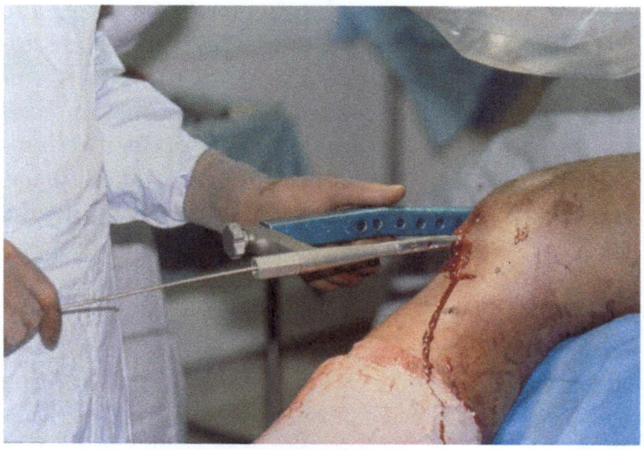

Fig. 4.3.6. With percutaneous nailing as shown here there is no soft tissue dissection and healing is generally rapid

duced – some had three holes proximal and two distal and others two proximal and three distal. The hole spacing, however, was the same for all supracondylar nails, so one guide worked for all of them. At the same time, longer nails were produced – 250, 300, and even 350 as well as a stouter 13-mm nail. In clinical practice nailing became a more frequently used method for the treatment of fractures of the lower femur shaft – not just for fractures in the supracondylar region.

The technique also evolved with increasing emphasis on percutaneous insertion [8]. The first nails had been placed using a medial parapatellar arthrotomy with direct and fluoroscopic visualization of the entrance point. The first patient with a percutaneous nailing was memorable. At the time of this nailing, specimens of fractures with internal fixation were being collected. Mr. F. had fallen and underwent patellectomy. His patella was in a jar in the office. After he fell again and sustained a supracondylar fracture, the nail was placed through a stab wound. The whole operation went quickly and the fracture rapidly healed. Increasingly operative fracture reduction and fixation was achieved through limited incisions (Fig. 4.3.6).

The problem of screw purchase in the condylar block was clinically important, particularly for older patients with osteoporosis [28]. Although Dr. Henri Matheson of Dunkirk, France developed a nail with 6.5-mm holes in the condyles and 5-mm holes in the shaft, the manufacturer thought the use of two screw sizes would be too complicated. To increase screw purchase, screws with a 5-mm thread at the tip and a 6-mm thread under the head (step screws) were tried. The step screws were not satisfactory since the bone in the distal femur really did not give good purchase. Various bolts with washers were also tried. Finally, a locking bolt similar to the one proposed by Küntscher was developed. With the triangular cross-section of the distal femur and the tendency for settling as the patient began to weight-bear, fixation in the distal femur of the elderly still posed a problem, since the bolts could become too prominent under the skin.

Inevitably, as longer and longer nails were introduced, nailing from the knee for diaphyseal fractures, not just retrograde nailing for supracondylar fractures, became an accepted technique in fracture surgery. The supracondylar nail was a straight implant with a bend near the driving end. Fixing the guide to the nail in the supracondylar region, the proximal holes were relatively easy to find with short nail sizes. Using longer, full-length femur nails, and with curved nails the guide no longer worked and locking screws had to be inserted using the free-hand technique under fluoroscopic control. Nails became available with one slotted hole either proximal or distal to allow some settling at the fracture and decrease the problem of subsidence of the implant into the knee.

Supracondylar Nailing Today and Tomorrow

Today the features of the intramedullary supracondylar nail have evolved. The modern nail is manufactured from a solid bar of stainless steel or titanium alloy, which is gun drilled the length of the nail with a cannulation large enough to pass the standard 3-mm ball-tipped reamer guide. The nail is tapered from the driving end to the tip. The larger end in the condyles has holes for interlocking 6.4-mm coarse threaded screws. These screws lie a few degrees out-of-plane to increase their hold in the distal condylar block (Fig. 4.3.7). The screws are placed with locking washers so they have better angular stability and cannot migrate in or out. The holes in the shaft are smaller; 5-mm cortex screws are used for interlocking. The more distal of the two proximal holes is a slot so that with axial loading the nail settles 5 mm when only a single screw is used in the femur shaft. The guide puts the screw proximal in the slot. The tip of the nail is conical so it can easily pass by the flange of a total knee prosthesis (Fig. 4.3.8). There will doubtless be further enhancement of the nail and guide, but the basic concepts remain the same. Results depend greatly on patient selection, performance of the procedure, and postoperative routine. The best use of this implant is still for the treatment of low-energy distal femoral fractures with and without ar-

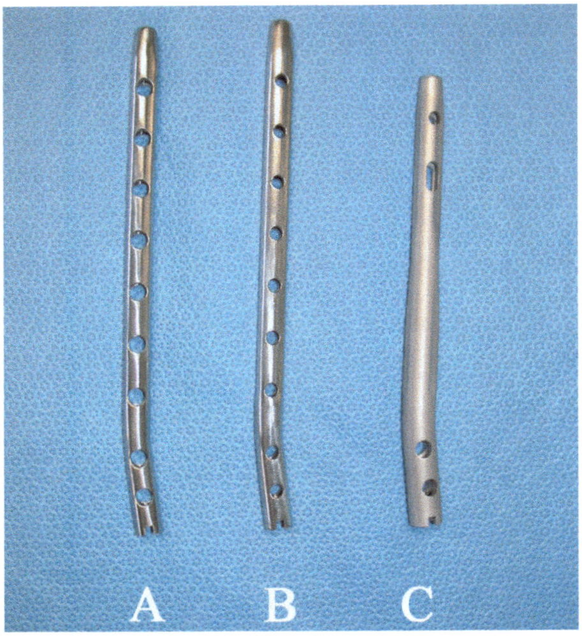

Fig. 4.3.7. The development of the supracondylar nail. The original nails had 6-mm holes for interlocking the entire length of the nail (A). To reduce nail breakage, hole size was decreased (B). Current nails have no holes in the fracture locus and are tapered with 6-mm holes distally and 5-mm holes proximally (C)

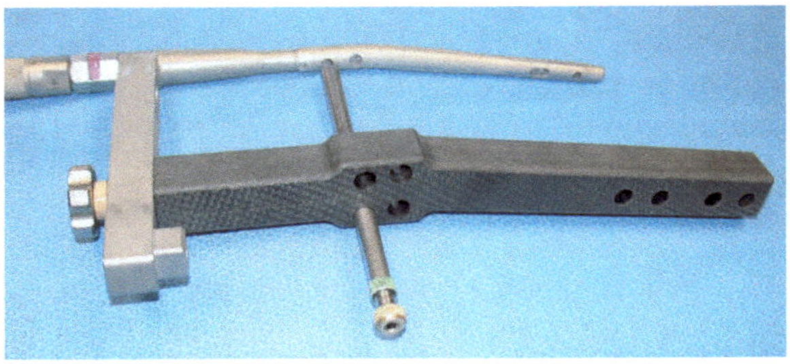

Fig. 4.3.8. In the current version of the nail and guide the 6-mm supracondylar screws are not in the same plane. The guide has been modified so that distal off-plane screws can be placed. At the proximal end of the nail there is a slot so the fracture, if stable, can settle around the nail

ticular extension in patients with limited activity demand and poor-quality bone.

The next substantial advance in the twenty-first century will be the introduction of biologic and chemical fracture-healing enhancers and stabilizers that work. Consider that the traumatologist has successfully reduced the fracture and placed an intramedullary supracondylar appliance with locking screws. The nail of the future is fabricated from absorbable materials and introduced using navigation with minimal X-ray exposure. It is a thin implant that is inflated after insertion. Now comes the exciting part. A nozzle is fitted to the end of the supracondylar internal stabilizer and foam that becomes hard and stable in the medullary cavity is evenly extruded into the distal femoral construct. This osteoconductive matrix fixes the implant in bone and provides good mechanical stability until fracture healing takes place. Healing is enhanced by a genetically engineered stem cell stimulator in the foam. This bone-healing peptide ignites and facilitates fracture healing until the bone is restored and the supportive matrix and the implant are absorbed. Damaged cartilage is regenerated by the instillation of another specially developed polypeptide into the knee joint. All the ingredients for this recipe are being introduced into clinical practice today. Doubtless as much progress will be made in coming decades in the treatment of fractures of the distal femur as was made in the last 20 years.

References

1. Brunner CHF, Weber BG: In: Special Techniques in Internal Fixation. Berlin, Springer-Verlag, pp 172–173, 1982.
2. Frederick D, Seligson D: Developments in locked femoral nailing. Orthopedics 13:1141–1145, 1990.
3. Green SA: Distal intramedullary fixation of supracondylar fractures of the femur. Techniques in Orthopedics 3:71–76, 1988.
4. Henry SL, Green S, Seligson D: Management of supracondylar fractures with the GSH supracondylar nail. American Academy of Orthopedic Surgeons 57th annual meeting, scientific exhibit # 3015, New Orleans, Louisiana, February, 1990.
5. Henry SL, Trager S, Green S, Seligson D: Management of supracondylar fractures of the femur with the GSH intramedullary nail: preliminary report. Contemp Orthop 22:631–640, 1991.
6. Henry SL, Iannacone WM, Born CT, Dalsey RM, Jamieson J, DeLong Jr., WG, Seligson D: Management of supracondylar fractures of the femur with GSH intramedullary nail (Abstract). Orthop Transactions 15:775, 1991.
7. Henry SL, Seligson D, Trager S: Management of supracondylar fractures of the femur with the GSH intramedullary nail (Abstract). Orthop Transactions 15:775, 1991.
8. Henry SL: Supracondylar femur fractures treated percutaneously. Clinical Orthopaedics and Related Research, No. 375, pp 51–59, June 2000.
9. Iannacone WM, Bennett FS, DeLong WG, Jr., Born CT, Dalsey: Initial experience with the treatment of supracondylar femoral fractures using the supracondylar intramedullary nail: a preliminary report. J Orthop Trauma 8:322–327, 1994.
10. Johnson EE, Marroquin CE, Kossovsky NIR: Synovial metallosis resulting from intra articular intramedullary nailing of a distal femoral nonunion. J Orthop Trauma 7(4):320–324, 1993.
11. Klemm K, Schellmann WD. Dynamische und Statische Verriegelung des Marknagels. Monatsschr Unfallheilkd 75:568–575, 1972.
12. Kuis W, de Ridder VA: Reversed gamma-nail: preliminary results of a new intramedullary implant. Injury 24:253–256, 1993.

13. Lambotte A: L'Intervention Opératoire dans les Fractures Récentes et Anciennes, Bruxelles: Lamertin, 1907.
14. Lambotte A. Chirurgie Opératoire des Fractures. Paris: Masson et Cie, 1913.
15. Lewert AH, Modney MT. Transfixion rod in condylar and intercondylar fractures of the femur. Orthop Rev 16:310–316, 1987.
16. Lucas SE, Seligson D, Henry SL: Intramedullary supracondylar nailing of femoral fractures. Clin Orthop 296:200–206, 1993.
17. Modny MT, Bambara J. The perforated cruciate intramedullary nail. J Am Geriatr Soc 1:579–588, 1953.
18. Moed BR, Watson JT: Retrograde nailing of the femoral shaft. J Am Acad Orthop Surg 7:209–216, 1999.
19. Mize RD, Bucholz RW, Grogan DP: Surgical treatment of displaced, comminuted fractures of the distal end of the femur. J Bone Joint Surg 64A: 871–879, 1982.
20. Müller MF, Allgöwer MM, Willenegger H: Manual of Internal Fixation, Translated by J. Schatzker. New York, Springer-Verlag, 1970.
21. Rush LV: Dynamic intramedullary fracture fixation of the femur. Clin Orthop 60:21–27, 1968.
22. Sárváry A, Berentey G, Feczkó J: Behandlung Supra- und diakondylärer Femurfrakturen mit retrograder Verriegelungsnagelung. Operative Ortho und Traumatologie 6:30–37, 1994.
23. Schatzker J, Lambert DC: Supracondylar fractures of the femur. Clin Orthop 60:21–27, 1968.
24. Seligson D: Supracondylar femur fractures: intramedullary nailing. In: Master techniques in orthopedic surgery, pp. 321–333, Wiss DA, ed. Lippincott-Raven, 1998.
25. Seligson D, Been JN, Howard PA: Supracondylar fractures: an historical perspective. Techniques in Orthopedics 9:180–188, 1995.
26. Umansky AL: Blade-plate internal fixation for fracture of the distal end of the femur. Bull Hospital Joint Dis 9:18–21, 1998.
27. Voor MJ, Verst DA, Mladsi SW, Khalily C, Seligson D: Fatigue properties of a twelve-hole versus a five-hole intramedullary supracondylar nail. J Ortho Trauma 11(2):98–112, 1997.
28. Wozasek GE, Seligson D, Durgin R, Voor M: Distal interlocking screw fixation strength in femoral intramedullary nailing: influence of bone quality and supplemental buttress nut. Osteosynthese International 2:123–127, 1996.
29. Zickel R, Fietti V, Lawsing J et al: A new intramedullary fixation device for the distal third of the femur. Clin Orthop 125:185–191, 1977.

Retrograde Nailing of the Femur: Contemporary Indications and Technique

R.A. Probe, T.R. Lewis

Introduction

The stabilization of femoral fractures with an intramedullary implant has proven itself to be a valuable clinical tool over the last half century [28]. Traditionally, nail insertion has been performed in an antegrade fashion; however, there are certain clinical situations where proximal to distal introduction is challenging. These circumstances include combined neck and shaft fractures, combined pelvic/acetabular trauma, obesity, polytrauma, pregnancy, distal fractures, and floating knee injuries.

In each of these circumstances, the placement of a nail in a retrograde fashion offers distinct advantages. With associated secondary fractures about the hip, it allows for femur stabilization without a proximal incision; in obese patients, a collinear starting point is much easier to obtain distally; in multiple trauma, several procedures may proceed simultaneously; and with a floating knee, intramedullary stabilization of both fractures may be made with a single incision. In considering the challenges presented by a combined neck and shaft fracture, Swiontkowski was the first to report on the use of a rigid nail inserted in a retrograde fashion [25]. His technique called for a starting point over the medial femoral condyle. Because of poor reductions with this off-axis starting point, technique pioneers soon moved the starting point into the intercondylar notch. This has greatly simplified the management of many of these complex fractures. Subsequent literature from the last decade has solidified the use of retrograde femoral nailing as a treatment alternative. This chapter will describe the variations in surgical technique, the relative indications for this procedure, and discuss complications that are unique to the technique.

Surgical Indications and Contraindications

Virtually all fractures of the femoral shaft that are distal to the lesser trochanter are amenable to retrograde fixation. Those factors listed above all provide relative indications for the use of this technique. As the fracture approaches the subtrochanteric zone, caution must be used. Once the fracture becomes proximal to the femoral isthmus, there is increasingly little endosteal contact to provide for alignment; and varus malposition becomes a concern [7, 22]. Additionally, the subtrochanteric zone experiences large cyclic bending forces. With retrograde insertion, interlocking screws and the associated weakened portion of the nail are placed in proximity to these forces, increasing the potential for hardware failure. Open fractures and fractures associated with soft tissue injury about the knee are also relative contraindications, because the intercondylar starting point is intra-articular. Should the fracture site become infected, the direct communication would place the knee at risk of septic arthritis.

Preoperative Planning

Integrity of knee ligaments and vascular supply should be assured by systemic physical examination. Quality radiographs of the entire femur should be obtained. Particular attention should be placed on examination of the femoral neck with an anteroposterior (AP) radiograph of the proximal femur being obtained in internal rotation to rule out an associated fracture of the femoral neck. A preliminary estimate of femur length and canal diameter may be made from these films. Should a delay of surgery beyond 24 h be anticipated, a tibial traction pin should be placed to prevent muscle shortening and resultant difficulties in reduction. Once anesthetized, the patient is placed supine on a completely radiolucent table. A small bump beneath the involved greater trochanter will partially correct for the external rotation commonly seen in the proximal segment. The uninvolved side should be used as a template for estimating nail size and determining the patient's normal leg rotation. It can be very helpful to perform a fluoroscopic examination of the intact femur, with the predicted nail positioned just above the intercondylar notch. A fluoroscopic image of the hip would then allow for precise determination of appropriate nail length and diameter. The normal leg may also be used as a rotation check. While fluoroscopically viewing the proximal femur, the limb is internally rotated until the lesser trochanter is eclipsed by the femur. The foot position at this point is noted, with the intent of reproducing this rotation during the procedure on the fractured side.

Surgical Procedures

The lower limb is prepared with an antiseptic solution circumferentially, from the iliac crest to the lower leg. If a traction pin has been placed (Fig. 4.4.1 a), this may be prepared into the sterile field as it is useful for intraoperative traction and manipulation (Fig. 4.4.1 b–j). The leg is placed on sterile supports to allow for 45° of knee flexion. This will allow for straight access into the femoral canal, between the anterior proximal tibia and the inferior pole of the patella.

Two options exist for surgical exposure. In the more extensive approach, a formal, medial parapatellar arthrotomy is created, incising the medial retinaculum from the lower portion of the patella to the tibial plateau. The patella tendon is then retracted medially, allowing for direct visualization of the femoral articular surface. The advantage of this approach is that the starting point may be easily visualized and all of the intramedullary debris that is returned from reaming may be removed. Alternatively, a percutaneous approach may be utilized. To do this, a guide wire is laid upon the skin and superimposed on the intramedullary axis. This is confirmed with fluoroscopy in both AP and lateral projections. The intersection of these two lines will be a point over the midportion of the patellar tendon (Fig. 4.4.2 a, b). At this crossing, a 2-cm longitudinal split in the patellar tendon is made. This approach is very simple; however, the surgeon must be vigilant in removing bone debris from the knee with the use of cannulated reaming guides. This percutaneous method is the author's preferred technique to utilize, unless there is concomitant head injury where there is concern over intra-articular heterotopic bone formation. In those cases, an open technique with thorough joint lavage is preferred.

Once the intercondylar notch is accessed, a 3-mm guide pin is used to identify the correct starting point. Cadaveric work, in which the axis of the medullary canal was extended to the joint surface, has demonstrated that in the frontal plane, the optimal starting point is 2.6 mm medial to the center of the intercondylar notch and, in the sagittal plane, 6.2 mm anterior to the insertion of the posterior cruciate ligament [5]. Using this point in 26 cadaveric knees, no instances of violation of the patellofemoral joint were noted. Other investigators [13] have suggested a more anterior point as ideal but this is to be avoided because of concerns over the patellofemoral joint (Fig. 4.4.2 c). Practically, this point can be identified by placing the guide wire 6 mm anterior to the termination of Blumensatt's line in the lateral projection and just medial to the deepest portion of the intercondylar notch on AP projection (Fig. 4.4.3). Once this position is identified, the guide wire is advanced, while aiming for the center of the medullary canal in both planes.

With the guide wire centered in the medullary canal, a cannulated drill is advanced over this wire, creating a 12-mm channel through the distal metaphysis. This is followed by the placement of ball-tipped guide wire into the distal medullary canal. If surgery is performed within 24 h, it is usually a simple matter to apply manual traction, manipulate the distal segment and pass the wire across the fracture under fluoroscopic control. If these measures prove unsuccessful, intramedullary reduction tools or mechanical distractors can be applied. If a femoral distractor is necessary, it may be attached via a pin into the greater trochanter and a second pin into the femoral condyle. Caution must be exercised in the placement of the distal pin so as to avoid the path of the subsequent nail. This is usually best accomplished by placing the distal pin from the mid-lateral condyle into the anterior medial condyle. This will allow the nail to pass posterior to this pin.

Mechanical distractors become useful in cases where restoration of anatomic length proves difficult. If a femoral distractor is necessary, it may be attached via a pin into the greater trochanter and a second pin into the femoral condyle. Caution must be exercised in the placement of the distal pin so as to avoid the path of the subsequent nail. This is usually best accomplished by placing the distal pin from the mid-lateral condyle into the anterior medial condyle. This will allow the nail to pass posterior to this pin.

Once the guide wire has been passed, it is seated into the metaphyseal bone above the lesser

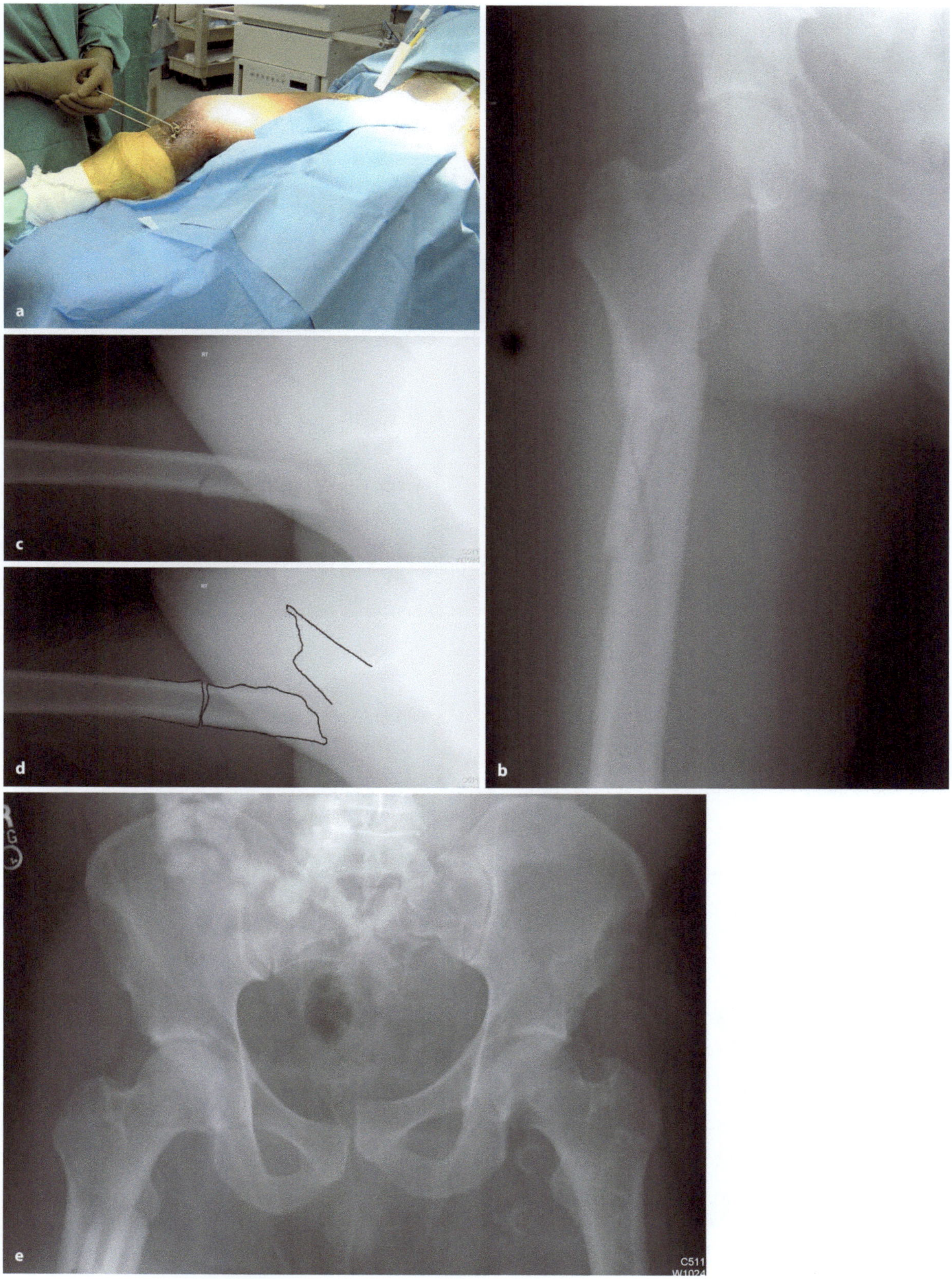

Fig. 4.4.1. a The draping of the lower limb for surgery. A tibial traction pin is inserted to facilitate intraoperative manipulation. b Preoperative frontal plane radiograph demonstrating a subtrochanteric femoral fracture. Relative contraindications to antegrade nailing included a displaced pelvic fracture as well as extensive soft tissue injury in the gluteal region. c, d Lateral views demonstrating significant flexion of the proximal segment. e Pelvic film demonstrating unstable

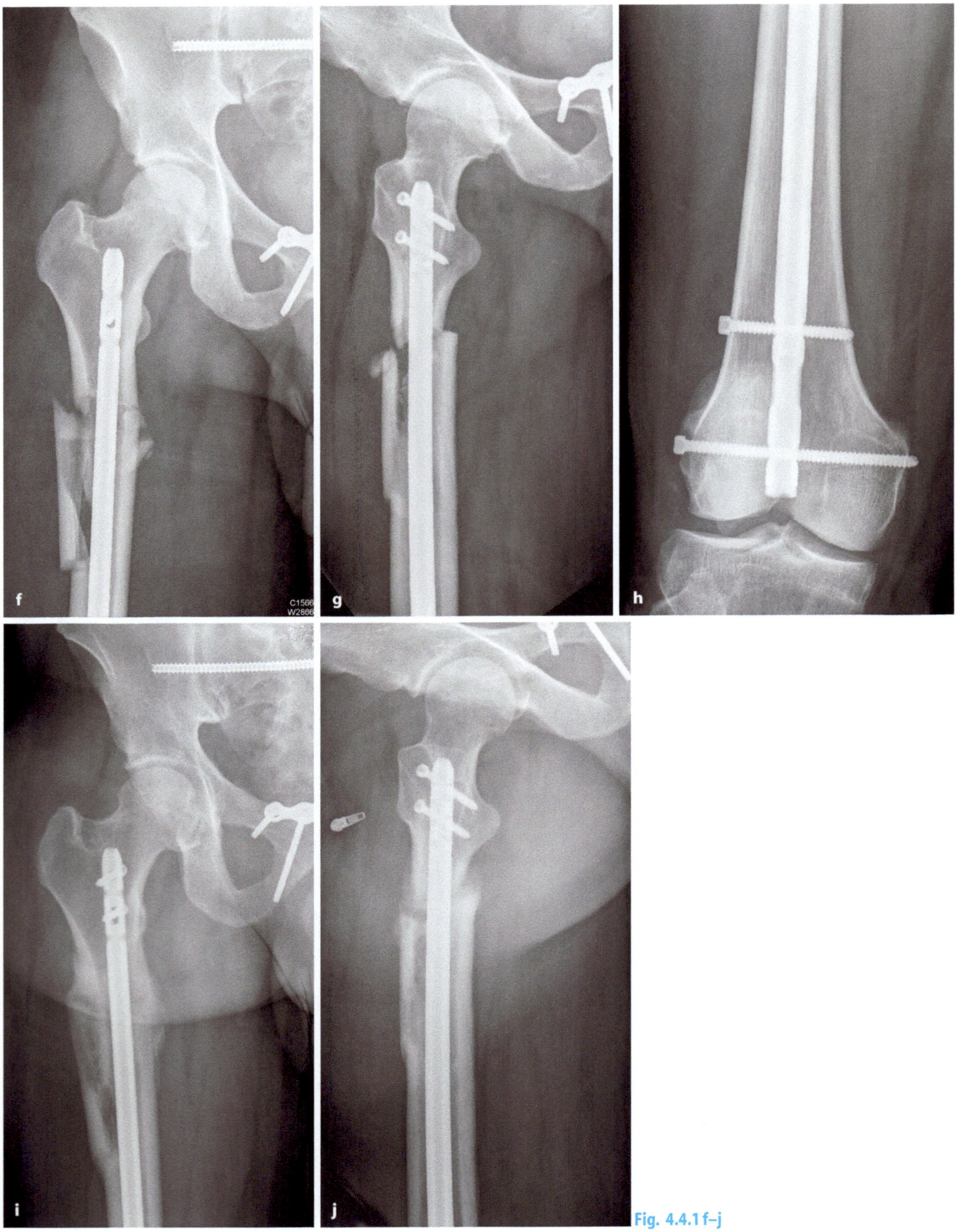

Fig. 4.4.1 f–j

pelvic fracture in combination with a subtrochanteric fracture. The pelvic fracture is a relative contraindication to a fracture table, making retrograde nailing attractive. f Postoperative frontal plane radiograph. When treating proximal fractures with retrograde nailing, it is imperative to seat the nail deeply into the proximal metaphysis and to avoid varus reduction. g Postoperative lateral radiograph. h Distal interlocking. i Healed frontal plane radiograph. j Healed lateral plane radiograph

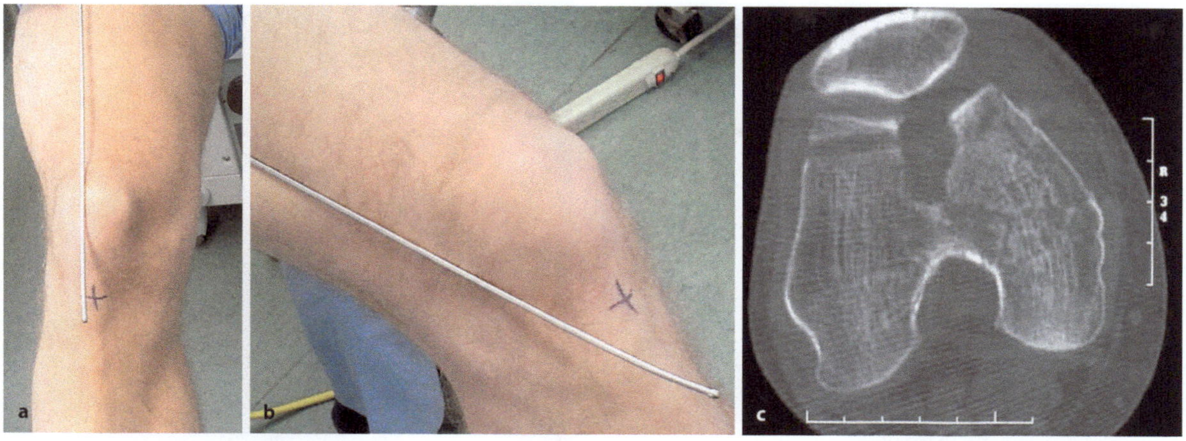

Fig. 4.4.2. a In order to place a percutaneous incision precisely, the fluoroscope is used to position a guide wire in the center of the medullary canal in the frontal and b sagittal planes. c The intersection of these two axes is the correct position to place a 2-cm vertical incision. A more anterior point with concern over the patellofemoral joint

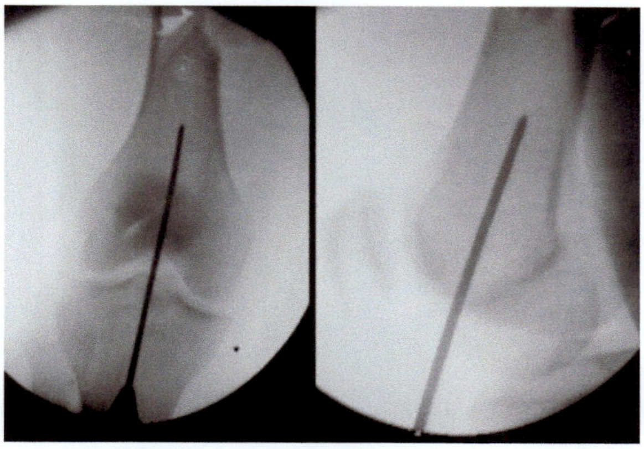

Fig. 4.4.3. Guide wire placed collinear with the medullary canal

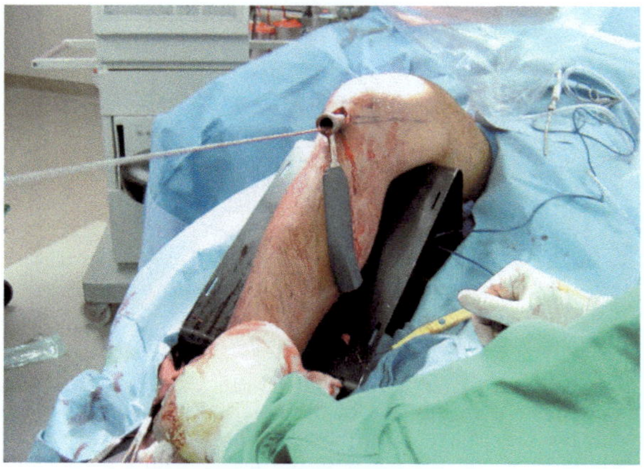

Fig. 4.4.4. Reaming is performed through a cannulated sheath to prevent debris from entering the joint

trochanter. Although these nails may be placed unreamed, it is the author's preference to perform reaming, as this allows for larger implants, more stable fixation and improved osteogenesis [21]. Reaming is performed in 0.5-mm increments, until cortical chatter is perceived. It is imperative to remove debris from the knee with the use of cannulated sheaths (Fig. 4.4.4). Following canal preparation, the nail of predetermined length is inserted to the level suggested by the preoperative plan. This should be at least to the level of the lesser trochanter. Once this proximal position is reached, the knee is fluoroscopically examined to assure that the junction of the rod and driving mechanism is below subchondral bone (Fig. 4.4.5). This is a critical step, as any intra-articular extension beyond the subchondral bone by the implant will interfere with the patellofemoral articulation [19]. Finally, the fracture site is fluoroscopically examined to assure that appropriate restoration of length has been achieved.

With the nail appropriately positioned, static locking is carried out in the vast majority of cases. If the fracture is contained within the isthmic portion of the femur, then a single interlocking screw is sufficient, because of the reduced bending load on the screw. Once the fracture extends beyond the isthmus, either proximally or distally, then additional screws should be placed. Distal locking is easily performed, utilizing the hole alignment instrumentation. If only one screw is to be used, the most proximal screw is preferred for several reasons. It does not leave an open stress riser, it gains purchase in strong cortical bone and the screw is unlikely to be symptomatic, because it will be deeply buried. If one

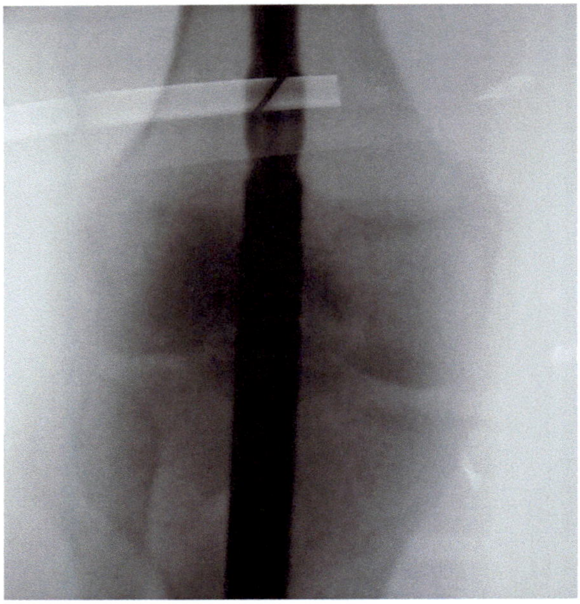

Fig. 4.4.5. The nail is seated well beneath the subchondral bone surface

of the more distal screws is to be utilized, accurate depth measurement is imperative. If these screws are left too long, the irritation to the knee capsule will limit postoperative knee function. If there is concern about the density of distal bone, medial washers and lateral nuts should be considered. Following distal locking, the driving mechanism may be removed and the knee extended. With the driving guide removed, the distal orifice of the nail may be covered by a cap. This diminishes access of the medullary canal into the knee joint and protects the nail threads from tissue ingrowth. Prior to proximal locking, a final assessment of length and rotation is made. Length is checked clinically and fluoroscopically. Any necessary adjustment may be made by traction or impaction applied to the leg. Rotation is verified by internally rotating the proximal segment until the lesser trochanter is eclipsed by the femur. In this position, the direction of the foot is noted and compared to the direction of the foot on the normal side. Proximal locking is begun by extending the leg and fluoroscopically finding the desired sagittal hole. The receiving portion of the C-arm is positioned on top and this is raised as high as possible, to provide magnification and space for the surgeon. Utilizing "free-hand" technique, the axis of the locking hole is reproduced by the C-arm, established when the hole is visualized as a perfect circle. This is accomplished in two steps. First the C-arm is rotated in the sagittal plane until the axis of the ellipse is perpendicular

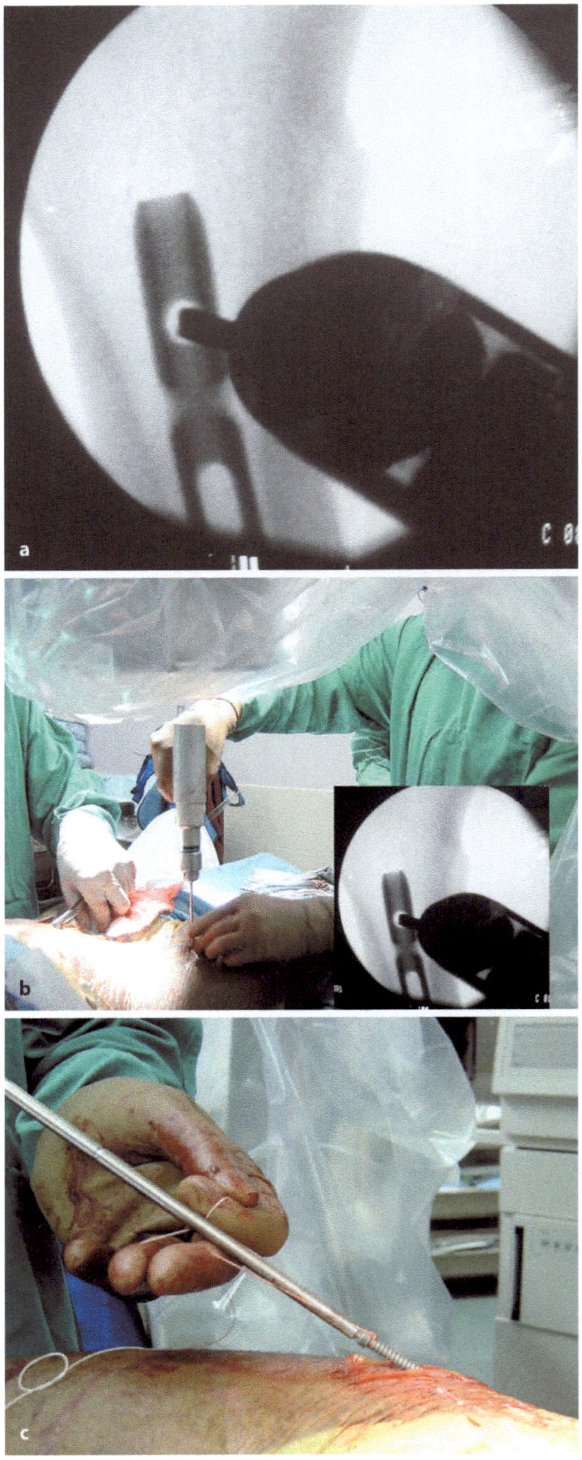

Fig. 4.4.6. a A perfect circle will indicate that the C-arm axis is collinear with the axis of the hole. b The drill is aligned with the C-arm axis. c In percutaneous placement it can be helpful to secure the screw to the driver with a suture tied beneath the screw head

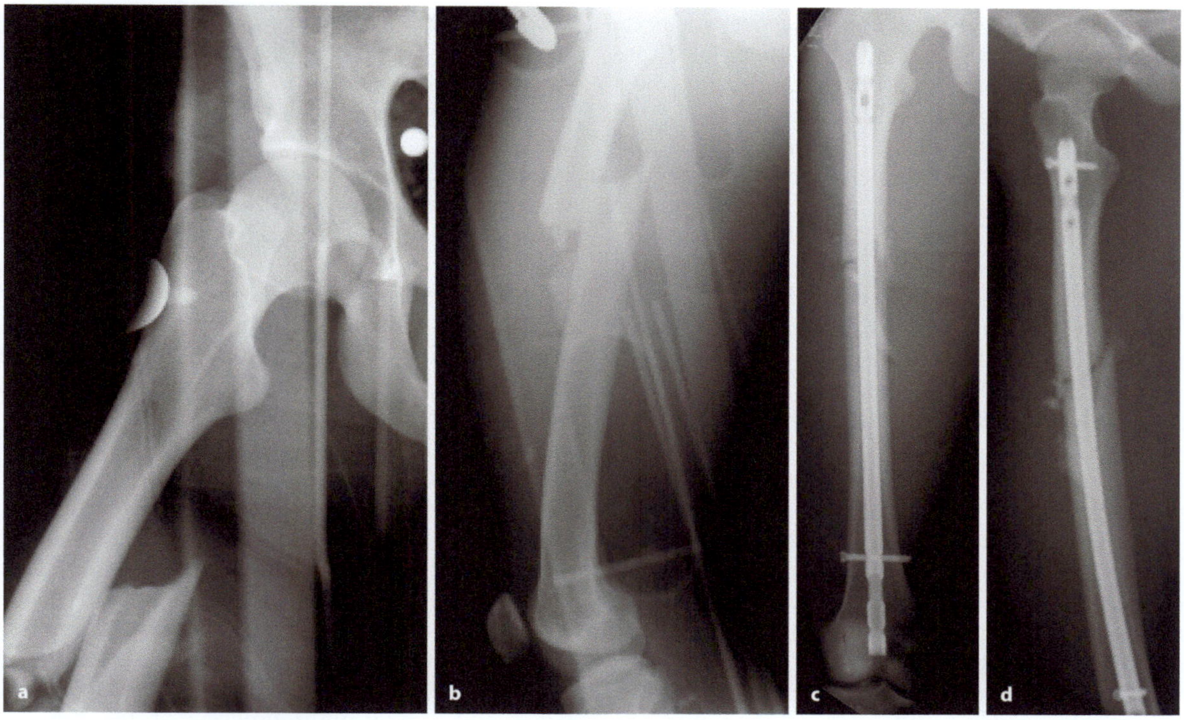

Fig. 4.4.7. a, b. Preoperative radiographs of an isthmic femoral shaft fracture. c, d Treatment with a retrograde femoral nail. Note proximal locking at the level of the lesser trochanter, the restoration of femoral length and the use of the proximal distal interlock to avoid subcutaneous prominence about the knee

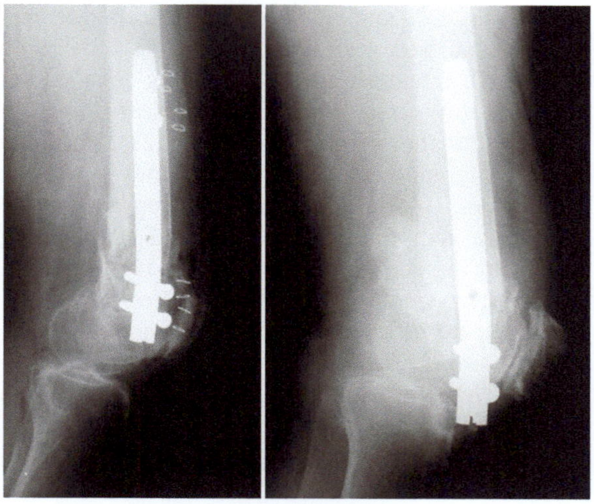

Fig. 4.4.8. In osteopenic bone, distal fixation may be lost allowing for implant migration

to the axis of the femur. Second, the C-arm is rotated in the frontal plane until this ellipse becomes a circle. With the axis identified, a fluoroscopically located skin incision is made and the appropriately sized drill placed in the center of the circle (Fig. 4.4.6 a–c). The pilot hole is drilled, depth measured, and the screw inserted. This process is repeated, if necessary, for a second screw.

Following implantation, the knee is thoroughly lavaged, to remove any remaining medullary debris, and the wounds are routinely closed. Radiographs, including the neck of the femur, are repeated and reviewed (Fig. 4.4.7 a–d); and, finally, the knee is checked for ligamentous stability. Vascular integrity is also verified before leaving the operating room. Postoperatively, patients are begun on immediate physiotherapy, with knee range of motion exercises and progressive weight-bearing. Exceptions to this protocol are made for patients in whom distal osteopenia places the construct at risk of migration (Fig. 4.4.8).

Discussion

There are certain clinical situations in which traditional antegrade nailing of the femoral shaft is problematic. Perhaps the best example of this is a combined fracture of the femoral neck and shaft. Searching for solutions to the problem, Swiontkowski et al. [25] were the first to report on the use of retrograde femoral shaft nailing. Their approach included preliminary screw fixation of the femoral neck, followed by retrograde femoral nailing from a medial condyle starting point. In their series of 13 patients, all fractures healed with outcomes that were improved over historical controls. The polytraumatized patient also presents with reasons to avoid fracture table positioning and antegrade nailing. Moed [16] reported the use of an unreamed retrograde technique in 20 polytraumatized patients. The average operative time was 75 min and these procedures were often performed coincident with other procedures. The authors were favorably impressed by the value of this technique; however, three of 22 fractures developed nonunions. Based on the concern over nonunion, the same authors instituted a protocol of early, planned dynamization that resulted in a reduction in the nonunion rate to 6% in 35 fractures [17].

Another cited indication for retrograde femoral nailing has been the presence of femoral and tibial shaft fractures in the same limb. Through a single approach, both can be stabilized. Gregory et al. [8] reported 22 limbs with diaphyseal fracture of both femur and tibia, treated with reamed retrograde femoral nailing and unreamed tibial nailing. In this series, secondary procedures were commonly required and final function was only good in 68% of limbs. Despite these compromised results, 85% of the femur fractures healed and femoral stabilization was expediently accomplished in these severely traumatized patients, without adverse sequela related to the femoral starting point. Other authors have also found this technique useful, to allow for simplified stabilization of these complex injuries [14, 20].

Early investigators also explored the performance of retrograde nails in the treatment of extra-articular and intra-articular distal femur fractures. Based on several mechanical studies, intramedullary stabilization has demonstrated comparable axial strength and stiffness but is notably less stiff in torsion when compared to plate constructs [9, 11, 15]. Fortunately, torsional loads are usually minimal in the distal femur and the mechanics of retrograde intramedullary fixation appear to be adequate to allow sufficient relative stability during healing. Clinical reports suggest that results of both short and long retrograde stabilization are capable of producing results comparable to traditional plate fixation, but in a less invasive fashion [2]. In considering the common problem of supracondylar fractures in elderly patients, Janzing [12] reviewed 24 patients over the age of 65 years, who were treated with a short retrograde intramedullary nail. Results were favorable; however, migration of the construct through the distal osteopenic bone was recognized as a problem. A sub-set of this group of patients are those in which a supracondylar fracture occurs adjacent to a knee prosthesis. Most modern prostheses have sufficient space between the condyles to allow for placement of a retrograde nail. This may be confirmed preoperatively with a notch view. Clinical series have suggested that this is effective treatment; however, the difficulties of fixation into osteopenic bone persist [27]. As more clinical experience is gained with locked plating and less invasive plating techniques, it is anticipated that treatment recommendations will become clearer in these increasingly common fractures [4].

Other series have confirmed the theoretic value of retrograde nailing for indications such as pathologic fracture, proximal existing implants, obesity, pelvic trauma, and pregnancy [1]. Consistent among these reports is the absence of significant detrimental effects to knee function. This allayed fear in combination with the relative simplicity of the surgical procedure has led some traumatologists to examine the role of retrograde nailing in femoral shaft fractures without secondary indications. In a prospective randomized trial of 69 fractures, Tornetta found similar union times and similar joint function at the time of healing; however, immediate postoperative pain was greater in the retrograde group and there was a 33% incidence of shortening in the retrograde group in unstable fractures compared to none in the antegrade group [26]. Ostrum, in a prospective randomized series, compared 40 retrograde nails to 37 antegrade nails. By placing canal filling nails, union rates of 97% were seen in both groups after the primary procedure [21]. The only other differences noted in this study included slightly less blood loss in the retrograde group and more symptoms from the distal interlocking screws in the retrograde group. In a retrospective, comparative study of 198 patients, Ricci et al. [23] identified no differences between groups, with regard to union, delayed union, nonunion or malunion. They did, however, identify an increased incidence of knee pain in the retrograde group and an increased incidence of hip pain after antegrade nailing.

As this group of studies suggests, there are few differentiating outcomes that dictate an antegrade or retrograde approach to femoral nailing. In light of this, it is appropriate to consider retrograde nailing in the routine treatment of femoral shaft fractures; however, there are complications specific to the retrograde technique that the surgeon should be aware of in making treatment decisions. While the incidence of heterotopic bone at the hip insertion site of antegrade femoral nailing has ranged from 24 to 60%, this rarely interferes with joint function. With a retrograde approach, cases of severe intra-articular heterotopic bone formation have been reported in patients with head injury that have led to severe joint dysfunction [10]. The proximal interlocking of retrograde nails is also potentially problematic. Riina et al. [24] have demonstrated that the femoral artery is only 1 cm medial to the usual trajectory of proximal locking. Of additional concern is the fact that an average of 1.7 branches of the femoral nerve will pass over the femur proximal to the lesser trochanter. In cases associated with pelvic trauma, these safe zones may become fewer as fracture displacement and hematoma may change the usual anatomic position of these structures. Vascular injury associated with retrograde nailing has been reported during proximal locking [6] as well as during fracture reduction [3], indicating that the surgeon must maintain awareness of this potential.

Despite the fact that several reports do not suggest an increased incidence of knee pain following this approach [18, 21], Tornetta has reported increased knee symptoms in the early postoperative period and Ricci [23] has demonstrated increased symptoms both early and late, when compared to an antegrade group. Also concerning is the fact that the follow-up in these studies is less than 3 years. The long-term effects of this transarticular approach remain unknown.

From our existing knowledge and experience, it can be concluded that retrograde femoral nailing is an effective method of treating diaphyseal and distal metaphyseal fractures of the femur. When there are factors that would make antegrade nailing difficult, it is reasonable to conclude that retrograde nailing is a preferred method of treatment. With more information on the long-term effects on the knee, it may prove that it is also a preferred method of treatment for routine femoral fractures.

References

1. Anup K, Mehra MM (2002) Retrograde femoral interlocking nail in complex fractures. J Orthop Surg (Hong Kong) 10(1):17–21
2. Armstrong R, Milliren A, Schrantz W, Zeliger K (2003) Retrograde interlocked intramedullary nailing of supracondylar distal femur fractures in an average 76-year-old patient population. Orthopedics 26(6):627–629
3. Barnes CJ, Higgins LD (2002) Vascular compromise after insertion of a retrograde femoral nail: case report and review of the literature. J Orthop Trauma 16(3):201–204
4. Bong MR, Egol KA, Koval KJ, Kummer FJ, Su ET, Iesaka K, Bayer J, Di Cesare PE (2002) Comparison of the LISS and a retrograde-inserted supracondylar intramedullary nail for fixation of a periprosthetic distal femur fracture proximal to a total knee arthroplasty. J Arthroplasty 17(7):876–881
5. Carmack DB, Moed BR, Kingston C, Zmurko M, Watson JT, Richardson M (2003) Identification of the optimal intercondylar starting point for retrograde femoral nailing: an anatomic study. J Trauma 55(4):692–695
6. Coupe KJ, Beaver RL (2001) Arterial injury during retrograde femoral nailing: a case report of injury to a branch of the profunda femoris artery. J Orthop Trauma 15(2):140–143
7. DiCicco JD 3rd, Jenkins M, Ostrum RF (2000) Retrograde nailing for subtrochanteric femur fractures. Am J Orthop 29(9 Suppl):4–8
8. Gregory P, DiCicco J, Karpik, DiPasquale T, Herscovici D, Sanders R (1996) Ipsilateral fractures of the femur and tibia: treatment with retrograde femoral nailing and unreamed tibial nailing. J Orthop Trauma 10(5):309–316
9. Hora N, Markel DC, Haynes A, Grimm MJ (1999) Biomechanical analysis of supracondylar femoral fractures fixed with modern retrograde intramedullary nails. J Orthop Trauma 13(8):539–544
10. Horne LT, Blue BA (1999) Intraarticular heterotopic ossification in the knee following intramedullary nailing of the fractured femur using a retrograde method. J Orthop Trauma 13(5):385–388
11. Ito K, Hungerbuhler R, Wahl D, Grass R (2001) Improved intramedullary nail interlocking in osteoporotic bone. J Orthop Trauma 15(3):192–196.
12. Janzing HM, Stockman B, Van Damme G, Rommens P, Broos PL (1998) The retrograde intramedullary nail: prospective experience in patients older than sixty-five years. J Orthop Trauma 12(5):330–333
13. Krupp RJ, Malkani AL, Goodin RA, Voor MJ (2003) Optimal entry point for retrograde femoral nailing. J Orthop Trauma 17(2):100–105
14. Lundy DW, Johnson KD (2001) “Floating knee” injuries: ipsilateral fractures of the femur and tibia. J Am Acad Orthop Surg 9(4):238–245
15. Meyer RW, Plaxton NA, Postak PD, Gilmore A, Froimson MI, Greenwald AS (2000) Mechanical comparison of a distal femoral side plate and a retrograde intramedullary nail. J Orthop Trauma 14(6):398–404
16. Moed BR, Watson JT (1995) Retrograde intramedullary nailing, without reaming, of fractures of the femoral shaft in multiply injured patients. J Bone Joint Surg Am 77(10):1520–1527
17. Moed BR, Watson JT, Cramer KE, Karges DE, Teefey JS (1998) Unreamed retrograde intramedullary nailing of fractures of the femoral shaft. J Orthop Trauma 12:334–342
18. Moed BR, Watson JT (1999) Retrograde nailing of the femoral shaft. J Am Acad Orthop Surg 7(4):209–216
19. Morgan E, Ostrum RF, DiCicco J, McElroy J, Poka A (1999) Effects of retrograde femoral intramedullary nailing on the patellofemoral articulation. J Orthop Trauma 13:13–16
20. Ostrum RF (2000) Treatment of floating knee injuries through a single percutaneous approach. Clin Orthop 375:43–50
21. Ostrum RF, Agarwal A, Lakatos R, Poka A (2000) Prospective comparison of retrograde and antegrade femoral intramedullary nailing. J Orthop Trauma 14(7):496–501
22. Ricci WM, Bellabarba C, Lewis R, Evanoff B, Herscovici D, Dipasquale T, Sanders R (2001) Angular malalignment after intramedullary nailing of femoral shaft fractures. J Orthop Trauma 15(2):90–95
23. Ricci WM, Bellabarba C, Evanoff B, Herscovici D, DiPasquale T, Sanders R (2001) Retrograde versus antegrade nailing of femoral shaft fractures. J Orthop Trauma 15(3):161–169
24. Riina J, Tornetta P, Ritter C, et al. (1988) Neurologic and vascular structures at risk during anterior-posterior

locking of retrograde femoral nails. J Orthop Trauma 12:379–381

25. Swiontkowski M, Hansen S, Kellam J (1894) Ipsilateral fractures of the femoral neck and shaft: a treatment protocol. J Bone Joint Surg 66(2):260–268
26. Tornetta P, 3rd, Tiburzi D (2000) Antegrade or retrograde reamed femoral nailing. A prospective, randomized trial. J Bone Joint Surg Br 82(5):652–654
27. Weber D, Pomeroy DL, Schaper LA, Badenhausen WE Jr, Curry JI, Smith MW, Suthers KE (2000) Supracondylar nailing of distal periprosthetic femoral fractures. Int Orthop 24(1):33–35
28. Winquist RA, Hansen ST Jr, Clawson DK (2001) Closed intramedullary nailing of femoral fractures: a report of five hundred and twenty cases. 1984. J Bone Joint Surg Am 83-A(12):1912

Antegrade Femoral Nailing Without the Aid of a Fracture Table

R. A. Probe

Introduction

The preferred treatment for fractures of the femoral shaft has become the antegrade insertion of a femoral nail. Multiple authors have demonstrated high union rates, restoration of limb function and low complication rates utilizing this technique [5]. One of the few drawbacks to this procedure is that most surgeons perform the surgery with traction being applied via a fracture table. Although this set-up provides mechanical traction that aids in realignment, there are a number of complications that have been reported with the use of a fracture table. These include pudendal nerve palsy [2], transient impotence and compartment syndrome of the opposite leg [3]. Some surgeons attempt to minimize these complications by performing this procedure with traction being applied with the patient in the lateral position; however, this position is difficult to set up and potentially compromising to patients with multiple injuries. In addition to these potential complications, a skeletal traction pin is required and there is significant amount of time spent positioning a patient on a fracture table.

These drawbacks have led some to perform this procedure without the use of a fracture table. In appropriate circumstances this can facilitate starting point creation, save time and eliminate the potential for complications related to the technique [4, 6].

Technique

Patient Preparation

The reduction of a femoral shaft fracture is easiest if surgery is performed soon after the fracture has occurred. Delays can lead to muscle spasm, which makes length restoration difficult. Ideally, surgery is performed on the day of injury after "advanced trauma life support" protocols have ruled out concomitant injury. If delays of 24 h or more are anticipated prior to surgery, it is helpful to place a skeletal traction pin with one-fifth of the patient's body weight attached. This will prevent muscle shortening and will facilitate subsequent reduction. Muscle-relaxing anesthesia is administered as well as prophylactic antibiotics. Prior to positioning, it is of great value to determine nail length from the intact femur. This is done with fluoroscopic examination of the opposite knee and hip with varying length rods held adjacent to the leg. The nail length that most closely extends from the piriformis fossa to the distal physeal scar is chosen. Alternatively an electrocautery cord can be fluoroscopically visualized and used to measure the length of the medullary canal. The opposite leg is also examined to assess the patient's normal limb rotation so that this may be reproduced during surgery. This requires that the C-arm be aligned with a reproducible rotational femoral marker and the foot's rotational position noted in relation to this axis. The best marker in the proximal femur is the lesser trochanter. In an anteroposterior projection, the femur can be internally rotated until the lesser trochanter is eclipsed by the femoral shaft and no longer visible. This same radiographic marker can be used to check rotation in the fractured limb after nail interlocking to assure restoration of physiologic rotational position.

The use of a completely radiolucent operating table is strongly recommended as multiple oblique fluoroscopic projections will be required. Metal side-rails will interfere with some of these projections. Femoral nailing without a fracture table can be performed in a lateral position. This is particularly useful for subtrochanteric fractures because flexion of the fractured leg removes the deforming influence of the iliopsoas. In all remaining patients positioning with the ipsilateral buttock elevated 20 cm from the table surface with sheets is preferred because of simplicity and physiologic advantages (Fig. 4.5.1). Prior to skin preparation a fluoroscopic check is performed to ensure that coronal and sagittal imaging of the

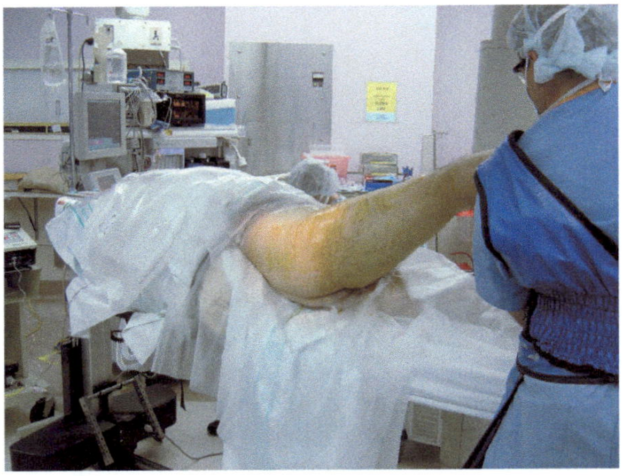

Fig. 4.5.1. Leg positioned to allow for adduction and access to the piriformis fossa

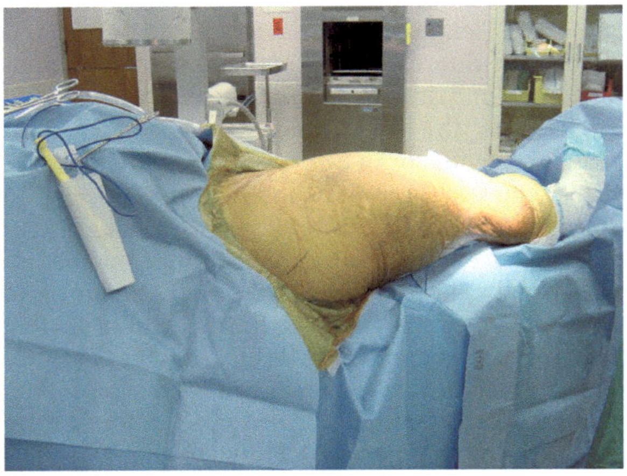

Fig. 4.5.2. The leg is draped to allow access proximal to the trochanter and free manipulation

entire femur is possible. In this position the limb is draped free with split-sheets applied in a fashion that leaves a large area of skin proximal to the greater trochanter exposed (Fig. 4.5.2).

Surgery

Controversy exists over the ideal starting point, with some surgeons preferring a trochanteric start position rather than one in the piriformis fossa. If a nail without a trochanteric bend is chosen, it is generally preferable to utilize the piriform fossa because this point is in line with the medullary canal. Deviation from this position will generate large hoop stress during nail insertion or lead to malunion. To gain access into the piriformis fossa, the hip is flexed, adducted and internally rotated. A 2-cm longitudinal skin incision is placed proximal to the trochanter in a spot that represents the virtual extension of the axis of the proximal femur. This should be confirmed fluoroscopically in both planes with a guide wire placed collinear with the femoral axis. This is typically one handbreadth proximal to the trochanteric tip. If adhesive drapes are used, they should be removed around the margin of the incision to ensure that they are not caught within the rotating reamers. The fascia of the gluteus maximus is incised and a finger is used to create a path through this muscle, exposing the underlying gluteus medius and trochanter. With the hip flexed it is possible to gain entrance into the piriformis fossa posterior to the gluteus medius with digital palpation. Staying posterior to the muscles minimizes insertion damage and postoperative abductor weakness. Once a path has been created, a 3.2-mm guidewire is drilled into the piriformis fossa and its position verified with biplanar image intensification. The wire is drilled down to the level of the lesser trochanter (Fig. 4.5.3) and then the hole is expanded with a 12-mm cannulated drill. It is critical that this channel be created exactly in line with the axis of the proximal segment. There is a tendency for inserting muscles to pull this segment into varus and flexion. This must be avoided or malunion will result, particularly in subtrochanteric fractures. Following channel creation a ball-tipped guide wire is introduced into the proximal medullary canal.

Passage of the guide wire across the fracture is occasionally challenging without the use of a fracture table and represents the greatest argument against this technique. The initial strategy is to match the axis of the proximal segment by bringing the distal segment to it. With assistants pulling on the leg, the surrounding musculature will often align the segments allowing for passage of the wire (Fig. 4.5.4). Sustained pulls are generally most effective in overcoming muscle shortening because of their viscoelastic properties. If several attempts fail, a number of alternative measures may prove helpful. One of these is to ream the proximal segment to 11 mm and then insert an intramedullary reduction tool (Fig. 4.5.5). This tool will allow for control of the proximal fragment and allow the surgeon to align this with the distal segment and subsequently pass the wire through the cannulated tool. Occasionally, fracture angulation or translation will prevent entrance into the distal segment. This can usually be corrected with application of strategically placed opposing forces through the skin. If a segment is posteriorly translated or the fracture angulated posteriorly, then sterile bumps placed posterior to

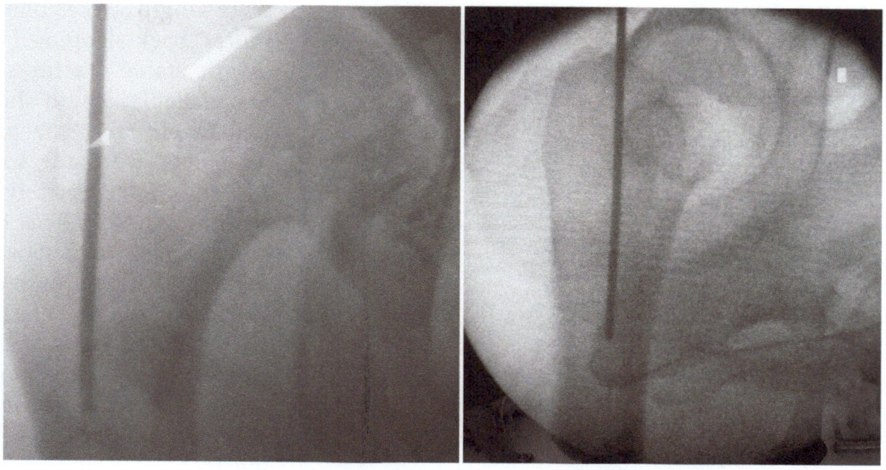

Fig. 4.5.3. Two-plane confirmation of guide wire placement

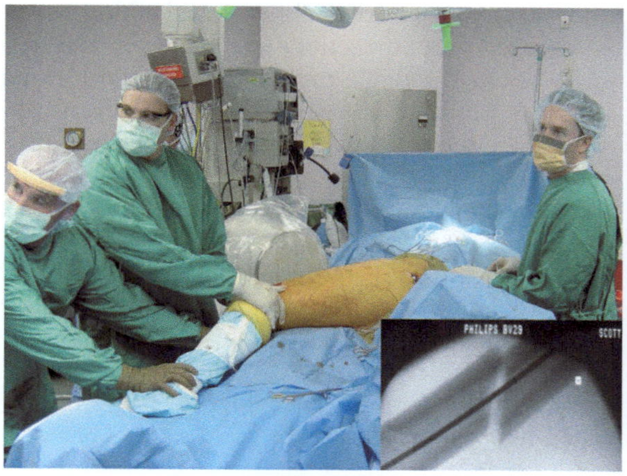

Fig. 4.5.4. Manual traction being applied, which allows for guide wire passage

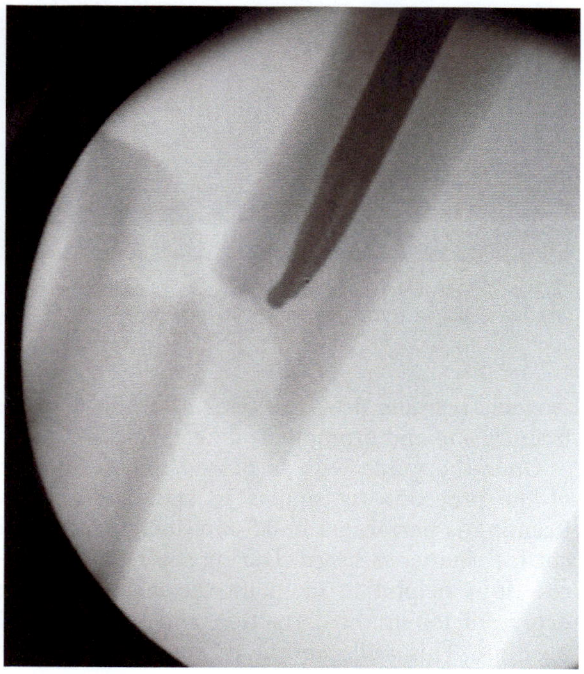

Fig. 4.5.5. This cannulated tool allows for proximal fragment manipulation

the deformity can provide a corrective force. This alignment can be augmented with a counter-force being applied to the anterior fragment manually. If these measures are not successful more invasive measures such as the placement of a percutaneous Schantz pin or bone hook for manipulation can also be helpful. If the principal impediment to reduction appears to be muscle contracture, application of a femoral distractor [1] may prove useful. The complexity of doing this is placing the anchoring pins in locations that are outside of the eventual nail tract. Distally this is not difficult as there is ample bone posterior to the nail tract to place a 5-mm pin from lateral to medial. Proximally, the pin can either be placed in the femur or the acetabulum. If the acetabulum is chosen, the supra-acetabular bone is ideal and has the advantage of not interfering with nail placement. In the femur, the best location is just above the calcar in an anterior to posterior direction. As great precision is required of this pin, it is recommended to place this under fluoroscopic control and to place the pin through sleeves so that the risk of neurovascular injury is minimized. On rare occasions, all of the adjunctive techniques for obtaining fracture reduction fail and opening of the fracture site may be required. With experience, this should occur in less than 10% of cases. If limited open reduction is required, it is performed with minimal stripping of bone so that the fracture biology is not disturbed. If fracture opening is required, this incision should be closed after guide wire passage. This will allow the os-

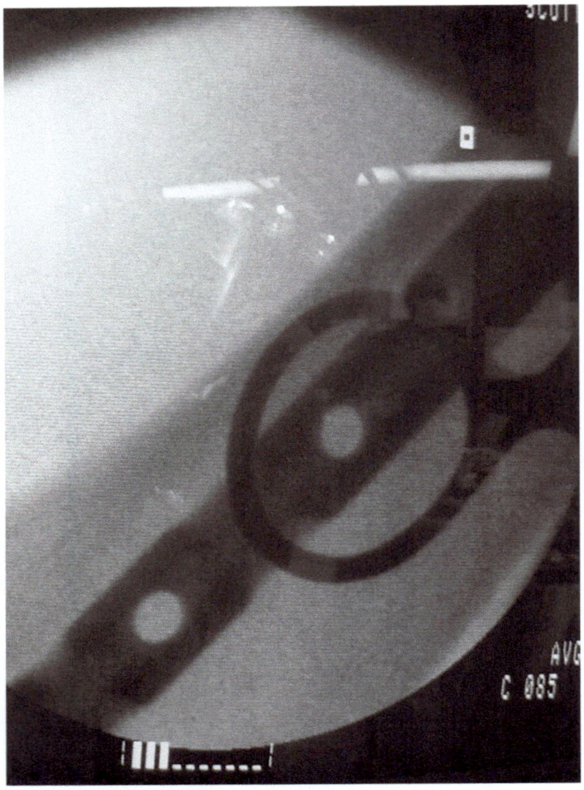

Fig. 4.5.6. Surgical instrument is used to identify the positioning of the skin incision for distal locking

teogenic reaming debris to remain localized at the fracture site and promote healing.

Once the guide wire is passed, the remainder of the procedure is similar to standard nailing. Reaming is performed in 0.5-mm increments until cortical chatter is heard. During the reaming process it is helpful to maintain the leg with some degree of longitudinal traction and in a reduced position. This will prevent eccentric reaming of the distal fragment. A nail diameter 1 mm less than the reamed diameter is chosen. With the driving rod and screw guides assembled, the accuracy of the proximal screw guides is checked prior to nail insertion. The nail is inserted over the guide wire with progress being verified with fluoroscopy. Once the distal end of the nail has reached the position determined by preoperative planning, it is locked with traditional "free-hand" technique. The image intensifier is rotated into a position that allows for the holes in the nail to be seen as perfect circles (Fig. 4.5.6). Through percutaneous incisions the pilot hole is drilled and the screw placed. With the distal rod now locked in its predetermined position, final length adjustments are made. If the fracture pattern allows for cortical contact, the fracture gap is useful to estimate length. Occasionally, the driving rod will require "back-slapping" to gain cortical contact in length stable fractures. If no cortical references are available, length should be estimated based on nail length from the preoperative plan. Final adjustments are made so that the proximal end of the nail rests precisely where it was planned on the normal limb. This can be done by driving the nail forward or backward assured that the distal segment will be moved because of interlocking. Once length has been restored, proximal locking is performed through the available guides. With a single locking screw both proximal and distal, rotation is checked to be certain that it is comparable to the opposite side. This is done by checking foot rotation against the hip rotation markers that were assessed preoperatively. Should significant discrepancy exist, either interlocking screw is removed and corrections are made. In the majority of cases a single proximal and distal locking screw is all that is required. If a fracture approaches either end of the femur or healing difficulties are anticipated, consideration should be given to the addition of the second interlocking screw.

Wounds are irrigated and routinely closed. At the completion of the procedure it is imperative to examine the knee for concomitant ligament injury. It is also necessary to review quality radiographs of the femoral neck to rule out an associated femoral neck fracture.

Discussion

Femoral nailing without a fracture table has many potential advantages when compared to traditional nailing. Time savings have been shown during positioning, surgery and for total anesthesia [4, 6]. From a surgical standpoint, access to the piriformis fossa is easier, injury to the gluteus medius may be avoided and correct rotation may be easily assessed. Importantly, it also removes the potential for complications directly related to the fracture table. The incidence of pudendal palsy has been reported between 10% and 15% [1, 6]. Fortunately those cases reported in the literature have been transient but nonetheless, disconcerting to patients. Additional advantages include the ability to perform other procedures simultaneously as well as providing a means of femoral nailing in those patients with unstable pelvic and spine trauma who would be potentially compromised with the use of a fracture table.

Despite these advantages there are limitations to this technique. Patients presenting for surgery after 24 h often have excessive shortening, which is difficult to overcome. Because of soft tissue tension, shortening of comminuted fractures is problematic and transverse, isthmic fractures in muscular individuals can also be very difficult to reduce without the aid of the sustained traction provided by the fracture table. Perhaps the most significant negative is the need for additional knowledgeable scrubbed personnel to assist with fracture reduction. In many cases three individuals are required: one for traction, one for fracture alignment and a third for manipulation of the guide wire. Even though these factors can make this procedure challenging, in certain circumstances it is clearly of benefit in the management of the trauma patient.

References

1. Baumgaertel F, Dahlen C, Stiletto R, Gotzen L (1994) Technique of using the AO-femoral distractor for femoral intramedullary nailing. J Orthop Trauma 8(4):315–321
2. Brumback RJ, Ellison TS, Molligan H, Molligan DJ, Mahaffey S, Schmidhauser C (1992) Pudendal nerve palsy complicating intramedullary nailing of the femur. J Bone Joint Surg Am 74(10):1450–1455
3. Meldrum R, Lipscomb P (2002) Compartment syndrome of the leg after less than 4 hours of elevation on a fracture table. South Med J 95(2):269–271
4. Reynders P, Broos P (1998) Unreamed intramedullary nailing of acute femoral shaft fractures using a traction device without fracture table. Acta Orthop Belg 64(2):175–179
5. Winquist RA, Hansen ST Jr, Clawson DK (1984) Closed intramedullary nailing of femoral fractures. A report of five hundred and twenty cases. J Bone Joint Surg Am 66(4):529–539
6. Wolinsky PR, McCarty EC, Shyr Y, Johnson KD (1998) Length of operative procedures: reamed femoral intramedullary nailing performed with and without a fracture table. J Orthop Trauma 12(7):485–495

The Operative Technique for the Latest Generation Gamma Nail (the Gamma3)

G. TAGLANG

As described in Chapter 4.7, the latest generation nail comes with some modifications in its features and, in particular:

- A change in the proximal diameter from 17 to 15.5 mm
- A reduction in diameter of the lag screw from 12 to 10.5 mm, with a change in its shape – notably the removal of the abrupt taper from the shaft to the beginning of the threads
- A modification in the lag-screw thread design, which improves its performance, especially with regards resistance to cut-out
- A modification in the shape of the distal locking hole that is now oblong, which allows either locking in a static or a dynamic mode
- A drop in diameter of the distal locking screw from 6.28 mm to 5 mm, and whose measured length includes the distance from the top of the head to the tip of the screw
- The targeted angle is now equivalent to the head-neck-shaft angle, since it now takes into account the medial/lateral curvature of the upper part of the nail.

These different improvements were made in order to achieve a better fit of the nail to the different types of femora, but without changing its biomechanical performance (Fig. 4.6.1).

Just as the implant has changed in some of its features, the same is true for the nail insertion guide – one unique device for all nail angles (Fig. 4.6.2). Of course, in its new design, it permits either static or distal cross-locking (short nails) and takes into account the changes in diameter of the lag screw and the distal cross-locking screw. Note that the previous instruments, for the first-

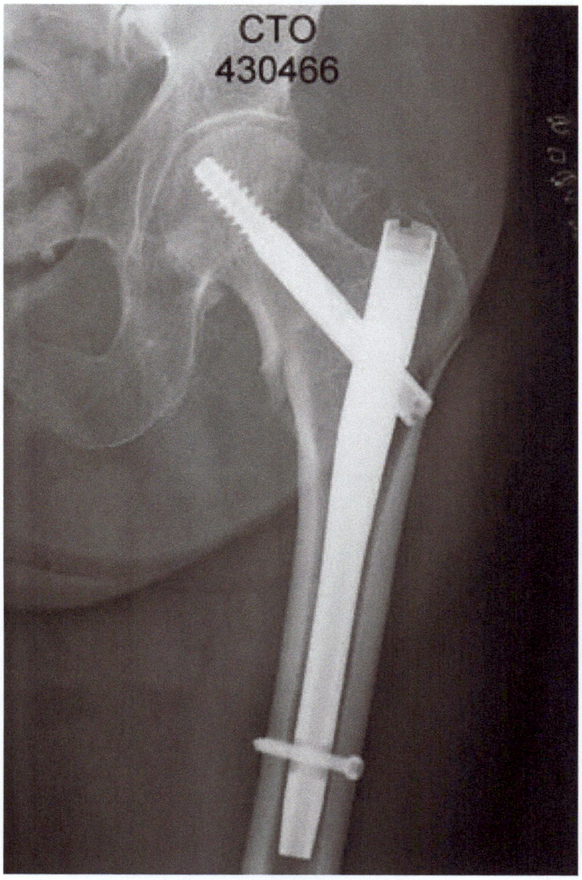

Fig. 4.6.1. Postoperative X-ray of titanium Gamma3 in a basi-cervical fracture

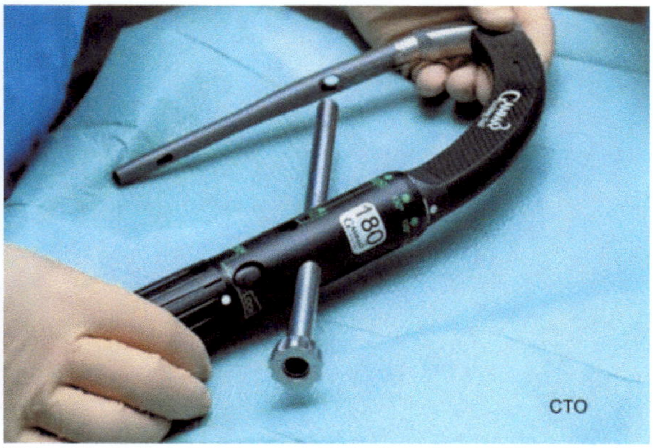

Fig. 4.6.2. The new target device for all nail angles

and second-generation nails, are not compatible with the newest generation nail.

The technique described will be that for the nail 180 mm in length (nails 170 mm in length are used in Asia).

Operative Technique

Patient positioning and fracture reduction is identical to that described in *Practice of Intramedullary Locked Nails*, Vol. 1.

The incision, made in relationship to the greater trochanter, can usually be shorter, given the decreased impingement of the nail insertion guide on the proximal part of the incision. Also, the use of fluoronavigation techniques permits even greater accuracy for determining the incision. The starting point of the incision is located at the junction of two lines, perpendicular to each other:

- The first of these lines is vertical, located at the tip of the greater trochanter. It can be determined with the aid of a metal tool as a marker, by taking an anteroposterior (AP) view with the image intensifier
- The second of these lines is horizontal and follows the diaphyseal axis of the femur (it may also be located using a drill held in alignment with the lateral cortex).

A first dot is marked on the horizontal of these two lines, located 2 cm cranial to their intersection; then, a second dot is marked 2 cm proximal to the previous one (Fig. 4.6.3). The incision is made between the two marked points, which can only be 2 cm long!

The opening of the tip of the greater trochanter is now accomplished ideally by the use of the cannulated awl. This same awl can equally be used with fluoronavigation and can be positioned perfectly. In all cases, it makes the insertion of the reaming guide wire easier, especially in the obese patient. Care must be taken to use a 3-mm diameter guide wire, to insure that it will pass through the cannulation of the awl (Fig. 4.6.4).

Alternative techniques may be used, particularly that using a rigid, conical reamer (Fig. 4.6.5). This conical reamer will prepare just the proximal part of the femur. It is inserted after the guide wire for reaming has been placed in the traditional manner, or after having placed a Kirschner wire in the tip of the greater trochanter. This reamer should be used with the T-handle and not

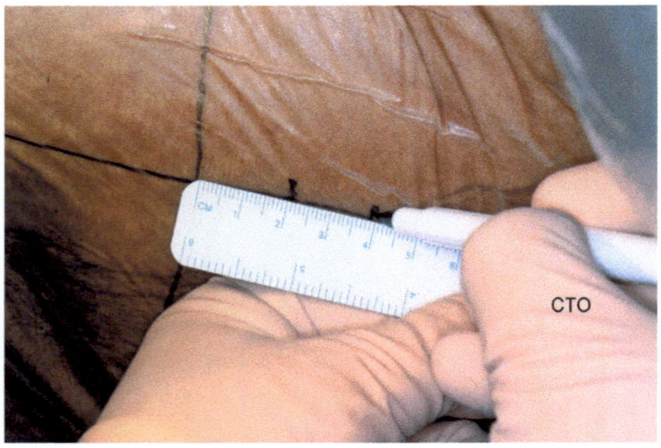

Fig. 4.6.3. Preparation for the 2-cm long incision

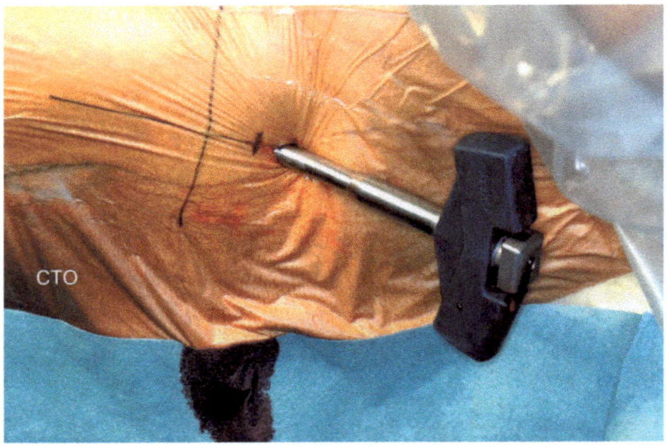

Fig. 4.6.4. The use of a cannulated awl for the opening of the greater trochanter

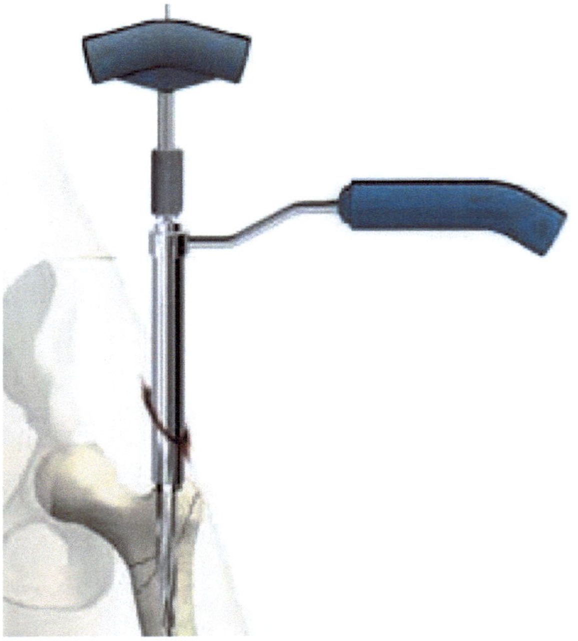

Fig. 4.6.5. The rigid conical reamer as an alternative technique to open the medullary canal

with a power tool, in order not to risk damaging the anterior or posterior regions of the greater trochanter (Fig. 4.6.5).

This technique is recommended only for elderly patients with very large canals.

Reaming is carried out in the classical fashion, i.e., to a diameter 2 mm greater in the diaphyseal area than the diameter of the nail to be used (e.g., reaming to 13 mm for a nail diameter of 11 mm). The proximal part should be reamed to at least 15.5 mm, to avoid nail incarceration upon insertion, especially in young patients, in whom the cancellous bone is still quite dense.

Assembly of the nail guide should be done in a very precise sequence, beginning with knowing that the locking part of the device must first be affixed onto the intermediate section of the device, with all targeting parameters, before attaching it to the rest of the assembly.

Nail insertion is done by hand, without the use of a mallet, in order to reduce the risk of creating additional fractures or damaging the targeting device. The nail is inserted to the correct level when the proximal hole for the lag screw aligns with the inferior part of the neck on the AP view. Two additional techniques can help in achieving this alignment:

- One is the use of an additional guide made of carbon fiber, with metal markers embedded (OneShot device), clipped onto the proximal sleeve and which indicates the eventual location of the Kirschner wire (Fig. 4.6.6).
- The other is targeting with the assistance of fluoronavigation, which gives precision in millimeters in the two planes sent to the computer and screen. This system also permits measuring the length of the lag screw. The big advantage, of course, is being able to adjust the future position of the lag screw, without being obligated to use the image intensifier at each device position change, thanks to the digitization of the images, which are stored in the computer's drive (Fig. 4.6.7).

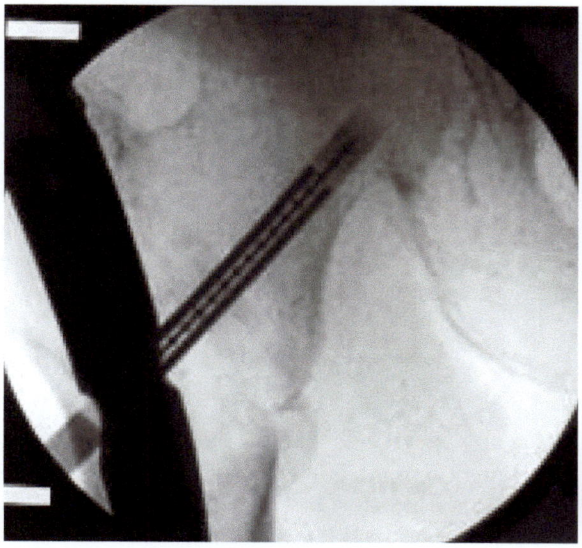

Fig. 4.6.6. AP view control on the image intensifier of the OneShot device

Lag-screw insertion starts with the opening of the lateral cortex (prior to this step, be sure that the reaming guide wire has been removed!). Unlike the old techniques, where the opening was achieved with a large pointed awl, the new technique uses a guide sleeve and a 4.2-mm diameter drill. This facilitates the opening of the cortex, especially if the lateral cortex is thick; and what is more, the use of the drill avoids secondary displacement of the nail insertion guide.

Insertion of the (Kirschner) lag-screw guide wire is then done, once the appropriate guide sleeve has been exchanged. It is best to do the insertion using the universal handle rather than with a power tool, the latter being potentially dangerous if it tends not to stop upon trigger release. Remember that the ideal position of the Kirschner wire is that of the inferior part of the neck, as seen on the AP view, and in the midline, as seen on the lateral view. The tip of the guide wire must be placed in the subchondral bone.

The measurement for the lag screw is done with a ruler, from which a direct reading is taken (Fig. 4.6.8). The reference point for this new ruler is the outer lag-screw targeting sleeve. This means that the measurement can be taken with or without having removed the smaller, k-wire sleeve. The one measurement taken indicates: (1) the set-

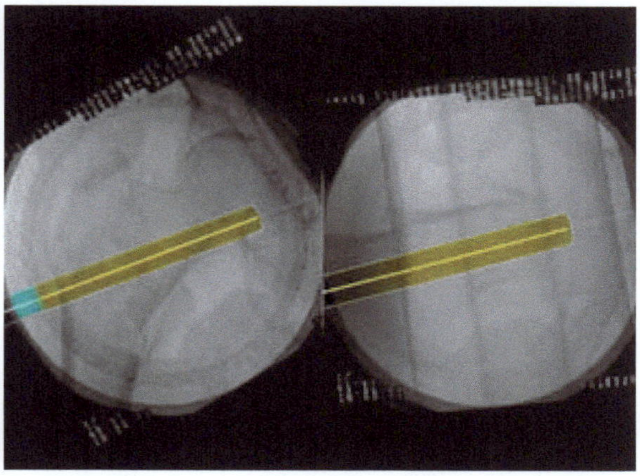

Fig. 4.6.7. Use of the navigation system to prepare to position the Kirschner wire

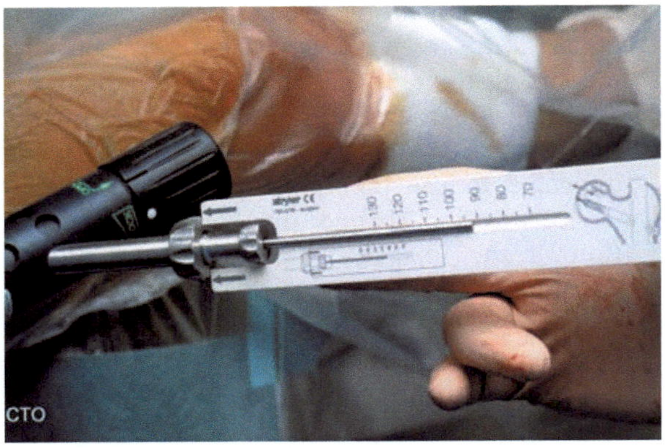

Fig. 4.6.8. The new ruler for lag-screw measurement

ting for the lag-screw reamer, as well as (2) the length of lag screw to be inserted. There is no longer the need to add or subtract from the measurement taken. Remember that the Kirschner wires are one-use only, since they may be damaged/deformed during insertion. If even slightly bent, they can be advanced into an intrapelvic position by the lag-screw reamer.

Reaming for the lag screw is done after setting the reaming depth, the measurement being read from the ruler. A new feature in the reamer is the presence of a "window" that helps to verify the position of the Kirschner wire and to keep an eye on any migration thereof. The reamer should be inserted by hand using the T-handle; again, this is preferable to using a power tool. The reaming is complete when the stop on the reamer comes into contact with the lag-screw sleeve.

Lag-screw fixation is done using a 10.5-mm diameter lag screw, passed over the Kirschner wire, after the reamer has been removed. Screw fixation is more easily achieved, compared to that with earlier implants, thanks to modifications incorporated into the design of the lag-screw threads. The lag-screw insertion is complete when the circumferential groove on the inserter is at the level of the lag-screw sleeve.

The handle of the lag-screw inserter must be either perpendicular to or in line with the nail targeting device, to ensure that the grooves in the lag screw are positioned to receive the set screw. The set screw is introduced through the nail targeting device by using a straight or, according to the patient's anatomy, a flexible screw driver.

Distal cross-locking can be carried out in a static or dynamic fashion. In fact, the distal locking hole is oblong and the position of the locking screw in this hole will determine the type of cross-locking achieved.

If the screw is located in the most proximal part of the hole, the cross-locking will be static. On the other hand, if the screw is placed in the distal part of the hole, one can expect a dynamization effect of the order of 5 mm. Dynamic cross-locking is indicated if there is a persistent diastasis at the level where the fracture starts, especially if the fracture focal area level is situated in the high, subtrochanteric region.

The targeting device is, therefore, set according to the type of cross-locking desired.

Once the distal targeting sleeve is put in place, the 4.2-mm drill will be used. This drill is graduated, allowing one easily to determine the length of the distal locking screw. Determine screw length:

- by taking a reading on the drill, once it has come into contact with the medial cortex (but not through it) and adding 5 mm to the reading,
- by taking a direct measurement from the drill, once it has slightly passed through the medial cortex, or
- one can equally use a conventional depth gauge.

The screw to be put in place is a fully threaded screw that is 5 mm in diameter and whose length is the full length of the screw itself, including the head.

An end-cap can optionally be put onto the end of the nail. Its theoretical advantage of making extraction of the nail easier has not been shown in our service.

Removal of the implant can be carried out using the same incisions. We prefer first to locate the lag screw and to place a Kirschner wire in its cannulation. This makes it easier to attach the lag-screw driver. Then the set screw is removed, followed by the lag screw.

The extractor for the nail itself is inserted. Finally, the distal cross-locking screw is removed, followed by the extraction of the nail. We prefer to put the nail extractor in place while the nail is still locked distally, in order to prevent pushing the nail deeper into the canal, which could make the removal more difficult.

Long Gamma Nail

The long Gamma nail was also modified. While the proximal portion of the nail is identical to its shorter counterpart, the distal part has two cross-locking holes:

- one round hole (the more proximal of the two)

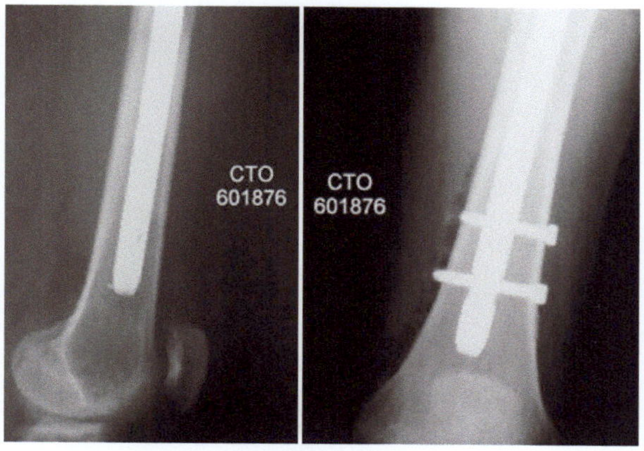

Fig. 4.6.9. Distal locking features of the long Gamma3 nail

- one oblong hole (the more distal of the two), which allows for the insertion of a cross-locking screw in either static or dynamic mode (Fig. 4.6.9). It is evident that the latter mode is possible only with the use of the oblong hole.

The most significant modification is found in the radius of curvature of the nail, which is now 2 m (compared to 3 m in previous generations). This radius has a better conformity to the curvature of the femur. This is of interest during prophylactic nailing of the femur for metastasis.

The operative technique is the same as for the first part of the surgery of the short nail. The distal cross-locking can be done either using freehand techniques or, equally, by using fluoronavigation techniques.

Evolution of Implants for Trochanteric Fracture Fixation: The Engineer's Point of View

H. Müller-Daniels

Trochanteric Intramedullary Fixation Devices

More than 65 years ago, in November 1939, Gerhard Küntscher implanted his first intramedullary nail in a shipyard worker who had fallen off the dock and broken his femur. This implant had been developed by Küntscher and manufactured by Ernst Pohl in Kiel, Germany. This initial treatment was the beginning point for the breakthrough of closed intramedullary nailing, which today is accepted as "state of the art" in fracture treatment.

Starting with this initial experience, Gerhard Küntscher was constantly refining and improving the implants. He was constantly working on new ideas for implants to treat more and more different types of fractures.

For the treatment of proximal femur fractures he developed the Y-nail in 1960. At that time Küntscher recognized that intramedullary fracture fixation in proximal thigh bones significantly improves the biomechanical stability in comparison to a conventional side plate construct. This was due to the shorter lever arm, as measured by d<D, especially in terms of load-bearing (Fig. 4.7.1).

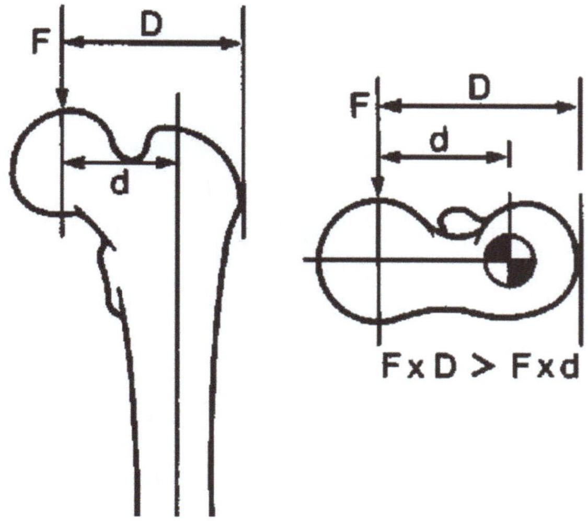

Fig. 4.7.1. Biomechanical advantage of intramedullary fixation versus extramedullary fixation

Nowadays side plates are called compression hip screws (CHS); the majority of them were not designed for the treatment of unstable proximal and subtrochanteric femur fractures and allowing full weight-bearing postoperatively. Treating these types of fractures with CHS as they were developed by McLaughlin in 1947 or Pohl in 1950 very often led to implant failures due to biomechanical overload. The dynamic hip screw, invented by Synthes in 1980, also did so [17–20].

Dr. Grosse at CTO in Strasbourg, France, as well as Dr. Halder and Mr. Gill in Halifax, UK, further developed in parallel and independent from each other the idea of intramedullary fixation at the beginning of the 1980s. After both designs were finalized in the Gamma nail, the so-called standard Gamma nail (SGN) was launched in 1988 (Fig. 4.7.2 a). This was the first intramedullary hip fracture fixation device allowing full weight-bearing because of its strong implant design. That is why it was able to treat all stable and unstable as well as ipsilateral and pathological femur fractures.

Clinical support for the Gamma nail was given by A. Grosse and G. Taglang from CTO, Strasbourg, France, from the beginning. Since the market introduction the product range was completed by long Gamma nails and special nail shapes for the Asian population, the so-called AP and AP-J Gamma nails.

In 1997, the second-generation nail, the trochanteric Gamma nail (TGN), was launched (Fig. 4.7.2 b). Its design was based on 9 years of clinical experience with the SGN. The TGN was improved by shortening the nail by 2 cm and reducing the medial-lateral bend from 10° to 4°. These changes led to an optimized shape of the nail and to an even better clinical outcome [9–15] of the implant. More than 750,000 Gamma nail implantations have been performed so far. This seems to be very clear evidence that this is the right direction for intramedullary treatment with Gamma nails [1–8] in trochanteric fracture fixation. In 2001, a full range of tita-

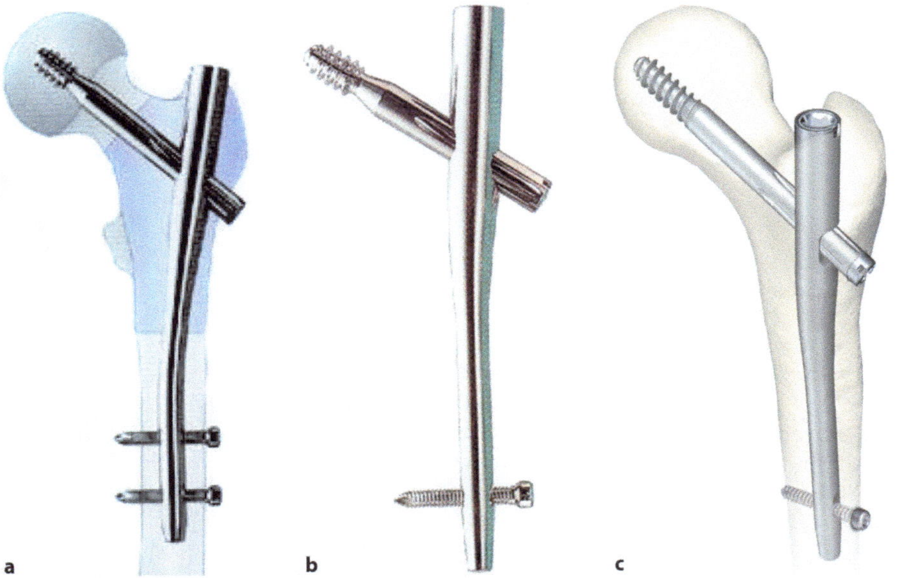

Fig. 4.7.2. Three generations of the Gamma nail: a SGN, 1988; b TGN, 1997; c Gamma3, 2004

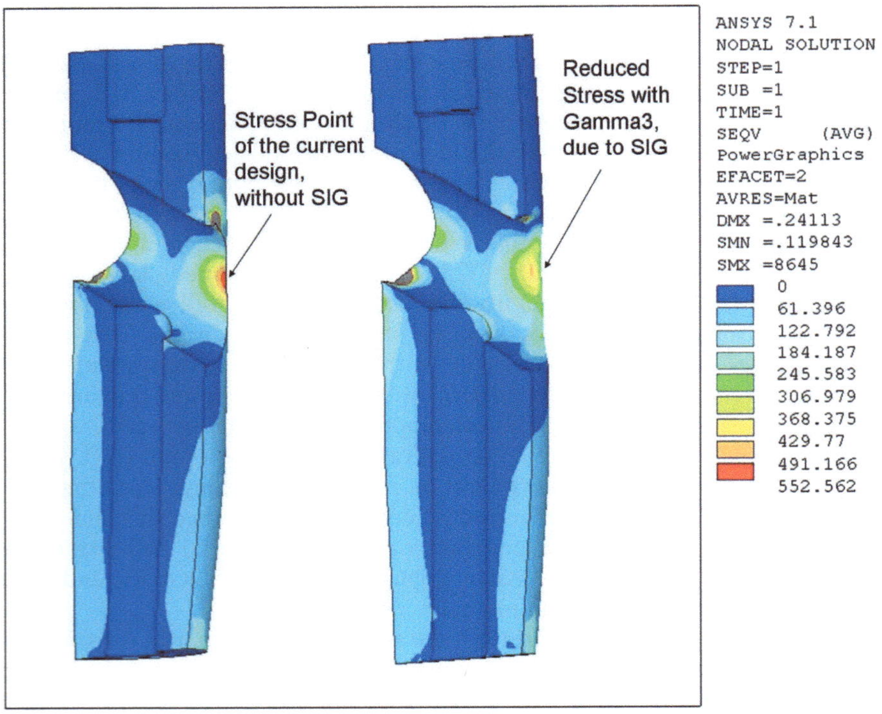

Fig. 4.7.3. Finite element analysis to reduce the proximal nail diameter

nium implants was launched under the name of Dyax-Asiatic and Gamma-Ti, mainly in Japan and Europe, to address surgeons' needs.

The concept of the Gamma nail has been copied by more than 20 orthopedic companies during the past decade.

After more than 15 years of clinical experience, the development of the third generation of Gamma nails started in the year 2001 with the contribution of leading surgeons of the AIOD and other trauma associations. Benchmarking the clinically successful TGN, the targets for the third genera-

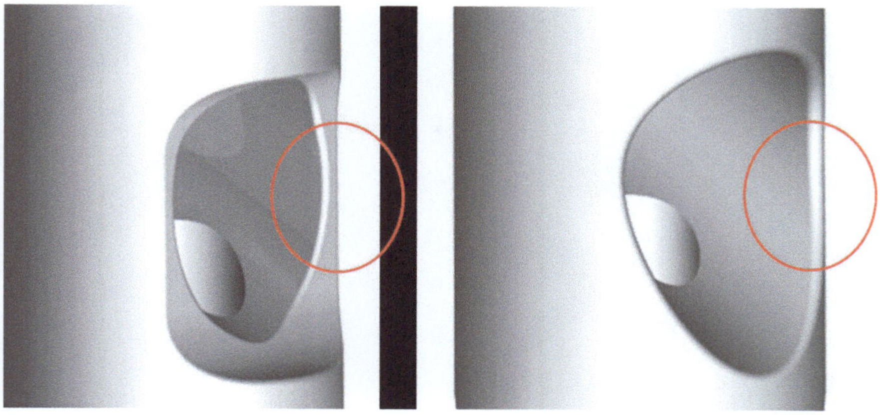

Fig. 4.7.4. Strength improvement groove (*left*)

tion of Gamma nails, the so-called Gamma3 nail system (Fig. 4.7.2 c), were as follows:

- Minimally invasive approach
- Offer lag-screw options for broader indications
- Develop operating room time-saving instruments.

The engineering part of the design of the new Gamma nail generation was clearly defined. These three major points gave the engineers of Stryker a difficult time to reach their target: minimizing the diameter of the implants without compromising the strength and the cut-out resistance of the implants and developing instruments to allow minimally invasive surgery.

Thanks to the support of high-end computer-aided finite element analyses programs (Figs. 4.7.3 and 4.7.4) and intense biomechanical dynamic laboratory testing, it was possible to reduce the proximal diameter of the nail to 15.5 mm, providing the same strength as the current 17-mm TGN. The patented shape of the strength improvement groove (Fig. 4.7.4) was the main factor allowing minimization of the proximal part of the nails.

The new implants of the Gamma3 nail system allow removal of approximately 16–20% less bone from the trochanteric region than other proximal femur nails with a proximal diameter of 17 mm and larger.

The Gamma3 nails are available in three neck shaft angles: 120° for coxa vara, 125° as standard nail angle and 130° for coxa valgus indications.

The diameter of the lag screw was minimized to 10.5 mm, at the same time increasing the cut-out resistance. This ambitious goal was realized because of the newly designed thread of the lag screw (Fig. 4.7.5) and verified by extensive biomechanical testing (Fig. 4.7.6), which confirmed the high cut-out performance.

However, minimally invasive surgery is not only related to the implant size – instruments also

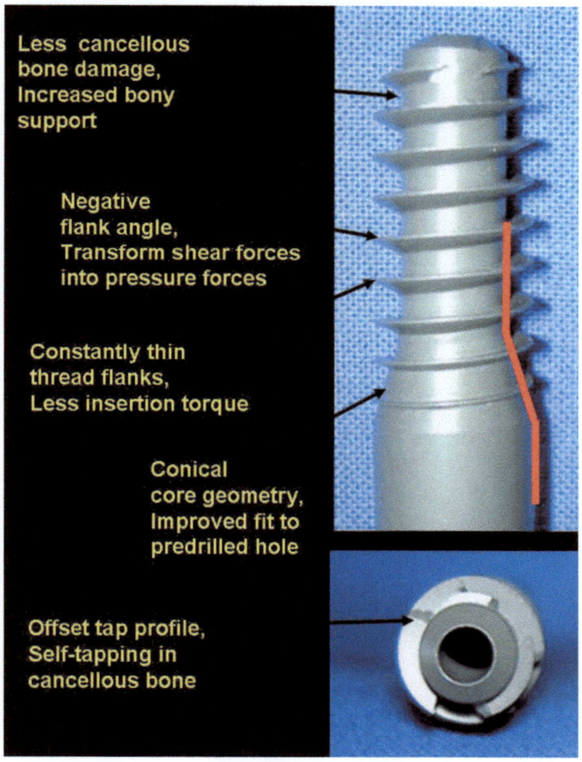

Fig. 4.7.5. New Gamma3 lag-screw geometry

play a big role in reaching this goal. The new generation of Gamma3 instruments work perfectly together with the implants (results of early product surveillance). They allow small skin incisions for implantation, which lead to less blood loss and less risk of infections (Fig. 4.7.7).

The instruments offer options for personal surgeons' preferences; the fragment control clip will provide additional fragment stability of the femoral head, for example (Fig. 4.7.8). That will stabilize the femoral head during lag-screw hole preparation and insertion, in cases of unstable and short head–neck fragments.

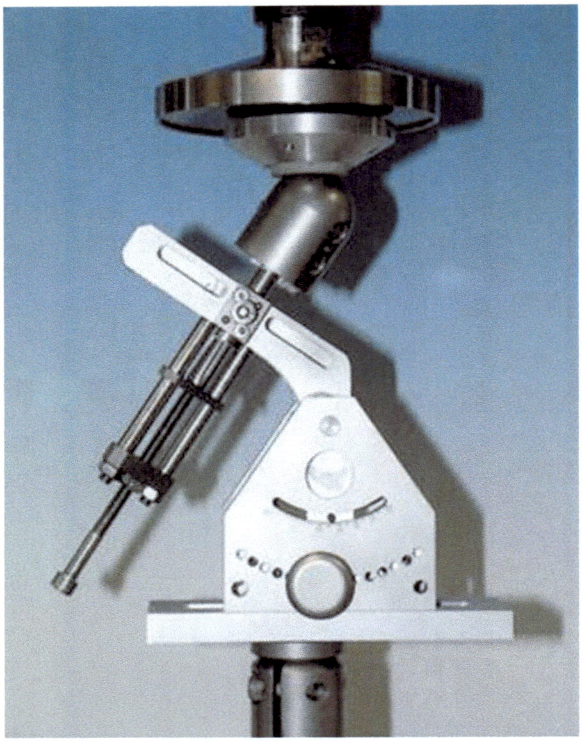

Fig. 4.7.6. Set-up for dynamic cut-out testing

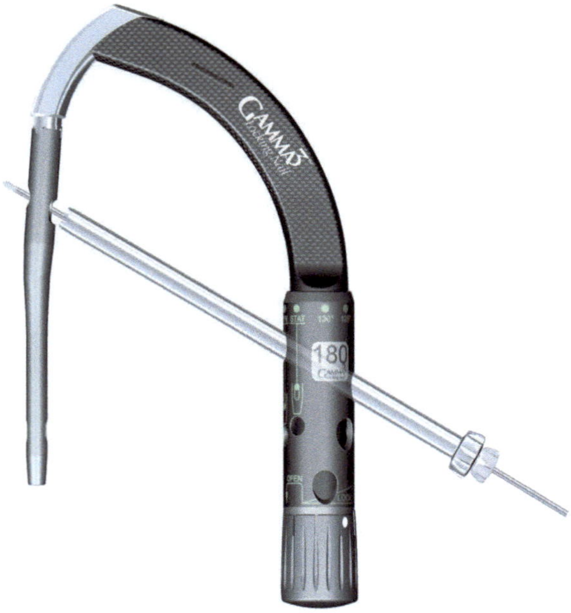

Fig. 4.7.7. Gamma3 targeting device

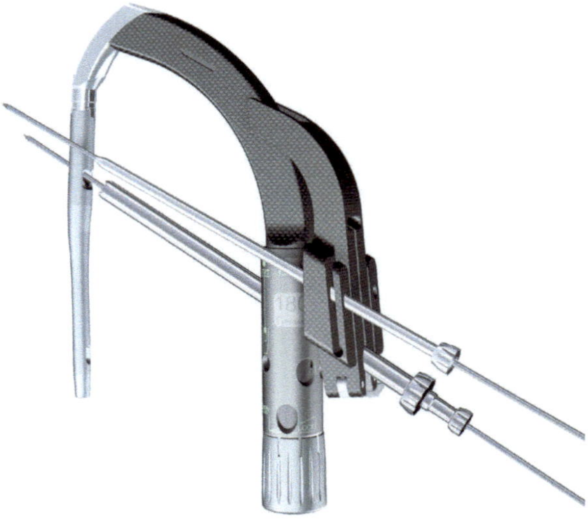

Fig. 4.7.8. Gamma3 targeting device plus fragment control clip

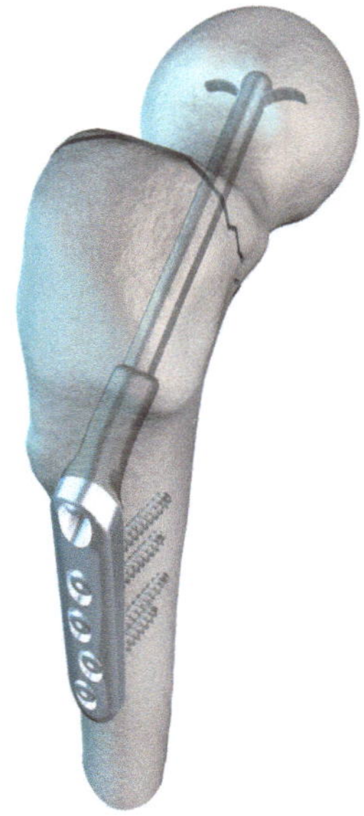

Fig. 4.7.9. Omega2 hip plate with twin hook fixation

Trochanteric Hip Screw Devices

Development in the CHS segment is not standing still either. In order to allow smaller incisions for treatment with CHS in stable situations, a new cephalic device was developed (Fig. 4.7.9). This new implant option was developed in Sweden and is called twin hook. It allows plate implantation before the cephalic part follows. Therefore it avoids rotational forces to the femoral head and provides additional rotational stability when it is implanted.

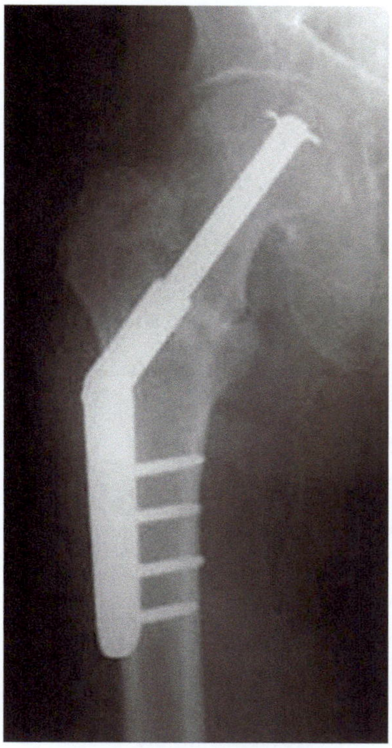

Fig. 4.7.10. X-ray of Omega2 hip plate with twin hook fixation

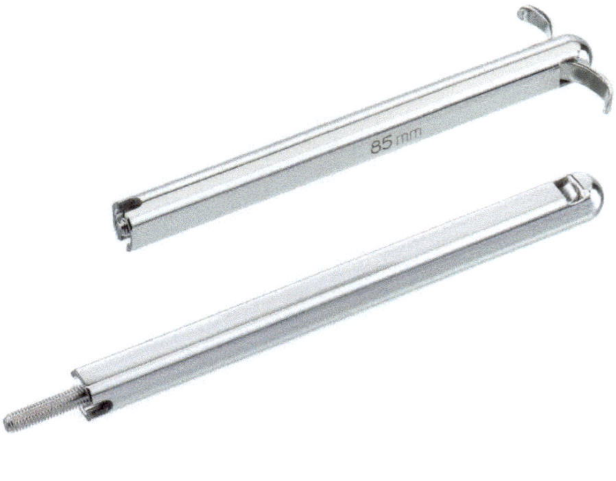

Fig. 4.7.11. Twin hook: *left* delivery status; *right* expanded hooks

The twin hook consists of two parts, an inner sliding tongue and an outer pin, which is 9 mm in diameter and compatible with the Omega2 hip plate. Fixing the twin hook in the femoral head is achieved by pushing the inner sliding tongue out through the proximal windows using a simple insertion device. By curling round and out about 10 mm on each side, the hooks give a durable fixation in the femoral head (Figs. 4.7.10 and 4.7.11).

A big clinical advantage of this design is the minimal invasive approach of the hip plate insertion because the plate can be implanted before the twin hook is placed. Even in cases of postoperative complications, the twin hook can be removed without removing the plate.

Clinically the twin hook is also used successfully in combination with the Medoff plate [16].

Navigation in Trochanteric Fracture Fixation

Navigation in trauma treatment is becoming increasingly important. A more precise implant placement improves surgical accuracy in order to minimize failure and complication rates. Especially in trochanteric fracture treatment, navigation will allow reduction of:

- X-ray exposure to surgeon and patient
- Cut-out rate, due to exact lag-screw placement and entry point determination
- Soft tissue damage, due to exact prediction of incision point
- Size and number of mechanical guidance instruments.

Furthermore it supports young and inexperienced surgeons in their training.

Due to the above-mentioned clinical advantages, navigation will play a much bigger role in terms of fracture treatment in the very near future.

Prospects

Evolution never stands still. Requests regarding product improvements and cost reductions in total patient care and treatment arrive nearly daily from the clinical and the economic side. Fracture treatment should be done in a way that ensures security and is cost-effective. Fracture treatment is expected to be done simply and fast using excellent working implants and instruments, while postoperative complications related to this and surgical techniques have to be reduced to a minimum.

Today most of the implant systems work mechanically with fixed guided instruments and target devices for the locking procedure. Therefore one of the most requested instruments for combined trochanteric and shaft fracture treatment is a reliable distal locking system for long nails. This device should also reduce X-ray exposure. A very promising distal targeting system will be available for the newest Gamma3 nail generation.

Navigation systems are evolving fast. In future trauma surgery they will allow the surgeons much better orientation and visualization of the anatomic situation.

Another breakthrough in the treatment of fractures will come with the further introduction of bioresorbable implants. Bioresorbable materials are going to become stronger and stronger. These new implants will probably take over a wide range of fracture treatment from conventional metal implants to bioresorbable implants. This may pave the way for further developments in the twenty-first century.

References

1. Parker MJ. Failure of femoral head fixation: a cadaveric analysis of lag-screw cut-out with the gamma locking nail and the AO dynamic hip screw. Injury 1998; 29 (7): 569.
2. Haynes RC, Poll RG, Miles AW, Weston RB. Failure of femoral head fixation: a cadaveric analysis of lag screw cut-out with the gamma locking nail and AO dynamic hip screw. Injury 1997; 28 (5/6): 337–341.
3. Leung KS, So WS, Shen WY, Hui PW. Gamma nails and dynamic hip screws for peritrochanteric fractures. A randomised prospective study in elderly patients. J Bone Joint Surg Br 1992; 74 (3): 345–351.
4. Guyer P, Landolt M, Eberle C, Keller H. The Gamma nail as a resilient alternative to the dynamic hip screw in unstable proximal femoral fractures in the elderly. Helvetica Chirurgica Acta 1992; 58 (5): 697–703.
5. Guyer P, Landolt M, Keller H, Eberle C. The Gamma nail in per- and intertrochanteric femoral fractures – alternative or supplement to the dynamic hip screw? A prospective randomized study of 100 patients with per- and intertrochanteric femoral fractures in the surgical clinic of the City Hospital of Triemli, Zurich, September 1989–June 1990. Aktuelle Traumatologie 1991; 21 (6): 242–249.
6. Dujardin FH, Benez C, Polle G, Alain J, Biga N, Thomine JM. Prospective randomized comparison between a dynamic hip screw and a mini-invasive static nail in fractures of the trochanteric area: preliminary results. J Orthop Trauma 2001; 15 (6): 401–406.
7. Mockwitz J, Ernst S. Operative Versorgung per- und subtrochantärer Femurfrakturen – Gammanagel oder dynamische Hüftschraube? Osteosynthese International 2001; 9: 211–215.
8. Haynes RC, Poll RG, Miles AW, Weston RB. An experimental study of the failure modes of the gamma locking nail and the AO dynamic hip screw under static loading: a cadaveric study. Medical Engineering Phys 1997; 19 (5): 446–453.
9. Lyddon DW Jr. The prevention of complications with the Gamma locking nail. Am J Orthop 1996; 25 (5): 357–363.
10. Friess P, Rader L. The Gamma nail. Indications, technique and early results. Zentralblatt für Chirurgie 1992; 117: 132–138.
11. Hotz TK, Zellweger R, Kach KP. Minimal invasive treatment of proximal femur fractures with the long Gamma nail: indication, technique, results. J Trauma 1999; 47 (5): 942–945.
12. Hotz TK, Breitenstein S, Di Lazzaro M, Keach KP. Trochanteric Gamma nail: a prospective clinical study on the treatment of peritrochanteric femoral fractures. OTA sat.10/20/01, Pelvis/Geriatrics, Paper #66, 11,30 AM; 179–180.
13. Rosenwasser MP, Sinicropi SM. Proximal femoral fractures. Orthopedic Special Edition, Vol. 6, 2000.
14. Bruce H, Ziran MD, Klatt B, Darowish M. Outcomes of Gamma nail fixation for peritrochanteric femur fractures. www.orthonet.upmc.edu/TraumDiv/Ziran/Gamma.html
15. Karich B. Probleme mit dem y-Nagel – Optimierungsmöglichkeiten, Trauma und Berufskrankheit 2003; 5 (Suppl 2): S175–S183.
16. Olsson O. Alternative techniques in trochanteric hip fracture surgery. Clinical and biomechanical studies on the Medoff sliding plate and the twin hook. Acta Orthop Scand 2000; 295 (Suppl): 1–31.
17. Landolt M. Comparison and presentation of technique and results of the Gamma nail and dynamic hip screw. Helvetica Chirurgica Acta 1993; 59 (5/6): 965–969.
18. Flahiff CM, Nelson CL, Gruenwald JM, Hollis JM. A biomechanical evaluation of an intramedullary fixation device for intertrochanteric fractures. J Trauma 1993; 35: 23–27.
19. Haynes RC, Poll RG, Miles AW, Weston RB. An experimental study of the failure modes of the Gamma locking nail and the AO dynamic hip screw under static loading: a cadaveric study. Medical Engineering Phys 1997; 19 (5): 446–453.
20. Leung KS, So WS, Shen WY, Hui PW. Gamma nails and dynamic hip screws for peritrochanteric fractures. A randomised prospective study in elderly patients. J Bone Joint Surg Br 1992; 74 (3): 345–351.

A New Concept in the Treatment of Fibular Fractures with Intramedullary Implants

W. Roth, M. Weber

Introduction

Closed intramedullary techniques have largely replaced the use of plates and screws in the treatment of long bone fractures. The goal in treating distal fibular fractures is either to reconstruct the ankle mortise, thereby achieving a functional, painless ankle as the final outcome, or, if the fracture is combined with a distal tibial fracture, to stabilize the distal tibia against rotation or valgus dislocation by reduction and fixation. Reduction of the lateral malleolus can be obtained in a closed or open fashion. Many methods of internal fixation of the distal fibula are advocated. These include tension band wires [3, 4, 11], malleolar or cancellous screws [1], cerclage wires [11], plates and screws [11, 13, 14], intramedullary fixation with Steinmann pins, Rush rods, Inyo or SST nails [14–16] and intramedullary screw fixation [5].

The classic technique of internal fixation with plates and screws, lag screws or both is a popular choice, as it provides stable anatomic fixation of the fracture and produces excellent results [6]. Nevertheless, several authors have criticized this method for the lateral paucity of overlying soft tissue and the fact that patients complain about painful prominent hardware [13]. Additionally, open reduction and internal fixation of the lateral malleolus may be difficult in elderly patients with bad skin conditions and osteoporotic bones and can lead to an increased risk of wound breakdown and infection [2, 12].

Intramedullary fixation of lateral malleolus fractures or distal fibular fractures has been associated with two major complications. Some reports described a shortening of the fibula during insertion that resulted in a widened ankle mortise [17]. A second complication involves implant migration, which results in patients suffering from painful prominent hardware (Fig. 4.8.1). Authors who therefore utilized a long intramedullary self-taping screw to counteract these problems were able to reduce these hardware complications [1,

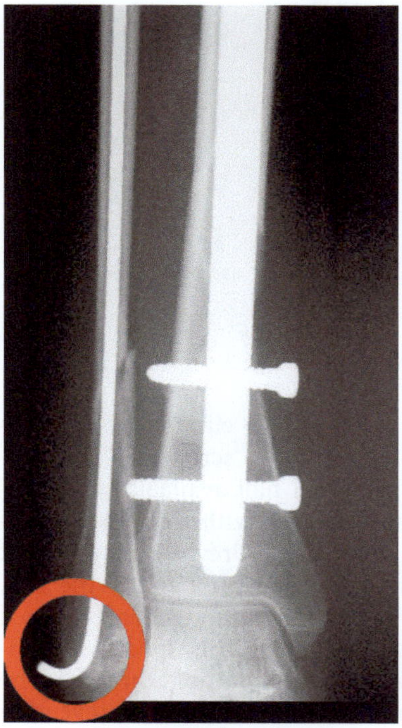

Fig. 4.8.1. Prominent hardware with painful soft tissue problems

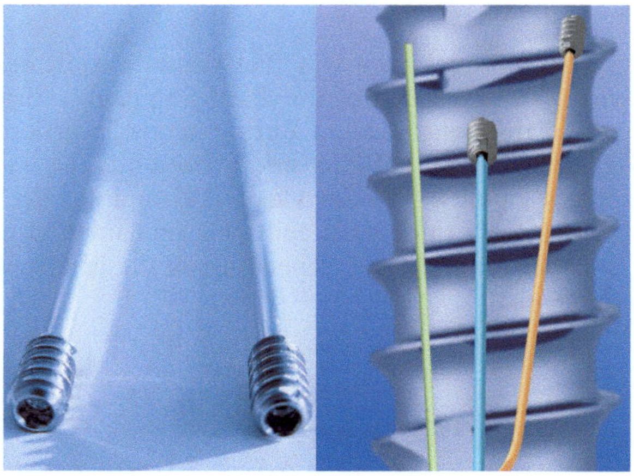

Fig. 4.8.2. Screw nail with turnable threaded head

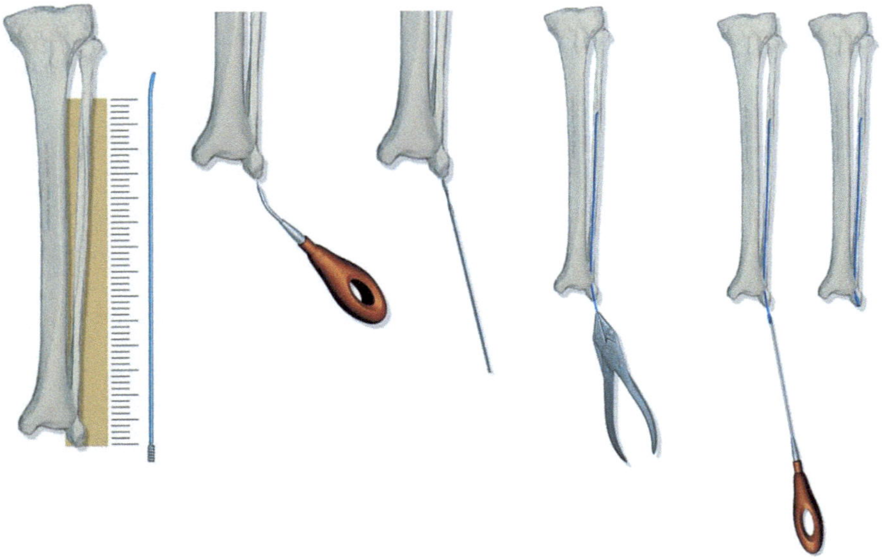

Fig. 4.8.3. Technique of the implantation of the screw nail

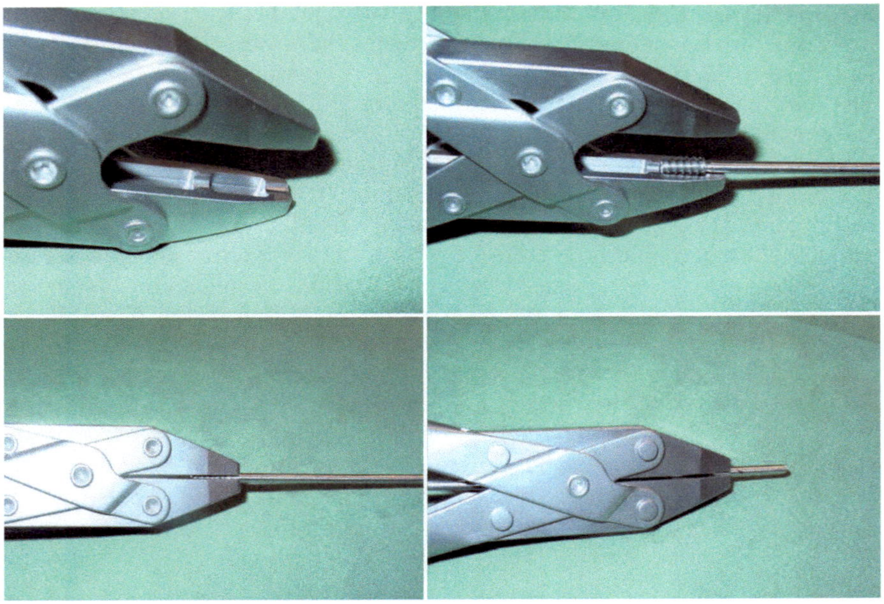

Fig. 4.8.4. Demonstration of the use of the pliers

5]. The disadvantage was that these fixation devices led to rotation of the distal fragment, which was mainly encountered during screw insertion. Another problem of long screw fixation is the implant's rigidity. The Inyo nail [14] and the SST nail [16] are thick nails and their implantation is not without problems, depending on the length of the fibula.

Materials and Methods

A new concept developed to eliminate the problems mentioned above is the "screw nail" or "thalon nail". It is a titanium nail available in diameters of 2.0, 2.5 and 3.0 mm with a pre-bent, flattened tip, and similar to the Prévot Nancy nail. A threaded head is positioned at the end of the nail, held in place by a circular running notch located on the nail shaft (Fig. 4.8.2). This special suspension design allows the self-cutting thread to be screwed in with a screwdriver while preventing rotation of the nail during insertion. Once inserted into the medullar cavity, the implant is

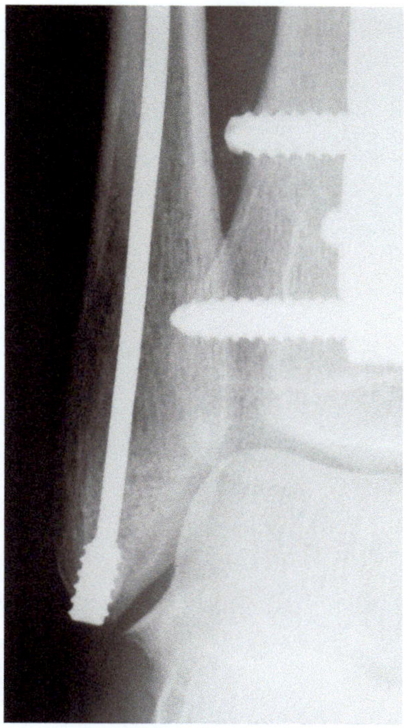

Fig. 4.8.5. Best position of the screw nail after implantation

fixed in the cortex and cannot dislocate during the course of fracture healing. Since the nail is inserted almost completely into the bone, soft tissue irritation is avoided. With this new nail design, the major complications associated with other devices mentioned above such as nail migration and soft tissue compromise are primarily avoided. Due to the graduation in length in 15-mm increments within a range of 90–300 mm, the screw nail can be used in long cortical bones as well as in cancellous areas near the joints.

Techniques and Positioning

Positioning of the new screw nail depends on the varying nature of the concomitant fractures, i.e., of the tibia. Under normal circumstances, the patient is placed in a supine position on a radiolucent table. The leg is prepped and draped above the knee. A small oblique incision is made distal to the tip of the fibula. The correct insertion point is lateral to the tip and is identified on an image intensifier (Fig. 4.8.3). The bone is opened with an awl. Subsequently, the cortex is reamed to allow the insertion of the threaded head. In oblique fibular fractures, reduction must be maintained with a towel clamp during nail insertion. The necessary length and thickness of the nail should be verified at this time either on the image intensifier or by placing the implant onto the extremity.

Now, the nail must be inserted by hand. Opening and closing the pliers facilitates gradual insertion of the nail; full insertion is achieved when the threads strike the end of the pliers' open jaw (Fig. 4.8.4). Then, the threaded head is advanced toward the bone with light hammer blows on the screwdriver until the first thread spiral has reached the cortex. Finally, the nail is screwed into the bone. The last thread spiral should be located outside of the bone and will make later location and removal of the implant easier (Fig. 4.8.5).

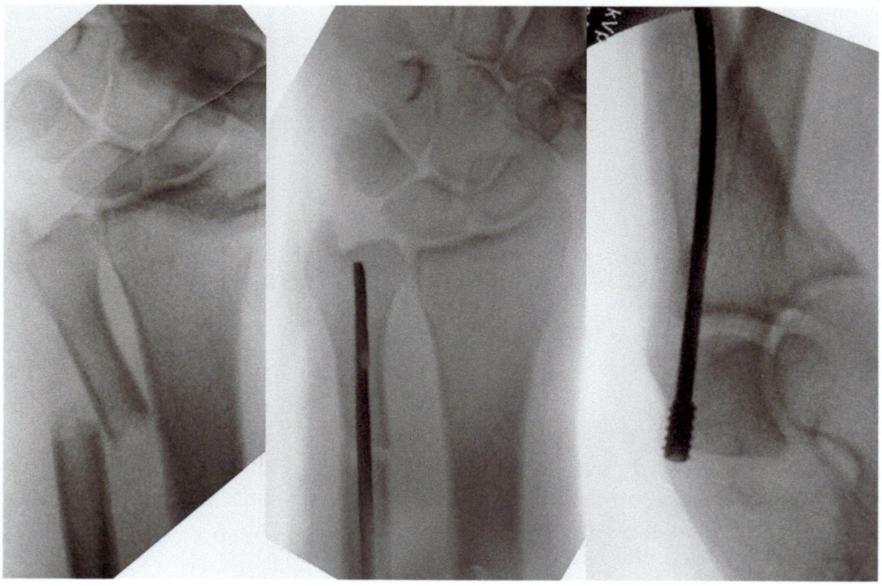

Fig. 4.8.6. Other indications of the screw nail include: isolated ulna fracture, fracture of the clavicle, fracture of the distal humerus

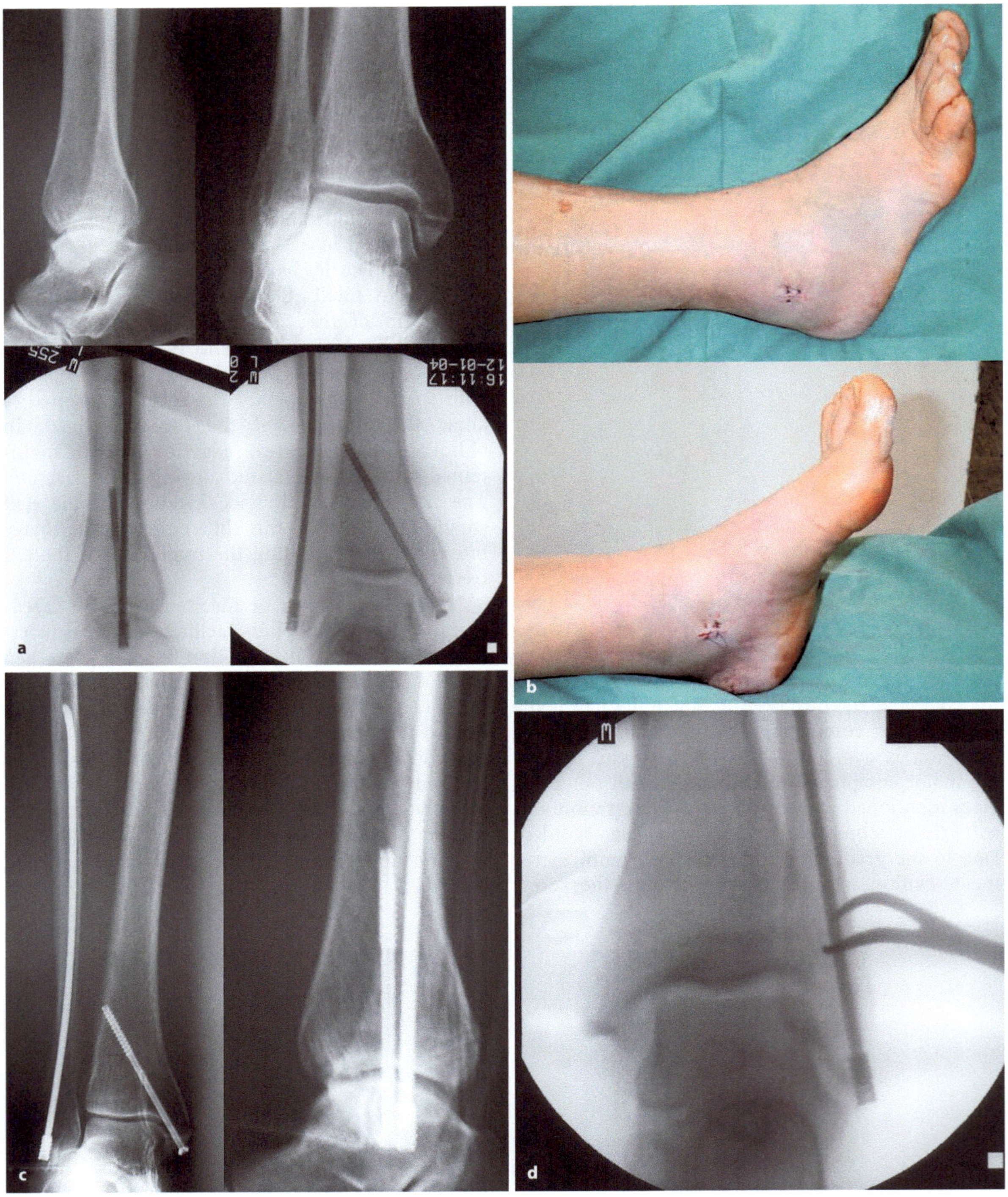

Fig. 4.8.7 a–d. Ankle fracture type Weber B, poor bone and skin conditions

Indications

The screw nail is indicated in all situations where minimally invasive procedures such as K wires, Rush pins, Prévot nails or other similar implants would otherwise be performed (Fig. 4.8.6). We have mostly used the screw nail for the treatment of distal fibular fractures such as ankle fractures, but also in combination with distal tibial fractures.

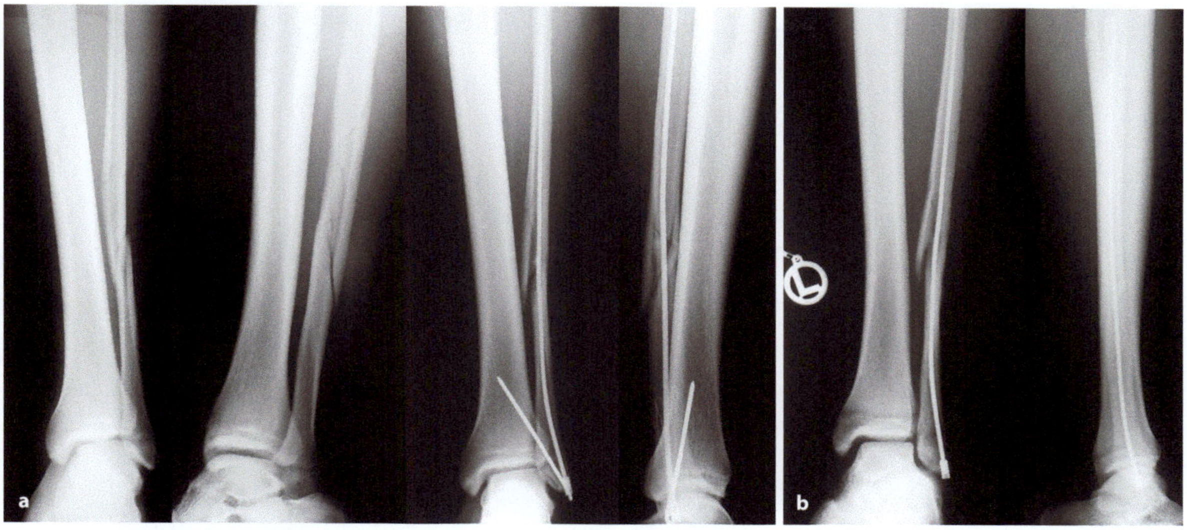

Fig. 4.8.8 a, b. Fibula shaft fracture with rupture of the tibio-fibular syndesmosis

Ankle Fractures

Elderly patients, particularly women, have poor skin and bone quality. Soft tissue damage can result in wound complications, and osteoporotic bone can contribute to fixation failure. The incision for nail insertion should not be made in an area prone to necrosis. The screw nail is an interlocking nail with distal static fixation and proximal dynamic situation. The nail is indicated in all kinds of Weber type B fractures and in all classifications of Weber type fractures in the elderly. Type C fractures additionally require tibiofibular fixation with a K wire to stabilize the syndesmosis. These are the only cases where an additional cast is needed (Fig. 4.8.7).

Advantages of fibula screw nailing for type B fractures in the elderly:

- Less invasive stabilization of the lateral column
- Better fixation in osteoporotic bones
- Minimal soft tissue dissection
- No additional cast needed.

If necessary, medial malleolar fixation should be performed with a cannulated screw and an additional K wire (Fig. 4.8.8).

A special indication is the treatment of the bimalleolar ankle fracture with luxation and fracture of Volkmann triangle in a patient with very poor skin conditions (Fig. 4.8.9).

Fibular Fractures in Combination with a Distal Tibial Fracture

When the tibia is intact, the fibula supports between 3% and 16% of the load transmitted through the lower extremity [7, 10, 18]. Therefore, when a tibial fracture is treated by fixation while the fibula remains intact, it is reasonable to expect that the fibula will assume some of this load-bearing role. Teitz et al. [19] found that an intact fibula may actually even delay healing in tibial fractures treated nonoperatively by distraction. However, little is known about the mechanical effect of the intact fibula on internally fixed tibial fractures.

As a result of their cadaver study, Kumar et al. [8] concluded that fibular plate fixation increased initial rotational stability secondary to distal tibial fracture compared with the initial rotational stability provided by tibial intramedullary nailing alone. When the applied torque was increased, no difference in rotational structural stiffness was observed between the specimens treated with and without plate fixation. Despite these results, the authors postulated that rotational stability in patients with ipsilateral distal tibial fractures treated with intramedullary tibial nailing can be increased by plate and screw fixation of the fibula, and that this method may also reduce the risk of valgus malunion.

In their study about the role of the fibular fixation in combined fractures of the tibia and fibula, Weber et al. concluded that fibular plating can decrease motion across a tibial defect but only when less rigid fixation (i.e., external fixation) of the

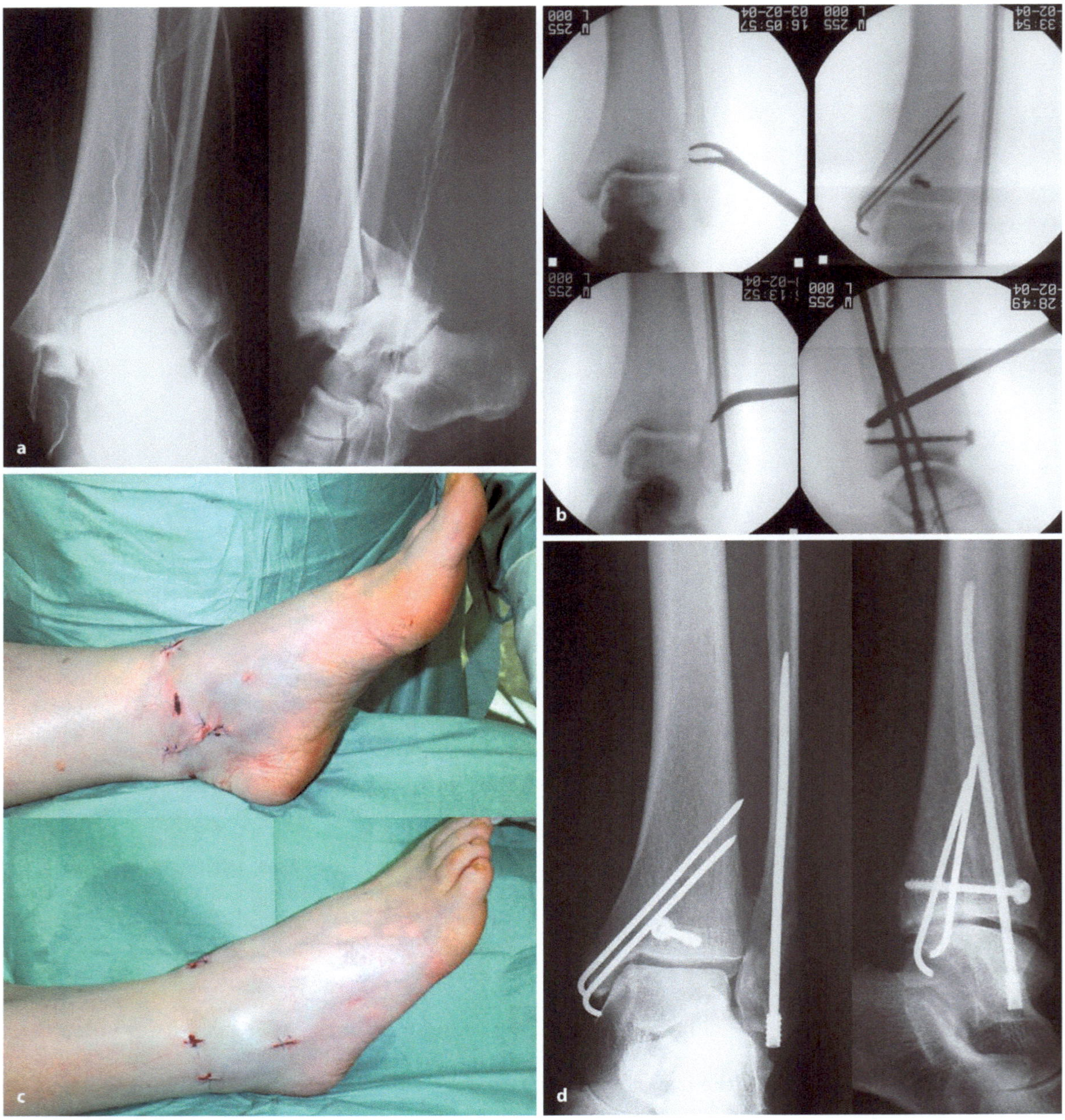

Fig. 4.8.9 a–d. Special indication: bimalleolar ankle fracture with luxation and fracture of Volkmann triangle with bad skin conditions

tibia is used [20]. The authors did not observe any difference between plate stabilization of the fibula and the use of an intramedullary rod, when the tibia is fixed with an intramedullary rod.

The first challenge posed by this technique is to achieve good closed anatomical reduction. The difficulty involved in holding the small distal fragment makes reduction of these distal fractures problematical [9].

The next challenge is how to maintain reduction. The disadvantage of the new locking nail generation designed with far distal locking holes is that the contact of the nail to the cortex is lost. There are several ways to solve the potential problems of achieving and maintaining reduction in these very distal types of tibial fractures. One solution to attain this aim is the fixation of the fibula using a plate or a nail.

For several years now at our hospital, we have routinely used intramedullary fixation to treat combined tibial and fibular fractures in the distal part of the leg.

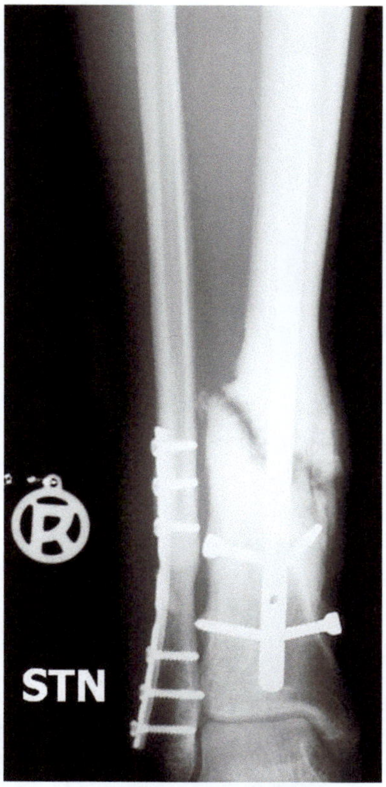

Fig. 4.8.10. Malunion: combined treatment with STN and fibular plate

We were able to achieve good outcomes with this type of treatment, particularly in fractures on the same level. We observed malunions and valgus deformities in some cases treated with tibial nail and fibular plate stabilization (Fig. 4.8.10). The reason was rigidity and stiffness of the fibular plate fixation. Most of these problems disappeared after we started using the method of fibular stabilization with an intramedullary implant (Fig. 4.8.11).

Krettek et al. [9] described an additional technique that relies on the use of blocking screws or Poller screws. By acting as a false endosteal cortex, these screws maintain fracture alignment by creating a "jamming" effect between screws and nail. In the early years of intramedullary fibular fixation, we used bent K wires. Once we switched to the new implant - the screw nail - with all the advantages we have illustrated above, we were able to avoid the soft tissue problems previously encountered at the distal fibula (Fig. 4.8.12).

Since then, our standard treatment for fractures of the distal tibia and fibula is only made dependent on the extent and nature of the soft tissue damage. In patients with open fractures or severe soft tissue injury, we first stabilize the tibia with an external fixator and the fibula with a screw nail (Fig. 4.8.13). After a couple of days, depending on the soft tissue situation, we change the instrumentation and stabilize the tibia with an interlocking nail.

Conclusion

The fibula screw nail is a new intramedullary implant effective in the treatment of small medullary bones. Compared with standard treatments employing plates and additional screws, this device is less invasive and minimizes soft tissue dissection, particularly in the fixation of distal fibular fractures. Patient comfort is enhanced and quicker fracture healing is promoted. Especially in osteoporotic bones, we have been able to achieve

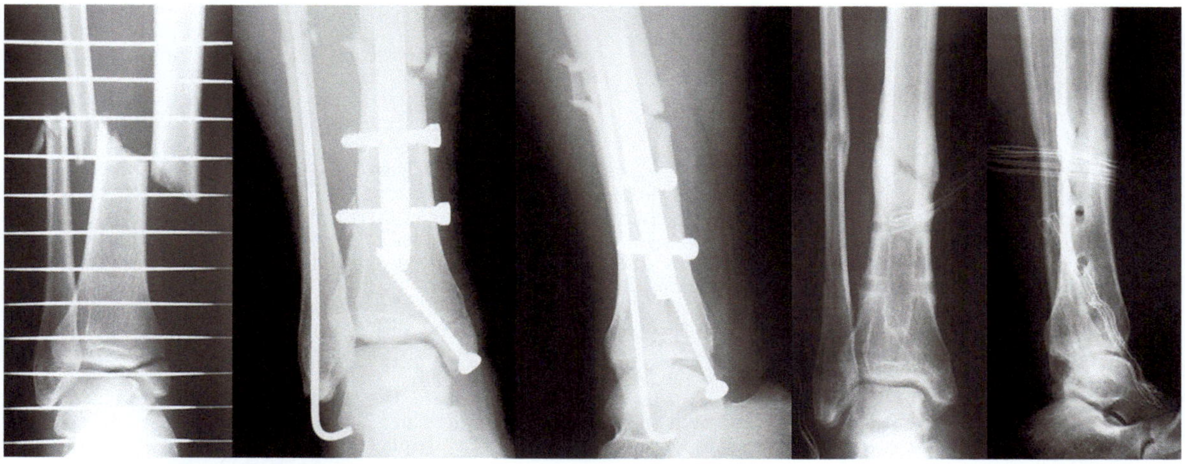

Fig. 4.8.11. Distal tibial and fibular fracture on same level combined with a medial malleolus fracture, treated with GK nail, K wire and screw

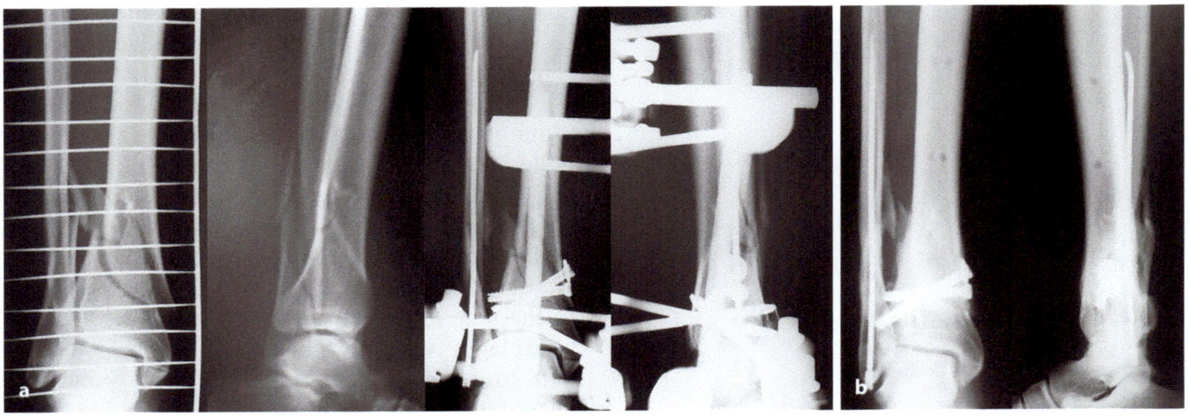

Fig. 4.8.12 a, b. Very distal combined tibial and fibular fracture treated with external fixator, fibular screw nail and cancellous screws

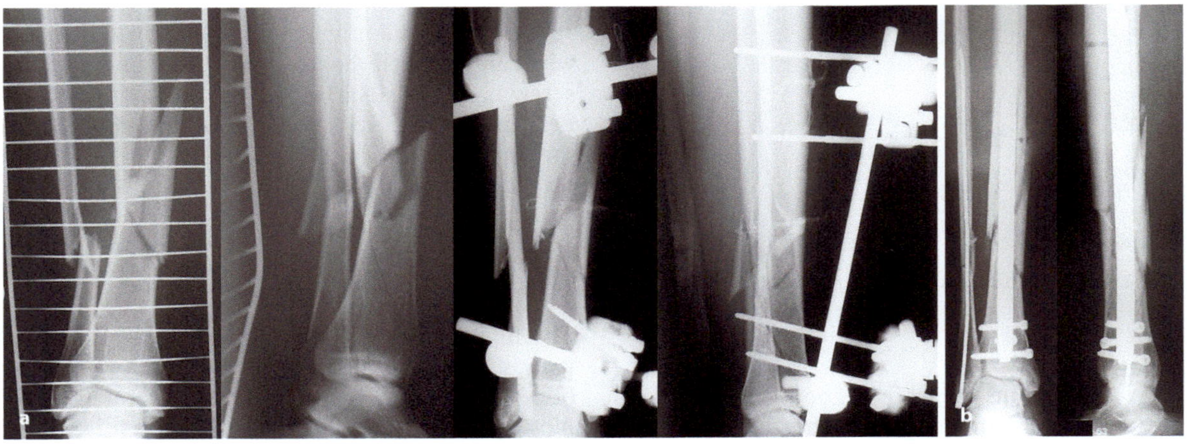

Fig. 4.8.13 a, b. Open distal tibial and fibular fracture first treated with external fixator. After 1 week, tibial nailing with locking nail and fibula with a screw nail

better fixation within a shorter operating time. Moreover, treatment of combined distal tibial and fibular fractures with an intramedullary dynamic implant is a more biological concept than the combination of plate and nail.

References

1. Bankston AB, Anderson LD, Nimityongskul P. Intramedullary screw fixation of lateral malleolus fractures. Foot Ankle Int 1994; 213:125–136
2. Benchamp CG, Clay NR, Thexton PW. Displaced ankle fractures operated with non-rigid internal fixation. Clin Orthopaed Relat Res 1986; 206:253–260
3. Burwell HN, Charnley AD. The treatment of displaced fractures at the ankle by rigid internal fixation and early joint movement. J Bone Joint Surg 1965; 47B:643
4. Cedell CA. Suppination – outward rotation injuries of the ankle. A clinical and roentgenological study with special reference to the operative treatment. Acta Orthop Scand 1976; 110(Suppl):83
5. Cools F, Martens C, Burssens P, Verdonk R. Osteo Trauma Care 2002; 10:27–32
6. Denham RA. Internal fixation for unstable ankle fractures. J Bone Joint Surg 1964; 46B:206
7. Goh JCH, Lee EH, et al. Biomechanical study on the load bearing characteristics of the fibula and the effects of fibular resection. Clin Orthop Rel Res 1992; 279:223–228
8. Kumar A, Charlebois SJ, Cain EL, Smith RA, Daniels AU, Crates JM. Effect of fibular plate fixation on rotational stability of simulated distal tibial fractures treated with intramedullary nailing. J Bone Joint Surg 2003; 85A(4):604–608
9. Krettek C, Miclau T, Schandelmaier P, Stephan C, Mohlmann U, Tscherne H. The mechanical effect of blocking screws (Poller screws) in stabilizing tibia fractures with short proximal or distal fragments after insertion of small-diameter nails. J Orthop Trauma 1999; 13:550–553
10. Lambert KL. The weight bearing function of the fibula. J Bone Joint Surg (Am) 1971; 53:507–513
11. Lauge-Hansen N. Fractures of the ankle. Arch Surg 1952; 64:488
12. Litchfield JC. The treatment of unstable fractures of ankles in the elderly. Injury 1987; 18(2):128–132
13. Mast JW, Teipner WA. A reproductive approach to the internal fixation of adult ankle fractures, rationale, techniques and early results. Orthop Clin North Am 1980; 11:661

14. McLennan JG, Ungersm JA. A new approach to the treatment of ankle fractures – the Inyo nail. Clin Orthop 1986; 213:125–136
15. Olerud C, Molander H. Bi- and trimalleolar ankle fractures operated with nonrigid internal fixation. Clin Orthop 1986; 206:253–260
16. Ramasamy PR, Sherry P. The role of a fibular nail in the management of Weber type B ankle fractures in elderly patients with osteoporotic bone – a preliminary report. Injury 2001; 32(6):477–485
17. Ray TD, Nimityongskul P, Anderson LD. Percutaneous intramedullary fixation of lateral malleolus fractures: technique and report of early results. J Trauma 1994; 36(5):669–675
18. Takebe K, Nakagawa A, et al. Role of the fibula in weight bearing. Clin Orthop 1984; 184:289–292
19. Teitz C, Carter DR, Frankel VH. Problems associated with tibial fractures with intact fibulae. J Bone Joint Surg Am 1980; 62:770–776
20. Weber TG, Harrington RM, Henley MB, Tencer AF. The role of fibular fixation in combined fractures of the tibia and fibula: a biomechanical investigation. J Orthop Trauma 1997; 11(3):206–211

Hydraulically Expandable Nailing in the Treatment of Long Bone Fractures and Pseudarthroses

D. Seligson, P.J. Buecker, J.S. Ogden

Introduction

In 1973, while studying the effects of intramedullary instrumentation on the endosteal microcirculation in healing fractures, Friedrich Rhinelander stated that "the ideal type of intramedullary fixation would be provided by a nail that firmly supported all quadrants of the endosteal cortex and also had wide external channels along which medullary blood vessels could regenerate" [1]. Recently, a nail matching these specifications has been introduced (Fig. 4.9.1).

The stainless-steel hydraulically expandable nail (HEN) features four equally spaced, longitudinally oriented flanges that, when expanded, grip the endosteal cortex along their entire length. Expansion is afforded by a thin-walled reservoir underlying the flanges that is filled with pressurized saline intraoperatively, allowing the nail to assume the shape of the patient's medullary canal as it expands up to 175% of its reduced diameter (Fig. 4.9.2). The nail can be placed with or without reaming.

While conventional nails rely on a few points of fixation provided by interlocking screws, the HEN provides literally limitless points of fixation along the entire length of the nail by the aforementioned mechanisms. The long segment of fixation provided allows for distribution of bearing forces along the entire length of the bone when the extremity is loaded [2]. Additionally, Shasha et al. [3] reported improved bending, torsional and axial stability with the HEN when compared to conventional interlocking nails. These features would seem to favor the use of this implant in situations where fixation with interlocking devices could prove tenuous, particularly in patients with abnormally mineralized or otherwise weakened bone.

Franck et al. [4, 5] reported on the use of the HEN in patients with osteoporotic and pathologic fractures of the humerus. In both series, they noted immediate stability of the fractures, allowing early physiotherapy and reliable return to activities of daily living. All 25 fractures healed by week 16. Operative times were found to be 32–35 min, and fluoroscopy exposure times were 1.4–1.5 min. They concluded that the HEN offered a simple, reliable surgical alternative for fractures in this cohort.

Use of this nail in the lower extremity also has been examined. Pascarella et al. [6] reported early weight-bearing in 19 patients treated with the HEN, and all fractures went on to union at an average of 5 months for femora and 4 months for tibias.

The hydraulic nail dramatically reduces the need for fluoroscopy since placement of interlocking screws continues to be the greatest use of im-

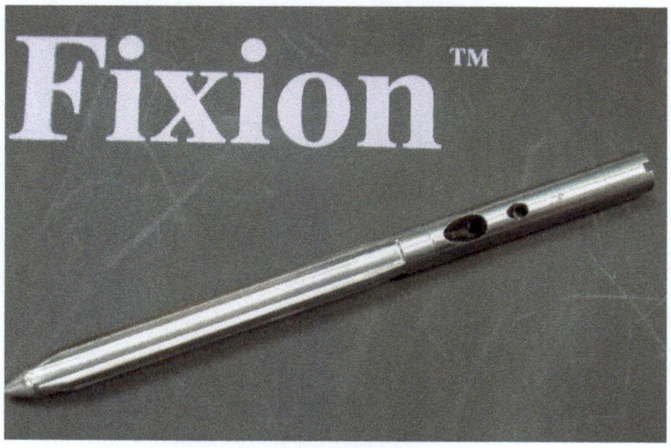

Fig. 4.9.1. The hydraulically expanded nail

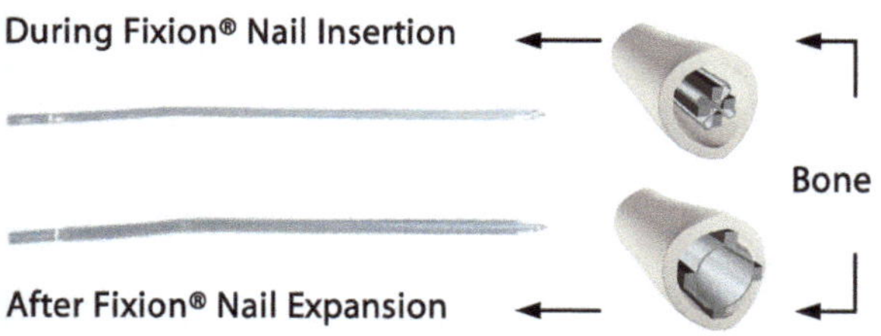

Fig. 4.9.2. Cross-section of the nail. The nail is constructed with four flat plates connected by a thinner membrane of steel, which deforms under pressure. It expands like an umbrella

age intensification in the practice of medullary nailing. Averaged over the entire case load in a trauma center, the use of HEN nails is practical in about 30% of the cases, with a concomitant reduction in X-ray exposure to patients and staff. In contrast, if cases are honestly evaluated, as the caliber of standard locked nails increases, the potential for fracture site comminution also increases. These cortical comminutions may be underemphasized since in general fracture healing takes place. There are nonetheless many times when the postoperative recovery is delayed and/or bracing is required. Further problems with interlocking screws, particularly at the knee joint, are omnipresent. Certainly most of these problems can be assessed to relatively inexperienced surgeons who use locking screws that are too long. It is nonetheless true that this possibility can be avoided entirely with use of a HEN nail.

The best indications for the HEN nail are:

- Stable fresh fracture of the tibia, femur and humerus
- Fractures in osteoporotic bone
- Pseudarthroses
- Pathologic fractures.

There is no doubt that conventional interlocking nails can be applied to these problems with good results. The advantages and disadvantages of standard interlocking nailing as compared with hydraulically expanded nails need honest evaluation. On the side of the HEN is the achievement of good stability with minimal enlargement of the canal since a small caliber nail is inserted. Then arguments for the use of unreamed nails apply. Against the use of expanded nails is the potential in fresh fractures to increase occult comminution as the implant expands.

Technique

Hydraulically expandable nailing is performed in the same manner as conventional interlocking nailing. At our center, for the tibia the patient is placed supine on a radiolucent table. The knee is flexed over radiolucent metal triangles. Care is taken to keep the anterior superior iliac spine, patella and first web space in line to prevent rotational deformity. The femur is nailed on a fracture table. Antegrade nailing with a trochanteric starting point in line with the medullary canal is preferred. The few retrograde femur nailings have been successful. The humerus nailing is done supine on a regular operating table with a board supporting the arm and shoulder. The fluoroscopy unit is brought in from the same side as the fracture.

In each instance the same starting point as in conventional nailing is used. Fresh fractures without comminution (type A) are suitable for treatment with HEN nails. A Küntscher guide pin is placed across the fracture using fluoroscopy, and the medullary canal is reamed 1–2 mm greater than the diameter of the collapsed HEN nail.

Nail size is selected based on the patient's bone. Femurs in old patients who have osteoporosis and large medullary canals are fitted with thicker nails than those in young patients who have narrow canals and stout cortices. Since the procedure is used mostly for patients with low energy, stable transverse and short oblique fractures without comminution, stability is adequate. We also do not use this nail in patients with polytrauma and a good prognosis where concomitant injuries would impose excessive loads on the construct during fracture healing, for example bilateral femur shaft fractures.

The usual tibia can be nailed with the 8.5-mm nail, which expands to 13.5 mm, the femur with the 10-mm nail, which expands to 16 mm, and the humerus with the 7.4-mm nail, which expands to 11 mm (Fig. 4.9.3). The expansion of the nail is limited by the endosteal cortex. So as the nail is deformed under pressure, it roughly takes the shape of the medullary cavity. The fit of the nail is not exact, since the stout, flat plates of the nail only gently bend during expansion.

HEN nails are available with and without interlocking screws. The interlocking construct is useful occasionally in situations where nail migration

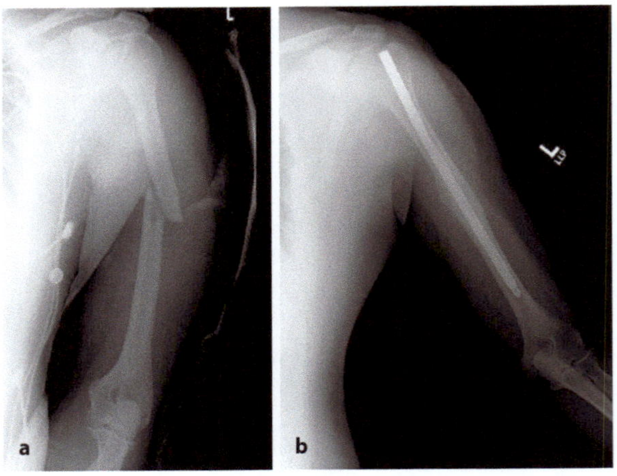

Fig. 4.9.3. a This 40-year-old man fractured his left humerus in a motor vehicle accident. b HEN was successful

might be a concern, such as in a retrograde nailing of the femur.

In pseudarthrosis, the nail relatively expands both proximal and distal to the narrow area through the nonunion. This gives good control of rotation and shear. However, if the area through the pseudarthrosis is too narrow relative to the canal proximal and distal to the nonunion, bending can occur. It is useful then to ream-up the pseudarthrosis so the hourglass configuration of the nail is not too extreme.

The nail is fitted with a hydraulic inflation device (Fig. 4.9.4). Saline is used to deform the nail with pressure. Once the nail has been expanded and the pressure relieved, the water inside the nail is no longer under pressure. In other words the nail is not inflated and it will not "deflate" if punctured. The steel is permanently deformed and will remain that way.

Rarely is there a problem with the valve breaking when nail inflation is attempted. Leakage from the valve occurs when the nail is driven rather than slid into the medullary canal. If too much hammering is needed, it is better to remove the nail, ream the bone up to a greater diameter and try with a new implant or use a smaller caliber nail.

The nail is expanded with a pump. The pump has a gauge graduated in bars. For fresh fractures the nail is expanded to the middle of the safe (yellow) zone or 60–65 bars. In cases with fragile bone or very thin cortices, it is prudent to limit nail expansion to 50–55 bars. After expansion the handle of the pump is backed down to retrieve the pressure on the wall of the nail. Leakage from the valve after insertion or infectious problems from the saline in the nail have not been observed.

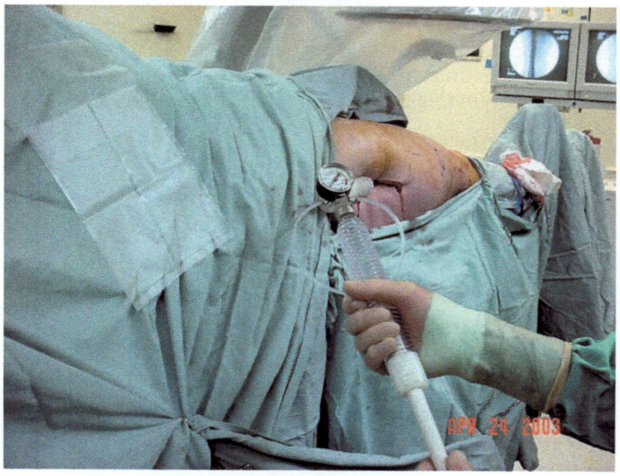

Fig. 4.9.4. Expansion of a femur nail with the water pump – operative set-up

The nails can be capped with a small end cap. This cap can be difficult to place and in practice can be omitted without consequence.

Rehabilitation after HEN nailing in stable cases is routine. We avoid rotational exercises for the humerus. Some patients are more comfortable in orthoses, some are not. Immediate progressive weight-bearing is usually prescribed. Straight leg raising is not permitted for femur shaft fractures. Active assisted knee range of motion and ankle dorsiflexion is encouraged.

In fresh fractures, healing is prompt since the cases that were selected for this method were the easy ones. In young patients the nails are removed in our practice. In the past, removal has been considered difficult, but with a new set of instruments this is no longer the case. The nail must be extracted back through the entrance hole, which means it must collapse some. The valve is relieved by the extraction bolt. It also usually helps to puncture the wall of the nail with a Steinmann pin. As the nail is drawn back through the entrance hole, it must again deform and this decrease in caliber repressurizes the water inside the nail. To find the end of a deeply buried nail, a guide pin can be placed under X-ray control and a cannulated drill used to make a channel for the extraction bolt.

Since its inception more than 80 years ago, intramedullary nailing for long bone fractures has enjoyed widespread acceptance. Current conventional implants achieve fixation through interlocking screws placed through fracture fragments and the nail. This allows for load-sharing; these points of fixation could prove tenuous. The HEN provides fixation throughout its length via equally spaced flanges that conform to the inner surface of the cortex and gain contact throughout their length. This has been shown to provide improved bending, torsional and axial stability when compared to interlocking constructs [3]. Additionally, the equal dispersion of bearing forces throughout the bone seen with the HEN [2] could prove advantageous over relying on a few points of fixation in weakened bone, as is the case with interlocking nails.

We have reviewed the clinical behavior of expandable nails in the treatment of diaphyseal fractures and pseudarthroses in patients with weakened or osteoporotic bone (Fig. 4.9.5). Early data are promising. A union rate of 96% has been achieved. This is consistent with prior studies of the HEN [2, 4–6]. Operating and fluoroscopy times were decreased by 50% when compared

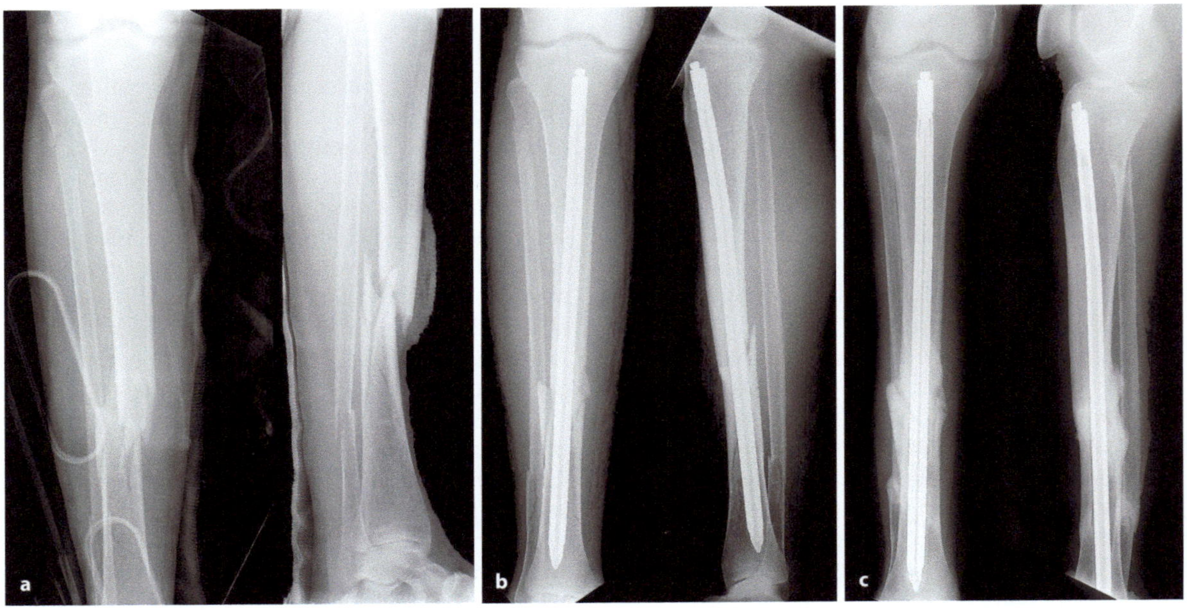

Fig. 4.9.5. a This 29-year-old man sustained a right tibia fracture in a fall. b Since he had osteoporia from endstage renal disease requiring dialysis, a HEN nailing was performed. c Despite some comminution and shortening, the fracture healed

with conventional interlocking devices, and patient satisfaction levels were quite high at 87% for lower extremities and 90% for humerus nail. It would appear from these data that the HEN shows great promise for treatment of fractures and nonunions in a subset of patients with compromised bone density or mineralization.

Future prospective studies with more statistical power may better define the role of this implant. Increasing use of this implant for fresh fractures and in patients with normal bone density also warrants further investigation.

References

1. Rhinelander FW. Effects of medullary nailing on the normal blood supply of diaphyseal cortex. Instructional Course Lectures 1973; 22:161–187.
2. LePore S, Capuano N, LePore L, et al. Preliminary clinical and radiographic results with the Fixion intramedullary nail: an inflatable self-locking system for long bone fractures. J Orthop Traumatol 2000; 3:135–140.
3. Shasha N, Blumburg N, Tauber M, et al. An expandable intramedullary nail for fixation in osteoporotic bone. In: An YH, ed. Internal Fixation in Osteoporotic Bone. New York: Thieme, 301–309.
4. Franck W, Olivieri M, Jannasch O, et al. Expandable nail system for osteoporotic humeral shaft fractures: preliminary results. J Trauma Injury Infect Crit Care 2003; 54(6):1152–1158.
5. Franck W, Olivieri M, Jannasch O, et al. An expandable nailing system for the management of pathological humerus fractures. Arch Orthop Trauma Surg 2002; 122(7):400–405.
6. Pascarella R, Nasta G, Nicolini M, et al. The fixion in the lower limb. Preliminary results. Chirurgia Degli Organi di Movimento 2002; 87(3):169–174.

Proximal Humeral Fractures

H. Seidel

Introduction

Proximal humeral fractures make up 4–5% of all fractures. The incidence increases with age, affecting 60% more women than men. The mean age is 74 years for women and 68 years for men in our patient group. The prognosis and outcome depend on the severity of the trauma, the fracture type, the success of stable reduction, and the compliance of the patients. The best results are seen in active patients and patients with compliance for the fracture and the treatment. For elderly patients, the proximal humeral fracture is often the beginning of loss of independence and the beginning of nursing conditions. The combination of osteoporosis and fragmentation of the fracture limits the success of treatment more than with any other fracture. Finally the fracture's destiny is dependent on the treatment, either orthopaedic or operative. The choice of the operative procedure and the implant has an influence on the success. Not every operative procedure is suitable for all fractures. Immediate operation has better results than secondary stabilisation. Modern therapy concepts improve the prognosis and outcome. The keys of success are stable fracture fixation, immediate functional treatment, short hospitalisation and adequate, sophisticated treatment postoperatively. Good and excellent results are achieved in 80% after operative treatment [48–50].

Classification

The clinical and anatomical diagnosis is simple using modern technical support – with X-ray amplifier, standard X-ray and CT. But the fracture classification is one of the most important steps of diagnosis to determine the optimal treatment.

The anatomical and functional background of different structures of the proximal humerus and the shoulder are the basis of every classification. The number of fragments, the displacement and dislocation, and the muscle lesions determine the functional circumstances of the proximal humerus and the blood supply of the humeral head. The oldest classification was described by Garre (1857–1928). He first distinguished the relevant anatomical and functional structures of the humeral head, tuberosities and humeral shaft. He distinguished fractures of the anatomical neck from those of the surgical neck. A similar classification was described by Codman [9]. The Neer classification, which is standard in clinical use, is generally accepted and facilitates the finding of the indication either for conservative or operative therapy [33]. The degree of displacement and dislocation depends on the muscle insertion. But the observer has to realise that the fracture is not static and that the classification type changes after the initial trauma. The Neer I fracture can change to a Neer IV fracture triggered by active or passive motion before the first therapy or during therapies. The opinion to treat the Neer I fracture conservatively with orthopaedic methods is correct, from the viewpoint of an anatomic classification. But the fracture can change in view of a functional classification to a more difficult fracture, if the treatment is not adequate. That fact shows the relativity and the problem of static diagnosis using the Neer classification. Another more specific problem is the reliability. In a retrospective study, the reliability has been as different as 30–32% in identical cases, between the first and second reviews of the radiographs.

The AO classification [32] is the most used classification. The differentiation of the fractures is visually performed using three types – A, B and C with subgroups. It is a static classification and has the same problems as the Neer classification. In addition, a very similar problem is described for the AO classification as for the Neer classification. The observer reliability is low and identical fractures are classified differently by the same observer, at first and second review, in 30% of instances [58]. Therefore the choice of treatment is different at the second run of diagnosis in 20% of cases, following the three-dimensional-

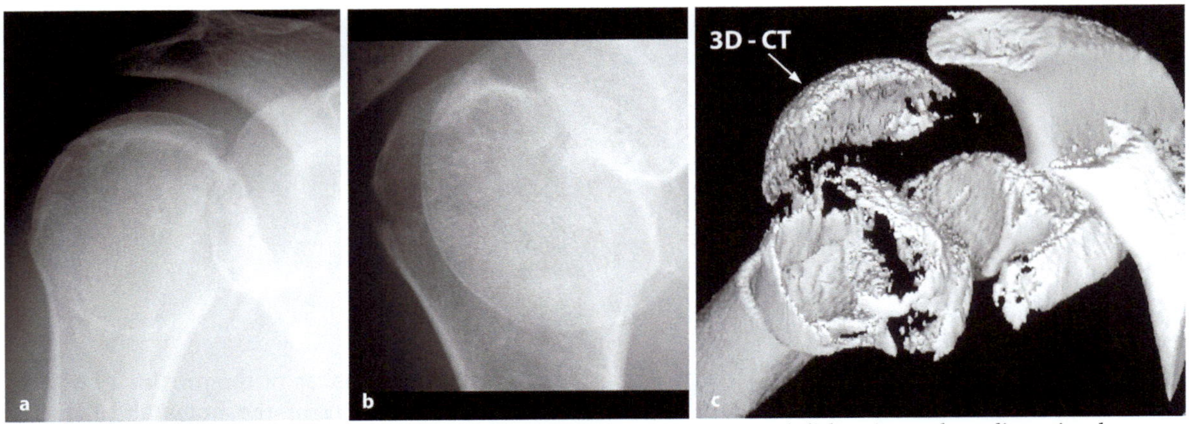

Fig. 4.10.1.1. Neer VI fracture: a anteroposterior view; b anteroposterior view, total dislocation; c three-dimensional scan

rendering diagnosis. It has been shown that the stereo visualisation changes the choice of therapy in 20% of cases, compared to the normal X-ray diagnosis [45]. In conclusion, the reliability of both the Neer and the AO classification is low and the consequence of choice of treatment is underestimated.

The correct diagnosis and classification is only possible by analysing the anatomical and functional structures of the fracture. If the normal X-ray diagnosis is not clear, CT is required (Fig. 4.10.1.1).

The proximal humerus is divided into three segments. Each segment represents special problems.

The Humeral Head

The humeral head allows the multidirectional motion of the shoulder. The problems with fracture of the humeral head are the vascularity, the degree of dislocation, and the splitting of cartilage, with the resultant necrosis of the humeral head. Humeral head necrosis develops if the vascularity is disrupted. Humeral head necrosis is observed in 30–100% of cases [17, 23, 26, 40, 44, 57] following three- and four-part fractures.

Humeral Tuberosities

The proximal humeral tuberosities are located between the anatomical and surgical neck. This osseous bloc is the anchorage point for the rotator cuff. The stable reconstruction of the rotator cuff is a precondition for the functional treatment of the shoulder.

An efficient cuff repair and tubercle stabilisation are often difficult. The osteoporotic bone usually gives insufficient support for normal screws or plates. On the other hand, safe fixation of the rotator cuff is essential and possible with special techniques.

The Humeral Shaft

The humeral shaft is the transmitter of multiple functional moments of the upper extremity and the shoulder. The functional problem of the humeral shaft, in proximal fractures, is the free motion in every direction, with the danger of soft tissue lesions. The functional fracture status, with accompanying tissue destruction, is more active after the fracture than radiographs demonstrate in the early stages of documentation. Displacement and dislocation continue at the fracture site after the fracture has occurred. If the connection of the shaft to the head fragment is interrupted, the proximal shaft is displaced in the medial direction by the muscles' traction. That displacement is a high danger for the axillary nerve and the axillary vessels.

The uncontrolled shaft motion provokes additional soft tissue lesions. The shaft provokes the dislocation of the humeral head and displacement of fragments. The humeral shaft penetrates and divides the tuberosities and destroys the anchorage of the rotator cuff. Three-part and four-part fractures need the stable reconstruction of the shaft and the humeral head. This stabilisation neutralises the negative bending and shortening moments between both shaft and head. Isolated wires or screws cannot stabilise the comminution of the humeral head. Osteoporosis increases the failure of those implants.

It is evident that functional problems have to be included in the classification and strategies of fracture repair. The anatomical classification alone is not suitable to decide the correct treatment. The anatomical classification has to be combined with the functional purpose to find the best treatment for the patient.

Habermeyer [16] recognised the importance of the functional considerations with his own classification. More recently, Gotzen did the same [14]. The same assessment was done by Weigand in 1984 [61].

Since 1985, we have used a basic classification that addresses the anatomic, functional lesion and its repair [50]. That basic classification is performed intraoperatively and documents every fragment, lesion, dislocation and displacement.

Conservative Treatment

The subcapital stable fracture on the surgical neck of the humerus is easy to treat. Orthopaedic treatment is possible if the fracture is stable.

Eighty-seven per cent of humeral fractures can be treated conservatively with good results according to Vrancken Peeters [59]. In 1906, Helferich [24] described orthopaedic treatment in detail. The old conservative treatment of Böhler [5] has been abandoned. Long immobilisation and long hospitalisation are typical for such procedures. Shoulder stiffness and loss of function were frequent. For the elderly patient, the fracture is often the loss of independence followed by further complications.

The functional treatment of proximal humeral fractures was discovered and introduced first by Poelchen, having himself had a subcapital fracture [38]. The method of early functional training was more sophisticated and developed by Specht [51] and later by Sarmiento and Latta [46]. For a short time, immobilisation is required, using a sling or a Gilchrist bandage. Functional treatment is assisted and trained by a physiotherapist; and, after a short time, training is performed independently. Controlled motion and muscle training are typical for the functional treatment. The fracture heals within 6–8 weeks, with good results. The hospital stay is very short.

The functional treatment has its limitations in the case of three- and four-part fractures. These fractures require open reduction with stable fixation. Fixation of the major and minor tubercle is imperative.

Operative Treatment

If instability occurs in proximal humeral fractures, surgical treatment is necessary. The advantage of operative treatment is anatomical reconstruction, immediate postoperative mobilisation, shorter hospitalisation and good functional results. Fractures of the humeral head remained an unsolved fracture for a long time, compared to medial femur neck fractures. Successful treatment of comminuted humeral head fractures is possible with new techniques that combine a humeral locking nail (HLN) with screws and washers and with new plates and new screws.

Wire Banding and Screws

Neer [33] proposed the wire-banding technique to fix the tuberosities with the rotator cuff. He demonstrated the limits of the wiring technique with regard to four-part fractures, for which he recommended hemiarthroplasty. The same experience was had by Tanner [57], Habermeyer [16] and Damanakis [12].

Resch [40] preferred the closed reduction of three- and four-part fractures and fixation with simple or cannulated screws. Speck [52] performed the wiring technique with resorbable sutures, using anchorage screws on the humeral shaft. He obtained good results with open reduction for three- and four-part fractures. On the basis of this experience, he recommended osteosyntheses instead of prosthetic replacement. That technique was also recommended by Szyskowitz [56] and the AO for B3 and C3 fractures, using additional screws for humeral head fixation. In the same way, Ochsner [37] stabilised three- and four-part fractures using resorbable PDS sutures, comparing that with a group in which he used metal banding wires. The results were sufficient comparing pain, function and motion, even in those cases with partial humeral head necrosis. This necrosis appeared in 50% following the use of metal wires and 50% after PDS sutures. Ochsner still recommended that procedure instead of prosthesis. The same experience was published by Lahm [27].

Plates

Old plating techniques have been abandoned for B and C fractures of the AO classification. The old concept of Müller and the AO [31], with plates and big spongiosa screws, is used in cases of A2 fractures [55]. Generally that technique was not successful for more difficult fractures [23]. Screw loosening and screw cut-out led to a loss of stability and revisions were necessary. Lill [28] observed impingement pain in 63% following T-plate osteosyntheses. With this plate and big screws, a secondary loss of reduction is due to the osteoporotic bone [7]. That event is normal in the elderly patient and better techniques are required to stop these complications.

These bad results stimulated the development of new plating techniques, using angle stable plates with smaller screws [23]. At first, Bothworth [6] introduced the angle stable screw plate. Bartsch [3] had good results with that new technique and proposed it as an alternative to hemiarthroplasty. Similar good results were reported by Hente [22] for three- and four-part fractures with the angle stable internal fixator. The angulated, 1/3 tubular plate published by Albrecht [2] did not have long-term success. Also, the double plate suggested by Wanner [60] did not fulfil hopes for durable results. Hessmann [23] recommended axial stable fixed plates, such as the clover leaf plate, with diverging 3.5-mm screws and the Philos plate for difficult four-part fractures. Hente [22] reported good results as well with the Philos plate. He summarised that no humeral head necrosis was provoked with the open reduction and plating technique. The good results with open reduction of four-part fractures contradict the old opinion that humeral head necrosis will appear following open reduction.

Shoulder Prosthesis

Replacement of the shoulder in trauma surgery can be restricted to a very few fractures with humeral head splitting. The functional result following prosthesis is not better than osteosynthesis. In the meantime the fourth generation of prosthesis is in clinical use [16]. Long-term results are not yet available. Painless function is achieved in 80% [45], but the function is more restricted than following osteosynthesis. Humeral head replacement is the last indication before arthrodesis of the joint. Reich [39] recommended the immediate intraoperative change from osteosynthesis to prosthesis if osteosynthesis reconstruction was not possible. Boss [8] preferred the prosthesis to osteosynthesis for treating three- and four-part fractures in elderly patients. Habermeyer [17], like Heitkemper [21], pointed out that the fixation of the major tubercle has a key influence for shoulder function. The results without osteotomy of the major or minor tubercle are better than those following the procedure or prosthesis with osteotomy. Boileau [4], Dines [10], Healy [20], Norris [36] and Scheck [47] had the same experience. Habermeyer [16] introduced a new prosthesis with the possibility of lengthening or shortening and correction in three planes of the proximal prosthesis with the goal of better centring of the articulation and better muscle function of the shoulder. Generally the prosthesis is reserved for elderly patients without the possibility of reconstruction of the humeral head [8, 45]. Robinson [41] reported poor results in a group of elderly patients with neurological deficit. He noted the same problems of fixation and function of the tuberosities as Habermeyer [17]. Regarding that background and the cost of the prosthesis, Rüter [45] advised more restriction of the use of shoulder prostheses. The hopeful results using humeral prostheses observed in 1988 by Neumann [35] have not been generally confirmed. The application of the humeral prosthesis in trauma surgery is more restrictive than in the last century. In 1991, Habermeyer and Schweiberer [15] preferred osteosynthesis for four-part fractures, knowing the poor results and complications of prostheses. Doursounian [13] combined the shaft fixation of the prosthesis with humeral head fixation on the metal shaft with stapes plates of titanium. This technique combines the disadvantages of both prosthesis and osteosynthesis.

Intramedullary Nail

Küntscher introduced the first intramedullary nail for proximal humeral fractures. The late results of the Küntscher treatment are not available. But the general complications of the Küntscher nail were too frequent when used for proximal humeral fractures. In 1974, Kapandij [25] showed the first results with intramedullary pins, similar to the Hackethal method [18]. This operation was indicated for stable subcapital fractures only. The HLN was designed in 1984 by Seidel [48]. It was the first interlocking nail designed specifically for humeral fractures. It was the first nail with a threaded screw hole on the top of the nail to stabilise humeral head fractures. It showed good results for proximal humeral fractures. The good results with this nail stimulated others to develop new intramedullary nail designs. Rodosky and Flatow [42] used a modified Ender nail for fixation of two-part fractures, with closed or open reduction. The Ender nail, with an additional proximal hole, is sutured on the rotator cuff. The purpose of the suture was to prevent cut-out of the nail proximally.

The intramedullary interlocking nail technique more or less replaced other techniques. Szyskowitz [56] proposed, as had Rommens [43], the retrograde implanted interlocking nail for subcapital fractures, using the universal humeral nail (UHN). The UHN is introduced antegrade or retrograde and is locked with proximal and distal screws. Halder [19] developed his own nail to stabilise subcapital fractures, introducing the nail in a retrograde fashion. The Stedtfeldt nail [54] is a straight nail and has proximal interlocking screws in different directions with threaded holes in the nail. The distal screws are introduced from lateral to medial. This nail is similar to the Polarus nail published by Adedepo [1]. He found the method particularly useful in the management of combined proximal humeral and shaft fractures. Mouradian [30] had similar results in 1986 with a modified Zickel nail. In 1998, Lin [29] published results on the use of locked nails for displaced surgical neck fractures of the humerus. Hessmann [23] recently published good results for proximal humeral fractures with the UHN in combination with a spiral blade plate. The T2 nail offers a good solution for proximal humeral fractures, using polydirectional screws in the proximal segment of the nail. In 1996, Seidel [49] published the first 10-year results with the HLN. Three alternatives were used with the HLN: nail and screws, nail and cup washer, nail and lateral washer.

Author's Materials, Methods and Treatment with the HLN

Over the last 20 years, operative treatment has been the preferred treatment for unstable and multifocal fractures in the Seidel series. The treatment of humeral fractures was performed in three series:

- The first series was performed with the locking nail and the proximal cap washer
- In the second series, the nail was used in combination with proximal locking screws. For this technique, the first of three locking holes was threaded, to allow a better grip for the screw (Fig. 4.10.1.3)
- In the third series, the cap washer was moved from the top of the nail to the lateral side (Fig. 4.10.1.2).

The results show that difficult fractures of the humeral head can be treated and the humeral head is not compromised by necrosis. The functional late results are acceptable and even excellent (Fig. 4.10.1.2 c).

A short HLN is usually implanted for this technique, in contrast to diaphyseal fractures, where the longest nail possible is usually selected. Reaming is not necessary for the most part, because the medullar canal is large in the proximal section.

One-third of all fractures were treated immediately. The remaining two-thirds of the fractures were treated secondarily, within the first week.

Open reduction techniques and bone quality are the keys for stable reconstruction of these fractures. If the bone quality is good and the fragments are large enough, a nail with screws is the preferred method (Fig. 4.10.1.3). If the bone quality is poor and the fragments are too small for screw fixation, the washer technique is used in combination with the nail.

In 79 cases out of a total of 134 patients, the fracture's location was totally intra-articular; and in nine cases, the humeral head was completely split. In 68 cases, the fracture line ran from the intra-articular section to the proximal humeral shaft. In two cases, the range of the fracture was down to the section of proximal shaft. In 55 cases, the main fracture was in the section of surgical neck but extended to the greater or lesser tuberosities. In 108 cases, more than four fragments were observed. Simple fractures were exceptional.

Dislocation of the humeral head was complete in 86 cases. The mean age of females was 74 years. The oldest female was 100 years old. The oldest male was 88 years and the youngest was 20. The elderly patients were 40% of all patients. The fracture reduction was anatomic in 38% of cases, poor in 3%, fair in 2%, sufficient in 33%, and good in 24%.

The mean consolidation time was 10 weeks. Pseudarthrosis presented in two cases, while 12 cases had delayed union. Forty-nine patients did not want removal of the implant, and removal was performed in 85 cases. A total of 120 fractures consolidated in time. In 3% of cases, an early infection was observed, and 2% had a late infection. Two patients who had had an infection proceeded to necrosis of the humeral head with post-traumatic arthroses. Two pseudarthroses healed after operation with a HLN.

The results are judged using different parameters – using radiographic control and a measurement of the degree of motion. The functional criteria included isolated motion, combined motion and functional motion.

The 3-month postoperative results show an excellent result in 30% of the cases, 53% had a good

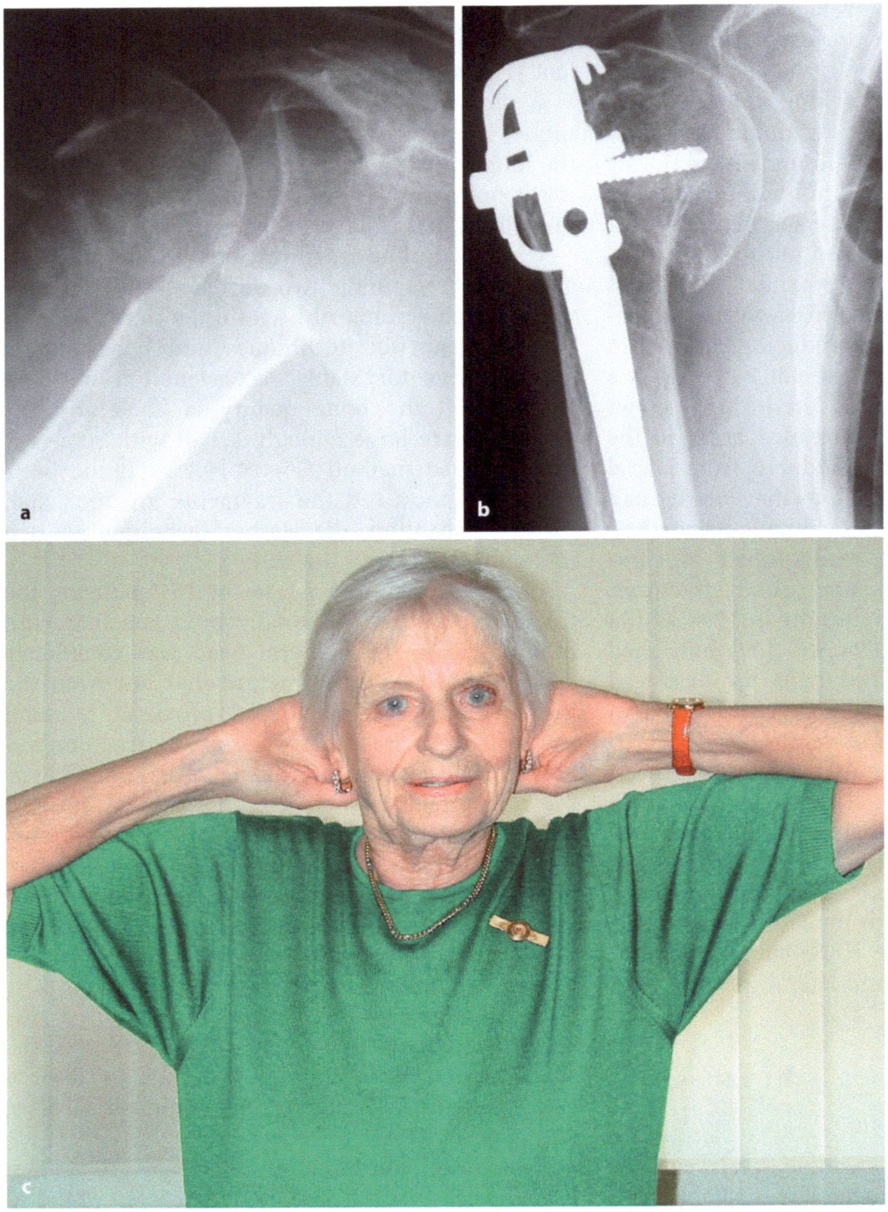

Fig. 4.10.1.2. Neer VI fracture: a total dislocation; b stabilisation with HLN and washer; consolidation after 6 months; c function after 6 months

result, and 12% had an adequate result, in terms of function and motion; 80% had a good or excellent result 12 months after the operation.

The series has shown clearly that continuous exercise and physiotherapy are important in improving the range of motion. Better results are seen in the late follow-up period, compared to those observed in the early postoperation follow-up.

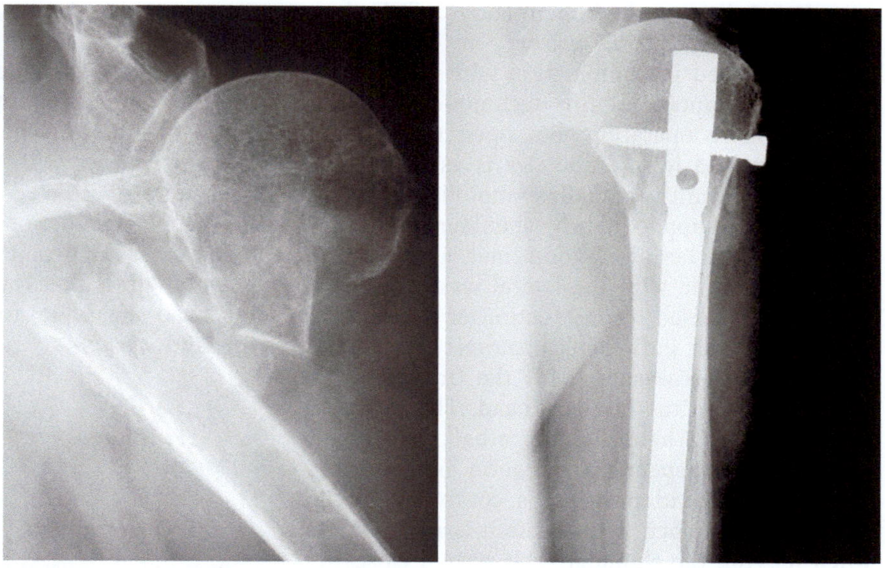

Fig. 4.10.1.3. Subcapital fracture: a total displacement; b stabilisation with HLN

Discussion

The treatment of humeral head fractures has generally changed over the last 20 years. The exclusively conservative treatment recommended by Böhler [5] is associated with the complications of shoulder stiffness and dysfunction. His recommendations have influenced more than five decades of fracture treatment in Europe. The first good results with operative treatment were reported by Neer [33]. In 1984, Stableforth [53] reported good results for displaced four-part humeral head fractures treated with non-operative reduction and stabilisation. Habermeyer and Schweiberer [15] recommended both non-operative and operative strategies. In 1969, the AO group published its first T-plates with spongiosa screws to stabilise proximal humeral fractures [32].

The critical problems of humeral head fractures are nutrition and continued blood supply of the humeral head. Every treatment has to consider that fact.

Non-operative treatment can hinder revascularisation. But the operative procedure can damage the last nutrient vessels with open reduction. The nutrition of the humeral head is provided by the vessels passing over the greater and lesser tubercles. Immediate reduction and stabilisation of fragments protect the vessels and stimulate regeneration of the vascularity. It is stimulated by bone and comes from within the bone. Anatomical repositioning of the humeral head fragments requires open reduction and is an important step to combat necrosis of the humeral head, which is caused by the disconnection of vascular supply. This is the most important aspect of any osteosyntheses. Anatomical reduction is often not 100% possible at the level of the greater and lesser tubercles. However, the functional fixation of these structures with the rotator cuff is more important than the 100% reduction of fragments. The impaction achieved with open reduction of the humeral head, the greater and lesser tubercle give the support needed for revascularisation.

The functional orthopaedic treatment and mobilisation of unstable fractures can produce more damage than the initial accident itself. With such techniques, the humeral shaft pushes the humeral head into dorsal dislocation. This effect was observed in 90% of our patients prior to secondary osteosyntheses. With our series it was pointed out that humeral head necrosis is not limited to three-part and four-part fractures. We found similar results for more difficult fractures, as reported by Neer [34] and Lahm [27], using wires for fracture fixation.

The array of different operative techniques and implants shows many unsolved problems. Recently the trend goes more toward osteosyntheses with small implants and screws. Hessmann [23] pointed out the differences of the minimally invasive technique with angle-stable plates and large, invasive, plating osteosynthesis.

Within my own HLN series, it was shown that a high percentage of dislocation and displacement of unstable fractures demand immediate stabilisation. Depending on the bone quality and the fragmentation, the lateral washer or interlocking screws are used in combination with the humeral nail. The advantage of this technique is a minimally invasive operation. But open reduction of the greater and lesser tubercles is essential. This procedure permits immediate mobilisation without external support. Early shoulder exercise is also one of the keys to a good final outcome.

The technique with the lateral washer allows a very individualised reconstruction of the fracture, modified to the individual, anatomic situation of the patient. The washer holds the fragments, the rotator cuff and the humeral head. The washer is comparable to a hand holding a ball. The stabilisation is not dependent on good bone quality. The humeral head position is controlled by the nail and the washer. A dislocation is not possible, when moving the shoulder. The system closes the rotator cuff and the capsule. Additional resorbable sutures solidify the montage of the rotator cuff with the circumnavigating washer.

Other techniques have been used by Stedtfeldt [54] more recently. He combined intramedullary nails with angle-stable screws. With the T2 nail, the stabilisation of fractures was the same. This static construct with an angle-stable screw is different to the washer technique. This type of construct can produce screw penetration in the articulation due to fracture retraction and dynamisation during fracture consolidation. Screw penetration can occur days or weeks after the operation. The reason for the penetration is the static coupling between nail and screws, without the possibility of dynamisation during fracture consolidation. The same results occur with plates and angle-fixed screws or nails in combination with twisted plates. The recent technique of combining an intramedullary nail and a twisted plate published by Blum [7] has the same disadvantage.

A shoulder prosthesis is the last treatment option. The four-part fracture is not the best indication. This fracture type has a better result with a reconstructive procedure. The indication for prosthesis in trauma surgery is when there is a split of the humeral head or a failed orthopaedic treatment, after weeks to months [57]. The immediate implantation of a prosthesis is not indicated. Immediate osteosynthesis has better results, as Speck [52] and many others have shown. The shoulder prosthesis is the last choice in the case of failed osteosyntheses.

The comparison of results and different techniques is difficult, because the reported series include and use different fracture types, different classifications and different scores. The Neer [33] score is very complex, as is the Constant [11] score, and their clinical use and relevance are critical. The disadvantage of these scoring techniques is the summing of many functions and the irregularities of grading. The rating and comparison of results are easier with separate scoring of unique parameters of isolated motion, combined motion and combined function.

The most important finding of our own experience is the fact that revascularisation of the humeral head was due to osteosyntheses with the HLN and washers.

References

1. Adedepo AO, Ikpeme JO (2001) The results of internal fixation of three- and four-part proximal humeral fractures with the Polarus nail. Injury 31: 115–121
2. Albrecht F (1983) Die abgewinkelte Drittelrohrplatte zur Osteosynthese dilozierter Humerusfrakturen durch das Collum anatomicum. Unfallchirurgie 9: 14–16
3. Bartsch S, Hullmann B, Hinrichs B, Giers R, Echtermeyer V (2001) Die Osteosynthese der dislozierten Oberarmkopffrakturen mit der winkelstabilen proximalen Oberarmplatte. Akt Traumatol 31: 64–71
4. Boileau P, Cligaris-Cordero B, Payer F, Tinsi L, Argenson C (1999) Prognostic factors during rehabilitation after shoulder prostheses for fracture. Rev Chir Orthop Reparatrice Appar Mot 85: 106–116
5. Böhler L (1964) Gegen die operative Behandlung von frischen Oberarmschaftbrüchen. Langenbecks Archiv klin Chir 308: 465–476
6. Bosworth CM (1949) Blade plate fixation. JAMA 141: 1111–1113
7. Blum J, Hessmann MH, Rommens PM (2003) Behandlung proximaler metaphysärer Humerusfrakturen mit Verriegelungsnagel und Spiralklinge – erste Erfahrungen mit einem neuen Implantat. Akt Traumatol 33: 7–13
8. Boss A, Hintermann B (1997) Primäre Versorgung der Humeruskopftrümmerfraktur beim älteren Menschen mit einer Kopfprothese. Der Unfallchirurg 100: 867–873
9. Codman EA (1934) The shoulder. Todd, Boston
10. Dines DM, Klarren RF, Altcheck DW, Moeckel B (1993) Posttraumatic changes of the proximal humerus: malunion, non-union, and osteonecrosis. Treatment with modular hemiarthroplasty or total shoulder arthroplasty. J Shoulder Elbow Surgery 2: 11–21
11. Constant CR, Murley AHG (1987) A clinical method of functional assessment of shoulder. Clin Orthop Rel Res 214: 160-164
12. Damanakis D, Schaal O, Mann J, Müller KH (1996) Ein modifiziertes Behandlungskonzept bei Humeruskopffrakturen des älteren Menschen. Unfallchirurg 99: 561–568
13. Doursounian L, Grimberg J, Cazeau C, Touzard RC (1996) Une nouvelle méthode d'ostéosynthése des fractures de l'extrémité supérieure de l'humérus: implant biobloquet. A propos de 17 cas revus à plus de 2 ans. Rev Chir Orthop Reparatrice Appar Mot 82: 743–752
14. Gotzen L, Bahrs CH, Leppek R, Schnabel M (2003) Suggestion for a modular topographic-morphologic classification of humeral fractures. Eur J Trauma 1: 31–41
15. Habermeyer P, Schweiberer L (1991) Konservative und operative Differentialtherapie. Unfallchirurg 94: 438–446
16. Habermeyer P, Ebert T (1999) Aktueller Entwicklungsstand und Perspektiven der Schulterendoprothetik. Unfallchirurg 102: 668–683

17. Habermeyer P, Schweiberer L (1990) Schulterchirurgie. Urban und Schwarzenberg, München, Wien, Baltimore
18. Hackethal KH (1961) Die Bündel-Nagelung. Springer-Verlag, Berlin
19. Halder S (1996) The Halder humeral nailing system. J Bone Joint Surg 78B: 61–66
20. Healy WL, Jupiter JB, White RR (1990) Non-union of the proximal humerus. In: Post M, Morrey BF, Hawkins R (eds) Surgery of the Shoulder. St Louis, Mosby: 59–65
21. Heitkemper S, Rickert M, Loew M (2004) Ergebnisse nach Schulterprothese bei der Behandlung Fehlverheilter Humeruskopffrakturen. Akt Traumatol 34: 117–122
22. Hente R, Kampshoff B, Kinner B, Füchtmeier M, Nerlich M (2004) Die Versorgung dislozierter 3- und 4-Fragmentfrakturen des proximalen Humerus mit einem winkelstabilen Plattenfixateur. Unfallchirurg 107: 769–782
23. Hessmann MH, Blum J, Hofmann A, Küchle R, Rommens PM (2003) Internal fixation of proximal humeral fractures: current concepts. Eur J Trauma 5: 253–261
24. Helferich H (1906) Frakturen und Luxationen 12: 142–159. JF Fischer Verlag, München
25. Kapandij A (1974) Le broches en palmiers. Techniques osteosynthese des fractures du col chirurgical de l'humerus. Communication orale aux Journees de printemps 1974 de la SOFCOT en Martinique
26. Kuhner EH, Siebler G (1987) Luxationsfrakturen des proximalen Humerus - Ergebnisse nach operativer Behandlung. Eine AO-Sammelstudie über 167 Fälle
27. Lahm A, Roesgen M (1991) Minimalosteosynthese mit Drahtcerclagen bei disloziierten Humeruskopffrakturen. Akt Traumatol 26: 22–28
28. Lill H, Lange K, Prasse-Bade J, Schmidt A, Verheyden P, Echtermeyer V (1997) Die T-Platten-Osteosynthese bei disloziierten proximalen Humerusfrakturen. Unfallchirurgie 23: 183–189
29. Lin J, Hou SM, Hang YS (1998) Locked nailing for displaced surgical neck fractures of the humerus. J Trauma 45: 1051–1057
30. Mouradian WH (1986) Displaced proximal humeral fractures: seven years experience with a modified zickel supracondylar device. Clin Orthop Rel Res 212: 209–218
31. Müller ME, Allgöwer M, Willenegger H (1969) Manual der Osteosynthese - AO Technik. Springer-Verlag, Berlin, Heidelberg, New York
32. Müller ME, Nazarian S, Koch P, Schatzker J (1988) The comprehensive classification of fractures. Springer-Verlag, Berlin
33. Neer CS (1970) Displaced humeral fractures. Part I: Classification and evaluation. J Bone Joint Surg Am 52: 1977–2089
34. Neer CS, Watson KC, Stanton FJ (1982) Recent experience in total shoulder replacement. J Bone Joint Surg 64A: 319–337
35. Neumann K, Ekkernkamp A (1993) Erfahrungen mit der Schultergelenkendoprothetik. Med Orthop Tech 113: 209–211
36. Norris TR, Green A, McGuigan FX (1995) Late prosthetic shoulder arthroplasty for displaced proximal humerus fractures. J Shoulder Elbow Surgery 4: 271–280
37. Ochsner PE, Hachmann Th (1991) Zuggurtungsosteosynthesen mit resorbierbaren Kordeln bei proximalen Humerusmehrfragmentbrüchen. Unfallchirurg 94: 508–510
38. Poelchen R (1930) Die Behandlung der Frakturen der oberen Extremität ohne Fixation, nur mit aktiver Extensionsbehandlung. Monschr Unfallheilkd 37: 193–219
39. Reich I, Lippert V, Otto W (2000) Aktuelle Behandlungsstrategien bei Mehrfragmentfrakturen des proximalen Humerus. Trauma und Berufskrankheit 2: 270–276
40. Resch H, Povacz P, Fröhlich R, Wambacher M (1997) Percutaneous fixation of three- and four-part fractures of proximal humerus. J Bone Joint Surg 79B: 295–300
41. Robinson CM, Page RS, Hill RMF, Sanders DL, Court-Brown ChM, Wakefield AE (2003) Primary hemiarthroplasty for treatment of proximal humeral fractures. J Bone Joint Surg 85 A: 1215–1223
42. Rodosky W, Flatow EL (1996) Two parts displaced surgical neck fractures. In: Flatow EL, Ulrich C (eds) Humerus, musculoskeletal trauma series. Butterworth-Heinemann, Oxford
43. Rommens PM, Blum J, Runkel M (1998) Retrograde nailing of humeral shaft fractures. Clin Orthop 350: 26–39
44. Ruchholtz S, Nast-Kolb D (2003) Die Oberarmkopffraktur. Unfallchirurg 106: 498–513
45. Rüther A (2001) Indikation und Technik der Schulterprothese bei der Frakturversorgung. Chirurg 72: 1246–1252
46. Sarmiento A, Latta LL (1981) Closed functional treatment of fractures. Springer-Verlag, Heidelberg, Berlin, New York
47. Scheck M (1982) Surgical treatment of the surgical neck of the humerus. Clin Orthop 167: 255–259
48. Seidel H (1989) Humeral locking nail: a preliminary report. Orthopaedics 12: 219–226
49. Seidel H (2002) Humeral fractures. Practice of intramedullary locked nails, Vol 1. Springer-Verlag, Heidelberg, Berlin, New York: 113–126
50. Seidel H (2002) Atlas of clinical cases: humerus. Practice of intramedullary locked nails, Vol 2. Springer-Verlag, Heidelberg, Berlin, New York: 154–158
51. Specht G (1976) Primäre funktionelle Behandlung der Oberarmschaftbrüche. Akt Prob l Chir Orthop 11: 227–234
52. Speck M, Reganzzoni P (1997) 4-Fragment-Frakturen des proximalen Humerus. Alternative Strategien der chirurgischen Behandlung. Unfallchirurg 100: 349–353
53. Stableforth P (1984) Four part fractures of the neck of humerus. J Bone Joint Surg 66B: 104–108
54. Stedtfeldt HW, Attmannspacher W, Thaler K, Frosch B (2003) Fixation of humeral head fractures with antegrade intramedullary nailing. Zentralbl Chir 128: 6–11
55. Szyskowitz R, Schippinger G (1999) Die Frakturen des proximalen Humerus. Unfallchirurg 102: 422–428
56. Szyskowitz R (2000) Humerus: proximal. In: AO Principles of fracture management. Thieme-Verlag, Stuttgart, New York: 271–290
57. Tanner MW, Cofield RH (1983) Prosthetic arthroplasty for fractures and fracture dislocation of the proximal humerus. Clin Orthop 179: 116–128
58. Treumann TC, Caspar U, Babst R, Schönhofen H, Strobel K, Allgayer B (2001) Stereovisualisierung von CT-Datensätzen bei komplexen Humerusfrakturen: Einfluss auf die Klassifizierung nach Neer und AO und Einfluss auf die Therapieplanung RoeFO 2001. Georg Thieme-Verlag, Stuttgart, New York, roefo@thieme.de
59. Vrancken Peeters MJTFD, Kastelein GW, Breslau PJ (2001) Proximal humerus fractures: a prospective study of the functional outcome after conservative treatment. Eur J Trauma 13: 133–136
60. Wanner GA, Wanner-Schmidt E, Romero J, Hersche O, von Smekal A, Trentz O, Ertel W (2003) Internal fixation of displaced proximal humeral fractures with two one-third tubular plates. J Trauma 54: 536–544
61. Weigand H, Müller A, Gutjahr G, Ritter G (1984) Einteilung der Frakturen des proximalen Humerusendes nach prognostischen und therapeutischen Gesichtspunkten. Unfallchirurgie 10: 221–236

Intramedullary Nailing of Proximal Humeral Fractures

A. ELSEN

Introduction

The treatment of proximal humerus fractures has undergone a large number of different concepts over the last years. Beside conservative measures, a variety of operative techniques have been proposed.

Decision-making is based on the specific fracture pattern, the quality of bone and the individual patient parameters such as biological age and functional needs.

Fractures with minimal or no displacement should usually be treated nonoperatively, as good functional outcome for this group of fractures has been reported [1]. Fortunately, 70–80% of all fractures of the humeral head can be treated conservatively, because they are not dislocated.

On the other hand, there is consensus that in displaced and highly comminuted four-part fractures and head-splitting fractures in the elderly, a primary hemiarthroplasty is recommended [2].

The treatment of displaced three-part and even four-part fractures of the proximal humerus remains controversial. The reported techniques show a wide range of different recommendations, such as percutaneous procedures using wires, pins or screws [3, 4], to open procedures with plate fixation or even joint replacement. The plate fixation of proximal humeral fractures is due to the introduction of angular stable locking plates, and reports show a good outcome [5, 6]. Nevertheless, plate fixation often needs an extended exposure of the fracture elements and can increase the risk of osteonecrosis of the humeral head by disturbing the blood supply. Bulky extramedullary hardware can lead to mechanical complications, as subacromial impingement, and loosening of the plate and screws in poor bone stock have been reported.

Therefore, minimally invasive techniques with closed and indirect reduction have been advocated to preserve the soft tissue envelope and the blood supply to the humeral head and fracture elements.

Intramedullary nailing is a common and usual therapy in the treatment of humeral shaft fractures. In proximal fractures, using intramedullary implants is associated with problems of secure fixation and achieving a rotational stability of the humeral head and its fragments. Therefore, because of the success of angular stable locking plates, angular and sliding stable locking nails have been developed [7–9].

These nails should provide multiplanar locking modes for a rigid fracture fixation, achieving a rotator cuff stability to allow early mobilization without the risk of secondary loss of reduction. Cadaver analyses have shown that the highest bone strength can be found in medial and dorsal aspects of the humeral head and that it decreases from cranial to caudal [10]. Implants should therefore provide secure fixation in this area.

Indications

Common classification systems for fracture typing of the proximal humerus are those from Codman, the AO system and the Neer classification [11]. Although limited inter- and intraobserver reliability is reported [12, 13], the Neer classification still represents the most used typing system in clinical practice.

As shown in Fig. 4.10.2.1, Neer describes four major fragments: the humeral head, the lesser tuberosity, the greater tuberosity and the humeral shaft. The classification is based on the presence or absence of significant displacement of one or more of these bone segments. If any of these fragments shows a displacement of more than 1 cm or is angulated more than 45°, the fracture is said to be displaced.

According to Neer: "Displacement defined arbitrarily as a guide for surgeons – 1 cm or 45 degrees, but no guarantee that those with less displacement will do well."

One-part fractures are nondisplaced fractures or fractures with minimal displacement. A two-

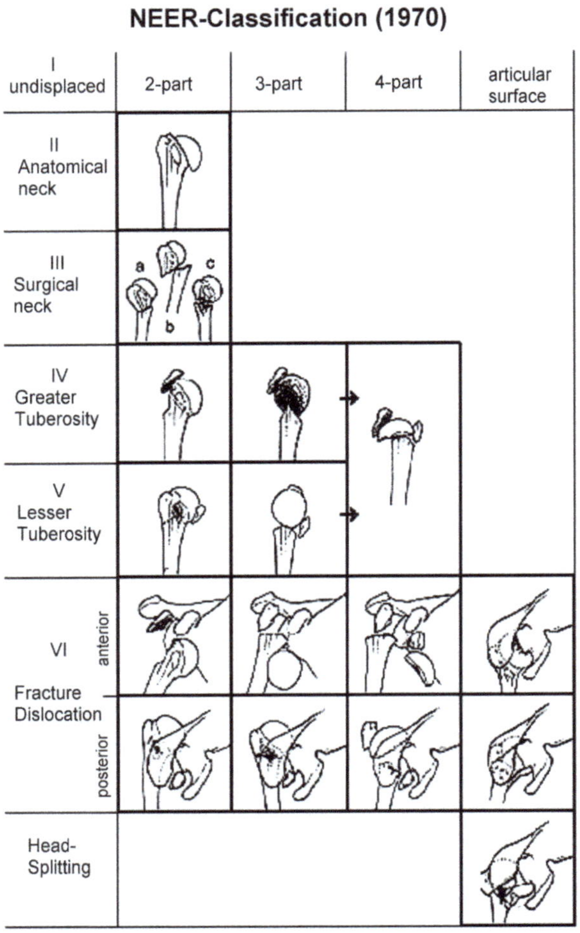

Fig. 4.10.2.1. Neer classification

part fracture is one in which only a single segment is displaced in relation to the other three. Three-part fractures occur when two segments are displaced with relation to the other two parts and a four-part fracture exists when all the humeral segments are displaced. Computed tomography scans allow an accurate determination of the Neer fracture pattern, particularly when the humeral fractures are complex.

This classification is not meant as a numerical classification but rather as a concept that makes it possible to describe a fracture or fracture dislocation with standard terminology.

According to this classification, we recommend intramedullary nailing for the following types of fractures:

- Neer type III
- Neer type IV three-part
- Neer type V three-part.

Additional indications are even four-part fractures but only with an intact head fragment. Special features of the T2 proximal humerus nail allow reliable fixation in the often poor cancellous bone, and additional fragments can be augmented by suture, using the locking screws as an anchor.

Proximal humeral fractures with diaphyseal extension can be treated by using special versions of intramedullary nails with a long diaphyseal stem. Furthermore we see an indication in very proximal humeral shaft fractures, where standard locking nails in retro- or antegrade technique do not achieve a secure fixation of the proximal locking screws in the humeral head.

Implant Features and Instruments

The following report is based on the use of the T2 proximal humerus nail (Stryker Trauma GmbH, Prof. Küntscher-Strasse 1–5, 24332 Schönkirchen, Germany).

The proximal humerus nail is made from type II anodized titanium alloy (Ti6AL4V) with its known mechanical advantages and biocompatibility. The material allows postoperative CT and MRI scans with minimized appearance of artifacts.

The nail has four proximal locking holes, thus enabling separate locking of fragments of the lesser tuberosity, the greater tuberosity and the humeral head. The proximal holes in the nail are threaded and have a nylon bushing to prevent screw back-out. The proximal 5-mm locking screws are in consequence of this feature axial and sliding stable fixated in the nail. Therefore the combination of the nail and the proximal screws performs mechanically as one firm construction.

The proximal humerus nail is manufactured in different versions. The standard short nail has a length of 150 mm and can be obtained in a left and right version with asymmetric positioning of the proximal locking screws to reduce possible lesions of the axillary nerve. Additionally long nails from 220 to 300 mm can be obtained for the left and right humerus to handle proximal humeral fractures with diaphyseal extension (Fig. 4.10.2.2). All nails have a proximal 6° lateral bend.

In both the short and long nail versions, the positioning of the proximal locking screws is guided by a target device. The distal locking for the short nail is done using the target device, whereas in the long nails a freehand locking is performed. The distal locking hole configuration allows either static or dynamic locking modes.

Proximal locking is always done using 5-mm screws; distal locking is performed with 4-mm

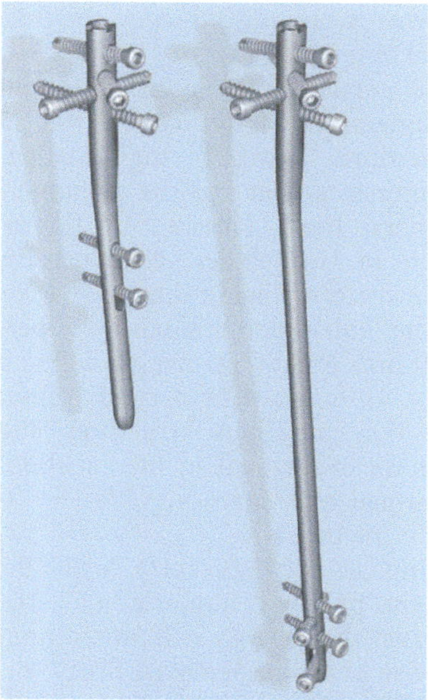

Fig. 4.10.2.2. T2 Proximal humerus nail

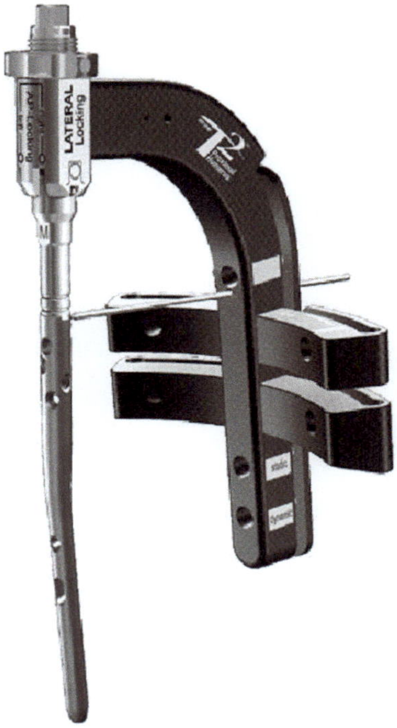

Fig. 4.10.2.3. Target device

screws. For both diameters, a 3.5-mm drill is used.

Additional to the screw fixation a supplementary hold in the humeral head is achieved by optimal fitting of the proximal nail end in the cortex. Therefore end caps of three different heights in 2-mm increments allow fine adjustment to the length of the nail and optimize the purchase of the nail in the entrance hole.

All nails have a proximal diameter of 10 mm, distal 8 mm. The long nails are cannulated and allow reaming of the medullary canal over a guide wire. The solid nail design of the short nail does not require additional reaming for nail insertion.

Most of the instruments are known from the T2 platform.

A specially designed carbon-fiber radiolucent targeting device (Fig. 4.10.2.3) allows placement of all proximal screws and distal locking screws of the short nail.

As described below in the operative technique, different features to secure the correct rotational alignment or the correct insertion depth of the nail are implemented in the target device.

Calibrated drill bits give correct measurements of screw length. Proximal screw holes should be drilled manually. This improves the surgeon's "feel" of the bone and helps to avoid penetration of the articular surface of the humeral head. The drill sleeves are held in position by a special friction locking mechanism. These sleeves, when locked into the targeting device, will also help to stabilize the nail and may temporarily stabilize fragments during fixation.

Operative Technique

The most important step before starting surgery is an accurate analysis of the fracture type and pattern. We therefore perform a CT scan in cases where classification with standard radiographic methods is uncertain or in complex fracture patterns.

We recommend placement of the patient in the "beach chair" position or supine on a radiolucent table supplemented with a standard arm rest. Prior to disinfection and draping, the correct placement of the patient should be checked to ensure that intraoperative fluoroscopy and access to entry side is possible (Fig. 4.10.2.4).

The skin incision should begin anterolateral to the acromion in line with the fibers of the deltoid muscle. The length of the incision depends on the fracture type and the need for an open reduction. The deltoid muscle is split to expose the subdeltoid bursa; the supraspinatus tendon is then incised in line with its fibers after identification of the bicipital groove by palpation. Reduction of the fracture can often be realized in "joy stick

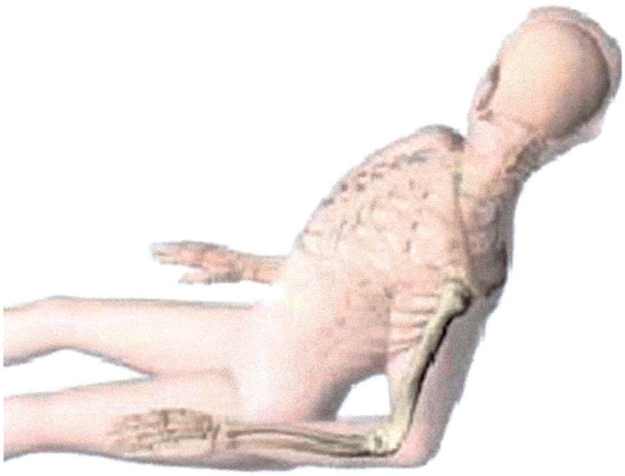

Fig. 4.10.2.4. Patient positioning

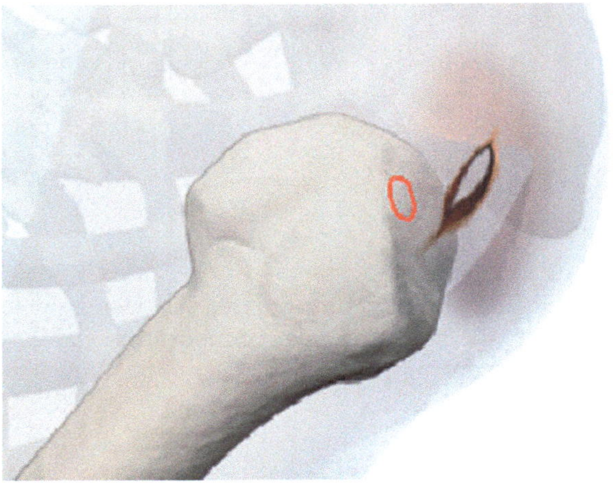

Fig. 4.10.2.5. Entry point

technique" using a 2.5-mm Kirschner wire to manipulate the fragments. As an alternative, sutures in the rotator cuff are used to achieve a valgus position of the humeral head fragment. Temporary fixation of fragments in four-part fractures can be realized with 1.5-mm Kirschner wires. If closed reduction is not possible, an open reduction should be performed.

The T2 proximal humeral nail should be inserted through a central entry point (Fig. 4.10.2.5). This entry point is located at the very top of the humeral head, in the articular surface, in line with the humeral axis. We would recommend this central access because of the supplementary hold of the nail in the cortex of the humeral head. An intermittently described lateral entry point is located just inside the greater tuberosity and aligned with the humeral axis. Apart from the decreased stability, in undislocated fractures of the greater tuberosity we have seen dislocation of fragments when introducing the nail through the lateral entry point.

Identifying the correct entry point in alignment with the humeral axis is the central step in the operative procedure. Control by digital palpation of the long biceps tendon and the circumference of the humeral head, followed by fluoroscopic verification in two planes, confirms the correct entry point before placing the guide wire. Preparation of the entry point should be performed with a 10-mm hollow reamer to define a clear-cut portal. A 10-mm awl or a rigid reamer may comminute the cancellous structures and weaken the purchase of the nail in the subchondral bone. For reamed techniques a guide wire is inserted across the fracture site.

Further reaming is not necessary with the short version of the proximal humerus nail. The nail may be inserted directly. As it is not cannulated, the guide wire has to be removed first.

For insertion of the long nail, reaming of the medullary canal may be necessary. Reaming is commenced in 0.5-mm increments. Final reaming should be 1–1.5 mm larger than the diameter of the nail to be used. An unreamed technique can be considered in cases where the medullary canal has the appropriate diameter. In these cases, the long nail can be introduced directly over the guide wire.

As the arrangement of the proximal locking screws is asymmetrical for the right and left version, the appropriate nail is chosen and mounted to the targeting device. Before inserting the nail, correct alignment should be checked by inserting a drill or K wire through the required holes of the targeting device.

The nail should be inserted only with manual pressure. Using a hammer may result in additional fractures or fragment displacements. If the nail does not advance easily, fluoroscopy should be used to identify the problem.

Depth of nail insertion may be determined with the help of two circumferential grooves on the nail adapter, which can be visualized with the image intensifier. The nail should be inserted at least up to the first groove on the adapter but not deeper than the second groove. Another option to determine nail insertion depth is performed with the target device. An inserted K wire (Fig. 4.10.2.3) indicates the exact top end of the nail.

Before proximal locking, the correct rotational position is checked. To achieve the correct anatomical 30° retroversion of the humeral head, a K wire is inserted through the targeting device. The wire should be parallel to the forearm to indicate the correct rotational alignment (Fig. 4.10.2.6).

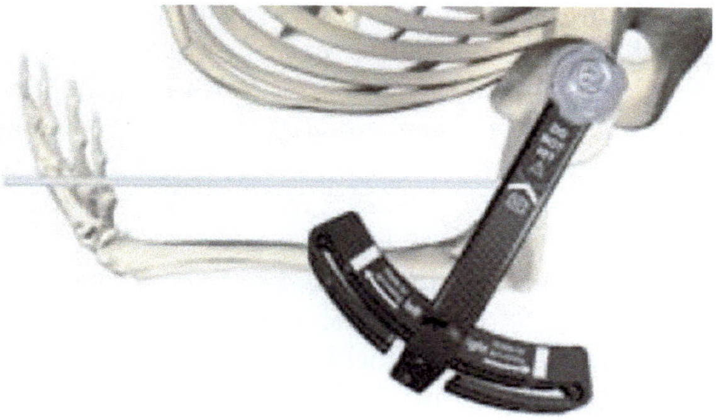

Fig. 4.10.2.6. Rotational alignment

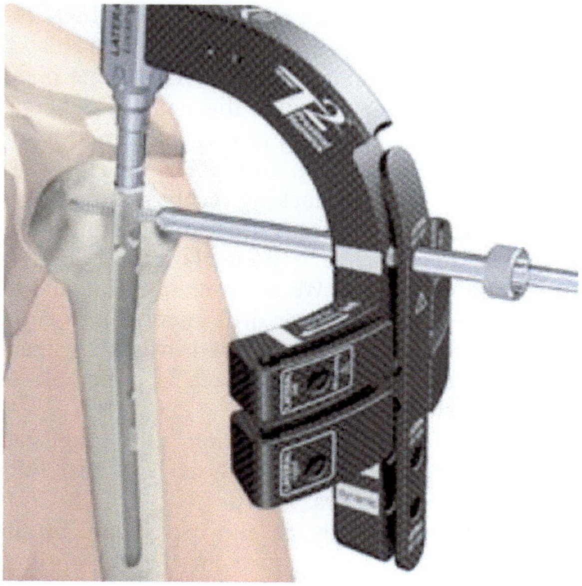

Fig. 4.10.2.7. Proximal locking I

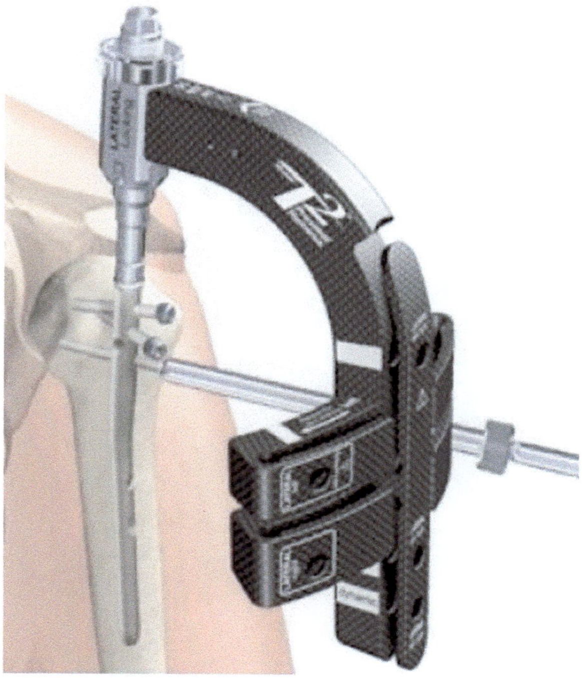

Fig. 4.10.2.8. Proximal locking II

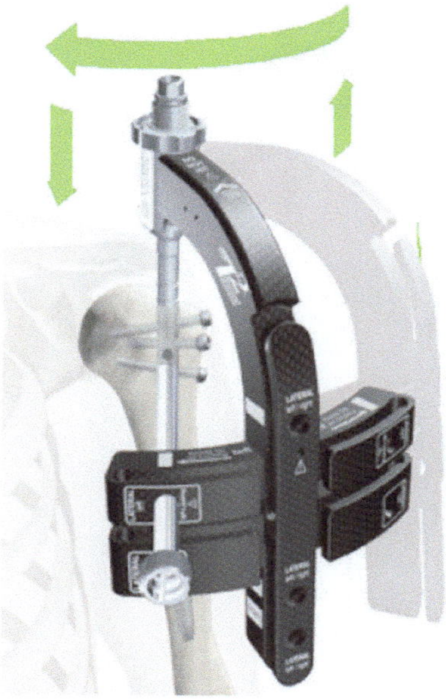

Fig. 4.10.2.9. AP locking

Except for the anteroposterior (AP) locking, all the proximal and distal locking procedures (short nail only) can be performed without changing the position of the targeting arm. Using sleeves inserted in the target device, manually drilling with a 3.5-mm drill is performed until it is in contact with the subchondral bone. The far cortex should not be injured. The correct screw length may be read directly off the drill at the end of the drill sleeve. The 5.0-mm screws are available from 25 mm to 60 mm in 2.5-mm steps. If in doubt about the appropriate screw length, the next shorter one should be used to minimize the risk of penetrating the articular surface (Fig. 4.10.2.7). The length of the locking screws should be checked with fluoroscopy. The next two screws are inserted in the same way using the target device (Fig. 4.10.2.8).

The AP screw is designed to fix the lesser tuberosity. To place this screw, the target device must be rotated (Fig. 4.10.2.9). After releasing the holding nut, the arm is pulled up and rotated anteriorly around the nail adapter.

We would recommend use of proximal locking options to achieve a secure fixation of the nail in

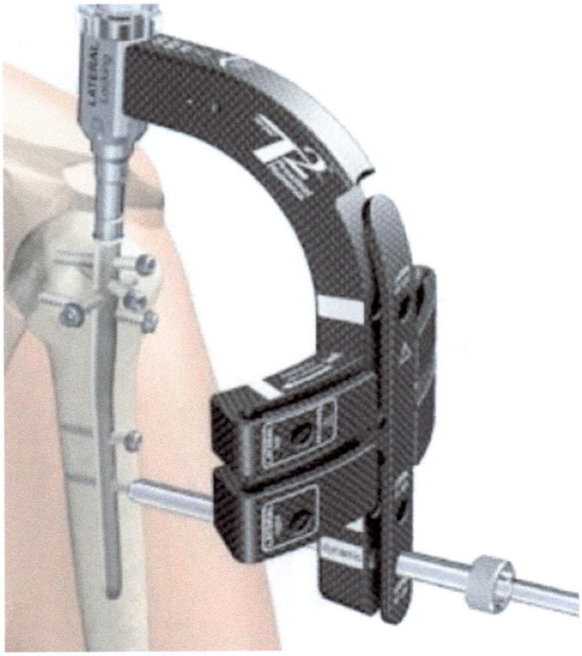

Fig. 4.10.2.10. Distal locking I

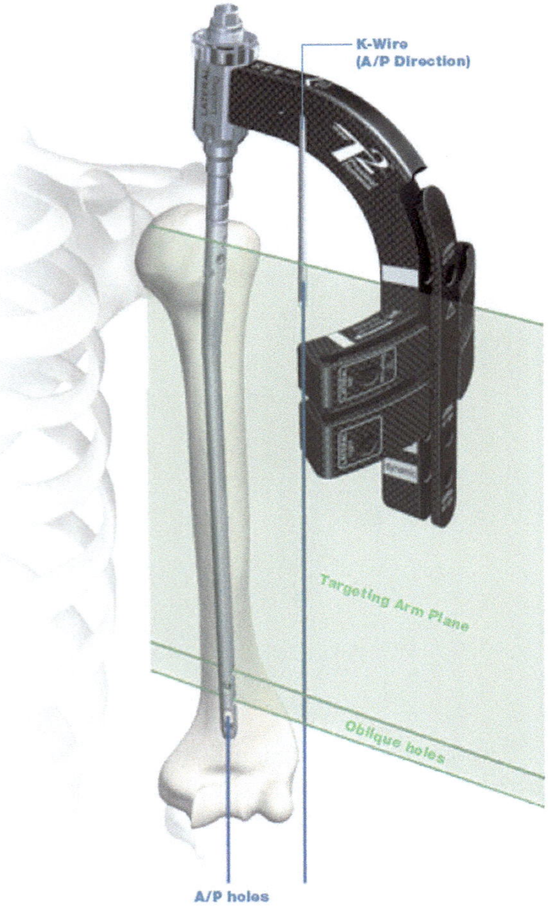

Fig. 4.10.2.11. Distal locking II

the humeral head and in consequence safe fragment fixation. Fractures of the tubercles can be fixed with the locking screws in cases with good bone structure. In a situation with comminuted fragments of the tubercles, tension band sutures fixed at the screw heads can provide further stability.

The distal locking with 4-mm screws can be done in static or dynamic mode. For static locking mode, two distal locking screws are used (Fig. 4.10.2.10). Dynamic locking is done with one screw at the bottom of the oblong hole.

The target device cannot be used directly for distal locking of the long nail versions. But leaving the targeting device attached can facilitate the freehand locking procedure. A K wire placed through the targeting device is in the same plane as the AP locking holes at the nail tip, whereas the plane of the targeting arm is the same for the distal oblique holes (Fig. 4.10.2.11).

There are multiple locking techniques reported. The critical step with any freehand locking technique is to visualize a perfectly round locking hole with the C-arm. We recommend using an angulated radiolucent power drill under fluoroscopy. In order to avoid lesions of neurovascular structures, the limited open approach is preferable to stab incisions.

Similar to the short version, the long nail should be locked distally with at least two fully threaded 4-mm screws.

After distal locking, an end cap should be inserted to adjust the height of the nail for optimal purchase in the subchondral bone. Additionally, the end cap locks and stabilizes the proximal locking screw. The length of the end cap must be selected accurately from three sizes (standard, +2 mm, +4 mm) to avoid subacromial impingement.

Clinical Cases

The first case is a 65-year-old woman with a three-part fracture of the right proximal humerus (Figs. 4.10.2.12 and 4.10.2.13). A closed reduction and osteosynthesis with the T2 proximal humeral nail was performed (Figs. 4.10.2.14 and 4.10.2.15). Nine months after primary surgery, the nail was removed (Figs. 4.10.2.16 and 4.10.2.17). Before removal of the implant, the patient showed a good clinical result and respectable range of motion (Figs. 4.10.2.18 and 4.10.2.19).

The second report is an 86-year-old male patient with a two-part fracture of the humeral head with a diaphyseal extension of fracture lines (Figs.

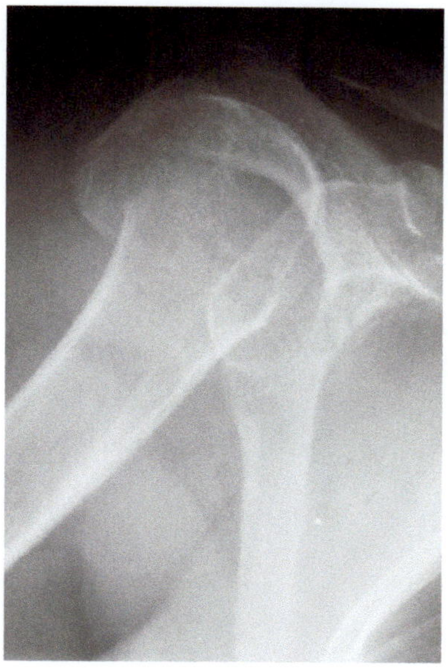

Fig. 4.10.2.12. Three-part fracture of the right proximal humerus

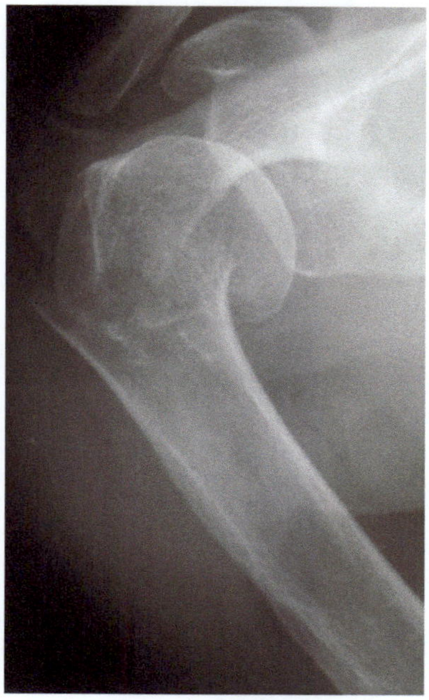

Fig. 4.10.2.13. Three-part fracture of the right proximal humerus

4.10.2.20 and 4.10.2.21). Stabilization was achieved with a long version of the T2 proximal humerus nail (Fig. 4.10.2.22). The patient underwent primary surgery at the time of finishing this chapter, in January 2005. Therefore no further radiological images are available.

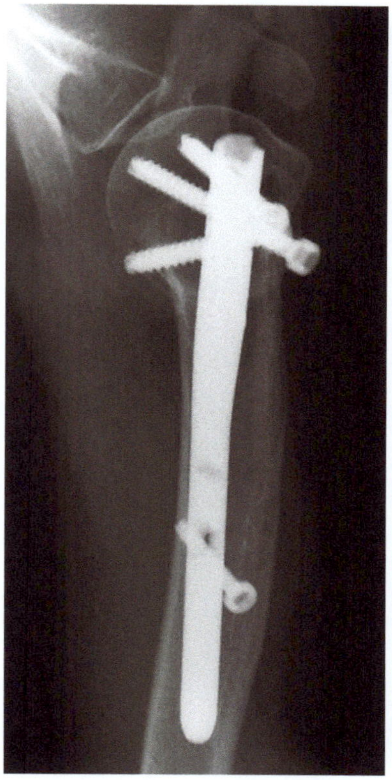

Fig. 4.10.2.14. Closed reduction and osteosynthesis with the T2 proximal humeral nail

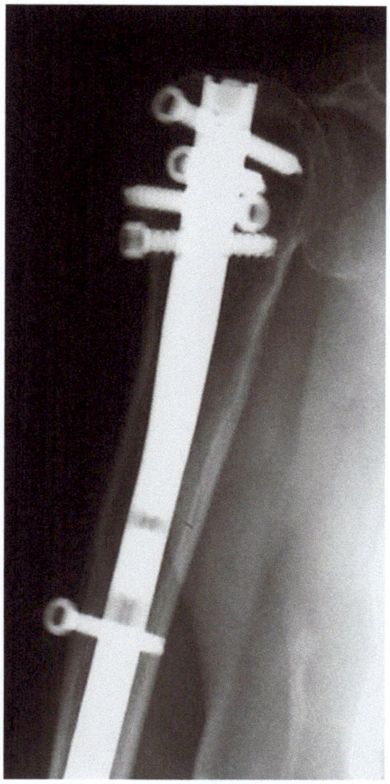

Fig. 4.10.2.15. Closed reduction and osteosynthesis with the T2 proximal humeral nail

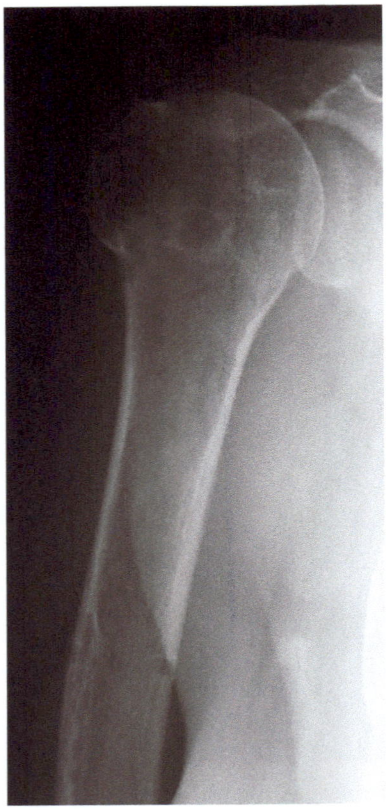

Fig. 4.10.2.16. The nail was removed 9 months after primary surgery

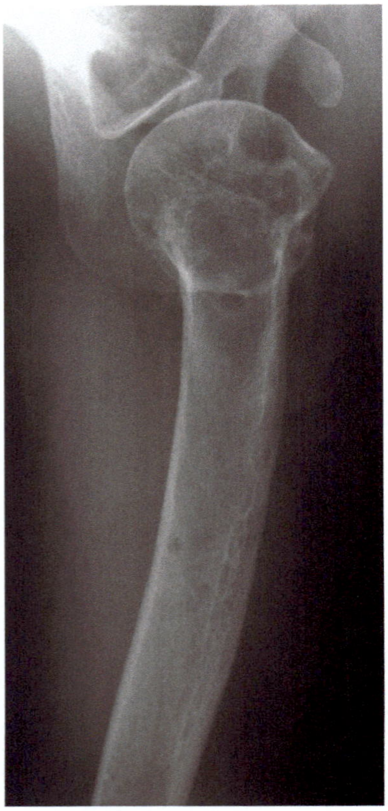

Fig. 4.10.2.17. The nail was removed 9 months after primary surgery

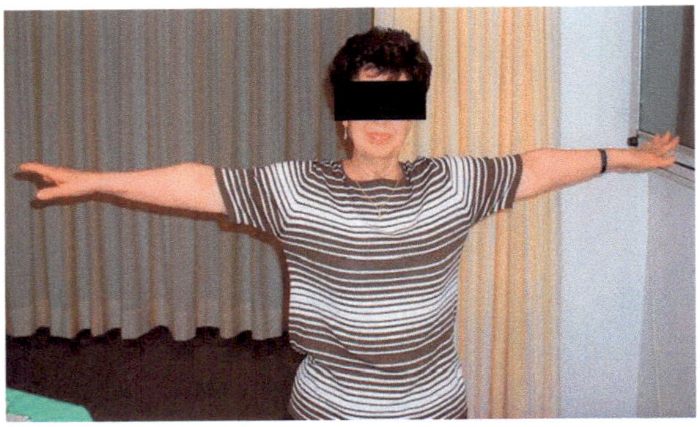

Fig. 4.10.2.18. Good clinical result and range of motion before removal of the implant

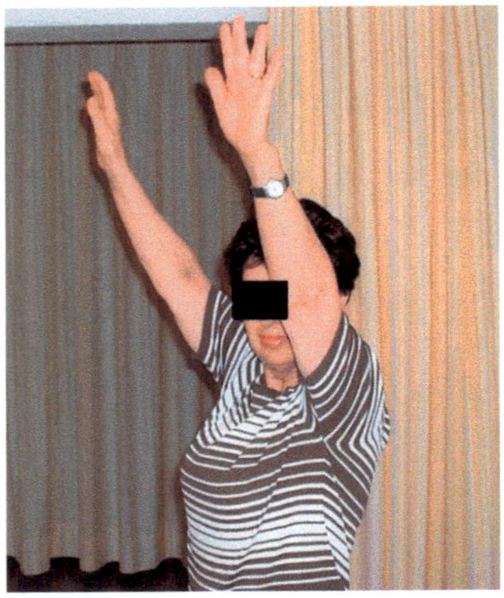

Fig. 4.10.2.19. Good clinical result and range of motion before removal of the implant

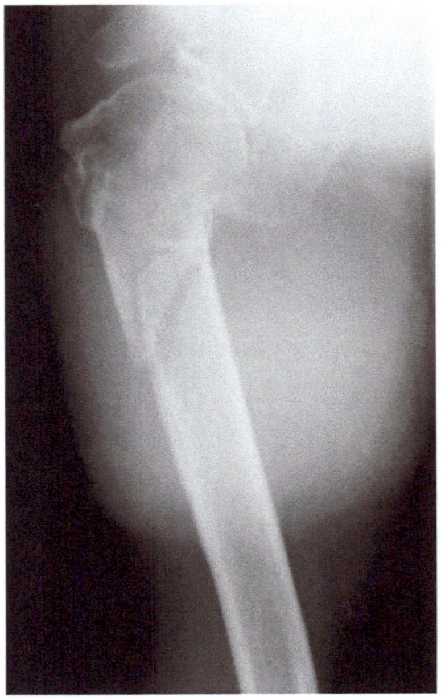

Fig. 4.10.2.20. Two-part fracture of the humeral head with a diaphyseal extension of fracture lines

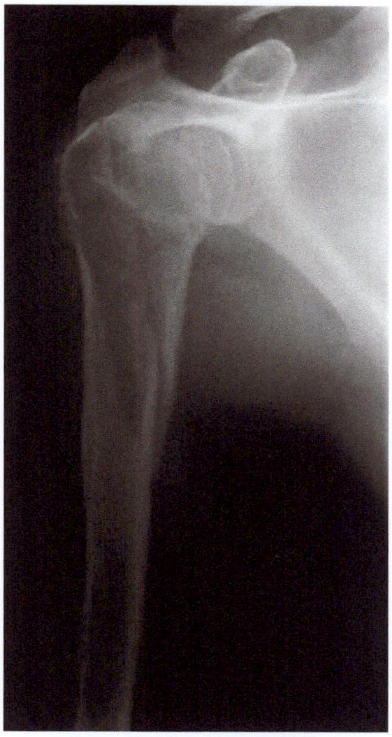

Fig. 4.10.2.21. Two-part fracture of the humeral head with a diaphyseal extension of fracture lines

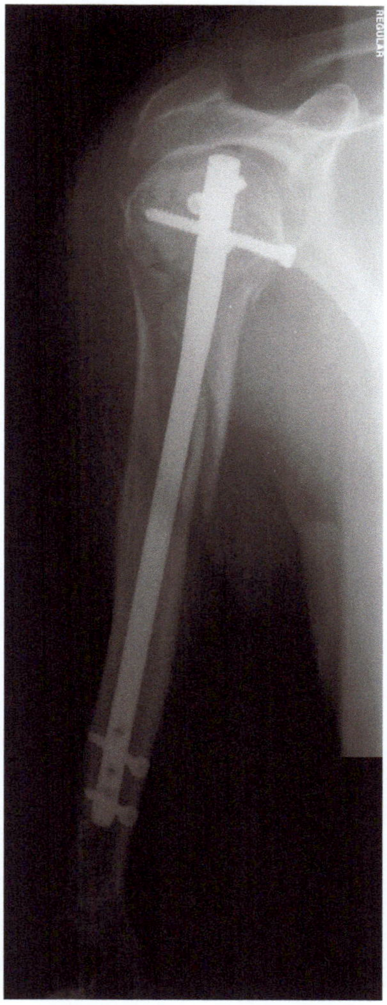

Fig. 4.10.2.22. Stabilization was achieved with a long version of the T2 proximal humeral nail

References

1. Szyskowitz R, Schippinger G. Fractures of the proximal humerus. Unfallchirurg 1999; 102(6): 422–428
2. Christoforakis JJ, Kontakis GM, Katonis PG, Stergiopoulos K, Hadjipavlou AG. Shoulder hemiarthroplasty in the management of humeral head fractures. Acta Ortop Belg 2004; 70(3): 214–218
3. Chen CY, Chao EK, Tu YK, Ueng SW, Shih CH. Closed management and percutaneous fixation of unstable proximal humerus fractures. J Trauma 1998; 45(6): 1039–1045
4. Resch H, Povacz P, Fröhlich R, Wambacher M. Percutaneous fixation of three- and four-part fractures of the proximal humerus. J Bone Joint Surg Br 1997; 79(2): 295–300
5. Hente R, Kampshoff J, Kinner B, Fuchtmeier B, Nerlich M. Treatment of dislocated 3- and 4-part fractures of the proximal humerus with an angle-stabilizing fixation plate. Unfallchirurg 2004; 107(9): 769–782
6. Köstler W, Strohm PC, Südkamp NP. Proximal humerus fracture in advanced age. Treatment with fixed angle plate osteosynthesis. Der Chirurg 2003; 74(11): 985–989
7. Rajasekhar C, Ray PS, Bhamra MS. Fixation of proximal humeral fractures with the Polarus nail. J Shoulder Elbow Surg 2001; 10(1): 7–10
8. Cuny C, Pfeffer F, Irrazi M, Chammas M, Empereur F, Berrichi A, Metais P, Beau P. A new locking nail for proximal humerus fractures: the telegraph nail. Technique and preliminary results. Rev Chir Orthop Reparatrice Appar Mot 2002; 88(1): 62–67
9. Mittlmeier WF, Stedtfeld HW, Ewert A, Beck M, Frosch B, Gradl G. Stabilization of proximal humeral fractures with an angular and sliding stable antegrade locking nail (Targon PH). J Bone Joint Surg Am 2003; 85A(Suppl 4): 136–145
10. Hepp P, Lill H, Bail H, Korner J, Niederhagen M, Haas NP, Josten C, Duda GN. Where should implants be anchored in the humeral head? Clin Orthop 2003; 415: 139–147
11. Neer CS. Displaced proximal humeral fractures. I. Classification and evaluation. J Bone Joint Surg Am 1970; 52(6): 1077–1089
12. Kristiansen B, Andersen UL, Olsen CA, Varmarken JE. The Neer classification of fractures of the proximal humerus. An assessment of interobserver variation. Skeletal Radiol 1988; 17(6): 420–422
13. Sidor ML, Zuckermann JD, Lyon T, Koval K, Cuomo F, Schoenberg N. The Neer classification system for proximal humeral fractures. An assessment of interobserver reliability and intraobserver reproducibility. J Bone Joint Surg Am 1993; 75(12): 1745–1750

Intramedullary Nailing of Humeral Shaft Fractures

J. Franke

Introduction

For the treatment of humeral shaft fractures, conservative treatment still competes with the operative approach to a much greater degree than is the case for fractures of the long bones of the lower extremity. The trend toward operative treatment continues unabated, however. Whereas Lorenz Böhler [4] could still write an article with the title "Gegen die operative Behandlung von frischen Oberarmschaftbrüchen" [Against the operative treatment of fresh humeral shaft fractures] in 1964, conservative treatment of humeral shaft fractures is now the exception at many hospitals. There are three main reasons for the preference now given to operative methods for the treatment of humeral shaft fractures: (1) the frequent absence of the necessary prerequisites for successful conservative therapy; (2) preferences expressed by patients; (3) the inherent advantages of surgical treatment as well as recent advances in surgical treatment (in particular, intramedullary osteosynthesis).

Indications

Assuming good patient compliance, an uncomplicated fracture of the humeral shaft represents an ideal indication for conservative treatment with the Sarmiento upper arm brace [12]. There are a number of situations, however, in which surgical treatment is required or in which an operative approach offers distinct advantages. In recent years, patient preferences – and the increasing demands that patients be rehabilitated quickly so they can return to work sooner – have played an increasing role.

For all of these reasons, the range of indications for osteosynthesis via intramedullary nailing has expanded markedly in recent years. In comparison with plate fixation, intramedullary nailing offers all the advantages of intramedullary implants for the treatment of humeral shaft fractures. The most important of these are: minimal surgical trauma, biological osteosynthesis, high stability of osteosynthesis, and short operation times [2, 5].

The classical indications for surgical treatment of humeral shaft fractures (Table 4.10.3.1) are quite naturally also ideal indications for intramedullary nailing.

Patients with multiple trauma profit primarily from the stabilization achieved by intramedullary nailing. Biomechanical studies have shown that the central load-bearing element in the humerus can withstand higher loads – such as those caused by the use of lower arm crutches – than fractures stabilized via plate fixation [5]. This can be a decisive advantage during follow-up treatment in patients with concomitant injuries of the lower extremity.

Two additional advantages of intramedullary nailing are that it is a rapid surgical method with minimal soft-tissue damage and thus less blood loss.

Primary treatment of open fractures of grades I–II° can be achieved via humeral shaft nailing. For higher-grade open fractures, intramedullary nailing can be carried out following initial treatment with an external fixation device. The advantage of intramedullary nailing in this situation is that it involves less soft-tissue trauma than plate fixation.

Fractures involving injury to nerves and/or blood vessels can be stabilized via intramedullary nailing without causing any substantial additional soft-tissue trauma in the area around the fracture.

Table 4.10.3.1. Classical indications for operative treatment of humeral shaft fractures

Multiple trauma
Open fractures
Nerve or vascular injury
Chain injury, bilateral fractures
Two-level fractures
Pathological fractures

The high stability of the intramedullary implant provides secure protection of the reconstructed blood vessels. Multilevel fractures can be treated by intramedullary nailing without the necessity of a long incision. Special reduction tools (Fig. 4.10.3.7) make it easier to rejoin the bone fragments.

The humeral diaphysis is frequently the location of pathological fractures. These fractures are usually caused by osteoclastic metastases of primary tumors in the kidneys, lungs or breasts. Fracture stabilization by intramedullary nailing represents an ideal method within the framework of (usually palliative) therapy [11]. The same applies, of course, to the prophylactic stabilization of impending fractures.

In addition to these classical indications, there are a number of relative indications for which intramedullary nailing is especially suitable.

Transverse fractures and short oblique fractures of the humerus are a risk factor for the development of pseudarthrosis. A high degree of rotational stability is achieved when these fractures are treated via intramedullary nailing. The fracture apposition or compression achieved by intramedullary nailing offers additional possibilities for the improvement of fracture healing in this situation.

As a rule, pseudarthrosis is still a classical indication for plate fixation in combination with spongioplasty. In cases where pseudarthrosis has developed after conservative therapy (with the exception of atrophic pseudarthrosis), fracture consolidation can be achieved by reamed intramedullary nailing. In this situation the reaming of the medullary canal serves as a kind of "internal spongioplasty." For certain types of fractures, the possibility of fragment compression offered by the intramedullary nail represents an additional advantage of this technique. In the literature good outcomes have been reported for the combination of intramedullary nailing and spongioplasty as a treatment for pseudarthrosis [9, 10].

Correction osteotomies are rarely indicated in the humerus. Intramedullary nailing represents an ideal technique for osteotomy stabilization, e.g. following derotation osteotomy.

Procedure Selection

Antegrade and retrograde procedures are basically equally suitable for the treatment of humeral shaft fractures. It is hard to decide which method is preferable since each of them has its own particular advantages and disadvantages. The following discussion has been provided to help the physician select the method most suitable for the particular case.

Implants and Instruments

The techniques described in this article are based on the use of the T2 humerus intramedullary nail system made by Stryker Howmedica GmbH (Fig. 4.10.3.1). This system is equally suitable for antegrade and retrograde intramedullary nailing. The nails are available in diameters of 7, 8 and 9 mm and lengths of 140–320 mm. To facilitate insertion and adaptation to anatomical configurations, the implants have a proximal curvature of 6° and a distal curvature of 4°. This permits eccentric insertion of the nail into the humeral head from proximal during antegrade procedures and gentle insertion into the distal humerus during retrograde procedures. The nails are manufactured from a type II anodized titanium alloy (Ti6AL4V) and cannulated. Locking is carried out with 4.0-mm fully threaded locking screws and partially

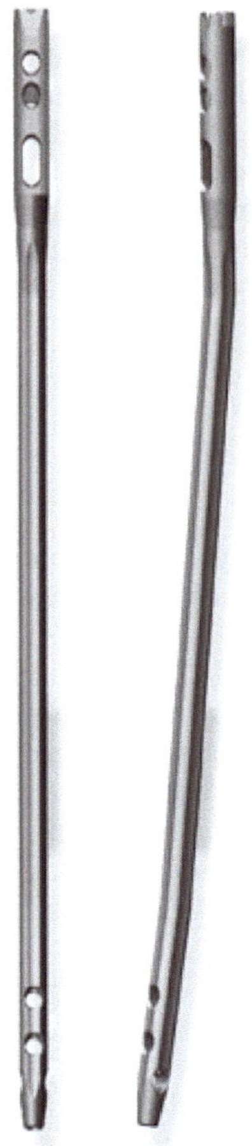

Fig. 4.10.3.1. T2 humerus intramedullary nail for antegrade and retrograde intramedullary nailing

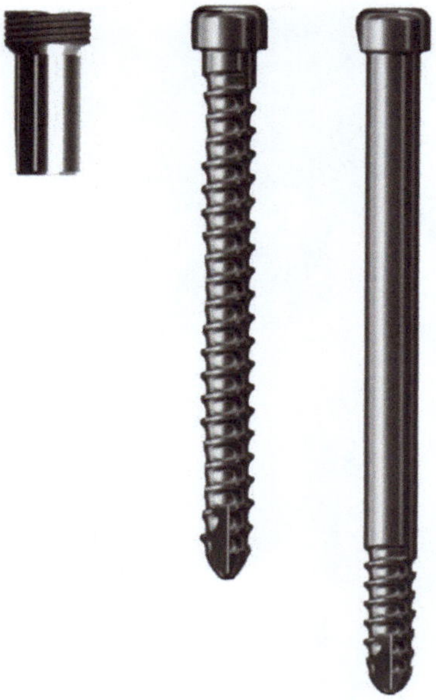

Fig. 4.10.3.2. From left to right: T2 humerus compression screw (diameter 6 mm), fully threaded locking screw (diameter 4.0 mm), partially threaded locking screw (shaft screw) (diameter 4 mm)

threaded locking screws (shaft screws). Compression locking can be carried out with the T2 compression screw (Fig. 4.10.3.2). End caps in various lengths and washers complete the system (Fig. 4.10.3.3).

Antegrade Intramedullary Nailing

During antegrade intramedullary nailing of the humerus, the intramedullary nail is inserted from

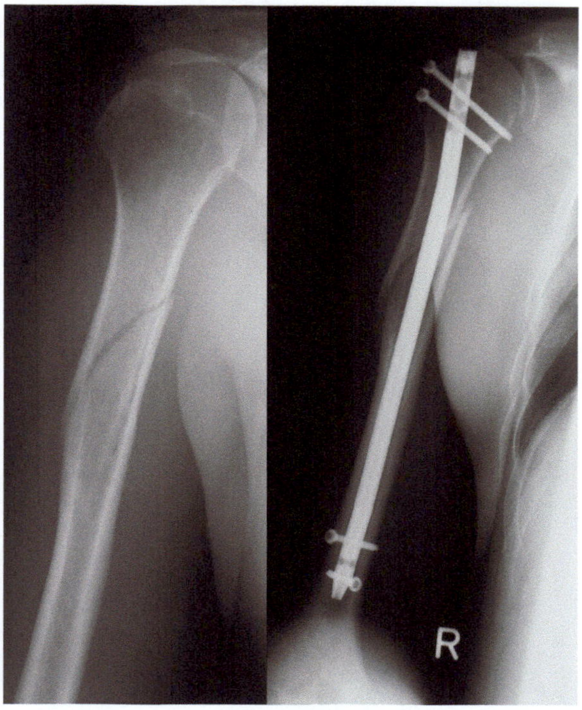

Fig. 4.10.3.4. Antegrade intramedullary nailing of the humerus with proximal diagonal locking

proximal toward distal (Fig. 4.10.3.4). The operative access is created via a deltoid split and incision of the rotator cuff. The negative effects on shoulder joint function associated with this access are sometimes considered a disadvantage of this method [1, 8, 13]. However, a search of the literature uncovers articles that report no difference in shoulder function following antegrade intramed-

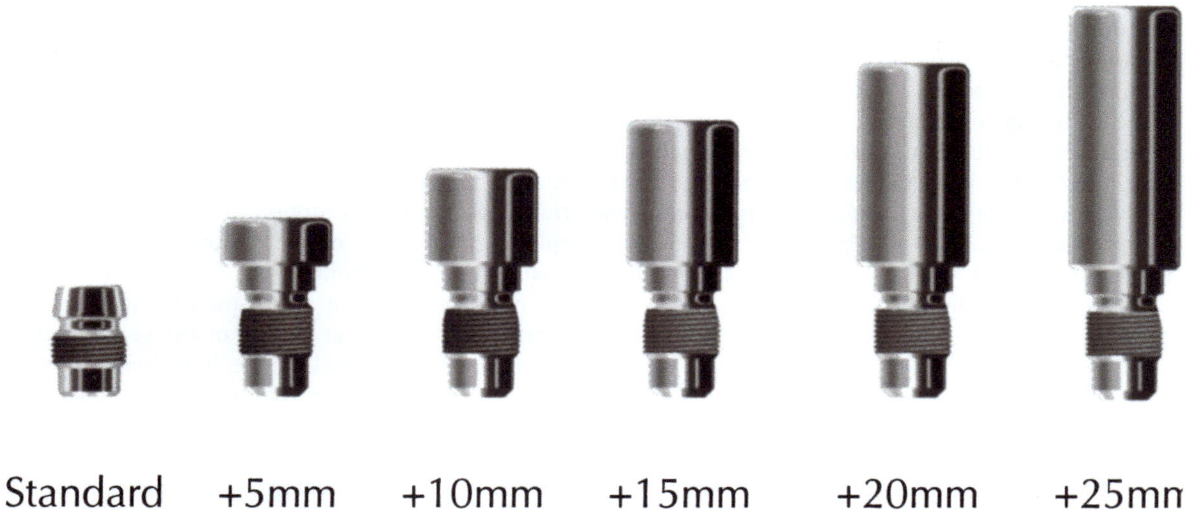

Fig. 4.10.3.3. End caps for the T2 nail in various lengths

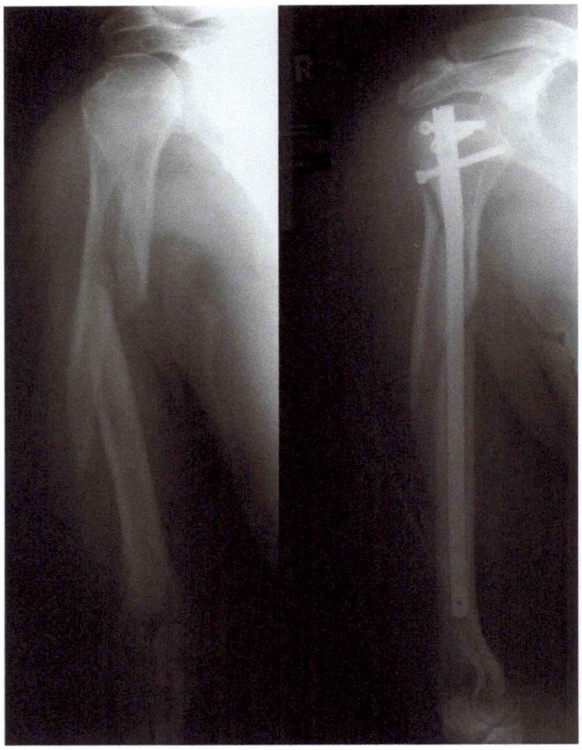

Fig. 4.10.3.5. Antegrade intramedullary nailing of the humerus with the T2 proximal humerus intramedullary nail system

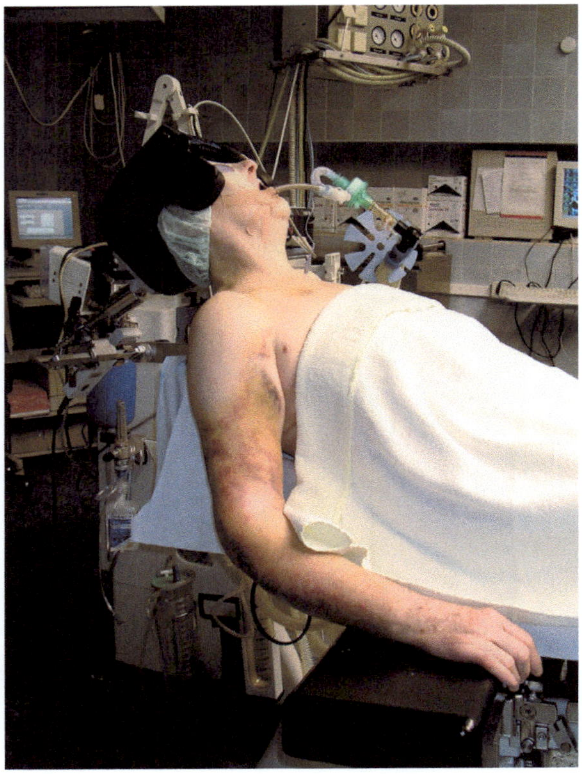

Fig. 4.10.3.6. Patient in the “beach chair position”

ullary nailing in comparison with a retrograde approach or plate osteosynthesis [2, 7].

At our hospital the antegrade procedure is performed most frequently because it offers several technical advantages: patient positioning is simpler and the nail can be inserted more easily and with fewer complications. Reduction and rotation can be checked without any difficulty. Distal locking can be performed more easily via a “freehand technique” because of the better possibilities for radiological visualization. On the other hand, finding the correct nail entry point can be more difficult, owing to the small incision.

Fractures of the proximal humeral shaft extending into the humeral head can be treated effectively via antegrade intramedullary nailing by using long versions of the proximal humeral intramedullary nail with locking options ensuring angular stability (Fig. 4.10.3.5).

Positioning

The patient is placed in the “beach chair position” (Fig. 4.10.3.6), i.e. in a semi-reclining position, on the shoulder table, and the image intensifier is placed so that the humeral head can be visualized during the procedure. The patient’s head is fixed in place on a head rest; cushions are placed under his/her knees and heels. X-ray control, which can be carried out without any difficulty, should be tested before the start of the operation. Special care should be exercised here that the entry point of the intramedullary nail in the humeral head can be visualized. The image intensifier is placed over the surgical field from the direction of the patient’s head.

Access and Entry Point

A continuous skin incision is made from the ventral edge of the acromion toward lateral. After splitting the fibers of the deltoid muscle and exposing the subdeltoid bursa, the surgeon makes an incision into the supraspinatus tendon. The correct entry point at the tip of the greater tubercle about 1 cm dorsal to the long biceps tendon can now be easily palpated. It is wise to check the chosen entry point via the image intensifier.

The medullary canal in the humeral head is opened with a cannulated awl, which can be advanced up to the zone of transition between the metaphysis and the diaphysis. Alternatively, the

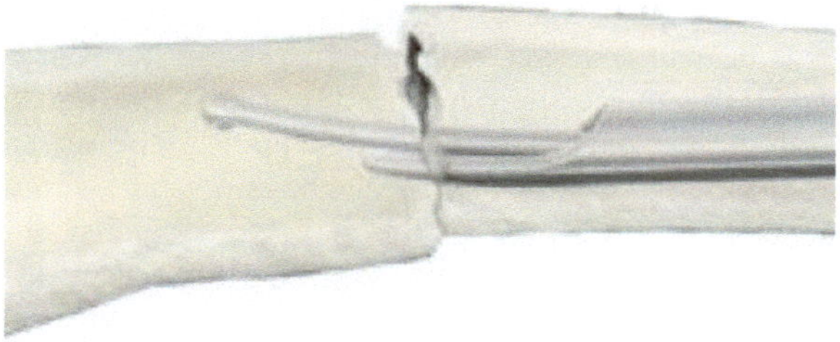

Fig. 4.10.3.7. Special reduction tool

entry point can be marked with a 3-mm Kirschner wire, which can then be forwarded in the medullary canal under image intensifier control. In this case the canal is opened with a cannulated 10-mm drill or, ideally, a special 10-mm reamer.

Reduction of the Fracture and Intramedullary Reaming of the Medullary Canal

Using the cannulated awl, it is now possible to advance a guide wire up to the distal humerus with image intensifier control. For reamed intramedullary nailing, the 2.5-mm ball tip guide wire is used. For unreamed intramedullary nailing, the 2.2-mm smooth tip guide wire is employed. In patients with multilevel fractures, in particular, special reduction tools can facilitate repositioning of the fracture fragments (Fig. 4.10.3.7). For reamed intramedullary nailing, the medullary canal is now reamed gently in increments of 0.5 mm with the guide wire.

Nail Selection and Insertion

First the appropriate nail length is selected. The intramedullary nail should be flushed with the cortex proximally and extend up to approximately 1 cm above the olecranon fossa distally. When selecting the correct nail length, the planned locking option (which depends on the type of fracture) should be taken into account (see below). Several types of rulers are available for determining nail length.

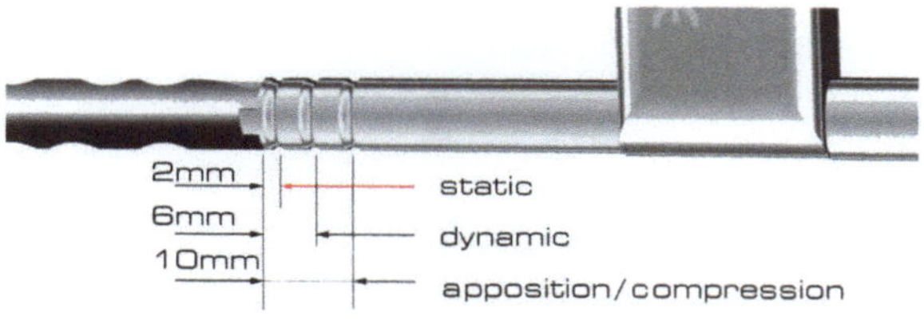

Fig. 4.10.3.8. Checking the insertion depth of the nail as a function of the locking option

The nail diameter can be determined with an X-ray template; alternatively, the diameter of the last reamer used can be taken as a guide value.

The nail selected is attached to the target device and inserted into the humerus with the 2.2-mm smooth tip guide wire. Insertion should be primarily manual. Problems may occur at the outset if the nail impinges on the medial cortex proximally and if it traverses the fracture zone. Aggressive advancement of the nail should be avoided here to prevent additional fracturing.

The correct insertion depth of the nail, which also depends on the locking option selected, can be checked using the markings on the target device (Fig. 4.10.3.8). The groove markings should be at the level of the cortex of the humeral head here.

When inserting the nail further toward distal, fracture dehiscence due to the nail should be avoided.

Locking and Compression

Proximal locking is carried out via the target device (Fig. 4.10.3.9). There are three different locking options – static, dynamic and apposition/compression – that can be selected to match the requirements for different kinds of fractures. In addition, the surgeon has the choice of a diagonal or a transverse screw posture (Fig. 4.10.3.10).

Static locking guarantees rotational and axial stability and is therefore indicated for instable fractures and comminuted fractures. The short tissue protection sleeve is inserted – along with the short drill sleeve and short trocar – into the static locking hole of the target device and posi-

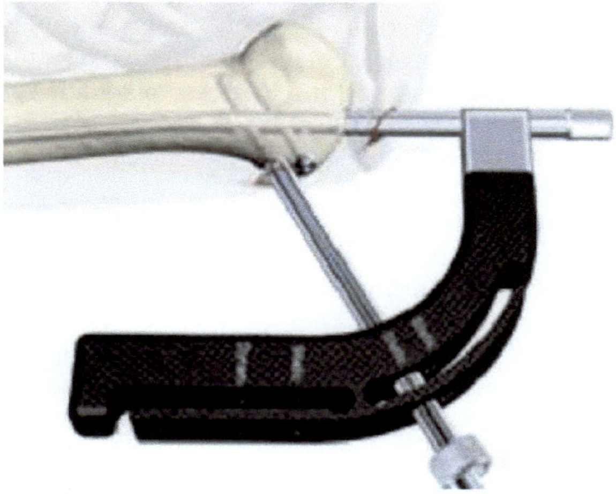

Fig. 4.10.3.9. Diagonal static locking proximally via the target device

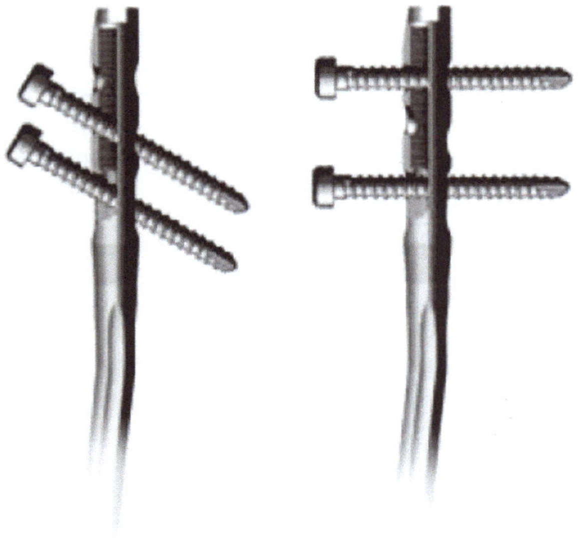

Fig. 4.10.3.10. Proximal locking options (diagonal and transverse)

tioned on the cortex of the proximal humerus via a stab incision. Drilling is carried out with a 3.5× 230-mm drill; screw length can be directly read off the scale on the drill. In addition, a screw gauge has been provided for the determination of correct screw length; this gauge is inserted over the short tissue protection sleeve. The 4-mm locking screw selected is then screwed in via the short tissue protection sleeve. When the transverse locking option is taken, care should be exercised not to perforate the opposite cortical substance in the interest of preventing an intra-articular screw position.

Consequently, in patients with poor bone substances in the humeral head, the diagonal locking option should be chosen, since, with this option, the opposite cortical substance can be drilled without the danger of screw perforation into the joint. The second locking screw is placed in an analog manner. Distal locking is performed using a freehand technique with a radiolucent drilling device.

Dynamic locking does not make much sense in the upper extremity. However, this locking option constitutes the technical prerequisite for compression or apposition locking. In fractures with axial stability, interfragmentary compression can increase fracture stability and improve fracture healing. First, distal freehand locking is carried out using the radiolucent drilling device. Prior to locking, the correct insertion depth of the nail (Fig. 4.10.3.8) and the rotational alignment should be rechecked. As a result of the compression, the nail is pulled out of the proximal fragment; for this reason it is necessary to insert the nail deeper in the humerus, paying attention to the markings on the target device. Subsequently, the proximal slot is occupied with a 4.00-mm shaft screw in the dynamic hole of the target device. For the purpose of inserting the compression screw, the nail-holding screw must be removed from the target device. Subsequently, the compression screw can be screwed in with the special screwdriver. There is a marking on the screwdriver shaft. When this marking reaches the target device, the compression mechanism starts. An image intensifier should be used to control the compression procedure in the fracture zone. Compression can also be detected indirectly by the bending of the shaft screw. If the compression screw is screwed in completely, a connection displaying angular stability will be created between the nail and the locking screw.

After compression locking, it is possible to achieve a complex compression locking affording additional stability and relief of the shaft screw by occupying the proximal transverse locking hole.

Compression locking can also be carried out in the form of fracture apposition in patients with dehiscence of the fracture. Since the aim of apposition locking is to bring the fracture ends closer together (and not to compress the ends), this technique can also be used to treat fractures with axial instability. The principle is identical to that of compression locking. The only difference is that the procedure of screwing in the compression screw is terminated as soon as bone contact has been achieved.

End Cap Insertion

Nail insertion is completed by screwing in the end cap. The end caps come in several lengths; they can thus be used to lengthen a nail that has been inserted too deeply. The option enables the surgeon to anchor the nail stably in the proximal cortex of the humeral head and facilitates material removal. Screwing in the end cap firmly creates a stable connection with angular stability between the intramedullary nail and the proximal locking screw that has been inserted transversally.

Follow-up Treatment

One of the main advantages of intramedullary nail osteosynthesis is the high stability achieved by the implant. As a rule this ensures early functional follow-up treatment and a speedy return of the patient to his/her everyday life. In patients who have undergone antegrade intramedullary nailing, for example, the disadvantage of the surgical trauma (with potential damage to the rotator cuff) can be minimized by starting physiotherapeutic exercise treatment as early as possible.

Retrograde Intramedullary Nailing

During retrograde intramedullary humeral nailing, the nail is inserted from distal toward proximal. The patient is placed in the prone position. For this reason, this method is of only limited applicability for patients with concomitant pulmonary and/or cardiac disease as well as for patients with multiple trauma including craniocerebral trauma and/or chest, abdominal or spinal column injuries.

An additional problem associated with this method is the relatively high rate of iatrogenic fractures in the vicinity of the nail entry point; in the literature this complication is reported in up to 8% of cases [1, 6]. In connection with proximal freehand locking, the dorsoventral locking option still poses the risk of injury to the axillary nerve [3].

Several authors report a higher incidence of pseudarthrosis in connection with retrograde intramedullary nailing. Since no cause specific for a particular method has been identified so far, we have to conclude that this complication is due to technical problems.

Numerous studies have been carried out to assess postoperative shoulder and elbow function in relation to the individual techniques used for intramedullary nailing. The researchers performing these studies conclude unanimously that, provided the nail is inserted correctly, there is no significant detrimental effect on elbow function after either antegrade or retrograde procedures. A comparison of the studies exploring functional outcomes in the shoulder joint, in contrast, reveals no uniform conclusions. The only point of agreement among the various authors is the early functional limitation of shoulder joint function observed after antegrade intramedullary nailing. After several months, however, there was no significant difference in shoulder function in patients treated with the different methods.

Retrograde intramedullary nailing of the humerus is the more complicated of the two methods and is, on the whole, associated with more complications.

Positioning

Surgery is performed with the patient in a prone position. The injured upper arm is supported on an arm board. The shoulder is abducted by 90°; the elbow joint is flexed by 90° (Figs. 4.10.3.11 and 4.10.3.12). Maximum elbow flexion is a prerequisite for inserting the nail without any difficulties.

In comparison with antegrade intramedullary nailing, patient positioning is distinctly more complicated here; in a number of patients with concomitant pathology or injuries, it is in fact im-

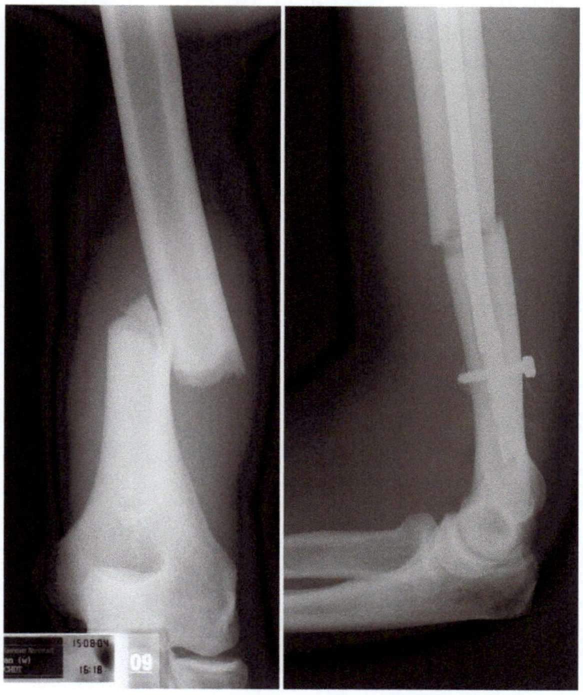

Fig. 4.10.3.11. Retrograde intramedullary nailing of the humerus

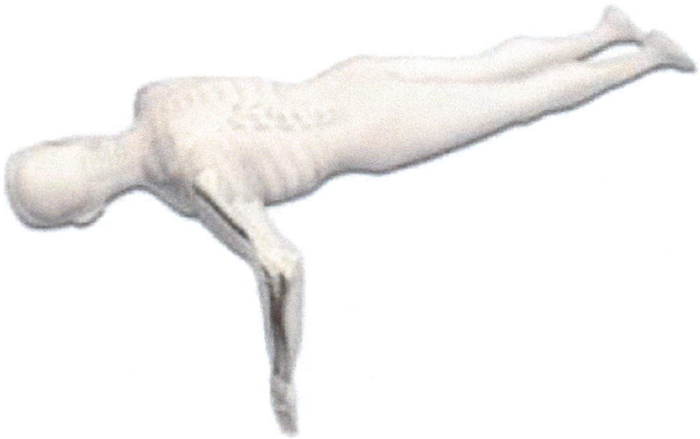

Fig. 4.10.3.12. Positioning of the patient for retrograde intramedullary nailing

possible. It must be possible to visualize with the image intensifier the nail entry point on the distal humerus and the region of the humeral head where proximal freehand locking has to be carried out. This can be difficult, especially in the humeral head, since the nail should be advanced far toward proximal.

Access and Entry Point

The main incision starts at the olecranon tip and proceeds in a proximal direction. The triceps tendon is split, and the distal humerus and the proximal part of the olecranon fossa is exposed.

The nail entry point is located 1 cm proximal to the olecranon fossa. The insertion template for the distal humerus is placed on the humerus; using a 3.5 mm drill, several holes are then drilled in the dorsal cortex (Fig. 4.10.3.13). The row of drill holes can now be expanded to form an oval window approximately 3 cm in length (Fig. 4.10.3.14). The preparation of this bone window is one of the most important steps during the operation. Even though the end of the nail exhibits a distal curvature of 4° to facilitate insertion, the entry point must be wide enough that the insertion of the nail does not provoke any new fractures of the humerus.

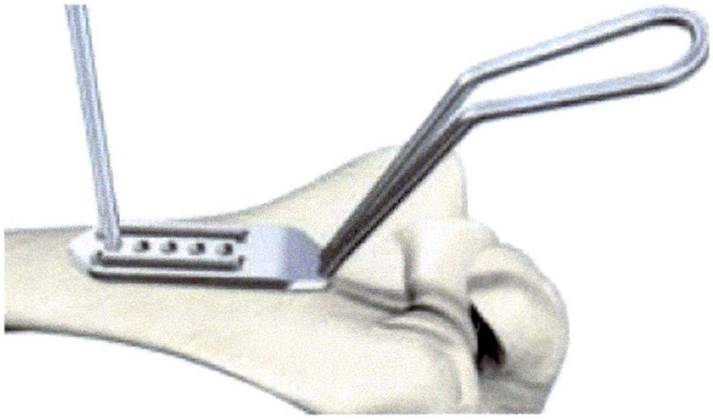

Fig. 4.10.3.13. Preparation of the nail entry point with drilling template and rigid reamer

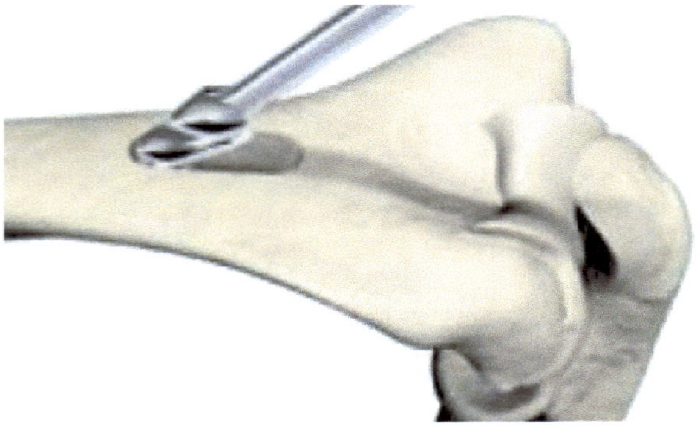

Fig. 4.10.3.14. Preparation of the nail entry point with drilling template and rigid reamer

Reduction of the Fracture and Intramedullary Reaming of the Intramedullary Canal

With the patient's arm supported on the arm board, fracture reduction can be carried out without any difficulty. The correct rotational alignment is established virtually independently by the vertically suspended lower arm.

Reduction and drilling are carried out in the same manner as during antegrade intramedullary nailing.

Here again the T2 nail can be inserted via a reamed method (which we personally prefer) or an unreamed method. A guide wire is used during both nail insertion procedures; during retrograde intramedullary nailing, this wire is advanced up to the center of the humeral head.

Nail Selection and Insertion

For surgeons planning a retrograde intramedullary nailing procedure, there are – as for the antegrade procedure – a number of tools available that facilitate the task of nail selection. The planned locking technique should be taken into consideration when deciding on nail length; this prevents impairment of elbow joint extension caused by impingement of an overly long nail. With regard to nail diameter, the thickest nail that can be inserted without difficulty should be selected.

Locking and Compression

The locking options available for retrograde intramedullary nailing do not differ from those used for the antegrade technique.

Owing to the oblong form of the entry hole in the distal humerus, there may not be a sufficient bone bridge to the drilled hole for the distal locking. In this case washers can be used for bridging.

Follow-up Treatment

Questions of functionality are also in the foreground in the follow-up treatment of patients after retrograde intramedullary nailing of the humerus. In view of the good results achieved with conservative brace therapy, load-stable osteosynthesis with good shoulder and elbow function is the prime goal of operative treatment.

Summary

The range of indications for operative treatment of humeral shaft fractures has expanded markedly in recent years. Whereas plate fixation is the procedure of choice for several special indications, e.g. pseudarthrosis, peri-implant fractures, and extremely distal shaft fractures, intramedullary nailing is becoming the standard surgical treatment for humeral shaft fractures for several reasons:

- The new intramedullary implants offering several locking options represent an ideal merger of the advantages of minimally invasive biological osteosynthesis with a high degree of stability in the treatment of fractures, even in osteoporotic bone.
- Interfragmentary compression and apposition are additional options as part of an optimal fracture treatment program aimed at minimizing delayed bone healing and pseudarthrosis formation.
- The implants lay the foundation for functional follow-up treatment, rapid restoration of weight-bearing capacity in the injured extremity, and thus a speedy return of the patient to his/her job and everyday activities.
- The range of instruments permits a safe surgical technique and short operation times.

At our hospital, antegrade intramedullary nailing of the humerus is now a standard treatment for humeral shaft fractures for several reasons:

- The uncomplicated positioning of the patient in the "beach chair position," which, in contrast to the prone position required for the retrograde approach, is also an option for patients with concomitant pulmonary disease, cardiac disease or multiple trauma.
- The proximal access to the humerus, which results in comparable functional results for shoulder and elbow function while minimizing the risk of iatrogenic fracture.
- The fact that extremely proximal fractures and combination injuries involving fractures of the humeral head and shaft are ideally treated via an antegrade procedure making use of the long versions of the proximal intramedullary humeral nail possessing angular stability.

References

1. Blum J, Janzing H, Gahr R, Langendorff HS, Rommens PM. Clinical performance of a new medullary humeral nail: antegrade versus retrograde insertion. J Orthop Trauma 2001; 15(5):342–349
2. Blum J, Rommens PM. Modern concepts of intramedullary nailing of the humerus. Osteo Trauma Care 2004; 12:121–129
3. Blum J, Rommens PM. Proximal interlocking of humeral intramedullary nails and risk of axillary nerve injury. Unfallchirurg 2002; 105(1):9–13
4. Böhler L. Gegen die operative Behandlung frischer Oberarmschaftbrüche. Langenbecks Arch Klin Chir Ver Dtsch Z Chir 1964; 308:465–475
5. Chen AL, Joseph TN, Wolinsky PR, Tejwani NC, Kummer FJ, Egol KA, Koval KJ. Fixation stability of comminuted humeral shaft fractures: locked intramedullary nailing versus plate. J Trauma 2002; 53(4):733–737
6. Fernandez FF, Matschke S, Hulsenbeck A, Egenolf M, Wentzensen A. Five years' clinical experience with the unreamed humeral nail in the treatment of humeral shaft fractures. Injury 2004; 35(3):264–271
7. Flinkkila T, Hyvonen P, Siira P, Hamalainen M. Recovery of shoulder joint function after humeral shaft fracture: a comparative study between antegrade intramedullary nailing and plate fixation. Arch Orthop Trauma Surg 2004; 124(8):537–541
8. Kropfl A, Naglik H, Niederwieser B, Hertz H. Unreamed antegrade humeral interlocking nailing. Unfallchirurg 2000; 103(5):348–354
9. Lin J, Chiang H, Hou SM. Open exchange locked nailing in humeral nonunions after intramedullary nailing. Clin Orthop 2003; 411:260–268
10. Martinez AA, Herrera A, Cuenca J. Good results with unreamed nail and bone grafting for humeral nonunion: a retrospective study of 21 patients. Acta Orthop Scand 2002; 73(3):273–276
11. Piatek S, Westphal T, Bischoff J, Schubert S, Holmenschlager F, Winckler S. Intramedullary stabilisation of metastatic fractures of long bones. Zentralbl Chir 2003; 128(2):131–138
12. Sarmiento A, Waddell JP, Latta LL. Diaphyseal humeral fractures: treatment options. Instr Course Lect 2002; 51:257–269
13. Scheerlinck T, Handelberg F. Functional outcome after intramedullary nailing of humeral shaft fractures: comparison between retrograde Marchetti-Vicenzi and unreamed AO antegrade nailing. J Trauma 2002; 52(1):60–71

A Fully Implantable, Programmable Distraction Nail (Fitbone) – New Perspectives for Corrective and Reconstructive Limb Surgery

R. Baumgart, P. Thaller, S. Hinterwimmer, M. Krammer, T. Hierl, W. Mutschler

Systems for Callus Distraction – Overview

Within the last few years distraction osteogenesis has become an established method for limb lengthening and for the treatment of large bone defects. Besides the original technique by Ilizarov [7] based on ring-fixators, monolateral fixators with special lengthening devices [10] are being used, especially at the femur. During the last few years intramedullary systems have gained increasing significance [1, 2, 4, 6].

Table 4.11.1 gives an overview of different systems for distraction osteogenesis at the lower limb. For the classical fixator devices, external fixation is necessary for the complete duration of treatment, i.e. for the time of distraction as well as for the whole consolidation period. Its advantages are relatively small surgical procedures and simple approachability concerning corrections. Especially at the thigh, ring-fixators are extremely incriminating. Monolateral fixators with special modulars provide almost the same corrective options and are therefore regarded to be more advantageous. However, due to pin-tract infections, pain and poor cosmetic results [8], external corrective systems barely seem to be justified for adults. There are considerably advantageous alternatives.

In order to reduce the time of external fixation, the fixator can be combined with an intramedullary nail. Thus the intramedullary nail provides internal stabilisation, both during the lengthening and consolidation period. The fixator itself is only necessary for lengthening and can be removed afterwards, when the nail is locked. This method is known as the lengthening over nail (LON) technique [9] and can be considered as a first important step on the way to fully implantable distraction systems. At the lower leg the LON technique appears to be justified for short distraction distances (<2 cm). For longer distraction distances and generally at the thigh, this technique is only a procedure of second choice.

Among the fully implantable systems, mechanical nails have to be distinguished from motorised distraction nails.

The Albizzia Intramedullary Nail

With this device, lengthening takes place mechanically by the patient himself or another person. A ratcheting mechanism is activated 15 times a day by internal and external rotation of 20° each at a time, causing a distraction of 1 mm per day [5, 6]. This procedure is regarded to be very painful, especially at the early stages of distraction, but often during the entire process. Often it cannot be tolerated without anaesthesia, which obviously decreases its acceptability. Preoperative planning was often reduced to the implantability of the nail into the bone without consideration of required corrections. Especially axis corrections can hardly be performed. The Albizzia intramedullary nail is only available for the femur with a starting length between 240 and 320 mm and diameters of 11, 13 and 15 mm. Lengthenings up to 100 mm are technically possible. In consideration

Table 4.11.1. Systems to perform distraction osteogenesis at the lower limb

External systems			Fully implantable systems		
Without intramedullary nail		With intramedullary nail	Mechanical systems		Motorised systems
Ring fixator	Monolateral fixator	Lengthening over nail	Albizzia	ISKD	Fitbone

of today's standards for corrective limb surgery with the demand to correct all deformities, this system does not bear quality control in the majority of cases. It can only be recommended for limb lengthening if there is no need for axis corrections and if the mentioned disadvantages are accepted.

The Intramedullary Skeletal Kinetic Distractor Nail

The intramedullary skeletal kinetic distractor (ISKD) works similar to an automatic clock. Internal and external rotations of about 6° are sufficient for activation of the installed mechanism [4]. Therefore, manual manipulation is no longer necessary. Referring to the manufacturer's instructions, "activities of everyday life combined with controlled ambulation and partial weight bearing" should be adequate to produce a rate of lengthening of 1 mm per day. As expected, this is not a very regular and continuous mechanism, leading to both rapid lengthenings of up to several millimetres per day (nickname: "run-away train") and standstills in distraction. An installed stick magnet and an external detector help control the achieved lengthening. For the thigh, the ISKD intramedullary nail is available as a straight model with diameters from 12.5 to 14.5 mm and a starting length of 255 mm. For the lower leg, ISKD nails with a Herzog bending are available in diameters from 12.5 to 13.5 mm and a starting length of 215 mm. Distractions up to 80 mm are technically possible. Apart from the poor control of the distraction rate, this implant again offers insufficient options for axis and torsion corrections.

The Fitbone System

In contrast to mechanical distraction nails, the Fitbone system enables lengthening through an integrated, hermetically encapsulated motorised drive. The power of the system reaches peak values of more than 2000 N. The required energy is sent from an external control unit via a transmitter to a subcutaneously placed receiver. Thus there is no direct connection from the implanted material to the outside. The skin can be closed completely after surgery (Fig. 4.11.1). The energy supply is provided by positioning the transmitter next to the skin opposite the subcutaneous receiver. Energy can be supplied either three to four times a day (90 s at a time) or continuously at night while the patient is sleeping. For the night-time distraction, the transmitter is fastened onto the skin similar to an electrocardiographic electrode.

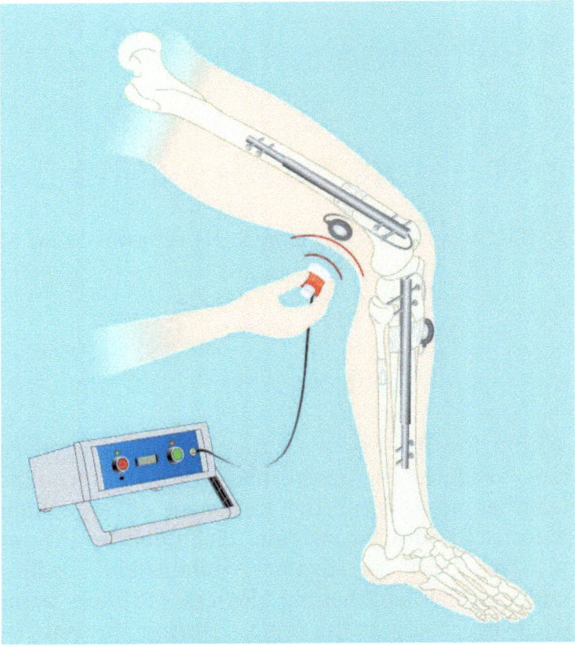

Fig. 4.11.1. Schematic view of the Fitbone system for lengthening the femur and the tibia. The energy for the integrated motor drive is transferred from outside by a high-frequency transmitter. There is no cable penetrating the skin

Two different types of Fitbone nails are available: the Fitbone slide active actuator (SAA) nail and the Fitbone telescope active actuator (TAA) nail.

The Fitbone SAA Nail

The SAA intramedullary nail has a longitudinal hole in its middle part and is currently only applicable to the thigh, due to its straight construction (Fig. 4.11.2). The modular conception facilitates implantation of the intramedullary nail first and bringing in the hermetically encapsulated drive afterwards at the end of surgery. According to this procedure, the drive and its complex technology can be removed separately after lengthening. The intramedullary nail has a diameter of 13 mm and is available in lengths between 260 and 520 mm. Extensions up to 85 mm as well as bone transport up to 200 mm are possible. The SAA intramedullary nail is almost exclusively implanted through an antegrade approach, although a retrograde approach is likewise possible.

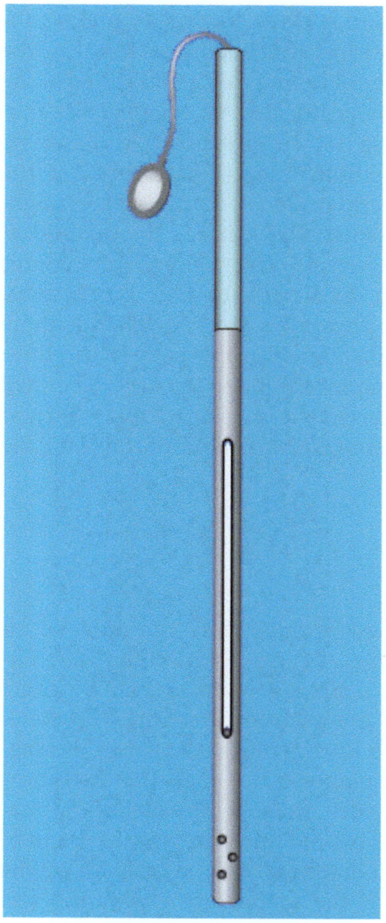

Fig. 4.11.2. The straight Fitbone SAA nail is a multifunctional correction tool for the femur. In the middle part of the implant a sliding hole is positioned, which allows lengthening and bone transport

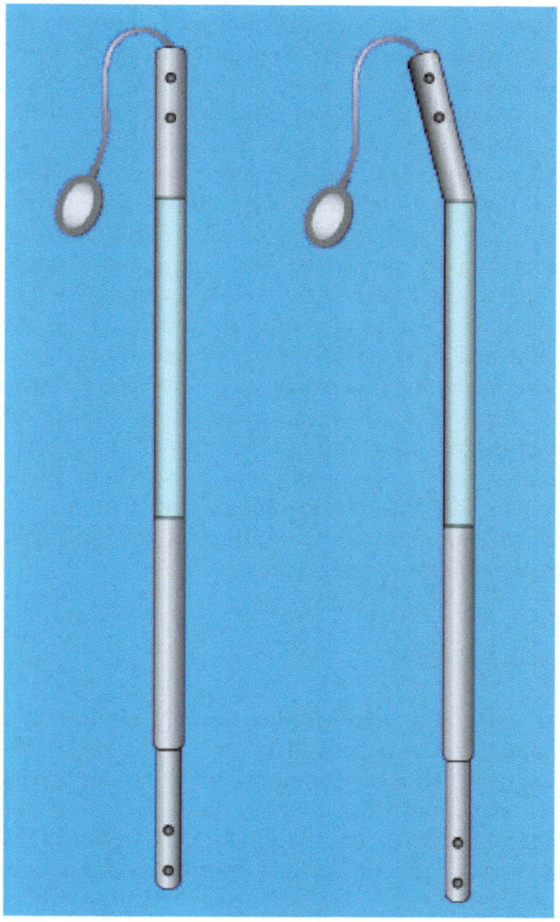

Fig. 4.11.3. The Fitbone TAA is available in a straight version for the femur and with a Herzog bending for the tibia

The Fitbone TAA Nail

The telescopic TAA intramedullary nail is developed in a straight variant for the thigh and a curved variant for the lower leg (Fig. 4.11.3). The motor drive is already integrated and therewith a firm component of the system. The diameter is 10 mm in the shaft area and 12 mm in the juxta-articular region. Furthermore there is a straight variant with a continuous diameter of 13 mm available. The surgical technique is easier than the SAA technique and allows extensions up to 55 mm at the thigh and 45 mm at the lower leg.

Indications and Surgical Techniques

Due to new surgical techniques, the range of indications for the fully implantable programmable Fitbone system has constantly extended in recent years. At the beginning of the development, only slight axis corrections were considered to be possible [2], whereas nowadays almost all corrections in the coronal as well as the sagittal plane can be performed. Axis deviations close to the ankle joint nevertheless constitute an exception. Furthermore torsion corrections are possible before locking the nail. Therewith the fully implantable Fitbone system enables us to perform for the first time complete corrections of all deformities (axis, torsion and length). Detailed analysis of the leg geometry and preoperative planning, taking the particular aspects of the intramedullary technique into consideration, are essential requirements. For this purpose a new method (reverse corrective planning) has proven to be exceedingly effective. First, it should be decided whether corrections of the femur, the tibia or both bones are necessary. Thereafter, the goal of the whole correction procedure including lengthening has to be defined as a starting point of the planning. From there, the planning of the different surgical steps is developed backwards (reverse) towards the preoperative findings, always considering the possibilities of the intramedullary nail. This ensures that the goal of the correction will be achieved, provided that the planning steps are fulfilled during surgery. However, this is only possible if the intramedullary cavity is reamed with rigid and straight reamers rather than with flexible reamers. The latter follow the line of minor resistance within the preformed intramedullary cavity and thus do not accomplish the requirements of the preoperative planning. Two different reamers (rounded or sharp-edged) and variable lengths of the tip are used to drill a straight canal into a bent bone. Thus a straight intramedullary nail can be implanted without tension and even complex axis corrections can be performed.

Femur Antegrade

The antegrade approach and the implantation of a Fitbone SAA intramedullary nail is the most efficient system for all complex corrections at the femur, especially when they are located close to the knee joint. With its special locking options, the SAA system offers optimal conditions for secure stabilisation of even very short supracondylar fragments. The reaming procedure can become very pretentious and may take a lot of time. If there is a remarkable antecurvation, a double osteotomy might be necessary. Corrective options result from the alignment of the distal metaphyseal fragment beneath the osteotomy. According to the preoperative planning, extreme angle corrections and even a lateral offset can be carried out. For simple lengthening procedures without any corrections, the femoral diaphysis offers best stabilisation options and a good bone formation can be expected. For implanting the intramedullary nail, a lateral skin incision of 2.5 cm above the greater trochanter is sufficient and cosmetically very advantageous.

Femur Retrograde

Although the retrograde approach opens the knee joint, the surgical technique is simple and causes only little damage to the soft tissue, including the intrinsic knee structures. In most cases a straight Fitbone TAA is used, again allowing correction of deformities located close to the knee joint. The osteotomy level can differ from the centre of rotation and angulation without having to make concessions to the correction result, as long as the rules for reverse planning are considered. The correction itself is performed by reaming the metaphysis according to the preoperative planning. Only small corrections can be performed at the diaphysis. The retrograde insertion of a straight TAA Fitbone intramedullary nail is the method of first choice for simple lengthening procedures with or without axis and torsion corrections. However, it must always be checked whether there are any contraindications on the part of the knee joint or the metaphyseal bone quality. The nail can easily be inserted via a cosmetically advantageous 2.5-cm transverse skin incision beneath the patella.

Tibia Antegrade

Intramedullary nails for the tibia can only be inserted by an antegrade approach. Only TAA Fitbone nails with a Herzog bending can be used. According to the preoperative planning, the metaphysis next to the knee joint is reamed in the sagittal and coronal planes. After that, the osteotomy is performed. Under manual antecurvating manipulation, the tibia is lined up in the sagittal plane, so that the diaphysis can be reached by the straight reamer. If the preoperative planning was correct, the curved intramedullary nail automatically aligns the main fragments in both planes and the bone can additionally be stabilised by the interlocking options.

Femur and Tibia Simultaneously

Using two Fitbone TAA nails, one for the femur and one for the tibia, simultaneous lengthening of the femur and tibia can be performed. Via a single 2.5-cm skin incision below the patella, both implants can be inserted. Thus congenital deformities with axis deviations and varus- or valgus-shaped genicular planes can be corrected completely by using this new technique. First, the distal femoral joint angle is restored to its physiological range according to the above-mentioned description for retrograde femoral nail implantation. Then both the stabilisation and the subsequent lengthening procedure are carried out by a straight TAA Fitbone nail. In the same way and by using the same skin incision, correction of the tibia is performed using a second but curved TAA Fitbone intramedullary nail for the tibia. This procedure offers complete alignment of the mechanical axis and the genicular plane, as well as length adjustment of both bones according to the opposite side. By lengthening 2 mm per day, this is a very time-saving and effective procedure.

Bone Transport at the Femur

The treatment of bone defects at the femur is particularly difficult. One reason is that the entire leg distal to the defect causes tremendous loads for the stabilisation system. The other reason is that all external fixation systems at the femur lead to irrigation of the large soft tissue. If the remaining juxta-articular main fragments are long enough, the stabilisation can be done with an SAA Fitbone intramedullary nail. The special locking options grant excellent stability. An intermediate fragment is osteotomised and automatically transported towards the corresponding main fragment by the integrated drive, generating new bone within the defect. Furthermore, using this method, lengthening can be performed immediately after bone transport without additional operation. The combination of "bone transport and limb lengthening" is only possible using custom-made implants and requires a sophisticated surgical technique.

Clinical Cases

Lengthening and Axis Correction of the Thigh with an SAA System

Figure 4.11.4 a shows the long radiograph in bipedal stance of a 23-year-old patient after osteosynthesis with a conventional intramedullary nail, having a 5-cm shortening of the femur together with a 13° supracondylar valgus deformity. After removal of the intramedullary nail, a new pathway inside the long proximal fragment was formed with straight reamers. According to the planning, osteotomy was performed 7 cm above the knee joint in the former fracture region. Afterwards the distal fragment was reamed. The preoperative planning even takes into consideration the lateralisation of the mechanical axis due to the lengthening procedure along the anatomical axis. That accounts for approximately 10% of the lengthening distance. With a Fitbone SAA intramedullary nail, the femur was lengthened within 50 days (Fig. 4.11.4 b). At the end of the treatment, complete length equality and correct axial alignment were apparent radiologically (Fig. 4.11.4 c) and clinically (Fig. 4.11.4 d).

Simultaneous Lengthening of the Upper and Lower Leg with Two TAA Systems

Figure 4.11.5 a shows the long radiographs in bipedal stance of a 16-year-old female patient with congenital hypoplasia of the left leg. Total shortening was 4.7 cm, distributed as 2.5 cm in the femur and 2.2 cm in the tibia. Two Fitbone TAA intramedullary nails were implanted, one into the femur and another into the tibia through a single 2.5-cm skin incision below the patella (Fig. 4.11.5 b). Postoperatively, the daily distraction rate amounted to 2 mm, achieving the correction goal within 30 days (Fig. 4.11.5 c). Four months postoperatively, the long radiograph shows the gaps consolidated and a perfect alignment (Fig. 4.11.5 d).

Distraction and Bone Transport with an SAA System

A seriously injured 18-year-old female patient with a primary bone loss of 10 cm at the thigh showed a remaining defect of 5 cm and a shortening of 5 cm after initial treatment (Fig. 4.11.6 a). With a Fitbone SAA intramedullary nail, the main fragments were stabilised and a segment was osteotomised from the distal fragment (Fig. 4.11.6 b). Subsequently an automatic closed bone transport from distal to proximal was performed, directly followed by leg lengthening within the same distraction gap (Fig. 4.11.6 c). The transition from bone transport to leg lengthening was done automatically without any further operation. No bone grafting was necessary at the docking side, which was currently set under pressure during the whole lengthening procedure (Fig. 4.11.6 d). Two years after the accident, the radiograph showed a bony consolidation (Fig. 4.11.6 e), equal leg length, full load bearing and a good functional result (Fig. 4.11.6 f).

Results

Worldwide, 297 Fitbone implantations (eight hospitals, 224 patients, 178 femurs, 119 tibias) had been performed by the end of 2003. Indications were post-traumatic (123 cases), congenital deformities (76 cases) and cosmetic reasons (25 cases). The average distraction length was 42 mm (20–85 mm). Replacement of the implant was necessary for extensions surpassing that length. Bone transport was performed in four cases, in two cases it was combined with limb lengthening. One hundred and eighty-one implantations (61%) were

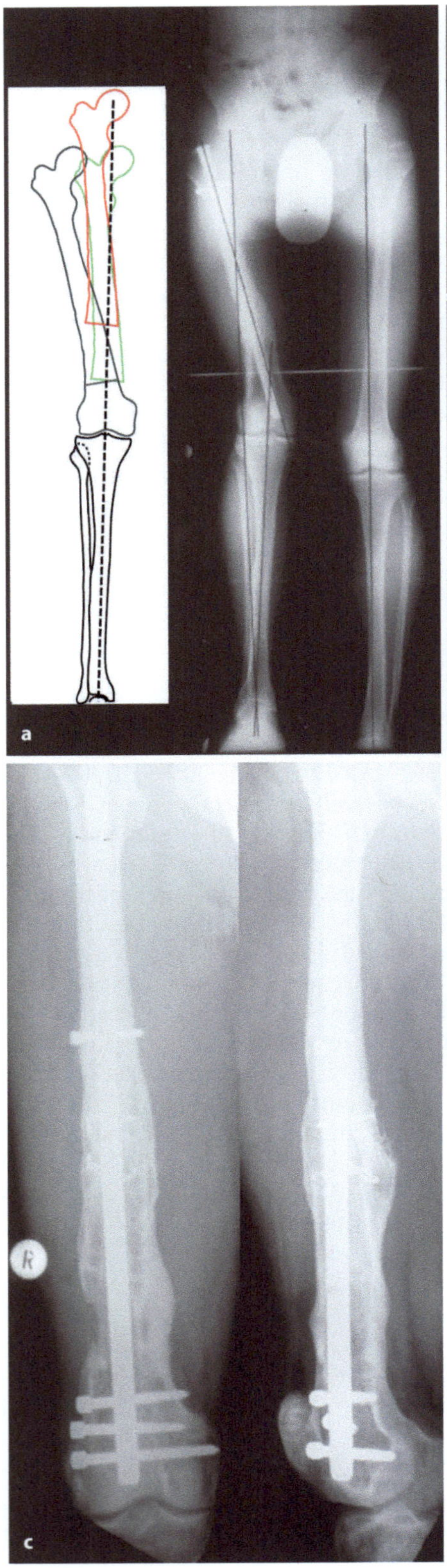

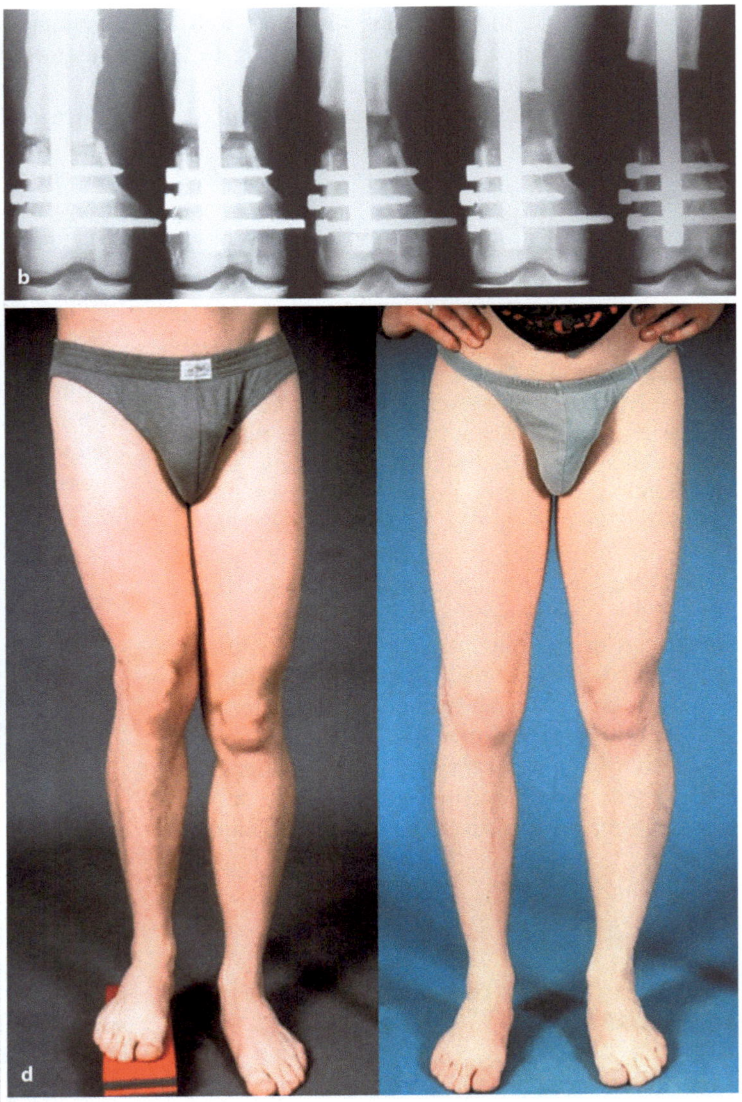

Fig. 4.11.4. a This patient had a 5-cm shortening and 13° supracondylar valgus deformity after nailing a femur fracture. The preoperative planning shows the status after surgery (*green line*) and after lengthening with the alignment of the mechanical axis (*red line*). b After intraoperative axis correction, lengthening takes place postoperatively at night time, with a rate of 1 mm/day, using a Fitbone SAA. c Radiograph after consolidation with the implant still in situ. d Clinical views of the patient before and after treatment

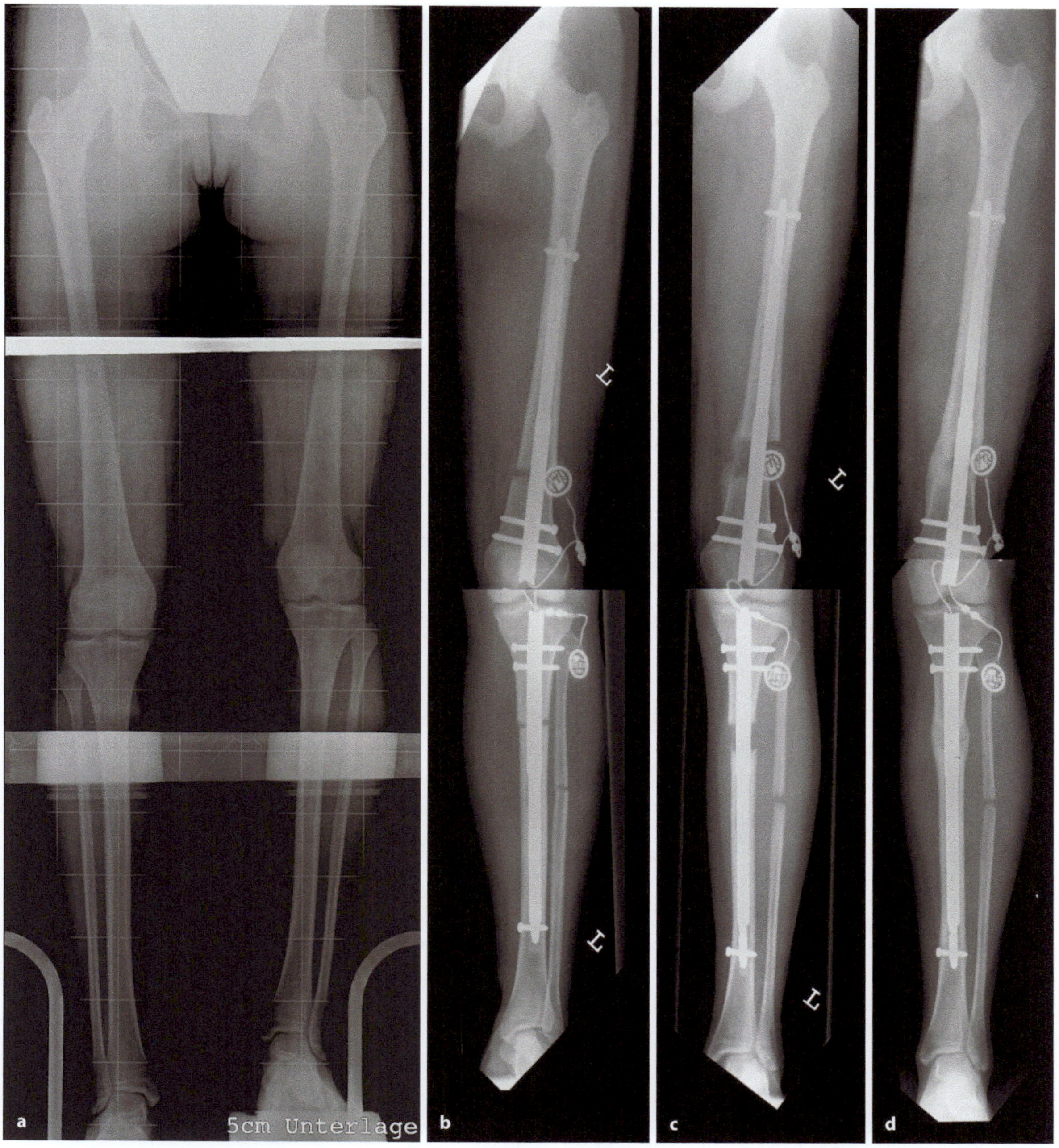

Fig. 4.11.5. **a** Radiograph in bipedal stance of a patient with a congenital shortening of both femur (2.5 cm) and tibia (2.2 cm). **b** After osteotomies at the femur and tibia, two Fitbone TAA nails were implanted. **c** Femur and tibia after lengthening was completed. **d** Femur and tibia after consolidation

done in the university hospital in Munich where the implant was developed, the rest were done in five other hospitals (2–65 implantations). One hundred and fifty cases have been evaluated by quality control sheets. The lengthening goal was reached in 144 cases (96%); all bone transports were successful. There was no infection. In three cases (2%), the intramedullary nail broke, in eight cases (5%) the achieved length of distraction was partially lost, in nine cases (6%) technical difficulties were reported. Altogether the implant had to be changed in only five cases (3%). Eighty-four patients were controlled by CT scan or long radiographs in bipedal stance. In 81 cases (96%), the remaining leg length discrepancy was less than 10 mm and in 72 cases (86%), it was less than 5 mm. The mechanical axis deviated was less than 5 mm from the centre of the knee joint in 79

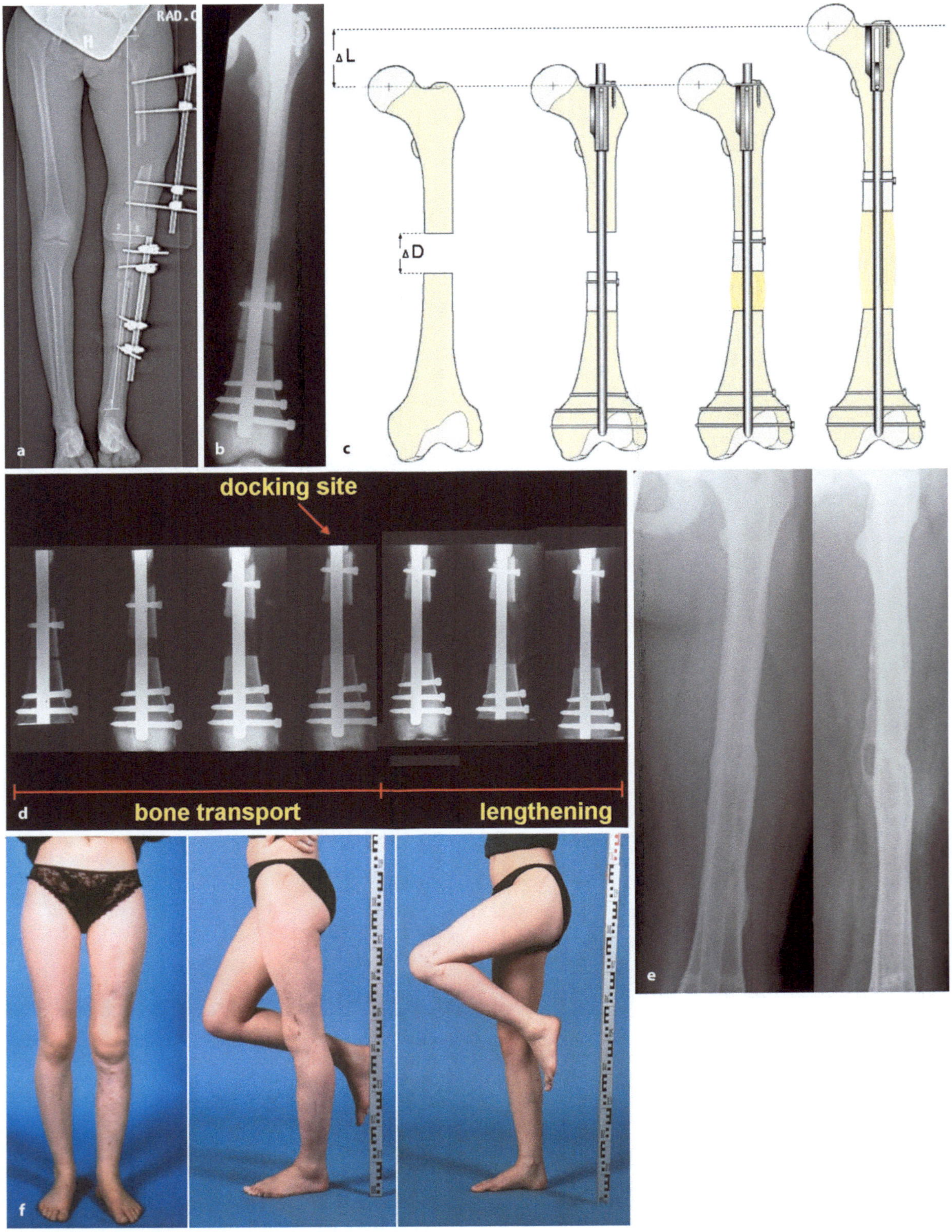

Fig. 4.11.6. a Post-traumatic primary bone loss of 10 cm at the femur. After external stabilisation, a defect of 5 cm and shortening of 5 cm resulted. b A custom-made Fitbone SAA implant stabilised the fragments. To perform bone transport, a segment in the distal part was osteotomised. c Schematic view of the treatment. At first the implant performs bone transport from distal to proximal, afterwards lengthening follows without further operation, setting the docking side under pressure. d Radiological follow-up: bone transport on the left side, lengthening on the right side. e Two years after the accident, the radiographs show bony consolidation. f Clinical follow-up: equal leg length, full load bearing and a good functional result

cases (94%). In clinical examination, torsion deviations were less than 10° in all cases.

The overall low complication rate can be traced to the fact that a distribution of the implants has been abdicated during the early stage of development. Technical difficulties initially mostly concerned the drive and wire breakages. These components have been improved in the meantime. In all cases, when the intramedullary nail broke, it was due to an overload caused by trauma or lack of compliance. Meanwhile the implants have been strengthened at the breakage site. In a few cases of the early use of the TAA type, a secondary loss of length was observed. After technical modifications, backtrack was not registered any more. Meanwhile, taking into consideration the learning process, the Fitbone system with its two variations has become an efficient, safe and versatile implant for corrections at the lower limbs.

Conclusion

Nowadays complex corrections of the lower extremity in various planes and combined with extensive lengthening procedures no longer make an external fixator indispensable. Exact evaluation of long radiographs and precise planning are the basics of all corrective procedures and thus help avoiding secondary corrections. Via suitable approaches similar to those used for laparoscopy or arthroscopy, most corrections with intramedullary nails can be performed with minimally invasive surgical techniques. Thus tissue damage can be reduced to a minimum, leaving barely visible scars. The advantages of intramedullary nailing procedures therefore obviously prevail compared to the classical external fixator technique. According to the guidelines of the Association for the Study and Application of the Method of Ilizarov [3] and the standard of operative deformity corrections [11], it is not sufficient to assess a system exclusively because of its successful distraction. Moreover all geometric parameters ought to be correct at the end of the treatment. This applies mainly to the mechanical axis but also to the joint angles and the torsion. Among all fully implantable distraction systems, only the Fitbone system complies with these requirements. With both the SAA and TAA systems, by courtesy of the accompanying surgical procedures, the technical requirements for pretentious and safe corrections are given for the first time. The reverse correction planning realises standardised procedures, guaranteeing a correct geometric result on the basis of correct surgical implementation.

At present, indications for intramedullary nailing are exclusively limited to the mature skeletal system, although first experiences with open growth plates have been made. The retrograde implantation at the femur with central penetration of the growth plate seems to be possible according to current knowledge. Within an observation period of up to 3 years, none of the performed cases showed disadvantageous effects. Although experience is still lacking for the tibia, first results are encouraging.

The clinical success of the Fitbone system is based on a 15-year development process without aiming for a fast distribution to a large number of surgeons. This avoids high complication rates, which empirically increase at the early stages of new developments. Although telemetric medicine is still at the beginning, remote monitoring of the Fitbone implants will furthermore increase treatment safety. First prototypes are currently in clinical testing. In order not to compromise the efficiency and quality of the system, only selected centres, guaranteeing a dedicated number of yearly operations, regularly undergoing a training programme offered by the centre in Munich, as well as participating in quality-control studies, can offer the Fitbone technique for the future.

References

1. Baumgart R, Betz A, Kettler M, Zeiler C, Schweiberer L. Perspektiven der Kallusdistraktion. Unfallchirurg (1996) 99: 84–91.
2. Baumgart R, Betz A, Schweiberer L. A fully implantable motorized intramedullary nail for limb lengthening and bone transport. Clin Orthop (1997) 343: 135–143.
3. Bianchi Maiocchi A, Aronson J. Operative principles of Ilizarov: fracture, treatment, nonunion, osteomyelitis, lengthening, deformity correction. Williams and Wilkins, Baltimore (1991) 245–262
4. Cole JD, Justin D, Kasparis T, DeVlught D, Knobloch C. The intramedullary skeletal kinetic distractor (ISKD): first clinical results of a new intramedullary nail for lengthening of the femur and tibia. Injury (2001) 32, Suppl 4: 129–139.
5. Garcia-Cimbrelo E, Curto de la Mano A, Garcia-Rey E, Cordero J, Marti-Ciruelos R. The intramedullary elongation nail for femoral lengthening. J Bone Joint Surg Br (2002) 84: 971–977.
6. Guichet JM, Deromedis B, Donnan LT, Peretti G, Lascombes P, Bado F. Gradual femoral lengthening with the Albizzia intramedullary nail. J Bone Joint Surg Am (2003) 85: 838–848.
7. Ilizarov GA. The principles of the Ilizarov method. Bull Hosp Jt Dis Orthop Inst (1988) 48: 1–11.
8. Paley D. Problems, obstacles, and complications of limb lengthening by the Ilizarov technique. Clin Orthop (1990) 250: 81–104.
9. Paley D, Herzenberg JE, Paremain G, Bhave A. Femoral lengthening over an intramedullary nail. A matched-case comparison with Ilizarov femoral lengthening. J Bone Joint Surg Am (1997) 79: 1464–1480.

10. Pfeil J, Heijens E, Gladbach B. Unilateral external fixators in the correction of deformities of the extremities. Orthopäde (2000) 29: 47–53.
11. Tetsworth KD, Paley D. Accuracy of correction of complex lower-extremity deformities by the Ilizarov method. Clin Orthop (1994) 301: 102–110.

A Novel Internal Callus Distraction System

U. Horas

Introduction

Leg-length discrepancies in the lower extremities have a static and dynamic effect on the entire postural and musculoskeletal system. Affected people often find that the associated cosmetic problem is just as debilitating as the functional limitations. It is hardly surprising then that, ever since the mid-1800s, attempts to lengthen pathologically shortened extremities have been made and described in detail. The causes of such differences in the length of the extremities can be congenital, enchondral, or deformities affecting either both sides or just one side of the body. Furthermore, the consequential resection of tumour tissue, performed within the accepted practice of tumour surgery, frequently calls for the removal of large sections of bone and soft tissue. More commonly today, however, differences in leg length arise because of a high-energy trauma with extensive loss of bone and soft tissue.

Conservative measures, such as shoe augmentations and orthotics to correct length, are clearly visible and are, therefore, mostly refused because they tarnish the external appearance. The option of surgically correcting the length of a leg by shortening osteotomy is likewise rarely accepted, despite the low risk involved, compared with surgery to lengthen limbs. The present-day ideal in the human mind as to what is aesthetically pleasing, which is associated with height as well as dominance and superiority, is often in direct contrast to this procedure. Spontaneous bridging of an extensive bone defect is a possibility [13], but this is seldom performed and is certainly not a routine therapeutic consideration.

Particular attention is thus paid to surgical techniques to lengthen the extremities or to bridge bone defects. In this respect, the contribution made by Ilizarov [14, 15] is undisputed. Through systematic basic research and extensive clinical application, taking into account all of the information available at the time, he introduced what he referred to as distraction osteogenesis as a standard technique.

To achieve the benefits of the generation of a load-bearing, autogenous and tube-shaped bone, by the methodical distraction of a self-forming callus, remains a challenging task, despite improved understanding of the biology of callus distraction and the availability of numerous technical devices and implants to carry out this procedure.

The main complications associated with callus distraction, such as infection, joint stiffening, soft tissue contraction, axial deviation and extensive scar formation, are due to the regularly used external components of the callus distraction systems (CDS) [16]. The few systems that are entirely implantable at the present time are not widely used because they are too limited in terms of function, are prone to complications and are difficult to finance, due to the complicated, time-consuming procedure involved. Furthermore, they are beset by more specific complications that prohibit wider application [3, 4, 8].

The aim to develop a device that is entirely implantable, without access via the skin during the distraction phase, was first achieved by a large, interdisciplinary working group at the orthopaedic clinic and outpatient department at the University of Munich, in conjunction with Messerschmitt-Bölkow-Blohm GmbH. They took up the idea of Schöllner's gliding splint, angular plate [18] and, using a great deal of technical expertise, constructed a drive unit, which the plate sits on and distracts. The drive unit comprises mechanical components, a battery and the corresponding electronics, and is small enough to be implanted beneath the lateral, femoral extensor muscles. The unit is operated externally by a transmitting device for wireless impulse transmission. The device is suitable only for lengthening the femur through callus distraction and was successfully implemented in 1978, in a 14-year-old female patient with a post-traumatic femoral shortening of 7 cm [19]. Twelve years later, an interdisciplinary working group from the surgical clinic and outpatient department of Maximilian University, Munich, reviewed the previously published ideas of Baumann and Harms [1] and Witt et al. [19]. At great technical and personal expense, as well as with the financial support of the Dr. Johannes Heidenhain foundation, they designed a medullary pin with a programmable drive for lengthening the femur. On the one hand, this system comprises an extracorporal, telemetric transmitter to guide the receiver implanted in the subcutaneous tissue, together with a control unit and battery pack. On the other hand, a telescopic medullary pin stabilises and distracts the femur as a tube-in-tube design with an interior electric motor, gears and spindle mechanism, including transverse interlocking screws. In a subsequent version of this nail, the battery pack is superfluous, since the necessary energy is transmitted by means of an extracorporal energy supply and control unit via high-frequency energy connection to a subcutaneously positioned energy receiver. This skilful solution to the energy problem in the specialist technical field must be viewed as an actual innovation regarding the nailing systems [2–4].

A design innovation was presented by Grammont and Guichet in 1995 with the "Albizzia nail". This telescopic nail is suitable only for lengthening the femur and works according to a straightforward, exclusively mechanical mode of action.

Both tubes of the telescopic nail, which are inserted one inside the other, allow step-by-step distraction via an interior ratchet by rotating the tubes against each other. The respective proximal and distal tube are fixed to the femoral bone with transverse interlocking screws such that the corticotomy position of the interlocking screws is incorporated. The ratchet mechanism can be activated externally by rotating the proximal section of the femur against the distal section. This manual twisting of the femur triggers the force required for the ratcheting manoeuvre involved [7]. Tests carried out to determine the material properties and the first clinical results have shown that the lengthening nail works convincingly in the femur to the extent that, up to 1999, over 150 of these nails were implanted by Guichet [8]. A theoretical further development of this nail also uses the ratchet mechanism for segmental transport, but there are no reports as to whether or not this modification has been tested [17].

Outside Russian-speaking areas, a femoral lengthening nail first came to the fore in 1997. Its design uses the active and passive movement of the hip joint to exert force onto an interior mechanical system. A telescopic lever arm, connected mechanically to the joint at the proximal end of the implanted lengthening nail, is passed through the gluteal muscle at the anterior iliac crest and fixed in position there with a screw. Via internal and external rotation of the hip joint, the femur is turned with the inlaying nail against the lever arm. This manoeuvre triggers the mechanism and, thus, the distraction of the lengthening nail. Over 174 femoral lengthening procedures using this device were reported between 1983 and 1995 at the Simferopol University Medical Centre, Ukraine [5, 6].

A new implant for callus distraction [9–11] is presented below, which overcomes many of the disadvantages of existing systems and helps to prevent the well-known complications. One essential feature of the CDS is that no external components are required and the system can be fully implanted. The problem of energy generation, which is essential for callus distraction, is solved with the CDS, without external components.

Given the particular biomechanical position of the lower extremity, the CDS has initially been developed for use in the femur and tibia. However, the indication for use can, in principal, be expanded to the upper extremities.

Design of the CDS as a Three-Component Implant

Solution Concept

The concept is presented only for segmental transport in the femur, although it can also be applied to the tibia or humerus. Basically, this concept can also serve to lengthen the long tubular bone through callus distraction by using the existing telescope system as a tube-within-a-tube implant via wire-pulling mechanics.

The CDS is made up of three individual components:

1. A locking intramedullary nail
2. A traction wire
3. The mechanism.

The interlocking intramedullary nail (*2* in Fig. 4.12.1) is introduced in a retrograde fashion into the femur. It stabilises the femoral fragments in terms of axis and rotation and holds the defective area open. At the distal end of the nail, a wire (*1*) is inserted before the momentary fulcrum of the knee joint. This wire, which passes through the lumen of the nail, provides the necessary strength for segment transport. The mechanism, once set in motion inside the nail's lumen (*3*), converts the force introduced via a threaded rod (*4*) and a bone segment connection (*5*) into segment trans-

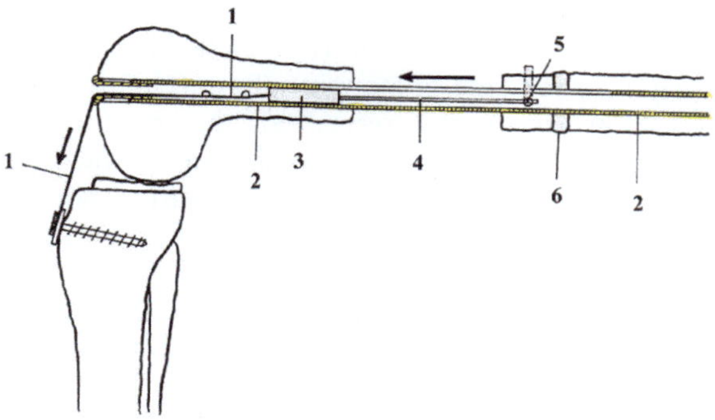

Fig. 4.12.1. Schematic drawing of the device

port. A constantly increasing callus (6), which bridges the defective area (Fig. 4.12.1), is produced by the distraction of the callus.

Component 1, the CDS Nail

The new CDS femoral nail is 340–420 mm long and has a maximum diameter of 14 mm. The external diameter, without longitudinal bulges to strengthen its walls, is 13 mm; and the internal diameter is 10.2 mm with a continuous strength wall with a thickness of 1.4 mm.

The nail has a 6-mm wide slit over a length of 216 mm; and transverse interlocking holes, with a diameter of 6 mm, are positioned both proximally and distally.

Component 2, the CDS Pull Wire

The strength needed for callus distraction in the femur is obtained by endogenous movement in the affected knee joint of the patient. The increasing distance, created by bending the knee, between the tibial tubercle and the ventral limitation of the intercondylar notch is crucial. This change in distance is determined by the functional change in length of a traction wire, attached to the tibia and femur and pulled ventrally with respective rotation of the knee joint (Fig. 4.12.2).

For callus distraction in the femur, the CDS traction wire is fixed to the tibial tubercle and introduced ventrally through the joint into the femoral medullary cavity, during rotation – in front of the end point of the intercondylar notch.

The CDS nail, introduced in a retrograde fashion into the femur, accepts the traction wire via its mechanical system located in the lumen. The functional change in the length of the pull wire in the intramedullary nail, occurring on passive or active movement of the knee joint, is converted via the mechanics of the system into callus distraction.

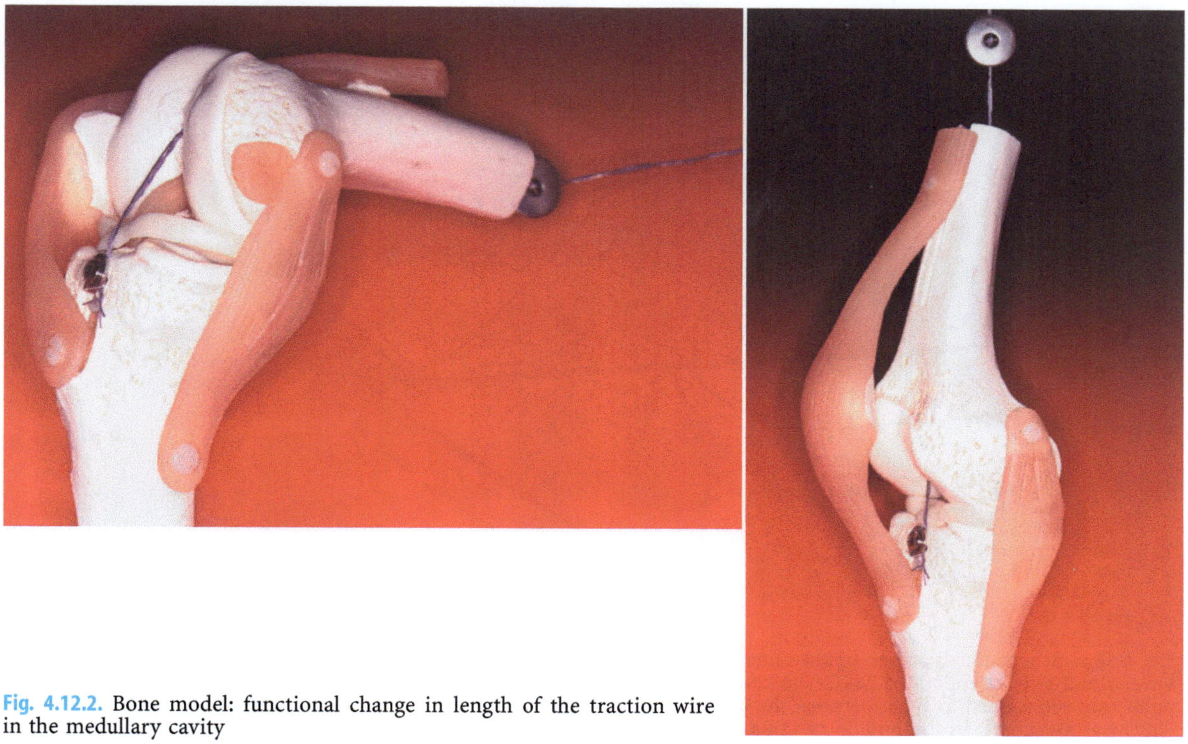

Fig. 4.12.2. Bone model: functional change in length of the traction wire in the medullary cavity

Component 3, the CDS Mechanics

The cylinder-shaped CDS mechanics system has an external diameter of 10.15 mm and is fully inserted into the CDS nail. The mechanics is produced by a straightforward screw gear, which converts the translational movement of the traction wire in the nail lumen into rotary movement of the threaded rod. The individual mechanical components are designed to withstand an axial force of 1400 N. This was done for safety, a multiple of 3.5 the anticipated transport load of 400 N that is seen during callus distraction.

Static Loading on the Knee Joint through the CDS Pull Wire

A traction force of 400 N is exerted on the traction wire under unfavourable conditions to trigger the mechanics. In addition, the total stoppage of the mechanics by increasing the traction force to up to 600 N as "maximum traction force" must be taken into account. Both these systems were used and assessed in relation to physiological routine knee joint exertion (reference load "squatting"). In the case of stopping the mechanism, the forces exerted in this respect via the traction wire do not place any more exertion upon the knee joint than that triggered during routine posture and movement.

Magnetic resonance images (MRI) of the knee joint of a male test subject were taken and evaluated in order to determine the moments and the resulting internal forces on the knee joint. The test subject was 185 cm tall and weighed 80 kg, with normal bodily proportions. The body axes of the test subject were established photogrammetrically, in order to establish the moment.

Relevant anatomical structures were basically taken into account for bearing the load. These are the femoral condyles and tibial plateau including the hyaline cartilage cover, the femoral and tibial axis, the anterior and posterior cruciate ligament and the extensor apparatus in the knee joint.

The joint geometry and the working axes in the individual, anatomical structures as well as those in the traction wire were determined from

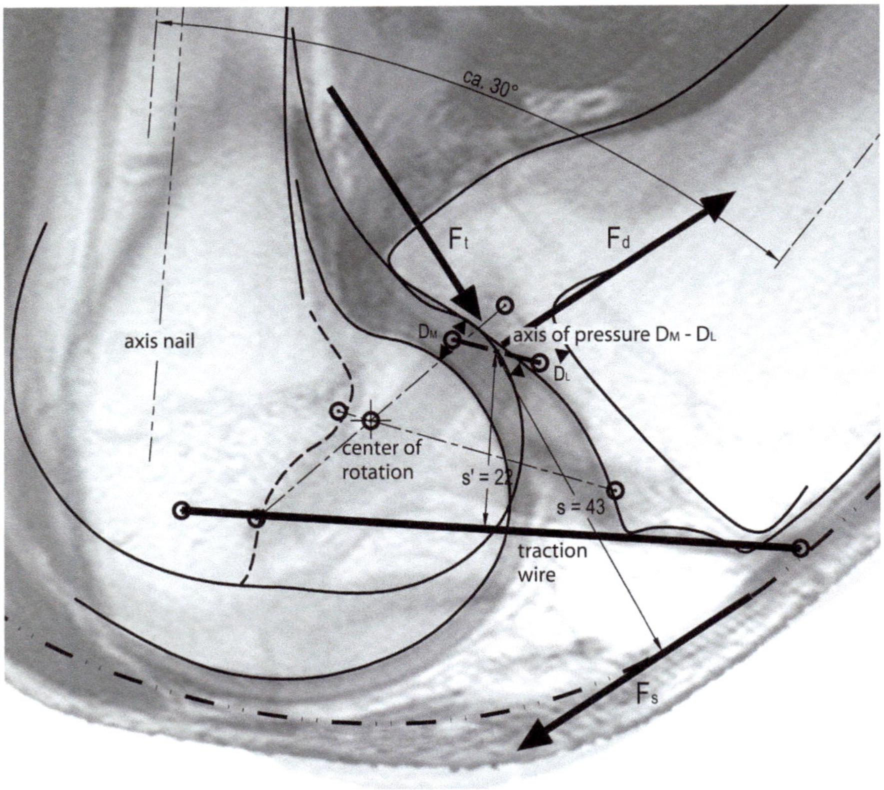

Fig. 4.12.3. Schematic drawings of the inner levers of the knee, s and s' on a calibrated MRI. The common pressure point was determined as lying between the medial and lateral pressure points, in the middle of the axis of pressure. F_t Tangential force, F_d compressive force on joint, F_s tensile force in the extensors, in this case, the traction wire, s inner lever arm of the joint, s' lever arm to the traction wire

calibrated MRI images of the coronal level at 90° and 150° positions. All of the intervals measured were projected onto the drawing for the purposes of simplification (Fig. 4.12.3).

Reference Load "Squatting"

In the squatting position, the physical focus is placed on the metatarsal head. The load axis runs vertically through this point. The bending moment in the knee joint is equivalent to the sum of full body weight, excluding the lower leg and the foot (G), multiplied by the distance of the rotation of the knee joint (lever arm *sx*).

In the case of the test subject, the moment is: $M = G \cdot sx = 650\ \text{N} \cdot 0.36\ \text{m} = 234\ \text{Nm}$.

The inner moment arm (s) is determined in the MRI-based knee joint geometry between the extensor tendon and the load axis.

The inner traction or pressure forces (Fs and Fd) combined amount to:

$$\frac{G \cdot sx}{s} = \frac{650\,\text{N} \cdot 0.36\,\text{m}}{0.043\,\text{m}} = 5440\,\text{N}$$

With equal load distribution, the force for each knee joint is 2720 N.

The transverse force (Q) is equivalent in the knee joint to the current body part weight of 650 N in the case of the test subject. The tibial plateau is ventrally inclined in this position with the semi-bending angle. A take-off force is generated in the tangential direction to the tibial plateau.

The tangential force F_t is:

$$F_t = Q \cdot \sin(\alpha \div 2)$$

where α is the flexion angle, Q is the transverse force at the knee joint and F_t is the tangential force in the pressure area (Table 4.12.1).

Table 4.12.1. Extent of the tangential forces in various bending positions

External angle	α	Q	F_t
90°	90°	650 N	460 N
120°	60°	650 N	563 N
150°	30°	650 N	628 N

Extent of the tangential forces in various bending positions

Load on Traction Wire

The traction force not exceeding 400 N in the wire must be distributed over the femoral condyles and on the tibial plateaus as an even pressure force. The latter is also 400 N; the line of force must run parallel to the traction wire. On bending the knee joint approximately 115°, the force vector of the pressure force (F_d) is perpendicular to the joint surface of the tibial plateau. With increased bending, the angle between the force vector and the joint surface is enlarged, so that take-off forces are triggered dorsally as tangential forces (F_t). This dorsally acting force component is partly absorbed by the posterior cruciate ligament, until it runs more or less perpendicularly to the posterior cruciate ligament (Fig. 4.12.4).

The force–angle relationships can be calculated as follows:

α = flexion angle
β = angle between the traction wire and tangential level of the pressure areas
γ = angle between the tangential level of the pressure areas and the posterior cruciate ligament
F_s = traction wire force
$F_{s'}$ = opposing reaction force to the traction wire force
F_d = pressure force components orthogonally on the tibial plateau
F_t = tangential force components on the joint pressure point
F_k = traction force components from Ft, working in the posterior cruciate ligament.

$$F_{s'} = -F_s \qquad F_t = \cos\beta \cdot F_{s'}$$
$$F_d = \sin\beta \cdot F_{s'} \qquad F_k = F_t \div \cos\gamma$$

The following values were calculated for squatting with flexion angles of 90°, 120° and 150° (Table 4.12.2).

Table 4.12.2. Overview of the angles and partial forces with various flexed postures

α	β	γ	$F_s/F_{s'}$	F_t	F_d
90°	65°	63°	400 N	169 N	363 N
60°	59°	71°	400 N	206 N	343 N
30°	47°	74°*	400 N	273 N	293 N

* Diversion of the posterior cruciate ligament via impact on the intercondylar notch during maximum flexion [20]

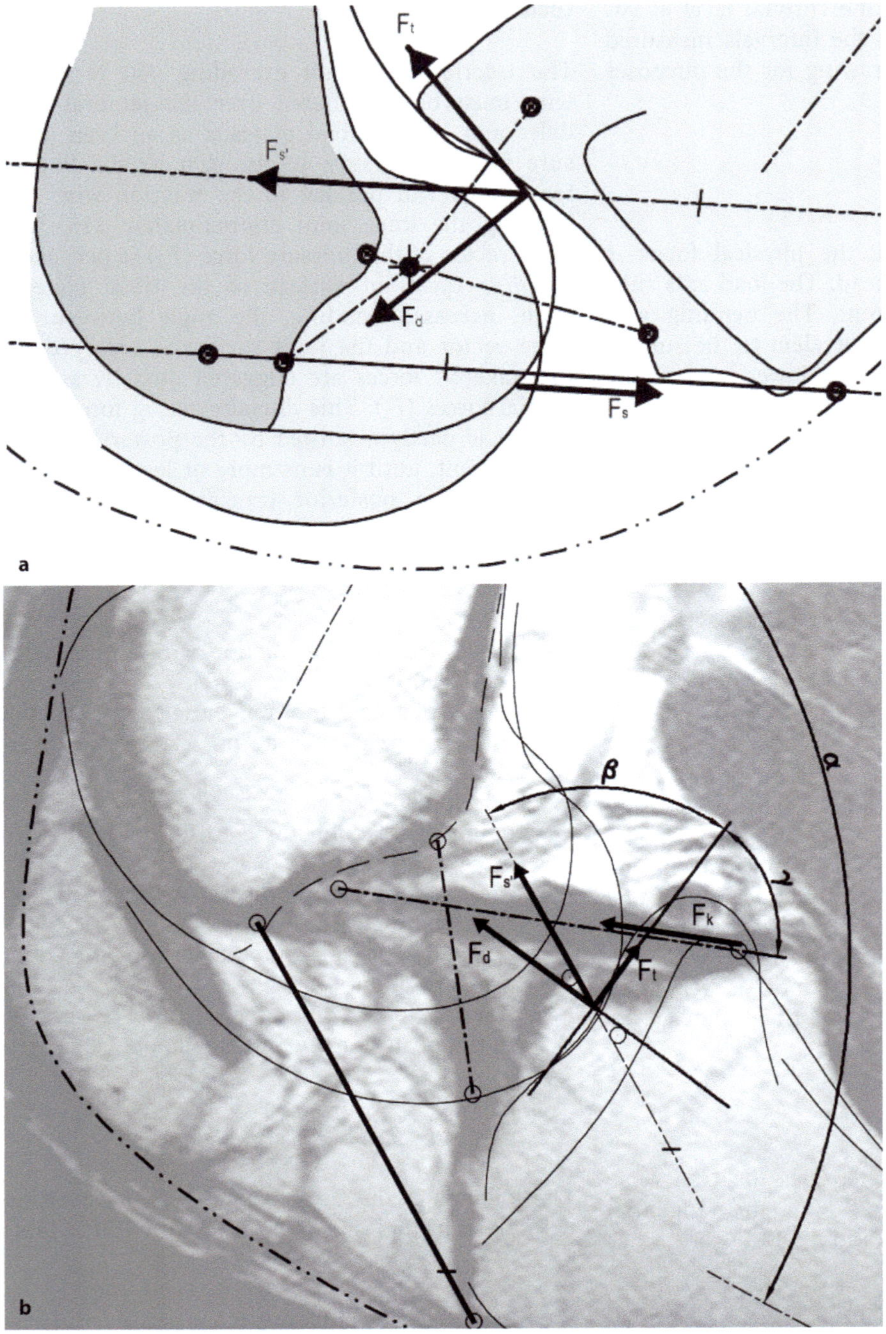

Fig. 4.12.4. a The parallel force of the traction wire is divided into an orthogonal pressure force and a tangential force. b Breakdown of the partial forces at the pressure point in a 90° flexion position

Load Case: Overload

If the functional change in length of the traction wire is impeded, for instance, by blocking the positioning mechanism, the traction forces that normally work against the transport forces become considerably larger than the 400 N assumed for the desired operating conditions. These forces are generated when the knee joint is bent further against the impeded traction wire.

External moments, by triggering forces in the lower leg, increase inner forces on the traction wire and knee joint, in accordance with the laws on leverage.

For this reason, the traction wire must be fitted with a theoretical break point at its fixation point

Table 4.12.3. Overview of the angles and partial forces in the case of impediment in various flexed postures. $F_{s'}$ is, in this instance, the defined rejection force of the pull wire

α	β	γ	$F_s/F_{s'}$	F_t	F_d
90°	65°	63°	600 N	254 N	544 N
60°	59°	71°	600 N	309 N	514 N
30°	47°	74°*	600 N	409 N	439 N

* Diversion of the posterior cruciate ligament by impact on the intercondylar roof in the area of maximum flexion [20]

on the tibial tubercle. The defined rejection force is set at 600 N. The resulting pressure on the joint works against this force.

The components are determined as in the traction wire application load (Table 4.12.3).

The calculated forces are given a 20% safety margin to establish the load multiples available in order to cover for simplification and the scatter of the biometric values. In a comparable case, i.e. squatting, the following maximum forces were thus determined:

Pressure force F_d: 2720 N·0.8 = 2176 N
Tangential force F_t: 628 N·0.8 = 502 N

The following were determined for the application load with a maximum of 400 N:

Pressure force F_d: 363 N·1.2 = 435 N
Tangential force F_t: 273 N·1.2 = 327 N

In the specific case of traction wire impediment, a defined rejection limit of 600 N was established:

Pressure force F_d: 544 N·1.2 = 653 N
Tangential force F_t: 409 N·1.2 = 491 N

All of the forces involved in the traction wire mechanism are lower than the physiological loads on the knee joint (Table 4.12.4).

The Material Properties and Functionality of the CDS

The CDS comprises the intramedullary nail with its transverse interlocking screws and the in-line mechanism, with threaded rod and the threaded spindle sitting on top, which produces the connection between the bone segment and the threaded rod. The longitudinally slit interlocking nail keeps the defective area open throughout callus distraction. The threaded spindle, lying within the nail, is connected with the bone segment to be transported through the nail slit by screws (Fig. 4.12.5).

The transported bone is moved in the direction of the desired callus distraction by rotating the threaded rod in a specific way. The mechanism turns the threaded rod by converting the translational movement of the traction wire. The wire is moved by flexing the knee joint; 30° of flexion in the knee joint is needed to trigger the mechanism. The length of the traction wire must be adjusted such that only the maximum potential flexion triggers the mechanism. Other movements in the knee joint do not affect the mechanism, thus allowing physiological movement of the limb by the patient.

Material Properties of the CDS Nail

Bending and torsion tests were carried out, comparing with the Klemm-Schellmann nail, while the results of the prolonged swing test and functionality of the mechanics were assessed by comparison to the anticipated load during clinical application.

The bending load was directed towards the nail slit, against the slit, and laterally to the slit. Compared with the average values of the proportional bending moments of both nail groups, 71.2 Nm compared with 78.1 Nm, the Klemm-Schellmann nail displayed elastic distortion, which was approximately 9.6% greater.

The overall result of the maximal bending moment of the CDS nail, at 144.6 Nm, is approximately 9.3% above that of the Klemm-Schellmann nail at 132.2 Nm. With 22.1 Nm/°, the greatest stiffness in the bending load for the CDS nail is measured laterally to the slit. Greater fluctuations were, however, observed in terms of load direction than with the Klemm-Schellmann nail.

Table 4.12.4. Pressure and tangential forces in relation to the reference load

	Load Applied		End Load		Squatting Force
	Force	Load-Factor	Force	Load-Factor	
Pressure Force, F_d	435 N	5.0	653 N	3.3	2176 N
Tangential Force, F_t	327 N	1.5	491 N	1.0	502 N

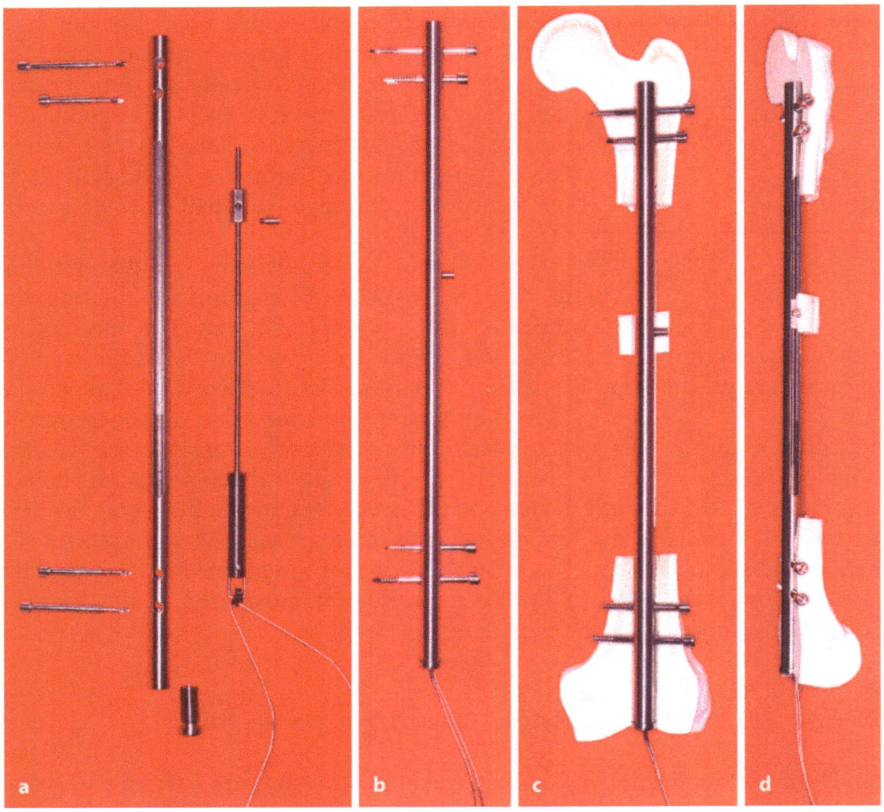

Fig. 4.12.5. Prototype of a CDS: a individual components; b nail completed mounted; c implanted in the femur – anteroposterior view; d implanted in the femur – mediolateral view

The CDS nail reacts to the load directed laterally to the slit with 56% more stiffness than to the load directed opposite the slit. Bending deformity was measured at 20.9° versus 22°, without any significant difference being observed between the two types of nail.

In the torsion test, the CDS nail at 0.293 Nm/° displayed twofold greater torsion stability than the Klemm-Schellmann nail at 0.151 Nm/°. The prolonged swing test produced a mean value of 41,850 load changes and, thus, exceeded the required threshold value of 30,000.

The Functionality of the CDS Mechanism

The CDS mechanism converts a translational axial wire pull into callus distraction, via segment transport. Thus, the force introduced via the traction wire is used to overcome the counter transport force. The disruption-free mechanical function is, therefore, of prime importance for CDS and was tested in a standard operating procedure (SOP), using the following parameters: the relationship between the traction force and transport force, force potential, the traction force–path relationship, maximum loading and the reliability of the mechanism. The SOP measures the traction force required on the traction wire, with increasing, defined transport forces to callus distraction via a defined piston stroke using a force-measuring device that is switched on intermittently. Moreover, the traction force is continuously measured in relation to the path travelled by the piston stroke.

With increasing transport force, the results show a linear rise in the mechanical traction force required. Furthermore, the mechanics trigger an approximate 50% change in force with favourable potentiation of the force involved. The maximum load is achieved with a transport force of 444 N with a traction force of 257 N and a traction force–transport force quotient of 58. The interpolated curves for various transport forces in the function test as a correlation between the traction force exerted [N] and the path [mm] highlight an extremely even curve formation (Fig. 4.12.6). This indicates that the mechanics are reliably set in motion with each individual measurement.

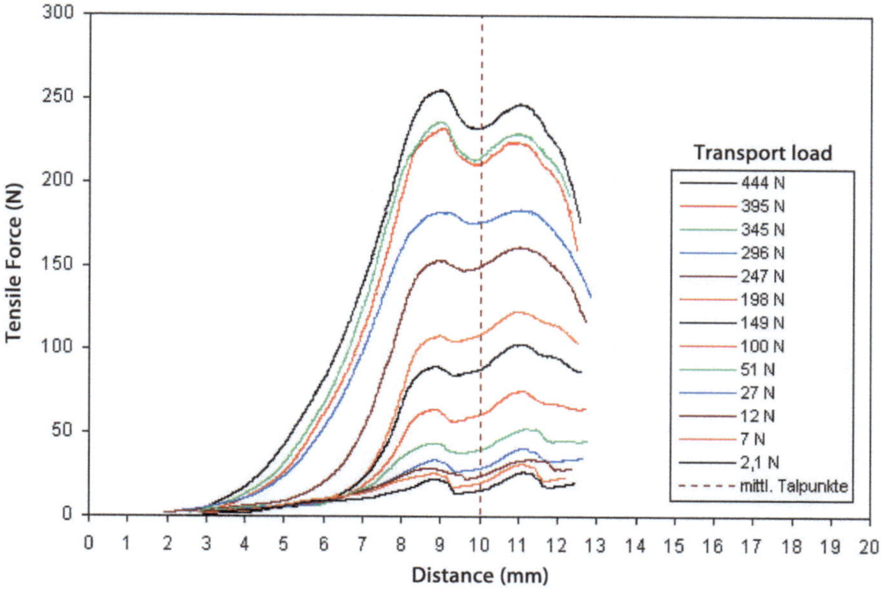

Fig. 4.12.6. Interpolated curves (n=30) of 13 varied forces during a functional study of the relationship between the tensile force and the distance of transport

CDS Implantation

The CDS is implanted in the femur via standard retrograde nailing access. Lengthening of the standard access by approximately 2 cm in the distal direction allows the traction wire to be fixed in the region of the tibial tubercle with a 6.5-mm diameter cancellous screw in a more anterior/posterior direction. This extension does not pose any risk to the functionally important structures. The mechanism is introduced into the positioned, intramedullary nail via a trans-ligament access. Corticotomy facilitates lateral access to the femur and the screwing of the threaded spindle to the bone segment to be transported. The proximal transverse interlocking of the CDS is carried out in a more anterior/posterior direction in the pertrochanteric region of the femur. Distal transverse interlocking is carried out from the medial to lateral and both fixes the mechanism in the nail and keeps the defective area open. With an assumed maximum range of movement of 0°–120° at the knee joint, the traction wire is firmly fixed to the tibial tubercle via a 6.5-mm cancellous screw. A lower leg splint is applied, with the knee joint flexed at 90°. Bending of the knee joint from 90° to 120° triggers the mechanics, while movement between 0° and 90° has no effect on the implant. The minimally invasive standard accesses selected, with less extension of the trans-ligament incision as far as the head of the tibia, are considered to pose few complications and risks.

CDS implantation does not, therefore, call for any notable change in terms of established access procedures.

Use in Cadavers

In four experimental implants in human cadavers, the CDS transported the respective bone segment over the entire defective area of 5 and 10 cm (two each), with X-ray control with the image intensifier. To trigger the mechanism between 80° and 120°, the knee joint was stretched and flexed passively over the entire range of movement from 0° to 120°. This was continued until the bone segment had reached the distal fragment of the femur (Fig. 4.12.7).

Segment transport ran smoothly. At the "docking site", interfragmentary compression of up to approximately 250 N could be achieved by further triggering the mechanism. No subluxation or luxation of the joint was observed, either in the X-ray documentation or on external examination, during passive movement in the knee joint to trigger the mechanism. Moreover, no traction-wire-related intra-articular complications were noted, such as displacement, jamming, loop formation or specific contact with the area of insertion of the cruciate ligament. The maximum intra-articular difference in the length of the traction wire, at 0° versus 120° positioning of the

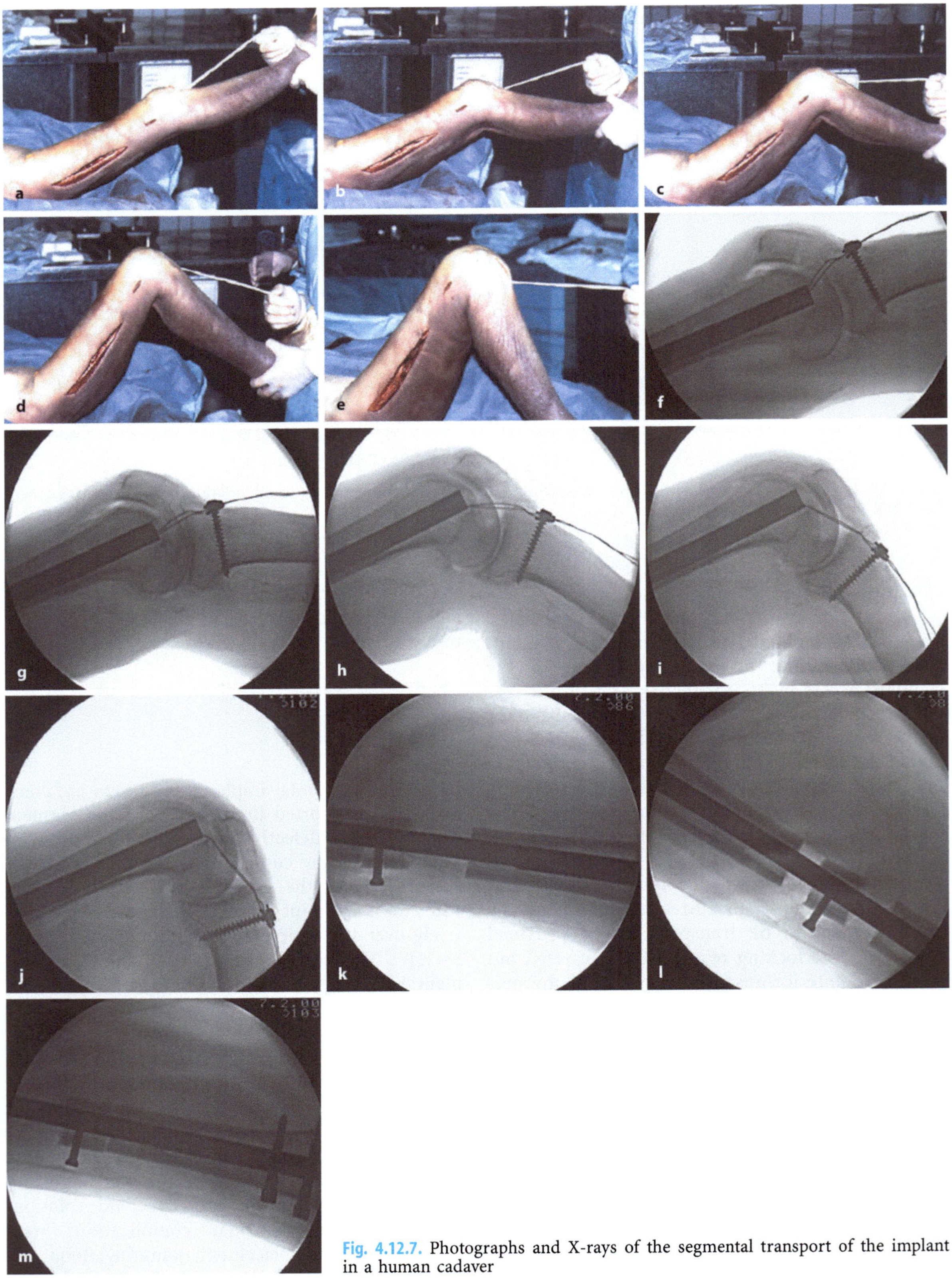

Fig. 4.12.7. Photographs and X-rays of the segmental transport of the implant in a human cadaver

knee joint, was 31.5 mm and 33 mm in the first and second implantations, respectively.

A force-measuring device, switched on intermittently at the traction wire, was used to determine a required maximum transport force of 55–61 N via the traction force–transport force relationship in all experimental cadaver implantations.

Summary

Acquired, prolonged bone substance losses or congenital differences in the length of the large tubular bones in the extremities have a negative statistic and dynamic effect on posture overall and on the entire musculoskeletal apparatus. For decades, reconstruction of the load-bearing bones using the principle of callus distraction has proven to be an established and tried-and-tested technique for correcting such bone defects. The fixation–distraction systems needed for this procedure are used clinically in various formats, external and internal apparatuses and implants. The obvious disadvantages of these systems are directly associated with the introduction of force required for callus distraction. This difficulty has not been resolved satisfactorily to date and attempts to find better solutions have been made over a number of years.

The hypothesis for the consideration of, planning and testing of the CDS technique presented was based on the fact that, through exerting endogenous force, by moving the large joints in an affected patient, force can be introduced into a suitable implant, thus overcoming the considerable disadvantages of distraction–fixation systems known and used to date.

Based on clinical observations and experience, a solution concept was devised for an implant as a callus distraction system, thus putting this hypothesis into practice. This is a three-component implant comprising a stabilising, intramedullary nail, internal mechanism for callus distraction and a traction wire that guarantees the introduction of the required force to trigger the mechanism via a special intra-articular layout. The aim was to use this particular concept technically to design an implant and then to test its properties and function. Analysis of the requirements of an appropriate implant led to the definition of framework conditions, which allowed concrete calculations to be made in relation to the technical composition of the individual components used in the new implant and the related loads of the human body.

Part of the technical objective associated with the new implant was achieved with the construction of a prototype based on the constructive draft that emerged from the calculations.

Both the physico-technical tests and the application-orientated, experimental implantation of the CDS in human cadavers highlighted a few defects in the first generation of prototypes, after analysing the measurements and the test observations. These defects could be completely eliminated by several technical amendments and supplements and by changing the actual surgical procedures. The partial objective, namely to test the properties and function of the new CDS, was thus achieved and led to the generation of a prototype that fully satisfied all requirements.

After assessing the tests, it is evident that the range of applications can be extended, risks minimised and procedures simplified with the newly developed implant compared with the earlier fixation–distraction systems. Clinical use of the CDS can lead to treatment optimisation, via callus distraction, and is thus recommended [12].

Pending the acquisition of a CE certificate for the new implant, prospective, controlled, clinical studies must be carried out, in order to assess the benefits of the new CDS even further. Particular attention will be paid in this respect to the tolerability of the CDS, which has not been fully elucidated to date.

References

1. Baumann F, Harms J (1977) Der Verlängerungsnagel. Eine neue Möglichkeit zur Verlängerung des Ober- und Unterschenkels. Arch Orthop Unfall-Chir 90: 139–146
2. Baumgart R, Betz A, Kessler S, Kettler M, Schweiberer L (1994) Möglichkeiten der Rekonstruktion von Knochendefekten. Orthopäde 23: 396–403
3. Baumgart R, Betz A, Schweiberer L (1997) A fully implantable motorized intramedullary nail for limb lengthening and bone transport. Clin Orthop 343: 135–143
4. Betz A, Baumgart R, Schweiberer L (1990) Erstes voll implantierbares System zur Callusdistraktion – Marknagel mit programmierbarem Antrieb zur Beinverlängerung und Segmentverschiebung. Chirurg 61: 605–609
5. Bliskunov AI (1983) Intramedullary distraction of the femur (preliminary report) (Russian). Ortop Travmatol Protez 10: 59–62
6. Bliskunov AI (1984) Method of dissecting the femur on the side of the medullary canal (Russian). Ortop Travmatol Protez 5: 53–57
7. Grammont P, Guichet JM (1995) Brevet: clou centromédullaire d'allongement progressif. Office européen des brevets. Date de publication 11.01.1995, numéro de dépôt 89420176.3; EP 0346 247B1
8. Guichet JM, Casar RS (1997) Mechanical characterization of a totally intramedullary gradual elongation nail. Clin Orthop 337: 281–290
9. Horas U (1997) Patentschrift: Verfahren zum Transport eines Knochensegmentes zur Überbrückung eines Kno-

chendefektes sowie Vorrichtung zur Durchführung des Verfahrens. Bundesrepublik Deutschland, Deutsches Patentamt Offenlegungstag 20.11.1997; DE 19618552 A 1
10. Horas U (2000) Patent: method for transporting a bone segment in order to bridge a bone defect and device for carrying out the method. USA, United States patent, date of patent May 2, 2000; patent number 6 056 755
11. Horas U (2001) Brevet: dispositif pour transporter un segment osseux destiné à réparer une lésion osseuse. Bone segment conveying device for bridging a bone damage. Vorrichtung zum Transport eines Knochensegmentes zur Überbrückung eines Knochendefekts. European Patent Office/Office Européen des Brevets/Veröffentlichungstag 01.08.2001 Patentblatt 2001/31; EP 0 902 658 B1
12. Horas U (2003) Ein internes neuartiges Kallusdistraktionssystem – Innovation, Konzeption, Entwicklung und Prototyp des Implantates, Physikalisch-technische und anwendungsorientierte Überprüfung. Habilitationsschrift aus dem Medizinischen Zentrum für Chirurgie, Anaesthesiologie und Urologie – Klinik und Poliklinik für Unfallchirurgie des Universitätsklinikums Giessen
13. Horch R, Dahl HD, Fery K (1989) Spontane Überbrückung eines ausgedehnten posttraumatischen Knochendefekts. Zentbl Chir 114: 257–262
14. Ilizarov GA, Soybelman LM (1969) Some clinical and experimental data concerning bloodless lengthening of lower extremities (Russian). Eksp Khir Anesteziol 4: 27–32
15. Ilizarov GA, Trohova VG (1973) Operative elongation of the femur (Russian). Ortop Travmatol Protezirov 34/11: 51–55
16. Paley D (1990) Problems, obstacles, and complications of limb lengthening by the Ilizarov technique. Clin Orthop 250: 81–104
17. Paley D (1995) Patent: bone fragment transport device. PCT intern pub date 21.09.1995, intern pub number WO 95/24870
18. Schöllner D (1972) Neue Möglichkeiten der operativen Verlängerung des Oberschenkels. Z Orthop 110: 971–974
19. Witt A, Jäger M, Bruns H, Küsswetter W, Hildebrandt J, Vogel A (1978) Die operative Oberschenkelverlängerung mit einem vollimplantierbaren Distraktionsgerät. Arch Orthop Traumat Surg 92: 291–296
20. Kummer B (1988) Morphologie und Funktion des Kreuzbandapparates des Kniegelenkes. Arthroskopie 1: 2–10

Callus Distraction with the Albizzia Nail

M. Hofmeister, C. Hierholzer, V. Bühren

Introduction

Differences in leg length of more than 3 cm of congenital, post-traumatic or post-infectious origin are generally viewed as an indication for continuous callus distraction [5]. Soft-tissue irritation caused by external fixation devices along with problems such as pin tract infection, pain, restricted mobility of adjacent joints, and cosmetically unsatisfactory scar healing [8] prompted the development of several intramedullary implants with an integrated lengthening mechanism. In 1984 the Albizzia intramedullary nail was developed by Grammont and Guichet at the University Hospital Dijon, Dijon, France [1–4] (Albizzia trees are known for their especially fast growth). This paper will discuss the technical principles of the use of the Albizzia intramedullary nail for femoral lengthening and the results obtained with this procedure over a 10-year period at the Murnau Trauma Center, Murnau, Germany.

Implant

The Albizzia nail (Fig. 4.13.1) is an intramedullary lengthening system made of stainless steel with a stable longitudinal axis. The nails are available in three sizes with a length of 240, 280, and 320 mm and diameters of 11, 13, and 15 mm. The nail is composed of two sliding tubes connected by a ratchet mechanism. The distal tube can be distracted over a maximum length of 100 mm via a double ratchet system that is anchored in the shaft of the telescopic nail. This lengthening effect is achieved by external and internal rotation of the distal femur through 20°. Each turn of the shaft lengthens the intramedullary nail by 0.07 mm. Stable anchoring of the nail in the medullary canal is achieved with a proximal 5.5-mm interlocking screw and two distal interlocking screws with diameters of 3.5 mm and 4.5 mm. Depending on specific indications, a lengthening distance of up to 100 mm is possible. To prevent overdistraction, the lengthening mechanism should be activated repeatedly prior to nail insertion until the intended distraction distance remains in the system. A blocking screw prevents overdistraction after the entire distraction length between the two sliding tubes has been expended.

Preoperative Planning

The correct nail is selected on the basis of femoral length, diameter of the femoral medullary canal, and the intended distraction distance.

Preoperative planning and nail templates are helpful to determine the position of the osteotomy. Parameters that need to be calculated include the initial length of the system, the intended distraction distance, and a minimal length for stable anchorage of the intramedullary nail into the distal diaphysis (Fig. 4.13.2).

Positioning

Surgery is performed with the patient lying in the supine or lateral position. We prefer the lateral position. During the operation it is necessary to visualize all sections of the femur in anteroposterior and lateral views using X-ray control.

Approach

The surgical approach is based on general recommendations for intramedullary femoral nailing. Attention should be directed to the reaming of the medullary canal in the line of the longitudinal femoral axis. The medullary canal is reamed by inserting a guide wire with flexible drill heads with a diameter of approximately 2 mm larger than the intended intramedullary nail size. To ensure correct axis alignment, rigid medullary drills are then used. The drill size should exceed the selected intramedullary nail diameter by approximately 1.5 mm.

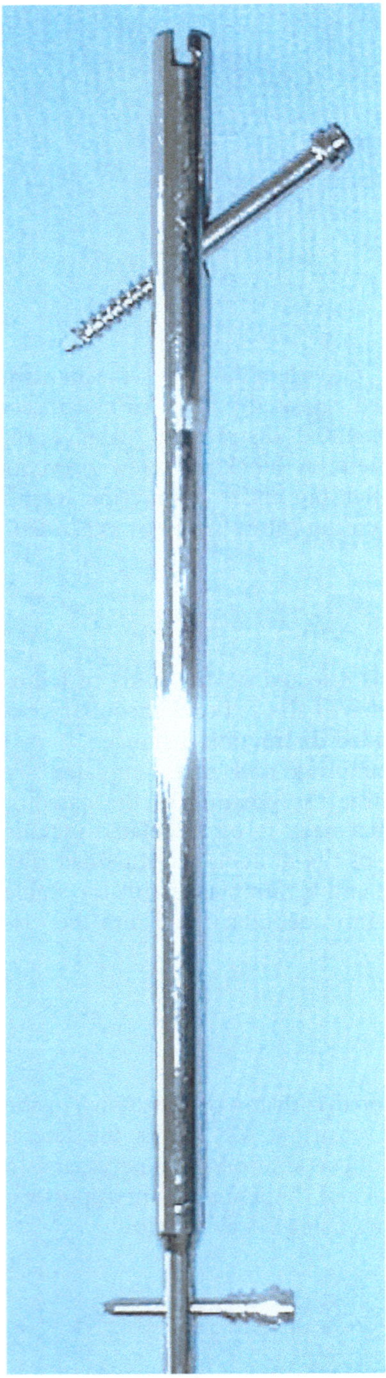

Fig. 4.13.1. The Albizzia intramedullary nail

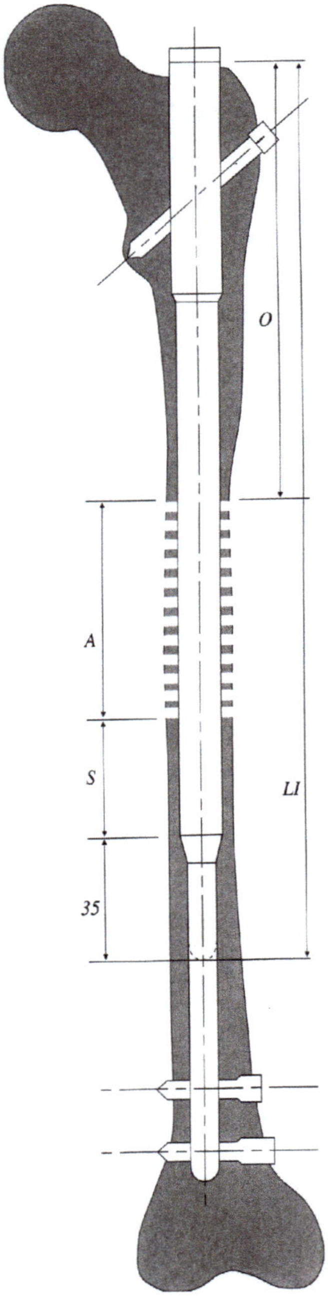

Fig. 4.13.2. Preoperative planning. *O* maximal height of the osteotomy measured from the trochanter major, *L* nail length (240, 280 or 320 mm), *A* intended lengthening, *S* 35-mm anchorage part (distal fragment). O = L–A–S–35 (mm)

Osteotomy

The osteotomy is performed according to preoperative planning and under X-ray control with an intramedullary saw by releasing the eccentric saw blade (Fig. 4.13.3). In patients with substantial thickening of the corticalis, completion of the osteotomy of the femoral diaphysis is performed using a lateral stab incision and drill or chisel (Fig. 4.13.4) [6]. Axis and rotational deviations can be corrected at this time [2].

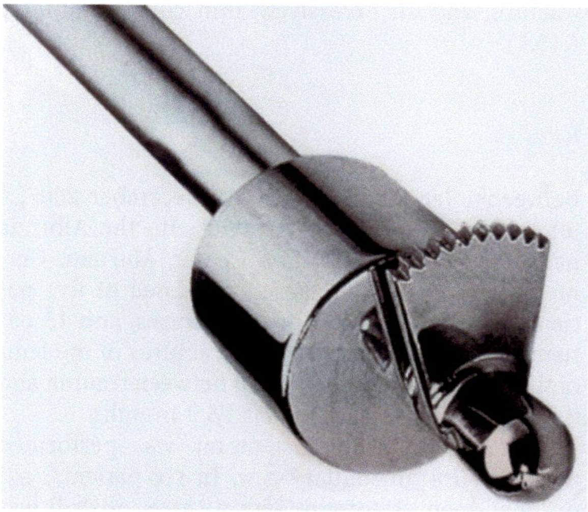

Fig. 4.13.3. Intramedullary saw for performing the osteotomy

Insertion of the Intramedullary Nail

The intramedullary nail implant is connected to the target device via a bayonet lock. Numerous technical details need to be followed for correct nail insertion.

Proximal locking of the implant with a 5-mm corticalis interlocking screw can be easily accomplished using the target device. However, distal locking may be difficult with this tool and experienced surgeons may perform this step faster and more reliably using a "freehand" technique.

During the operation, the lengthening mechanism is activated repeatedly by external and internal rotation of the distal femur through 20° until an initial distraction distance of 2–3 mm is gained. After routine closure of the surgical approach, the surgeon should document the initial position of the implant and the site of the osteotomy using X-ray control.

Starting on postoperative day 3, callus distraction of 1 mm per day is initiated. This lengthening mechanism is activated 15 times a day by performing external and internal rotations as described. During this procedure an audible "click-clack" sound is typically emitted by the double ratchet system.

Due to the intact periosteal cover, the rotation movement may initially be painful and administration of brief general anesthesia may be necessary. Alternatively, a regional psoas block can be administered.

The surgeon performs the initial ratcheting with the patient in a sitting or supine position. Continuous supervision is recommended in order to prevent uncontrolled activation of the lengthening mechanism by the patient. It is advisable to enter each lengthening procedure in a documentation sheet.

To control the distraction path and the expected callus formation, regular X-ray follow-up

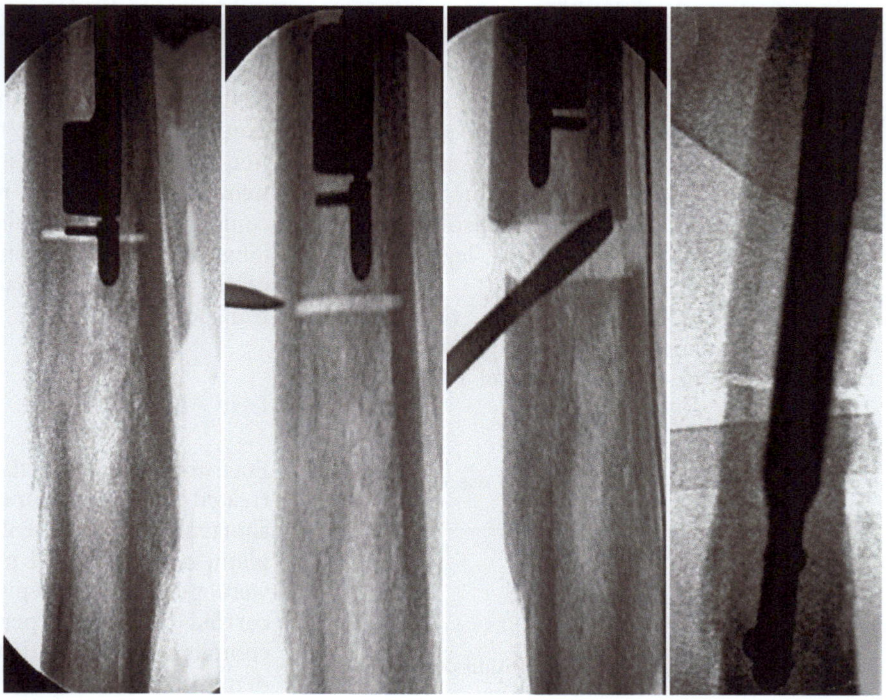

Fig. 4.13.4. X-ray control of the incomplete osteotomy. Completion of the osteotomy with a chisel

is necessary. In addition, sonographic three-dimensional measurement of the leg axis (e.g., Zebris with a measurement accuracy of 3 mm) can be performed during follow-up [7].

Until callus distraction is completed, weight-bearing is limited to toe-touch weight-bearing on the ipsilateral extremity. Depending on the quality and consolidation of the distracted callus as evaluated by X-ray, partial weight-bearing is required on the affected leg for approximately 6 weeks after the end of the distraction procedure.

The inserted intramedullary nail should not be removed until reliable evidence of callus consolidation is observed. Early removal of the intramedullary nail may cause loss of distraction due to soft tissue traction.

During callus distraction, intensive physical therapy must be performed daily. In addition, soft tissue stretching is essential as soft tissue traction may be a limiting factor for callus distraction.

Contraindications

Advanced age is considered a general contraindication since there is evidence for impaired callus formation in this group of patients. The success of callus distraction is dependent on the existence of preserved and functional periosteal cover.

In patients with congenital leg shortening, it is important to stabilize and limit motion of hip and knee joints. The rotation performed to activate the distraction mechanism may lead to dislocation of adjacent joints [2].

The leg-lengthening procedure requires treatment over a period of several months and may necessitate administration of general or regional anesthesia on several occasions. In addition, callus distraction mandates reliable and accurate handling of the ratcheting device on a daily basis. Therefore, patient compliance is absolutely critical for successful application of the leg-lengthening device.

Contraindications for the use of the intramedullary nail implant include overly contoured femoral axis, a large medullary canal resulting from fracture, and an excessively thin corticalis (Table 4.13.1).

Table 4.13.1. Contraindications for the use of the Albizzia intramedullary nail

Periosteum in poor condition
Elderly patients
Unstable knee or hip joint
Poor patient compliance
Increased femoral curvature
Narrowing of the medullary canal or thin corticalis

Results

Between 1 January 1994 and 31 December 2003, a total of 18 patients were treated with the Albizzia nail at the Murnau Trauma Center, Murnau, Germany. This study population consisted of five patients who had suffered open fractures, and 13 patients who had suffered closed fractures of the femoral shaft. The average interval between trauma and the distraction treatment was 78.9 months.

In 12 of 18 cases, osteotomy was performed using the intramedullary saw. In six patients, additional open osteotomy with a chisel or drill was necessary.

In all patients, callus distraction was performed using brief general anesthesia during the first 3 days of treatment. Thirteen of the 18 patients required no additional anesthesia after the first three distraction procedures. Twelve of the 18 patients were able to activate the lengthening mechanism independently with little pain following the initial distraction distance of 1 cm. The total distraction gain was 4.4 cm (3–7 cm).

In five of 18 patients, the intended distraction distance was not completely achieved. In these cases, a persistent leg-length discrepancy of less than 1.5 cm was observed.

The postoperative clinical and radiological follow-up did not reveal any rotational deformity.

In two of 18 patients, delayed consolidation of the distraction callus was found. Consequently, the intramedullary nail was exchanged according to the principles of nonunion treatment. Reoperation was necessary in three cases due to dislocation of proximal or distal locking screws. One patient insisted on early removal of implant prior to complete callus consolidation. This resulted in a longitudinal correction loss of 1.5 cm. In two cases, a nail was replaced because of a defective transport mechanism.

Case Example

Fracture healing of the distal femoral diaphysis treated with an intramedullary nail resulted in leg shortening of 4 cm. Following removal of the implant, osteotomy and insertion of an Albizzia nail were performed. Stepwise callus distraction was carried out over a period of 40 days. Following completion of the distraction phase, the callus demonstrated complete bony consolidation.

Implant Costs

The implant costs are approximately 4,000–4,500 euros. At the present time, reimbursement provided by the DRG system barely covers the implant costs. The total treatment costs – including preoperative and postoperative care, hospital stay, anesthesia and pain medication required during the initial period, in addition to physical therapy – are not entirely covered by any of the health insurance plans.

Summary

The Albizzia nail permits continuous callus distraction in the femur. With this method frequent complications associated with the use of conventional external fixation devices, e.g., pin tract infections or soft tissue irritation, are prevented as a result of the intramedullary position of the implant. For anatomical reasons, the use of the straight intramedullary nail is limited to the femur. The lengthening mechanism can be activated a few days after the operation by rotating the extremity by 20°. Osteotomy and insertion of the nail are technically challenging procedures that require surgical expertise. Activation of the lengthening mechanism generally causes severe pain in the first postoperative days. Therefore, brief general anesthesia is required during this period. In general, the lengthening mechanism is highly reliable and technical failure is rare. For successful application of the Albizzia nail, patient compliance is important because overdistraction and failure of the distracted callus may occur and need to be ruled out in consecutive follow-up visits. As in all distraction procedures, the soft tissue envelope is the principal limiting factor for maximum distraction distance. The high costs for implant and treatment are not entirely covered by any of the current health insurance plans.

References

1. Guichet J-M (1988) Clou d'allongement progressif. Bases théoriques – etude experimentale. Thèse de Médecine, Faculté de Médecine, Dijon, France (651 pp, 2 vol)
2. Guichet J-M (1997) Intramedullärer Verlängerungsnagel (Albizzia), Technik, Anwendung und Ergebnisse nach kontinuierlichen Verlängerungen von Femur und Tibia. In: Strecker W, Keppler P, Kinzl L (eds) Posttraumatische Beindeformitäten. Springer, Berlin, Heidelberg, New York, 251–264
3. Guichet J-M, Lascombes P, Grammont PM, Prévot J (1995) Gradual elongation intramedullary nail for femur (Albizzia). Results of the 52 first cases in 48 patients. J Jpn Orthop Assoc 69 (2) (3): S 310
4. Guichet JM, Deromedis B, Donnan LT, Peretti G, Lascombes P, Bado F (2003) Gradual femoral lengthening with the Albizzia intramedullary nail. J Bone Joint Surg Am 85-A(5): 838–848
5. Hankemeier S, Bastian L, Gosling T, Krettek C (2004) Prinzipien der Kallusdistraktion. Unfallchirurg 107: 945–958
6. Ilisarov GA (1990) Clinical application of the tension-stress for limb lengthening. Clin Orthop 250: 8–26
7. Keppler P, Strecker W, Kinzl L, Simmacher M, Claes L (1999) Die sonographische Bestimmung der Beingeometrie. Orthopäde 28: 1015–1022
8. Paley D (1990) Problems, obstacles and complications of limb lengthening by the Ilisarov technique. Clin Orthop 250: 81–104

Section 5 Intramedullary Fixation of Long Bond Fractures in Infancy and Adolescence

Intramedullary Stabilization of the Long Bones in Children with Osteogenesis Imperfecta

V. Topouchian, G. Finidori, C. Glorion

Since the initial description by Sofield [20] of intramedullary nailing of long bones for patients with osteogenesis imperfecta, palliative stabilization has not been contested. The concept of fragmentation, realignment and intramedullary rod fixation is an essential contribution in the management of long bone deformities. Segmental osteosynthesis in a delicate bone structure remains questionable. Fragmentation by multiple osteotomies, realignment and intramedullary rodding has been subject to multiple technical improvements, especially in children. The most significant advances were:

- The development of Bailey-Dubow extensible rods [2, 3].
- The expansion of intramedullary bipolar nailing with two bowed Kirschner wires described by Metaizeau [16].
- Recent advances are due to the development of closed intramedullary pinning techniques in children [17, 18].

Surgical progress accomplished in the last three decades has occurred within the framework of a better pluridisciplinary management of the pathology. Nowadays, improvements in rehabilitation techniques, casting, anesthesiology and bisphosphonate therapy have profoundly modified the prognosis of patients with osteogenesis imperfecta.

Kypho-scoliosis and respiratory restriction at adulthood is being managed by early surgical treatment for kypho-scoliosis and respiratory physiotherapy, especially in severe cases.

Living within the community with the support of associations [22] has contributed to better management of these patients and their family members. These associations are absolutely necessary to provide better information for patients and the medical professionals.

Prenatal screening tests have considerably reduced the number of severe forms of osteogenesis imperfecta frequently encountered in the past. Patients with moderate forms have less severe bone fragility at maturity. If treatment during infancy has been adequate with no significant deformities of long bones at adulthood, functional prognosis will be reasonable and these patients will have a nearly normal existence.

Aims of Osteosynthesis

Surgery must provide effective protection against bone fragility; it should prevent long bone bowing and reduce the total number of fractures.

Osteogenesis imperfecta can be considered as two separate ailments, constitutional and acquired. Genetic anomalies induced by the mutation of genes coding for collagen synthesis [6, 7, 14] are the basic reason for initial osseous fragility. Multiple fractures, bone distortion and frequent and long immobilizations contribute to secondary osteopenia and a tragic worsening of the disease. It is essentially to improve this secondary pathology that treatment and particularly surgery may be of use.

Surgical Methods and Techniques

Intramedullary rodding was first described by Sofield with a large subperiosteal exposure of bone shaft, and numerous osteotomies, and realignment has been much improved. Less aggressive techniques, with limited surgical approaches and subperiosteal exposures are preferred.

Bailey and Dubow introduced extensible intramedullary fixation devices to diminish the need for reoperation due to bone growth. Their telescoping rod can be elongated by being anchored to the epiphysis without damage to bone growth plate [2, 3]. Since their initial description, Bailey-Dubow extensible rods have been considered to be the best way to treat growing children suffering from deformity or multiple fractures. Telescopic rods comprise a sleeve portion with a detachable T-piece that can be screwed on at its extremity; the second component is the inner obturator with an incorporated T-piece at its extremity. This inner rod can telescope totally into the sleeve. The T-shaped ends are anchored into the epiphyses, and with longitudinal bone growth the telescoping rods elongate. Special instrument sets comprising a detachable drill and two nail guides are necessary.

Imaging in the anteroposterior, lateral and maximal deformity planes is used to plan the sites of osteotomies and determine the length and width of the bone in which the device is to be inserted. It is not advisable to cut the sleeve at the time of operation since this could produce distortion of the tube and loss of the sliding mechanism. Rods are prepared and cut by the manufacturer as previewed by the surgeon using the preoperative views.

Femoral Intramedullary Telescopic Rodding

Osteotomy and rod insertion can be carried out as has been initially described [2, 3, 9, 10]. The entire lower limb should be prepared and included in the operating field. Blood loss can be minimized with the use of an Esmarch band, especially during the distal femoral approach. Intramedullary reaming is performed starting at the intercondylar notch of the femur using an anterolateral approach and a parapatellar arthrotomy. The rod direction is perpendicular to the femorotibial space in the frontal and anteroposterior planes (Fig. 5.1.1). Classically the medullary canal is drilled toward the greater trochanter using a detachable drill bit screwed into the tubular sleeve of the rod until it impinges on the cortex at one site of the curve. Osteotomy is carried out at this site. It is better to use long and stiff drills rather than the sleeve part of the rod. This procedure is repeated until all shaft incurvation is corrected. The outer tubular sleeve of the device (with the T-piece detached) is driven into the upper femoral segment using a retrograde approach, through the medullary canal, exiting on the upper-lateral aspect of the femoral neck medial to the greater trochanteric notch. Through a separate small incision the upper end of the tubular sleeve is pushed out through the skin, the T-piece is screwed in and tapped into the superior aspect of the femoral neck. The inner obturator rod is driven upward through the intercondylar notch of the femur and fitted into the outer sleeve. The T-shaped end is tapped into the osseous part of the lower femoral epiphysis. The surgical approach to the bowed bone uses subperiosteal exposure. The deformed bone is osteotomized into the appropriate number of fragments so that they can be aligned for insertion of the rod. If femoral bowing is considerable, bone shortening may be necessary to ensure proper lining of the femoral shaft. To avoid this drawback it is best to rod earlier before severe incurvations occur. Infratrochanteric valgus osteotomy is performed to avoid secondary varus bending of the upper femoral extremity (Fig. 5.1.2).

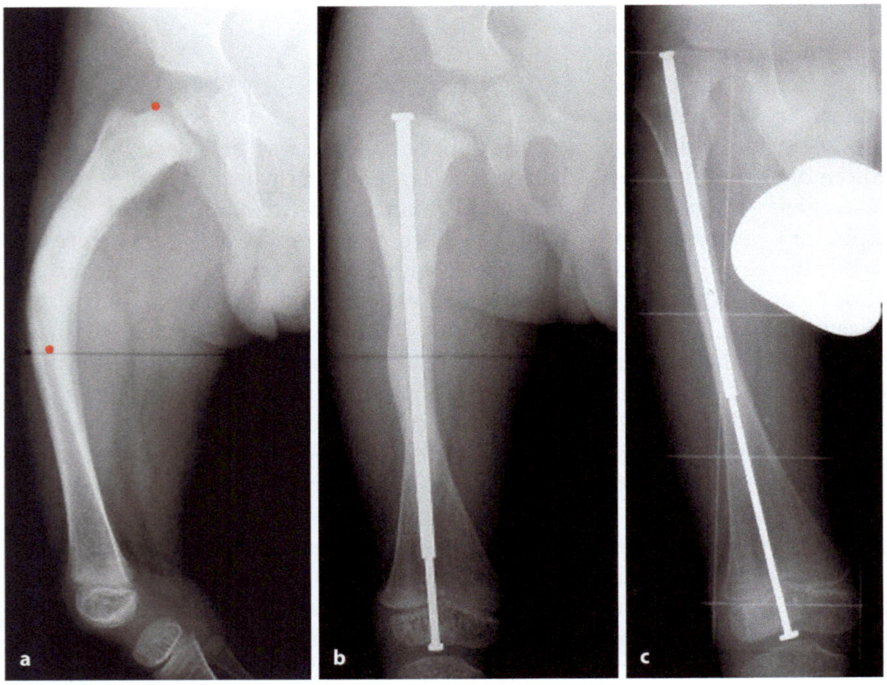

Fig. 5.1.1. Femoral telescopic rodding with Bailey-Dubow rods. a Preoperative radiograph; b 3 months and c 4 years postoperatively

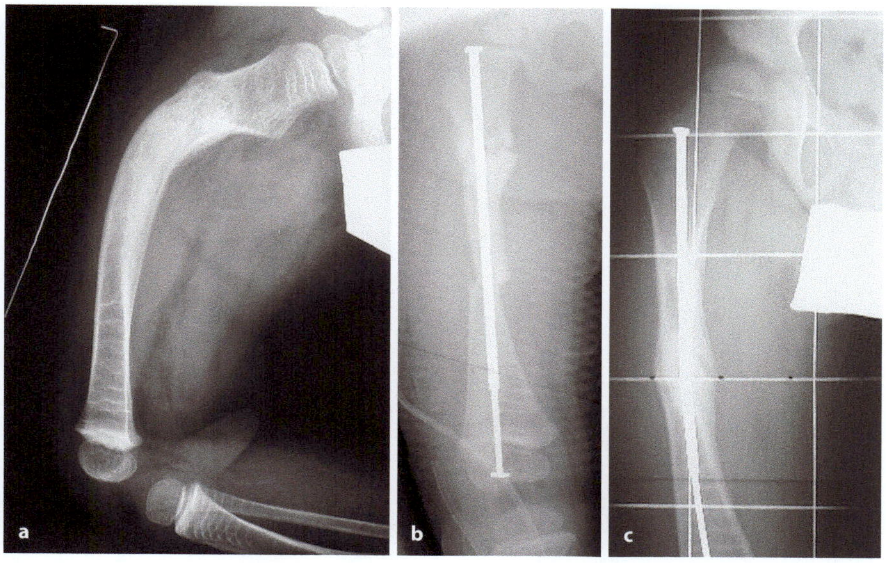

Fig. 5.1.2. Femoral bowing in a 4-year-old boy despite bisphosphonate treatment (distal sclerotic growth lines are produced by intravenous bisphosphonate treatment). a Initial radiograph. b Immediate postoperative radiograph. c At 2.5 years postoperatively with satisfactory extension of the rods

After the wounds are closed, the patient is immobilized, usually for 4 weeks, in a hip spica cast. Later on a rehabilitation program for upright posture and walking is established.

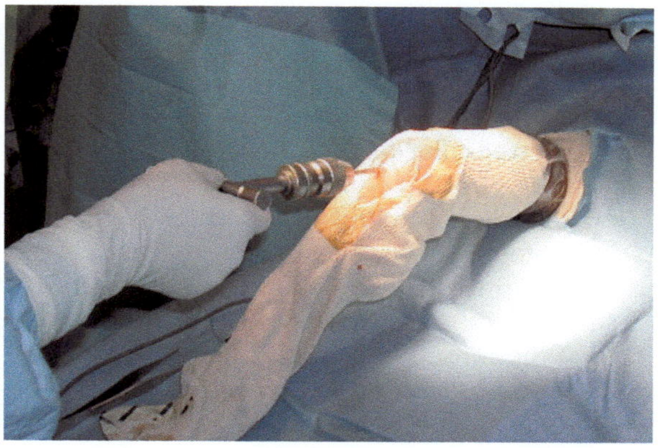

Fig. 5.1.3. Percutaneous femoral telescopic rodding with a midline incision through the patellar ligament

Percutaneous Femoral Telescopic Rodding

With these positive developments in technical and medical treatments, severe bone deformities with considerable bowing are less frequently encountered. It seemed possible to consider less invasive modalities of surgical treatment. F. Fassier [8] developed a new intramedullary rod and instrument set to provide percutaneous femoral telescopic rodding. In our institution we have developed an original technique of percutaneous femoral telescopic rodding. We use the original Bailey-Dubow implant because of its proven mechanical characteristics and low cost advantages. A special instrument set has been developed for percutaneous rodding. A long stiff drill with a diameter two-tenths greater than the rod to be inserted is introduced percutaneously with a midline short skin incision through the patellar ligament with the knee flexed to 90° (Fig. 5.1.3). Shaft reaming is performed upward starting at the intercondylar notch with fluoroscopic control. Multiple osteotomies can be performed percutaneously using the stamping technique and osteoclastic correction. As for classical rodding, infratrochanteric valgus osteotomy is performed to achieve a valgus position of the upper femoral extremity (Fig. 5.1.4). Once the endomedullary canal has been prepared and the different osteotomies have been performed, the drill is pushed toward the greater trochanter, and its upper end is driven out of the skin through a separate small incision. The tubular sleeve of the device is attached to the distal part of the drill and pushed upward with a metal guide till its proximal extremity comes out of the skin. The inner obturator rod is driven upward through the intercondylar notch and into the tubular sleeve. The T-piece is screwed in and tapped into the upper femoral epiphysis. The T-shaped end of the obturator rod is tapped into the distal epiphyseal bone under fluoroscopic control. Postoperative care and immobilization are the same as for the initial classical technique. Depending on difficulties with the osteotomy, short surgical approaches may be necessary, especially at the upper part of the shaft where bowing is often considerable. This percutaneous femoral telescopic rodding is only a variant of the traditional technique.

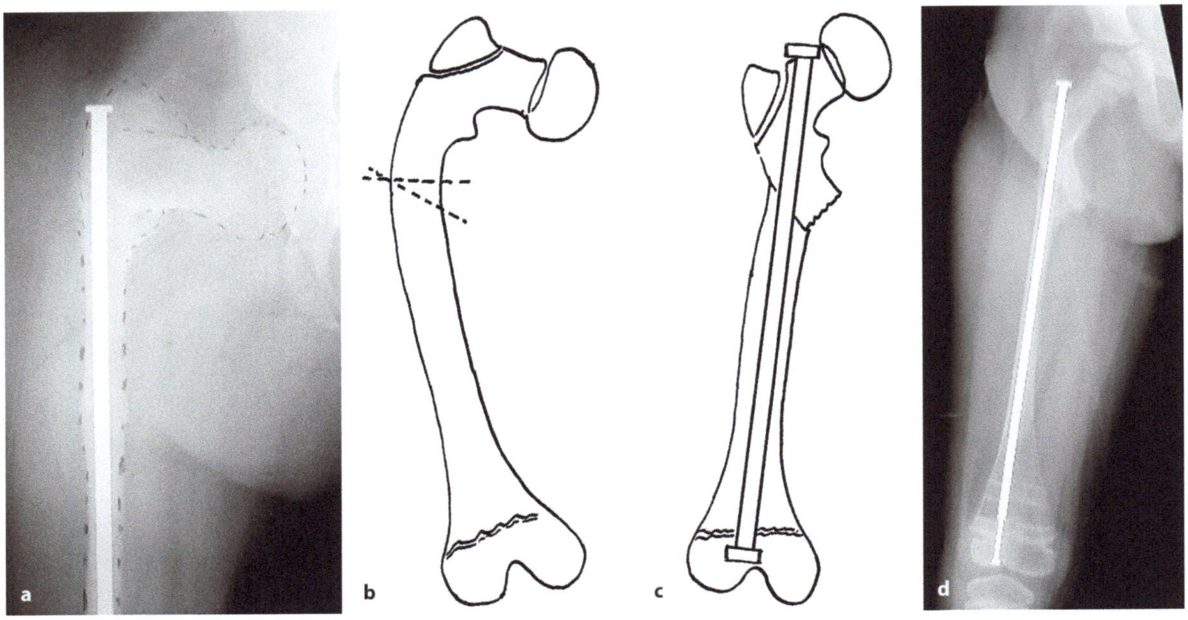

Fig. 5.1.4. a Incorrect position of the proximal end of the rod with persistent varus of the femoral neck in a 12-year-old girl. b–d Correct positioning after valgus osteotomy for the same patient

Tibia Telescopic Rodding

Tibia telescopic rodding is performed in the same way and follows the same principles as femoral rodding. The proximal tibia epiphysis is exposed with a short arthrotomy allowing drill insertion at the base of the anterior cruciate ligament. As for the femur, the rod direction is perpendicular to the femorotibial space. In patients with a genu recurvatum, a flexion osteotomy is performed at the proximal tibia segment. Reaming is performed downward with a long drill. Multiple shaft osteotomies are performed. No surgical approach is necessary for the fibula; simple osteoclastic correction is sufficient. The ankle joint is exposed through a large anterolateral incision and the talus is dislocated medially and posteriorly. The long drill is pushed downward through the medullary canal and lower distal epiphysis. A drill guide and a spatula allow for better positioning of the drill at the center of the ankle joint cartilage. It would be a technical error to use an anteriorly positioned insertion point of the rod at the distal tibia end. Since the long drill is more rigid than the definitive sleeve part of the rod, reaming is performed with no distortion, and the sliding between the two parts of the rod is not impaired. The T-piece is screwed in and the sleeve is tapped into the cartilage at the distal end of the tibia in the subchondral region. The inner obturator is driven downward and engaged into the sleeve, its T-shaped end is tapped into the proximal tibia epiphysis. The arthrotomy and tibiofibular ligaments are sutured. If multiple osteotomies are performed, prophylactic anterior compartment fasciotomy may be appropriate to avoid compartmental syndrome. Special care must be taken not to induce rotational anomaly with cast immobilization. An above-the-knee cast is applied for 3–4 weeks postoperatively. A short immobilization is essential to avoid secondary osteopenia.

Humeral Telescopic Rodding

Humeral rodding principles are the same as described above. The whole upper limb is prepared and included in the operating field. An Esmarch band may be used during the distal humeral approach. With a posterolateral incision, the elbow joint is exposed. The drill is introduced at the lateral margin of the trochlea perpendicular to the elbow joint area. Diaphyseal osteotomies are performed using a lateral humeral approach, taking care to avoid the radial nerve. Osteotomies are carried out through small incisions with limited subperiosteal exposure [5, 15, 21]. The upper end of the tubular sleeve is driven through the proximal epiphysis and pushed out of the skin anteriorly to the acromion. The inner obturator rod may be equally inserted at the proximal or distal segment of the humerus. T-pieces are tapped into the bone epiphysis. As for the femur and the tibia, care should be taken not to induce torsion anomaly during cast or bandage immobilization, usually applied for 4 weeks.

Telescopic Intramedullary Pinning

This technique is more and more frequently used. Pinning is often carried out percutaneously and surgical procedure if necessary is limited. The implantable material is not expensive. Pins can be put in place with epiphyseal anchorage in a telescopic mode allowing for long-lasting protection against bowing and fractures during child growth.

Femoral Telescopic Pinning

As for telescopic rodding, the first pin is introduced at the intercondylar notch of the distal femoral epiphysis. This pin is pushed upward into the neck of the femur. The second pin is positioned downward through the greater trochanter. Usually this pinning is carried out percutaneously. A small surgical procedure may be necessary for osteotomies, especially the valgus osteotomy of the proximal extremity of the femur (Fig. 5.1.5).

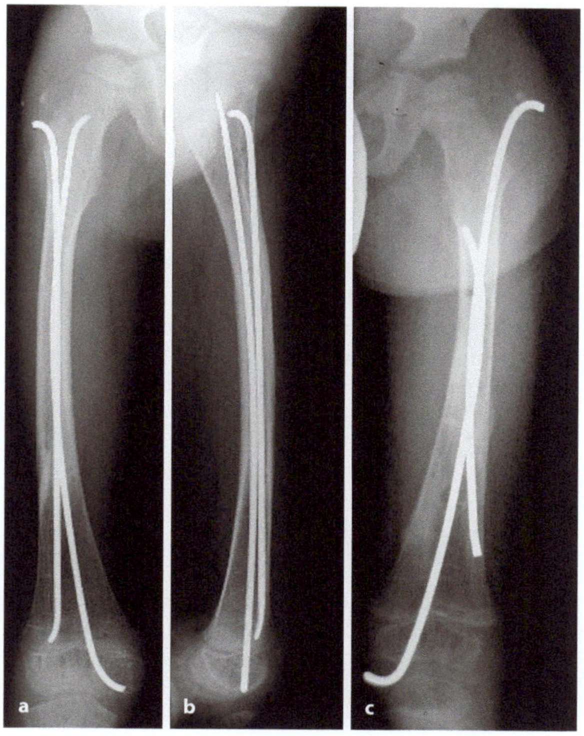

Fig. 5.1.5. a, b Anteroposterior and lateral radiographs of a femoral telescopic pinning. c Erroneous anchorage of pin extremities into the epiphysis, with protrusion into soft tissue limiting joint mobility

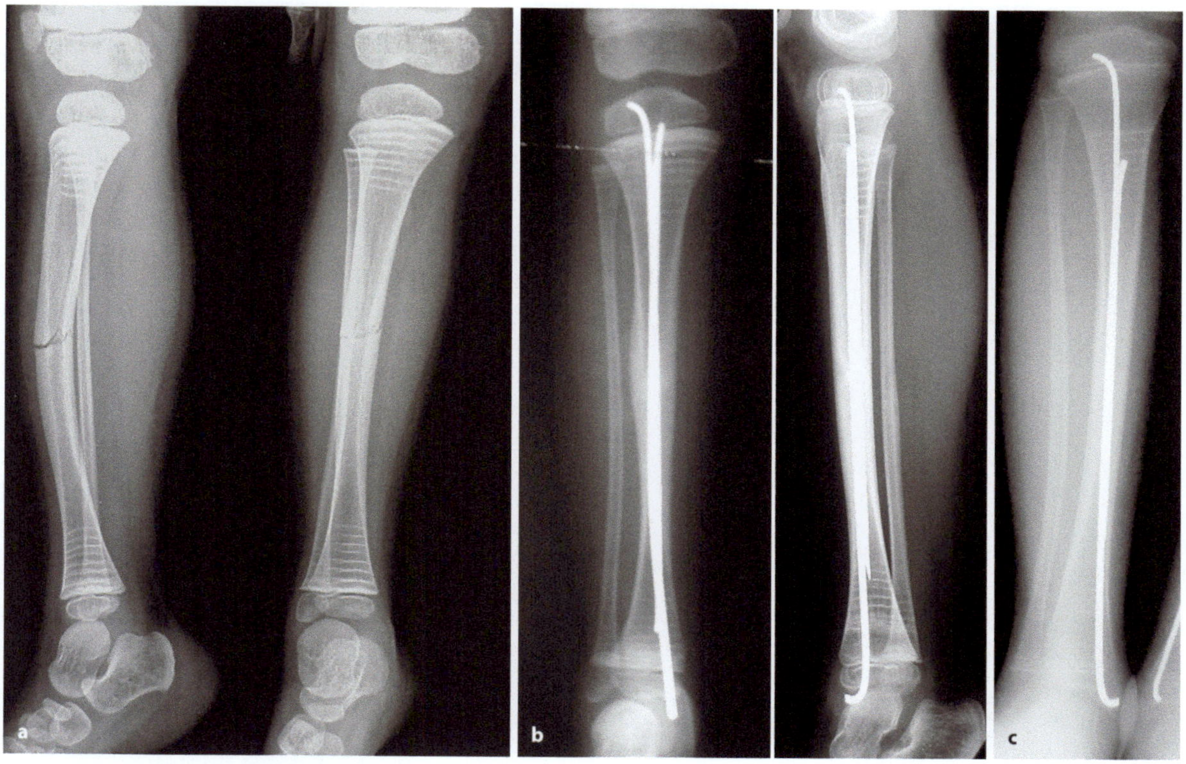

Fig. 5.1.6. a A 4-year-old girl who had type III osteogenesis imperfecta. Preoperative radiographs. b Anteroposterior and lateral views of the same patient 6 months following telescopic intramedullary pinning. c Same patient 2 years later demonstrating growth of the tibia, no recurrence of deformity and elongation of pins

Tibia Telescopic Pinning

Tibia telescopic pinning is a simple and attractive technique usually performed percutaneously. The first pin is inserted through the medial malleolus and directed upward into the proximal metaphysis. The descending pin is introduced in the prespinal space downward as far as the distal metaphysis. Into each epiphysis a pin is bent and tapped to obtain a telescopic effect. Whenever the femur and tibia need to be operated on it is technically more appropriate to start osteosynthesis of the tibia first, to protect the synthesis with a thick bandage and then to operate the femur (Fig. 5.1.6).

Humeral Telescopic Pinning

This technique is simple and effective (Fig. 5.1.7). The first pin is introduced laterally through the lateral condyle and driven up the intramedullary canal until just beneath the proximal epiphysis. The second pin is introduced through the proximal humeral epiphysis percutaneously anterior to the acromion and directed downward as far as the distal metaphysis. The extremities of the pin are bent and stuck into the epiphyseal bone to prevent the pin sliding and impairment of joint mobility. Epiphyseal anchorage allows a telescopic effect. As previously described for telescopic humeral rodding, multiple osteotomies are performed if necessary. Special care must be taken to prevent varus deviation of the elbow and internal rotation of the brachial segment.

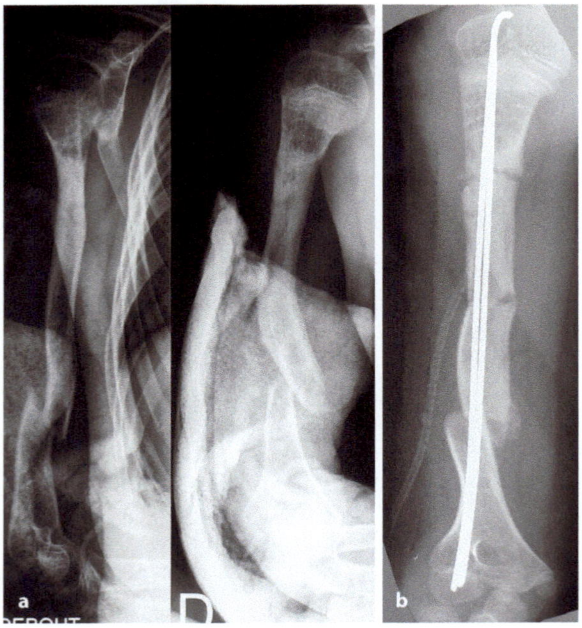

Fig. 5.1.7. a Preoperative and b postoperative radiographs showing humeral telescopic pinning. Note pin extremities bent and stuck into the epiphysis

Forearm Telescopic Pinning

Multiple fractures and significant bowing of the radius and the ulna require realignment and osteosynthesis. Telescopic rods have a wide diameter; they are not suitable for forearm osteosynthesis. Intramedullary pinning remains the most suitable technique (Fig. 5.1.8).

Osteosynthesis of the Ulna: the pin is introduced through the olecranon. Osteotomies are performed, depending on the degree of bowing and the pin is driven in as far as the distal metaphysis. The proximal part of the pin can be curved into a "Z" shape and stuck into the proximal epiphysis to have a secure purchase and to prevent the pin from sliding (Fig. 5.1.9). For patients with an almost inexistent medullary canal, the periosteum of the osteotomized segment is gently split longitudinally, the pin is placed underneath, and then the periosteum is sewn up again. Gradually the pin is pushed forward as far as the distal end of the ulna. This method ensures maintenance of the position without creating a solid osteosynthesis. The ossification of the periosteum will progressively incorporate the nail into the bone shaft. Pseudarthrosis of the ulna may produce disparity of bone length, with shortening of the ulna, and as a result limit rotational movements. For pseudarthrosis of the ulna, it is best to advise against operation. Secondary pseudarthrosis may follow radial head dislocation especially with hypertrophic callus formation. In such situations there is no hope of putting the radial head back into position; its excision is the best palliative operation.

Osteosynthesis of the Radius: radius osteosynthesis is difficult. The pin is introduced upward until it reaches the radial head. The pin must be bent to follow the normal curve of the radius. A straight radius impinges on the movement of the radioulnar joint and limits prono-supination. Osteosynthesis of the radius constitutes invasive surgery for the wrist joint. We prefer, whenever skeletally mature or nearly mature patients need no more forearm telescopic pinning, to carry out a solid osteosynthesis of the ulna with an intramedullary nail and multiple osteotomies of the radius with no synthesis.

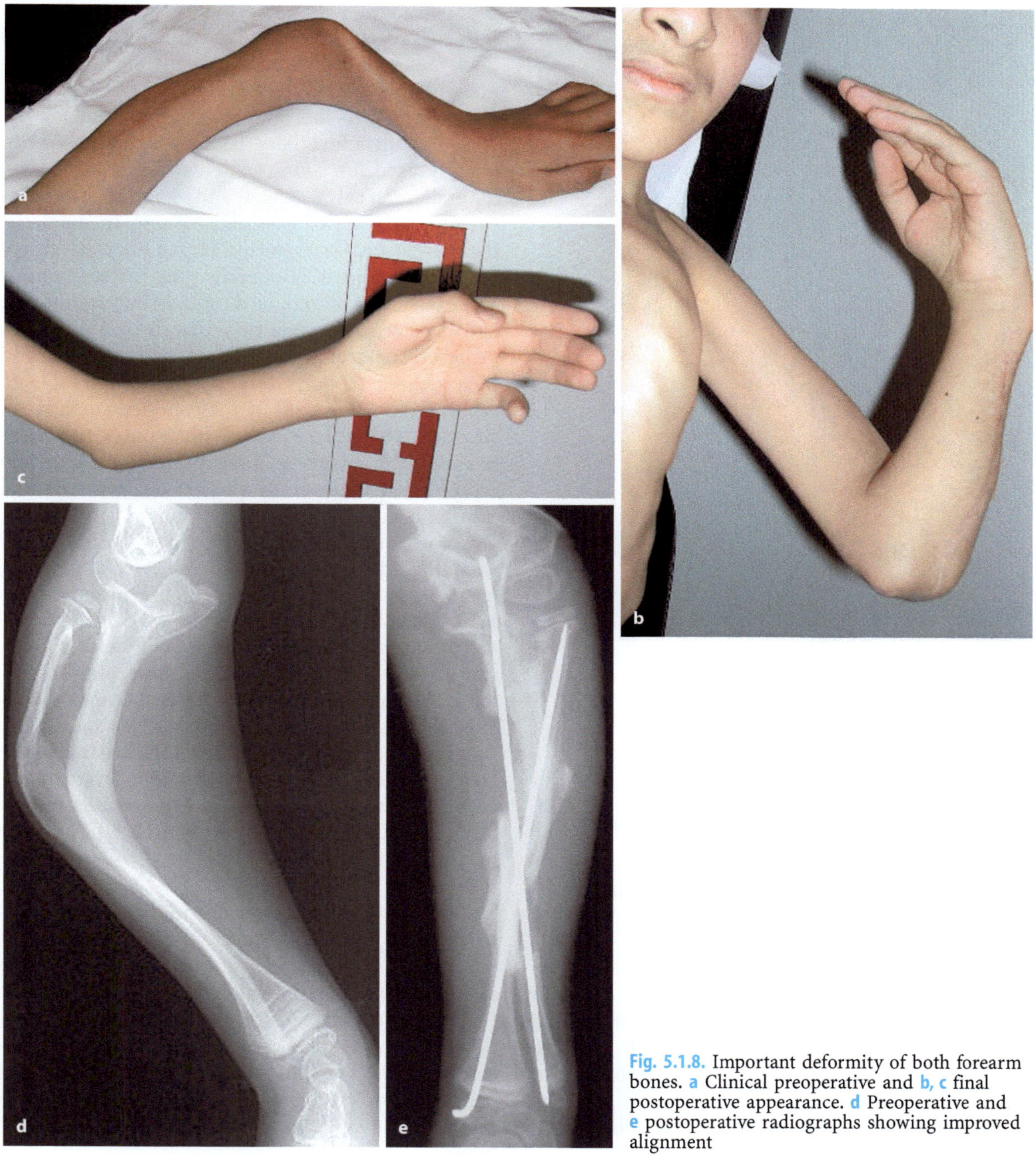

Fig. 5.1.8. Important deformity of both forearm bones. a Clinical preoperative and b, c final postoperative appearance. d Preoperative and e postoperative radiographs showing improved alignment

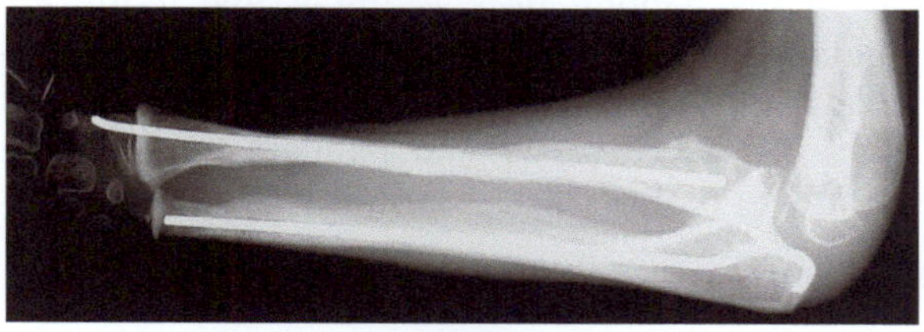

Fig. 5.1.9. Postoperative radiograph of the forearm. Note proximal part of the pin curved into a "Z" shape and stuck into the proximal epiphysis of the ulna

Technical Problems of Osteosynthesis

Limb surgery in patients with osteogenesis imperfecta is very tricky and requires appropriate techniques, particularly in severe cases. Bleeding may be limited with the use of an electrocautery during the surgical procedure and an Esmarch band. Fasciotomy is recommended whenever multiple osteotomies are practiced. For severe curvatures,

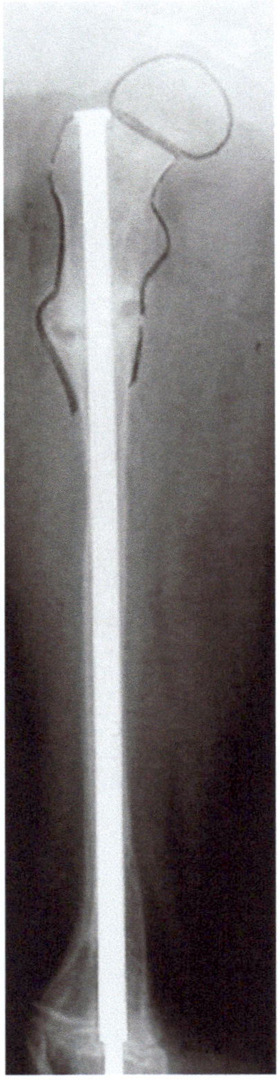

Fig. 5.1.10. Anteroposterior femoral radiograph showing bone resorption at femoral shaft due to a too large rod

osteotomies may be carried out first. Correction of the distortion without limb length shortening is obtained by progressive axial limb traction. Once the bone segments are aligned, osteosynthesis is carried out.

Reaming of the medullary canal and nail insertion are usually carried out manually. Motorized drills may induce bone cortex burst and growth plate damage. During surgery, care must be taken to avoid fractures in the operated limb, especially of the femoral neck. If some of the osteotomized segments are very compact with no medullary canal, pins may be slid under the periosteum and maintained in position with wires and periosteal suture. Periosteal ossification will gradually incorporate the pin into the medullary cavity.

The choice of pin or rod diameter to be inserted is made according to contradictory requirements (Fig. 5.1.10). If the osteosynthesis material is too thin, it will not provide sufficient protection to prevent fractures and bowing. Using too thick material will induce a stress shielding phenomenon with bone resorption and cause secondary fractures to the bone and intramedullary device. The intramedullary telescopic rods most frequently used for young patients in our institution have diameters of 3.5, 4 and 4.5 mm. The pins usually used are of 2, 3 and 3.5 mm in diameter. It is rarely necessary to use larger material except for adult patients. Generally, the osteosynthesis materials are not removed, and if they cannot be left in place, they must be replaced by a more appropriate device depending on patients' age and their degree of bone fragility. It is preferable to remove too thick rods if they induce cortical resorption and replace them with thinner and more flexible pins ensuring bone protection. This pin replacement is generally carried out once skeletal growth is achieved.

Lower limb length discrepancy is frequently encountered in osteogenesis imperfecta patients, particularly in severe forms of the disease. This may be avoided by limiting the shortening to the osteotomy site, especially in patients with significant bowing of long bones. Shortening osteotomies are not performed to correct length difference in this particular pathology because further fractures may still modify lower limb length. We have not attempted limb lengthening even in patients with moderate forms of osteogenesis imperfecta. This is to be taken into consideration in the future, particularly with the use of elongating rods.

Pelvis deformity is frequent in osteogenesis imperfecta, especially in severe forms (type III of Sillence) [19]. Acetabular protrusion leads to hip joint motion limitation and to an invalid posture (Fig. 5.1.11). Pelvis deformity with sacral distortion and acetabular protrusion occur progressively and are worsened once spinal fusion has been achieved and both femurs are nailed. At the present time we have no solution to prevent this complication.

Femoral neck fractures are frequently seen in patients with acetabular protrusion. Osteosynthesis of the femoral neck is impossible if the hip has severe limitation of motion and it is preferable to let pseudarthrosis become established. This will cause better and painless hip mobility even with patients who can walk.

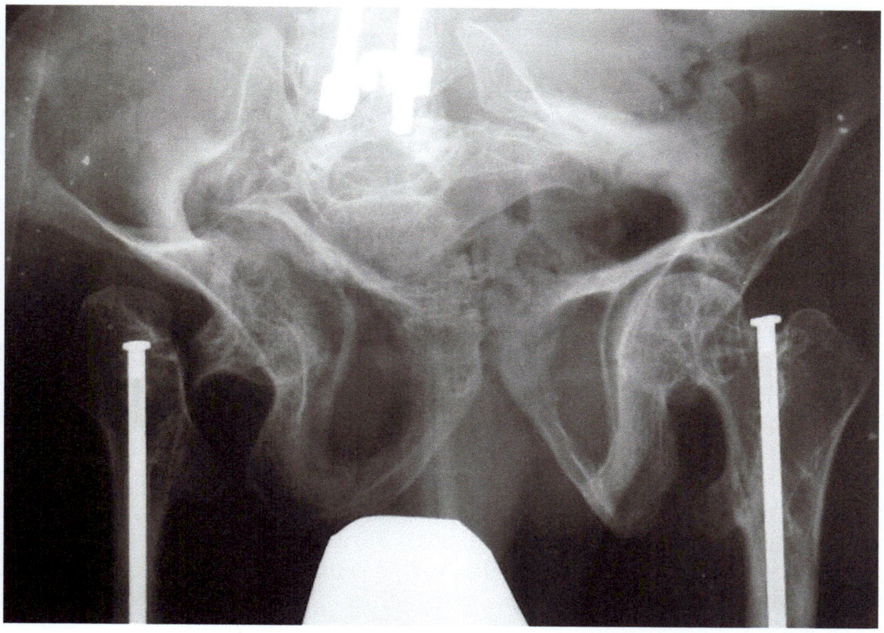

Fig. 5.1.11. Right femoral neck fracture in a patient operated from bilateral femoral rodding and spinal fusion. Note acetabular protrusion and pelvis deformity

Treatment Indications

Patients and their family must be informed about how the treatment will proceed and they must support the treatment program. Multidisciplinary management and coordination between physicians and the associations dealing with osteogenesis imperfecta are necessary for patients and their families to achieve the best medical and surgical results.

The primary concern of the orthopedic surgeon is to reduce fracture recurrences and to limit bone bowing.

Until walking capacities are acquired, surgery is rarely necessary, although in severe forms with significant bowing in very young patients osteosynthesis may be essential for the well-being of the patient. Bone protection will make nursing easier and will reduce pain and fracture recurrences. Telescopic rodding whenever possible is the preferred mode of osteosynthesis for the femur since it affords effective long-lasting protection. Pins in young patients with severe forms are less effective and may migrate through the cortical bone.

When walking is acquired, protective osteosynthesis should be practiced particularly in the femur. Delaying osteosynthesis is not a good idea since bone bowing will increase and secondary bone demineralization will be exacerbated due to repeated immobilizations. If that happens, surgery will be technically more difficult. In these conditions percutaneous surgery cannot be considered: more aggressive surgery is necessary, with shortening osteotomies.

Most often, fortunately, telescopic rodding and osteotomies can be carried out percutaneously in patients with satisfactory general treatment and as long as surgery is performed before the onset of severe deformities. Choosing between telescopic rods and pins may depend on the surgeon's experience and also on the availability of material. Pins are less expensive and widely available. Telescopic pinning is more appropriate than rodding for tibia osteosynthesis since it is easier to insert and is less aggressive and impairing to the knee and ankle joints. Humeral and forearm distortions are frequently seen with severe forms of osteogenesis imperfecta and especially in patients with hypertrophic callus [13]. These cases are best managed with multiple osteotomies and telescopic pinning. Upper limb curvatures must be operated on before significant deformities make surgery more difficult. In young adult patients this surgery will lead to frequent complications, such as delayed bone healing and pseudarthrosis.

Recurrent Surgery of Intramedullary Osteosynthesis

The occurrence of fractures despite intramedullary osteosynthesis is a frequent event. Fractures may be the result of persistent bone fragility and/or insufficient osteosynthesis. Fractures may also occur following a severe trauma in patients who have achieved a fair surgical result. In many cases osteosynthesis prevents fracture displacement and simple orthopedic immobilization can be enough to ensure bone healing. Occasionally bone fracture is associated with rod or pin bending; in such situations external manual correction avoids open surgery. If bending is considerable or the intramedullary device is fractured, open surgery will be necessary. Replacement of osteosynthesis in a fragile bone is often difficult. If fractures occur despite intramedullary osteosynthesis, this may be the result of technical errors or due to a real and major trauma.

Inadequate lining of lower limbs, with small anteroposterior, lateral or rotational distortions are well tolerated in children and they do not require immediate reoperation, which can be postponed till skeletal maturity is achieved. Surgery can be necessary in growing children if residual deformities compromise walking possibilities or they induce exacerbated risks of fracture.

Complications

Complications are not frequently encountered; they depend largely on the experience of the surgeon.

Operating complications are mainly technical difficulties due to bone fragility. There is a risk of additionally induced bone bursts. Bone manipulation must be carefully managed using nonaggressive instruments. Excessive bleeding can be avoided by using an Esmarch band as a tourniquet; the surgical approach will be carried out using an electrocautery. After intramedullary drilling of bone segments a guide is left in the medullary canal to limit bone marrow bleeding. In case of multiple surgical procedures, while operating on one site, the other wounds are closed with a slightly compressive bandage.

Compartmental syndrome and nerve palsy can be prevented by a nontraumatic technique with prophylactic fasciotomy and the correction of severe deformities avoiding excessive traction with elongation of vasculo-nervous bonds. The osteogenesis imperfecta fragile bone is well vascularized with very thin cortices and has a better resistance to infection. Although this fact is not reported in the literature, the incidence of postoperative infection seems particularly low in our experience.

Axial and rotational abnormalities are secondary to intraoperative misalignment, and a lack of correct postoperative immobilization. Secondary deviation can result from a noneffective epiphyseal purchase and fractures. These complications justify reoperation if they impair the possibility of verticalization and walking capacities.

Delayed bone healing and pseudarthrosis are exceptional in young patients with osteogenesis imperfecta. They can result from an inappropriate osteosynthesis. Bone healing can be more problematic in older patients.

The onset of epiphysiodesis with premature growth plate closure is not frequent. In Bailey-Dubow rods a lack of sliding of the telescopic device generally does not lead to growth plate damage. The same thing is observed for the pins. Although a limited amount of epiphysiodesis is observed in patients who have been operated upon, it is not clear that this is due to the telescopic device. Some nonoperated patients have spontaneous premature closure of the growth plate, probably because severe bone fragility also concerns the growth structure, which may also be impaired.

Surgery and Bisphosphonates

Bisphosphonate treatment was initially reported by F. Glorieux [11, 12]; since that time it has been widely used for children suffering from bone fragility due to osteogenesis imperfecta. Bisphosphonates are synthetic analogs of pyrophosphate and are potent inhibitors of bone resorption. In cohort studies, bisphosphonates have shown their effectiveness in improving bone mass in children with severe forms of osteogenesis imperfecta [1, 4]. This medical treatment seems to be effective since the pain is reduced, the bone is more dense and the conditions for physiotherapy are improved. Although the bone mass is increased, skeletal plastic bone distortion and fractures are still encountered. Surgery with multiple osteotomies and intramedullary osteosynthesis is still required with different technical problems. The bone is more compact, drilling requires the frequent use of a motorized drill, the shafts are less slender. In such situations it is often possible to use osteosynthesis of a larger diameter.

Conclusion

At the present time, better management of patients with osteogenesis imperfecta thanks to coordination between physiotherapy programs, bisphosphonate treatment and surgery leads to an improved functional outcome.

In patients with moderate forms of osteogenesis imperfecta (types I and IV of Sillence), if treatment during infancy has been adequate with no major deformities of long bones in adulthood, the functional prognosis will be good, and they can have normal autonomy and a nearly normal existence.

In severe forms (type III of Sillence), the prognosis is now improved with bisphosphonate treatment, intramedullary long bone stabilization and particularly with the treatment of severe kyphoscoliosis and prevention of respiratory restrictions. Major growth disturbances can cause severe dwarfism. Pelvic deformities with acetabular protrusions lead to hip joint stiffness, secondary articular degenerative alteration and therefore a limited functional outcome and ambulatory possibilities.

Young patients with osteogenesis imperfecta have normal intellectual capacities. Physical difficulties may lead these patients to excel intellectually in order to overcome their physical disability. Appropriate orthopedic management may allow these patients to have a normal social and professional existence.

References

1. Astrom E, Soderhall S. Beneficial effect of long term intravenous bisphosphonate treatment of osteogenesis imperfecta. Arch Dis Child 2002; 86(5):356–364.
2. Bailey RW, Dubow HI. Studies of longitudinal bone growth resulting in an extensible nail. Surg Forum 1963; 14:455–458.
3. Bailey RW, Dubow HI. Evolution of the concept of an extensible nail accommodating to normal longitudinal bone growth: clinical considerations and implications. Clin Orthop 1981; 159:157–170.
4. Bembi B, Parma A, Bottega M, Ceschel S, Zanatta M, Martini C, Ciana G. Intravenous pamidronate treatment in osteogenesis imperfecta. J Pediatr 1997; 131(4):622–625.
5. Cole WG. Early surgical management of severe forms of osteogenesis imperfecta. Am J Med Genet 1993; 45(2): 270–274.
6. Cole WG. Etiology and pathogenesis of heritable connective tissue diseases. J Pediatr Orthop 1993; 13(3): 392–403.
7. Eyre DR. Concepts in collagen biochemistry: evidence that collagenopathies underlie osteogenesis imperfecta. Clin Orthop 1981; 159:97–107.
8. Fassier F. Ostéogenèse imparfaite de l'enfant. Conférences d'enseignement 1999, pp. 235-252. In: Cahiers d'enseignement de la SOFCOT. Expansion Scientifique Française, Paris, 1999.
9. Finidori G. Treatment of osteogenesis imperfecta in children. Ann NY Acad Sci 1988; 543:167–169.
10. Finidori G. Ostéogenèse imparfaite. Indications thérapeutiques chez l'enfant. Conférences d'enseignement 1988, pp. 327–345. In: Cahiers d'enseignement de la SOFCOT, no. 31. Expansion Scientifique Française, Paris, 1988.
11. Glorieux FH, Bishop NJ, Plotkin H, Chabot G, Lanoue G, Travers R. Cyclic administration of pamidronate in children with severe osteogenesis imperfecta. N Engl J Med 1998; 339(14):947–952.
12. Glorieux FH. Bisphosphonate therapy for severe osteogenesis imperfecta. J Pediatr Endocrinol Metab 2000;13 Suppl 2:989–992.
13. Glorieux FH, Rauch F, Plotkin H, Ward L, Travers R, Roughley P, Lalic L, Glorieux DF, Fassier F, Bishop NJ. Type V osteogenesis imperfecta: a new form of brittle bone disease. J Bone Miner Res 2000; 15(9):1650–1658.
14. Kocher MS, Shapiro F. Osteogenesis imperfecta. J Am Acad Orthop Surg 1998; 6(4):225–236.
15. Li YH, Chow W, Leong JC. The Sofield-Millar operation in osteogenesis imperfecta. A modified technique. J Bone Joint Surg Br 2000; 82(1):11–16.
16. Metaizeau JP. Sliding centro-medullary nailing. Application to the treatment of severe forms of osteogenesis imperfecta. Chir Pediatr 1987; 28(4–5):240–243.
17. Middleton RW. Closed intramedullary rodding for osteogenesis imperfecta. J Bone Joint Surg Br 1984; 66(5):652–655.
18. Parsch KD. Modern trends in internal fixation of femoral shaft fractures in children. A critical review. J Pediatr Orthop B 1997; 6(2):117–125.
19. Sillence D. Osteogenesis imperfecta: an expanding panorama of variants. Clin Orthop 1981; 159:11–25.
20. Sofield HA, Miller EA. Fragmentation, realignment, and intramedullary rod fixation of the deformities of the long bone of children. A ten year approval. J Bone Joint Surg 1959; 42-A:1371.
21. Wilkinson JM, Scott BW, Clarke AM, Bell MJ. Surgical stabilisation of the lower limb in osteogenesis imperfecta using the Sheffield Telescopic Intramedullary Rod System. J Bone Joint Surg Br 1998; 80(6):999–1004.
22. Association de l'Ostéogenèse Imparfaite. BP 075. F 80082 Amiens Cedex 2, France. www.aoi.asso.fr

Intramedullary Fixation of Long Bone Fractures in Infancy and Adolescence

C. Karger, P. Gicquel, J.-M. Clavert

Until the early 1980s, the treatment of long bone fractures in children was essentially conservative, combining closed reduction and plaster cast immobilization. The main argument favoring this attitude was remodeling of malunions by future growth. It had also been demonstrated that adult fixation techniques, especially open reduction and plate fixation, could lead to severe leg length discrepancies, due to overgrowth by periosteal damage and growth plate stimulation. Furthermore, adult intramedullary nailing techniques were considered as contraindicated because of the potential risk of epiphysiodesis when crossing growth plates. The only adult technique that could be used safely in children was external fixation.

It is the merit of Jean-Paul Métaizeau [8, 11, 13] to have imagined and developed a new fracture fixation technique, specifically adapted to the pediatric population: elastic stable intramedullary nailing (ESIN). Currently, this method has become the standard treatment for all femur fractures in children over 6 years of age. It is also the primary indication for unstable forearm or radial head fractures. It can be used in selective cases of displaced tibia and humerus fractures.

Biomechanical Principles

Specific Biomechanical Properties of Long Bones in Children [6]

Pediatric bones are less mineralized but more hydrated compared with adult ones. Therefore, they are less resistant but more elastic and plastic, which explains the specific fracture types in this age group. The main difference is represented by the periosteum, which is thicker and more resistant, compared to adults. The biologic healing process of fractures is identical in children and in adults. However, children have a higher healing capacity, basically because of a thick and well-vascularized periosteum, which acts as a natural internal splint and produces the peripheral callus.

Mechanical Properties of Elastic Stable Intramedullary Nailing

The concept of the method is to stabilize fractured long bones with an intramedullary elastic frame. Except for the forearm, this frame is obtained with two steel or titanium flexible nails bent in opposite directions, in a double secant arc construct. Each nail achieves a three-point stability: the first point is represented by the introduction site of the nail into the metaphysis, the second point is obtained by the contact of the apex of the nail with the inner wall of the cortex close to the fracture site, the third point is realized by the anchoring of the tip of the nail into the opposite metaphysis. Under axial load, the two nails behave as a spring and tend to increase their curvature at the apex. The contact of the nail with the inner cortex will act against this elastic deformation, achieving the stability of the fracture. The same concept is applicable for the control of coronal deformations due to bending forces (Fig. 5.2.1a). Rotation and shear forces are equally controlled by a similar elastic mechanism. It is important to point out that this technique also uses periosteum and muscular structures as adjuvant for obtaining fracture stabilization. This is particularly important for the control of rotational displacements.

Biological Advantages of Elastic Stable Intramedullary Nailing

It is well known that primary periosteal callus formation, as described by McKibbin [10], is inhibited by rigid fixation, and on the contrary favored by micro movements at the fracture site [2, 6]. ESIN has been conceived as an elastic fracture fixation, ideal to enhance peripheral callus formation. The use of two intramedullary elastic nails, bent in opposite directions, allows a certain degree of micro movements at the fracture site, especially in axial loading, whereas shear and rotational forces are prevented.

The nails are introduced through percutaneous incisions into the metaphysis of the fractured bone segment. They never cross any growth plate, which is a major requirement for a method aimed to treat pediatric fractures. Furthermore, whenever possible, the nailing is performed closed, in order to respect soft tissues and fracture hematoma. Since no additional cast or splint is required, early muscular contractions improve the blood supply at the fracture site and enhance fusiform callus formation and rapid bone healing. Almost immediate joint mobilization and early weight-bearing prevent stiffness and muscle atrophy. These are all major advantages of this method over conservative treatment by cast immobilization.

Technical Aspects and Procedures

Nail Preparation

Elastic stable intramedullary nails are available in titanium or stainless steel. Biomechanical tests have demonstrated that steel nails are less elastic and more plastic than titanium nails, which makes contouring easier. On the other hand, titanium nails require a greater diameter to obtain a comparable stiffness than steel nails. In our experience, steel nails are preferred for fractures located on the lower limbs.

Selection of nail diameter is of major importance to obtain adequate stability. A rule of thumb is to calculate 40% of the narrowest part of the medullar canal to obtain the ideal nail caliber.

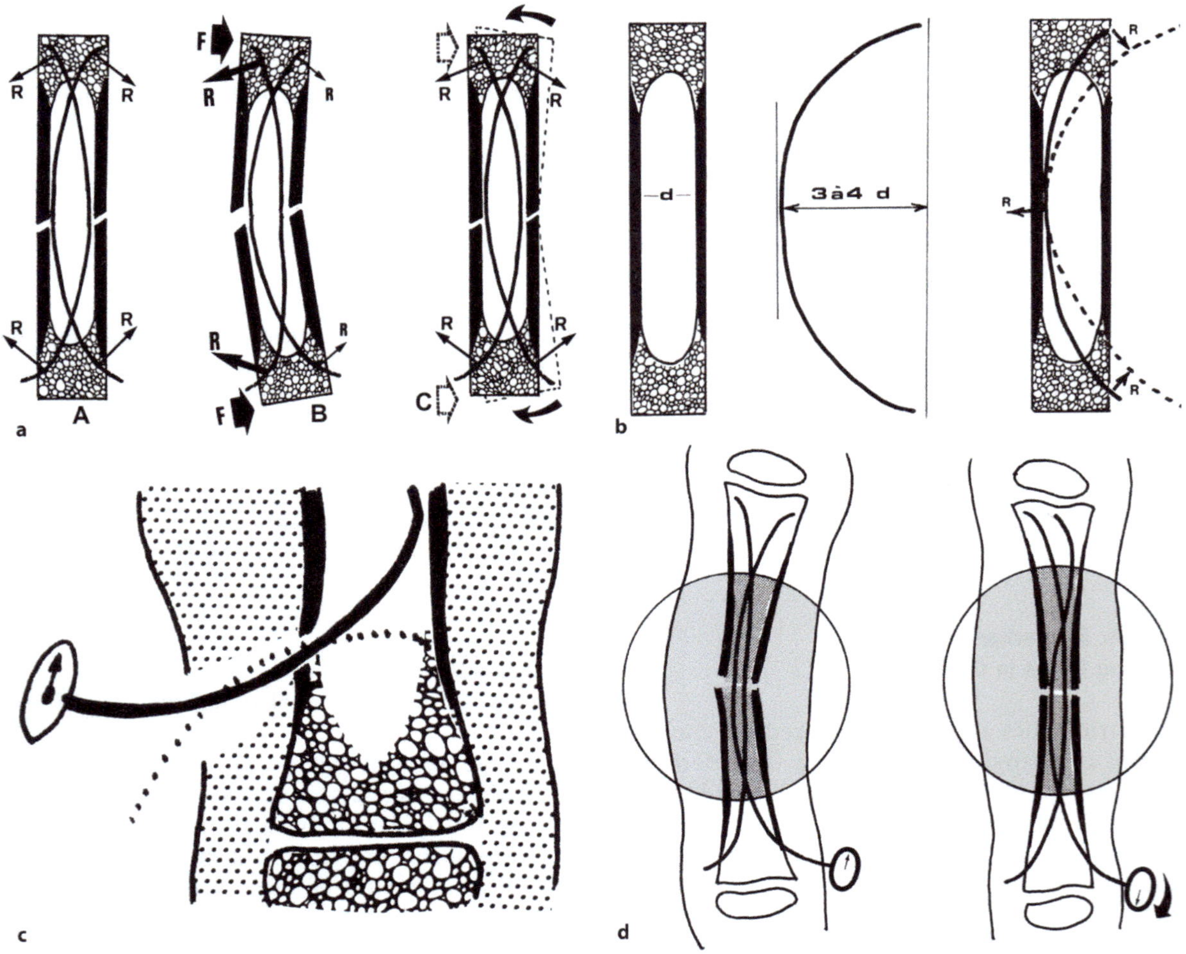

Fig. 5.2.1. Basic principles (courtesy of Dr. J.P. Métaizeau, reproduced with permission). a Double secant arc construct. The elasticity of the nails controls stability under bending loads. b The contoured nail should have a curvature with a radius four times larger than the diameter of the medullar canal. c Introduction of the nail into the metaphysis. The bent tip and the nail curvature avoid penetration into the opposite cortex. d Use of the nail curvature to improve the fracture reduction, by rotation of 180° of the concave nail

The nails are manufactured straight and before introduction, it is necessary to contour them and to angulate their tip over a length of 3–10 mm, depending on the canal diameter. The contoured nail will have the shape of a circle arc, the height or radius of which should be three or four times larger than the canal diameter, in order to allow the elastic recoil effect necessary for fracture stability (Fig. 5.2.1 b). The angulated tip and the curved shape of the nail will facilitate its introduction into the canal, by preventing a conflict with the opposite cortex of the bone.

Nailing Technique

Elastic stable intramedullary nailing is a closed procedure, therefore reduction maneuvers should be tested and practiced before nailing is started. Femur fractures are usually installed on a traction table, whereas all the other locations are reduced with manual traction and external manipulations. It is recommended to determine the nail entry point under image intensifier in order to make sure it stays a reasonable distance from the growth plate, at least 2 cm, to avoid the perichondral ring. The skin incision has a length of 1 or 2 cm, with a more distal extension than the bone entry point, to respect the oblique tract of the nail. The soft tissues are divided with scissors, as directly as possible to the bone level, always in an oblique direction. The entry point is prepared with a sharp pointer, again under image control, and then the curved nail is introduced into the metaphysis, with the tip oriented perpendicularly to the axis of the bone. After introduction, the nail is rotated 180° to orient the tip away from the opposite cortex of the bone (Fig. 5.2.1 c). Progression of the nail into the canal is achieved manually, by pushing on and gently rotating the nail holder. The convexity of the nail is applied to the opposite cortex, and it is sometimes necessary to increase the curvature of the nail to favor its progression. Crossing of the fracture site is made under image control. Rotation of the nail will help the angulated tip to penetrate the medullar canal across the fracture site. External reduction maneuvers may be required at this time, to facilitate crossing the fracture. The nail is then pushed forward until its tip reaches the opposite metaphysis. A second nail is then introduced in a symmetric manner, from the opposite metaphysis. After fracture crossing, the nail is rotated to obtain an opposite orientation compared to the first nail. The ideal fracture stability is obtained when both nails have a close contact with the inner cortices at the fracture site. Finally the two nails are pushed with a hammer in the dense part of the metaphysis, to obtain a stable distal fixation point. If at the end of the procedure the alignment of the fracture is not totally satisfactory, the curvature of the nail can be used to improve the reduction, by rotating one of the nails under image control (Fig. 5.2.1 d).

Trimming of Nail Extremities

Before closing the wounds, the extremities of the nails must be cut at adequate length, not too short in order to facilitate hardware removal, not too long to avoid skin irritation. The ideal length is different from one location to another, depending on the thickness of the soft tissues around the nail. Bending of the implant tip before cutting it is advocated by most authors, since it favors nail stability. However, the other option of leaving it straight may also have advantages, especially by avoiding skin problems.

Postoperative Care

In most cases, no additional immobilization is required. The only exception would be an unstable comminuted femur fracture, especially in adolescents, which could need skin traction for 2 or 3 weeks, in order to avoid fracture telescoping.

Adjacent joint motion is rapidly permitted, after postoperative pain relief. At the lower limb, weight-bearing is usually allowed after 2 or 3 weeks if the fracture has a spontaneous stability, like in transverse cases, and if muscle strength has recovered. For spiral or comminuted fractures, full weight-bearing may need to be delayed until bone healing.

Specific Aspects According to Fracture Location

Femur Fractures

Elastic stable intramedullary nailing can be considered as the standard treatment for all diaphyseal femur fractures in children over 5 years of age, and a recent multicenter study has confirmed that this technique has been accepted in many major trauma centers in Europe and North America [5]. However, particularly in this specific location, the results of this method are dependent on three basic principles: selection of adequate nail diameter, precise contouring of the implant to ob-

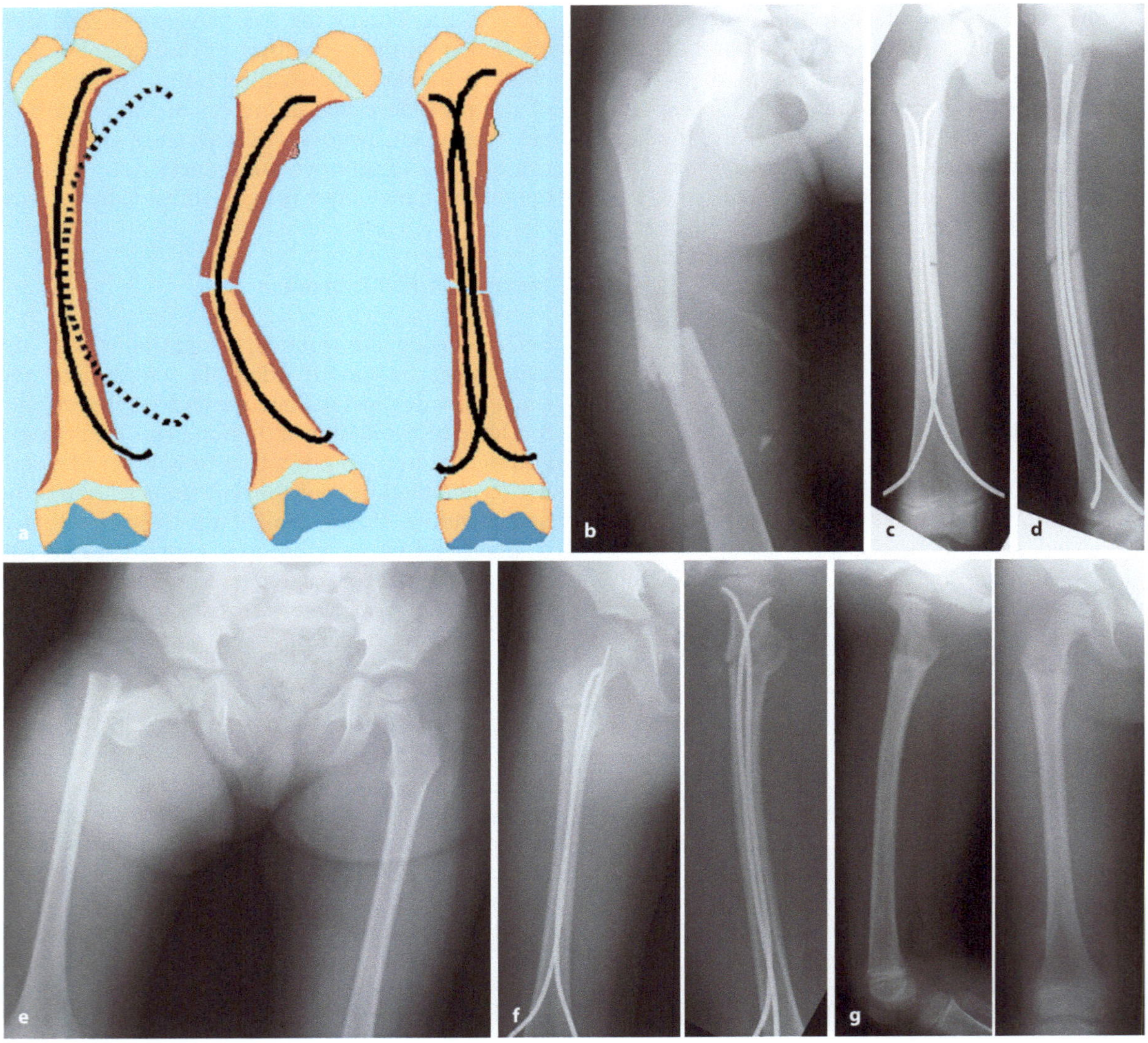

Fig. 5.2.2. Femur fractures. a Concept of femur fracture reduction and stabilization with two elastic nails curved in opposite directions (double secant arc construct) (courtesy of Dr. J.P. Métaizeau, reproduced with permission). b Transverse mid shaft fracture. c ESIN in anteroposterior view. d ESIN in lateral view. e Subtrochanteric fracture (case of Dr. Schnettler). f Anteroposterior and lateral view following ESIN. g Anteroposterior and lateral view after hardware removal

tain a close contact of its convexity with the bone cortex at the fracture site, and strong anchoring in the proximal metaphysis [9]. In most cases, the nailing is performed in a retrograde direction, from the distal metaphysis to the femoral neck (Fig. 5.2.2 a–d). This technique can also be used for proximal fractures, up to the subtrochanteric area (Fig. 5.2.2 e–g). For distal fractures, an antegrade technique may be used, with an introduction point of both nails into the lateral cortex, under the greater trochanter. In this case, one of the nails must be rotated 180° after introduction, in order to obtain a divergent construct into the distal metaphysis, or epiphysis if the growth plate has to be crossed to obtain sufficient stability.

The still unsolved problem is the unstable femur fracture in heavy adolescents, for which ESIN yields often poor results. In such cases, the use of rigid nails has been advocated [1], with a potential risk for avascular necrosis of the femoral head [3], especially if the entry point of the nail is too close to the piriformis fossa, instead of being located at the tip of the greater trochanter.

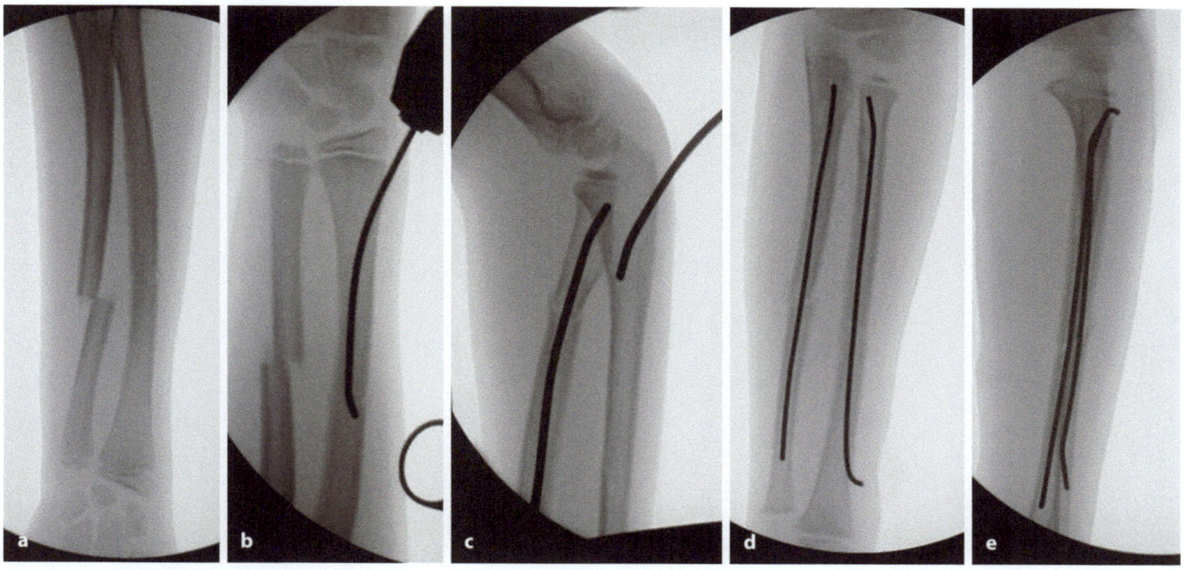

Fig. 5.2.3. Forearm fractures. a Transverse mid shaft fracture. b Introduction of the radius nail. c Introduction of the ulna nail. d Postoperative anteroposterior view. e Postoperative lateral view

Forearm Fractures

A large number of pediatric forearm fractures can be treated with closed reduction and cast immobilization. However, in older children and adolescents, the remodeling process is less efficient, and almost anatomical reduction is required to avoid functional problems. Therefore, unstable forearm fractures in this age group are best treated with ESIN [4, 7]. The stabilization concept is original in this location: each forearm bone receives only one nail, because of the small diameter of the medullar canal. Despite this particularity, the fixation obtained by ESIN can be considered stable, since radius and ulna are closely connected by ligaments and by the interosseous membrane, so that nailing of both bone segments restores the stability of the forearm frame, together with soft tissue connecting structures.

Nailing of the radius is always ascending (retrograde), with an entry point located at the lateral part of the distal metaphysis, 1 cm above the growth plate (Fig. 5.2.3 a, b). Care must be taken not to injure the sensory branch of the radial nerve. Nail diameter is usually between 2.0 and 2.5 mm, depending on the age of the child, and the implant must be bent in order to restore the pronating curvature of the radius. The nailing is best performed closed, but in about 10% of the cases, a "mini open" reduction is required, because of soft tissue interposition. Nailing of the ulna is most often performed in an anterograde descending direction (Fig. 5.2.3 c–e). The entry point is located either at the tip of the olecranon, or at its lateral border to avoid the proximal growth plate. The nail diameter is usually the same as for the radius, and the implant is left straight, as is the ulna. No additional cast is required and early motion is encouraged.

Tibia Fractures

A vast majority of tibia fractures continue to be treated conservatively in children, and ESIN is only selected for unstable fractures, usually after secondary displacement during cast treatment (Fig. 5.2.4 a). Open fractures can be treated with ESIN, especially Gustilo 1 and 2 types, after thorough debridement and high pressure rinsing. Nailing of type 3 remains controversial, and in most cases external fixation is preferred. Nailing of tibia fractures is most commonly performed in an anterograde direction, with entry points on the lateral and medial aspects of the proximal metaphysis (Fig. 5.2.4 b, c). Principles and technique are similar to those presented for the femur. For proximal fractures, a retrograde technique may be used. In the case of an isolated tibia fracture with intact fibula, there is a high incidence of varus displacement with conservative treatment [15]; therefore ESIN may be used as a primary treatment to avoid this complication. A special construct is recommended, using two parallel nails with their convexity oriented to the medial cortex of the tibia, to control the varus displacement forces.

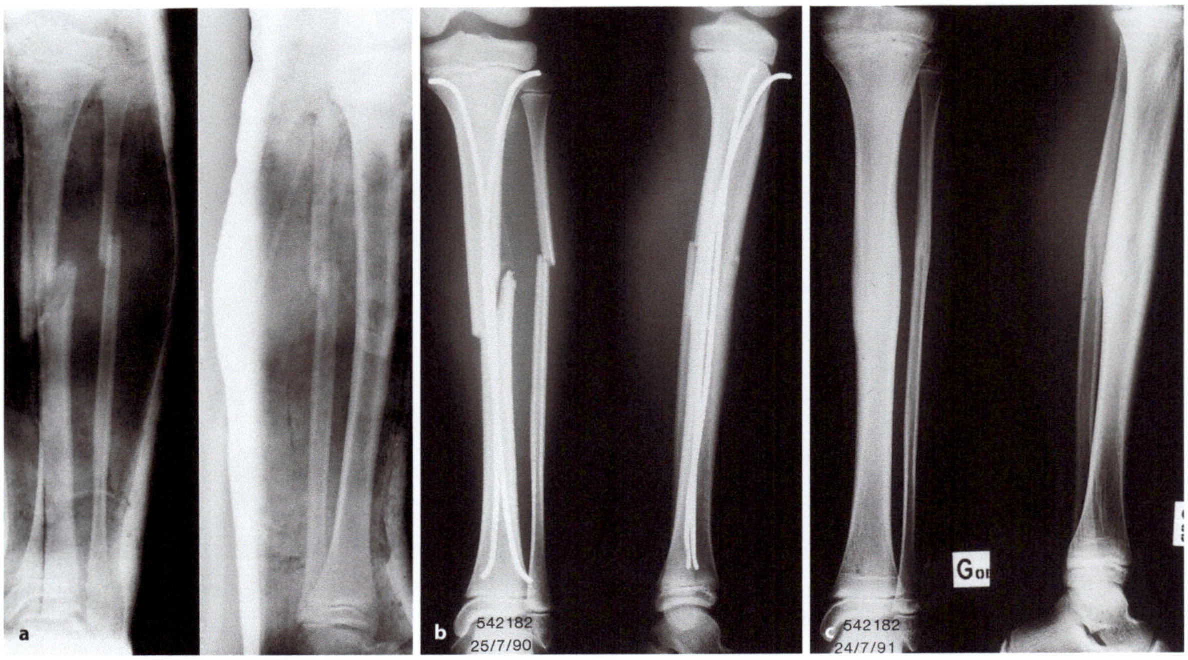

Fig. 5.2.4. Tibia fractures. a Secondary displacement during conservative treatment. b Postoperative anteroposterior and lateral views. c Anteroposterior and lateral views following hardware removal

Humerus Fractures

Again, most of the humerus fractures can be treated conservatively in children. This is particularly true for proximal fractures, which remodel rapidly and have a good tolerance for malunions because of the considerable range of mobility of the shoulder. Relative indications for ESIN are proximal displaced fractures in adolescents, since cast immobilization is not well tolerated and accepted in this age group (Fig. 5.2.5 a–f). Diaphyseal fractures do not remodel so well, therefore ESIN can be indicated in older children. In case of radial nerve palsy, it is usually recommended to verify the position of the nerve, even though entrapment in the fracture gap is rare in this age group. Nailing is generally performed in a retrograde direction, with an entry point for both nails located at the outer cortex of the distal metaphysis, above the lateral epicondyle (Fig. 5.2.5 c). To achieve a better distal anchoring effect, it is recommended to prepare two separate entry points, one for each nail. During nailing, one of the implants must be rotated 180°, in order to obtain a divergent position at the proximal metaphysis level. If the fracture is close to the growth plate, an epiphyseal anchoring may be required.

Other Indications

Radial Head Fractures

For the treatment of radial head fractures, open reduction should absolutely be avoided in children, because of the high risk for avascular necrosis. Therefore, ESIN has brought an interesting way of treating these lesions without opening the fracture site [12]. The technique is similar to other radius fractures, but it is recommended to use a special nail with a sharp upper extremity. This will help to penetrate the epiphyseal fragment, and then to replace it over the metaphysis by rotating the nail about 180° (Fig. 5.2.6 a–c). Sometimes this will not allow the correct tilting of the radial head, which can then be obtained with a percutaneous pointed awl.

Supracondylar Fractures

The inventors of the method have proposed to use ESIN for the treatment of displaced supracondylar fractures [14]. We have no personal experience of this specific indication.

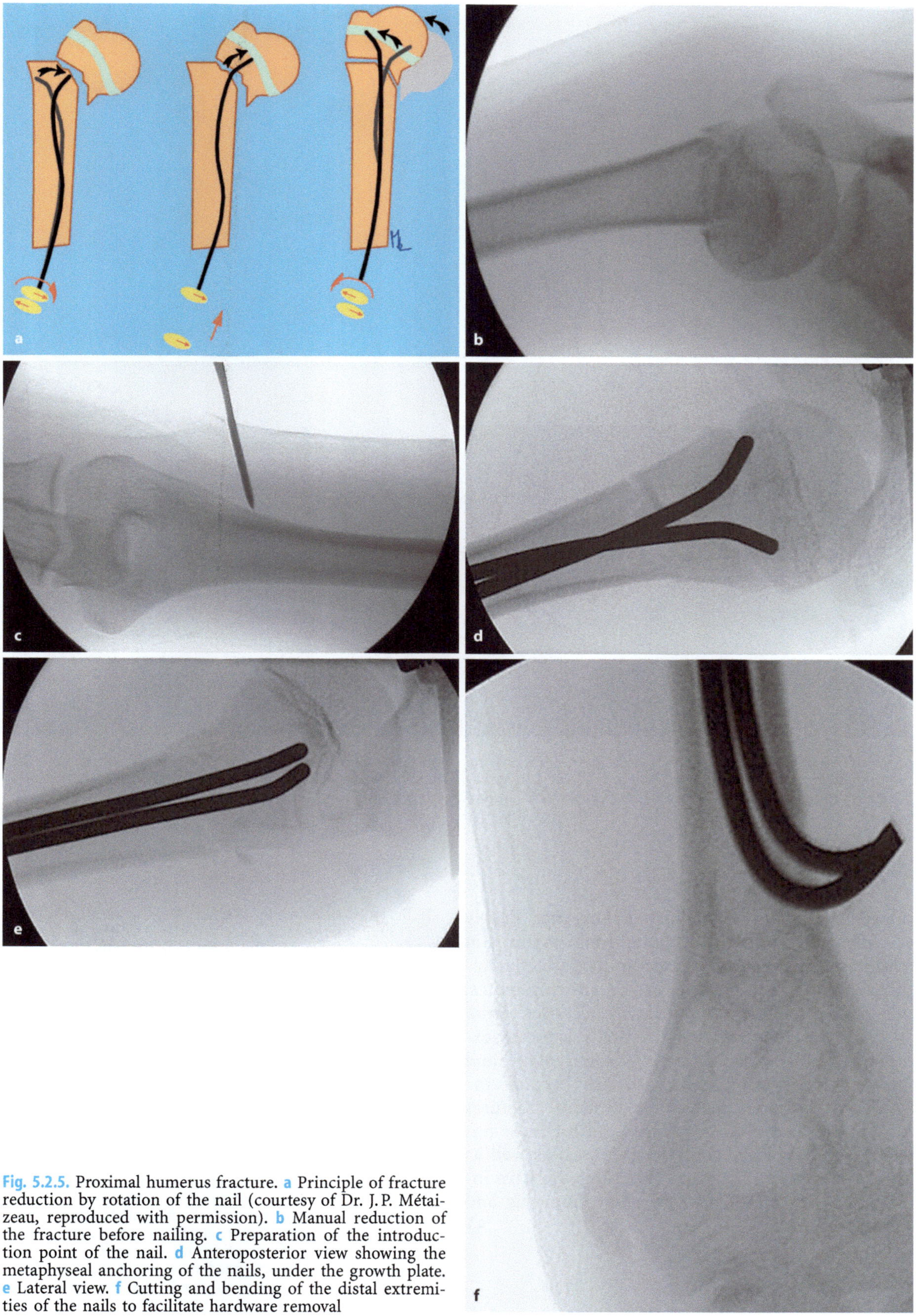

Fig. 5.2.5. Proximal humerus fracture. **a** Principle of fracture reduction by rotation of the nail (courtesy of Dr. J. P. Métaizeau, reproduced with permission). **b** Manual reduction of the fracture before nailing. **c** Preparation of the introduction point of the nail. **d** Anteroposterior view showing the metaphyseal anchoring of the nails, under the growth plate. **e** Lateral view. **f** Cutting and bending of the distal extremities of the nails to facilitate hardware removal

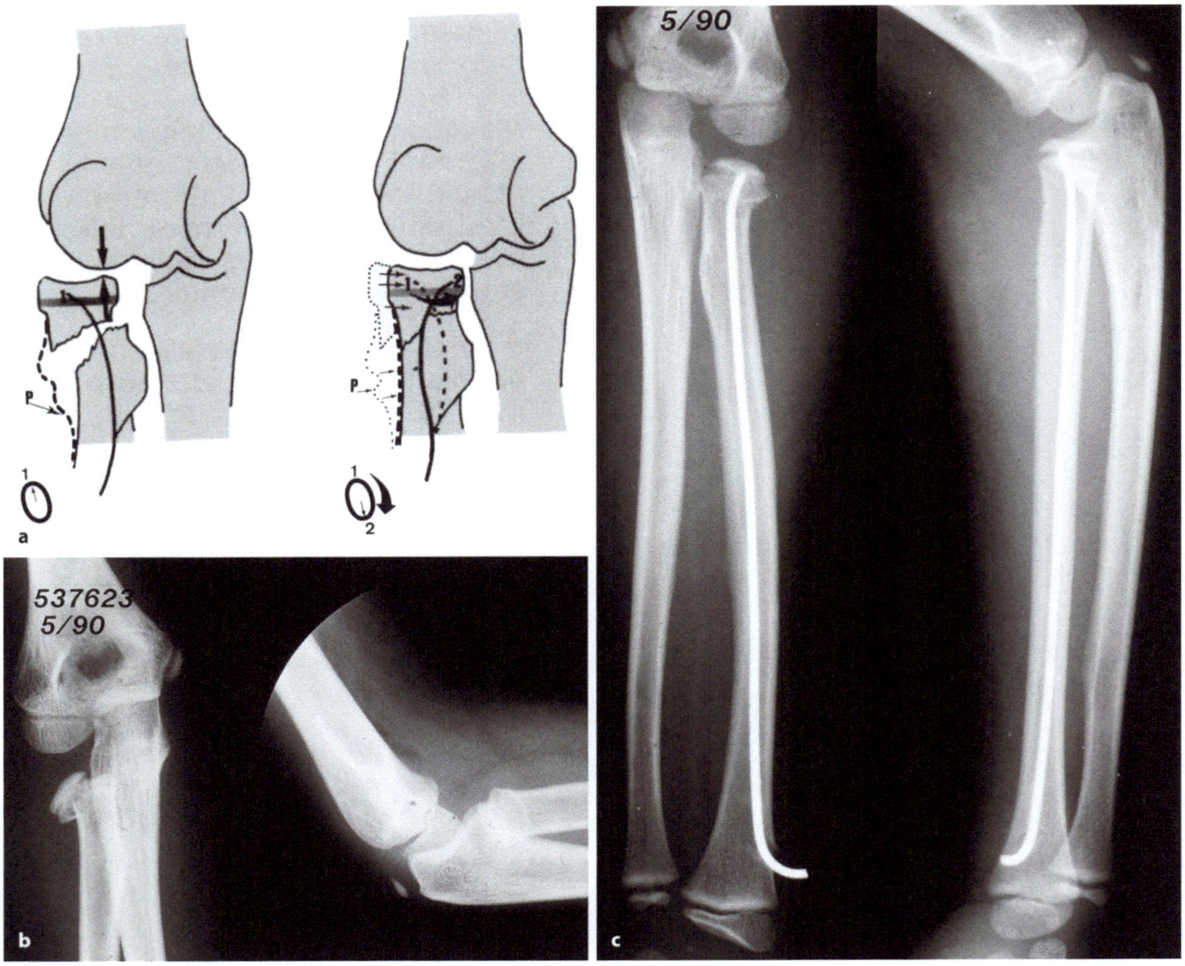

Fig. 5.2.6. Radial head fractures. a Principle of fracture reduction by rotation of the nail (courtesy of Dr. J.P. Métaizeau, reproduced with permission). b Preoperative anteroposterior and lateral views, showing a 60° tilt of the radial head. c Postoperative view, a nail fitted with a sharp tip has been used

Summary

Elastic stable intramedullary nailing has deeply modified the concept of treating limb fractures in children. This method, thanks to its perfect adaptation to the requirements of the growing bones, has gained general acceptance all over the world. It has been demonstrated that ESIN achieves excellent results with shorter hospital stays and quicker functional recovery. It has become the standard treatment method for all femur fractures in children over 5 years of age, and for most unstable and displaced forearm fractures, as well as for all displaced radial head fractures. Relative indications are represented by some humerus and tibia fractures.

References

1. Beaty JH, Austin SM, Warner WC, Canale ST, Nichols L (1994) Interlocking intramedullary nailing of femoral-shaft fractures in adolescents: preliminary results and complications. J Pediatr Orthop 14:178–183
2. Firica A, Popescu R, Scarlet M, et al. (1981) L'ostéosynthèse stable élastique, nouveau concept biomécanique. Etude expérimentale. Rev Chir Orthop 67 Suppl 2:82–91
3. Gordon JE, Swenning TA, Burd TA, Szymanski DA, Schoenecker PL (2003) Proximal femoral radiographic changes after lateral transtrochanteric intramedullary nail placement in children. J Bone Joint Surg 85A:1295–1301
4. Lascombes P, Prevot J, Ligier JN, Metaizeau JP, Poncelet T (1990) Elastic stable intramedullary nailing in forearm shaft fractures in children: 85 cases. J Pediatr Orthop 10:167–171
5. Launay F, Flynn J, Moroz L, Kocher M, Newton P, Frick S, Bollini G, Sponseller P (2004) An international multicenter analysis of complications of elastic stable intramedullary nailing of paediatric femur fractures. 23rd Meeting of the European Paediatric Orthopaedic Society, Geneva, 31 March–3 April 2004

6. Ligier JN (2002) Consolidation des fractures diaphysaires de l'enfant. Treatment orthopédique, osteosynthèses. In: Clavert JM, Karger C, Lascombes P, Ligier JN, Métaizeau JP (eds) Fractures de l'enfant. Monographie du Groupe d'Etude en Orthopédie Pédiatrique. Sauramps Médical, Montpellier, pp 29–32
7. Ligier JN, Metaizeau JP, Lascombes P, Poncelet T, Prevot J (1987) Traitement des fractures diaphysaires des deux os de l'avant-bras de l'enfant par embrochage élastique stable. Rev Chir Orthop 73 Suppl 2:149–151
8. Ligier JN, Metaizeau JP, Prevot J (1983) L'embrochage élastique stable à foyer fermé en traumatologie infantile. Chir Pediatr 24:383–385
9. Ligier JN, Metaizeau JP, Prevot J, Lascombes P (1988) Elastic stable intramedullary nailing of femoral shaft fractures in children. J Bone Joint Surg 70B:74–77
10. McKibbin B (1978) The biology of fracture healing in long bones. J Bone Joint Surg 60B:150–162
11. Metaizeau JP (1988) Ostéosynthèse chez l'enfant. Sauramps, Montpellier
12. Metaizeau JP, Lascombes P, Lemelle JL, Finlayson D, Prevot J (1993) Reduction and fixation of displaced radial neck fractures by closed intramedullary pinning. J Pediatr Orthop 13:355–360
13. Metaizeau JP, Ligier JN (1984) Le traitement chirurgical des fractures des os longs chez l'enfant. J Chir 121:527–537
14. Prevot J, Lascombes P, Metaizeau JP, Blanquart D (1990) Fractures supracondyliennes de l'humérus de l'enfant. Traitement par embrochage descendant. Rev Chir Orthop 76:191–197
15. Yang JPY, Letts RM (1997) Isolated fractures of the tibia with intact fibula in children: a review of 95 patients. J Pediatr Orthop 17:347–351

Section 6 New Technologies: Navigation and Targeting Devices

Basic Principles of Fluoro-Navigation

A. Sarvestani

Introduction

Fluoroscopic navigation systems allow localization of the position of a surgical instrument relative to the anatomy of the patient [1, 2]. By superimposing the instrument's geometry onto fluoroscopic images, the surgeon can follow live the progression of the intervention.

Navigation Technology

The most common navigation technology used is based on infra-red tracking. A camera is used, which is equipped with two infra-red image sensors, where each one produces a two-dimensional image. By synchronizing the two sensors (stereographic principle), the three-dimensional position of a tool can be localized.

Tools to be tracked emit infra-red light, which is detected by the camera. In order to track position and orientation, a tool is equipped with at least three infra-red sources. One distinguishes between active systems and passive systems.

Active systems consist of tools with light-emitting diodes. They actively send infra-red light, which is tracked by the camera. Passive systems consist of tools with infra-red reflecting balls. The camera emits infra-red light, which is reflected by the tool and again tracked by the camera.

The first generation of navigation systems had active tools, which were powered by cables, resulting in handling limitations. Passive tools were introduced with the second generation of navigation systems. They do not need cables but suffer from ambiguity by partially covered or overlapping reflecting objects and visibility problems when the reflecting surfaces are soiled or partially obscured. The latest generation of trackers is based on active and wireless tools, which are battery powered. They combine the advantages of both technologies. In addition, these trackers are equipped with on-board electronics and bidirectional communication with the navigation system, which allows for automatic instrument detection and software remote control.

Principle of Fluoro-Navigation

The basic components of a fluoroscopic navigation system are: infra-red camera, computer with monitor, patient tracker, instrument tracker, and C-arm tracker (Fig. 6.1.1).

Prior to the procedure, a C-arm tracker is attached to the image intensifier (Fig. 6.1.2). Beside tracking the position of the image intensifier, the C-arm tracker also compensates for image distortions and X-ray source shifts due to mechanical flex. Small metal balls are integrated into a plate (phantom), which is positioned in front of the imaging plane. In the acquired images the software detects the position of these balls, compares them with the measured positions and corrects for any image distortions.

During the procedure a patient tracker is rigidly attached to the bone that is going to be treated (Fig. 6.1.3). Different anchoring systems are available based on single or multiple screw fixations (Fig. 6.1.4).

As soon as a fluoroscopic image is taken, it is automatically transferred to the monitor of the navigation system via a standard video signal cable. At the same time, the camera localizes the position of both the image intensifier and the patient tracker. This allows the image reference to be transferred from the image intensifier to the patient tracker. This step is called registration. The uniqueness of fluoroscopic navigation is that registration is done automatically. The C-arm can now be removed from the surgical field without losing the image reference. Usually, two images from two perpendicular views are taken (e.g., anteroposterior and lateral), which allows for a three-dimensional determination of the instrument's position.

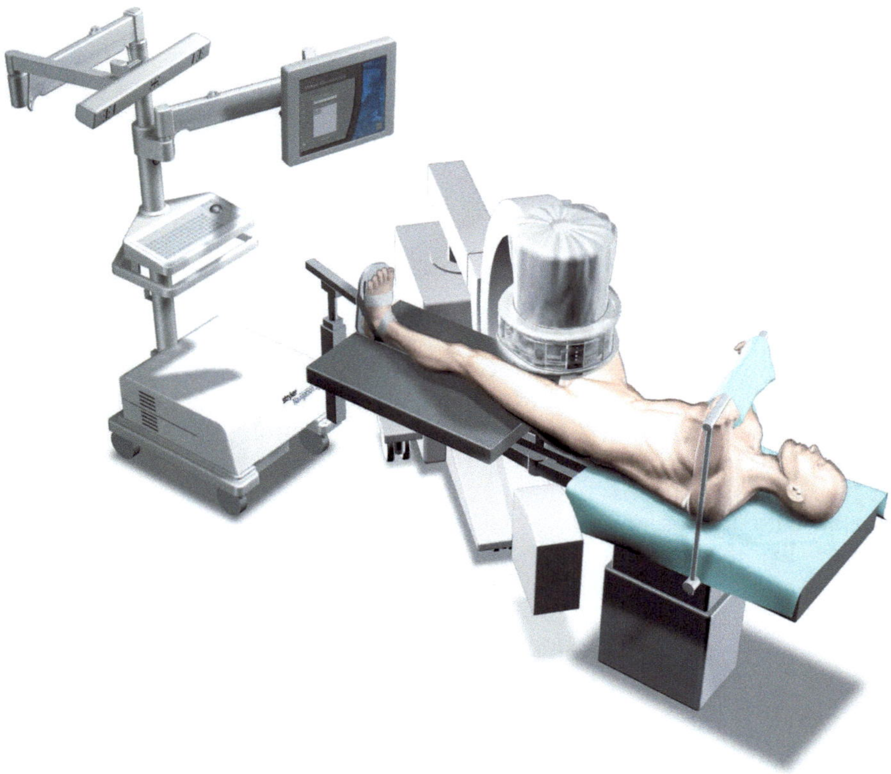

Fig. 6.1.1. Components and setup for a fluoroscopic navigation surgery (infra-red camera, computer with monitor and C-arm tracker)

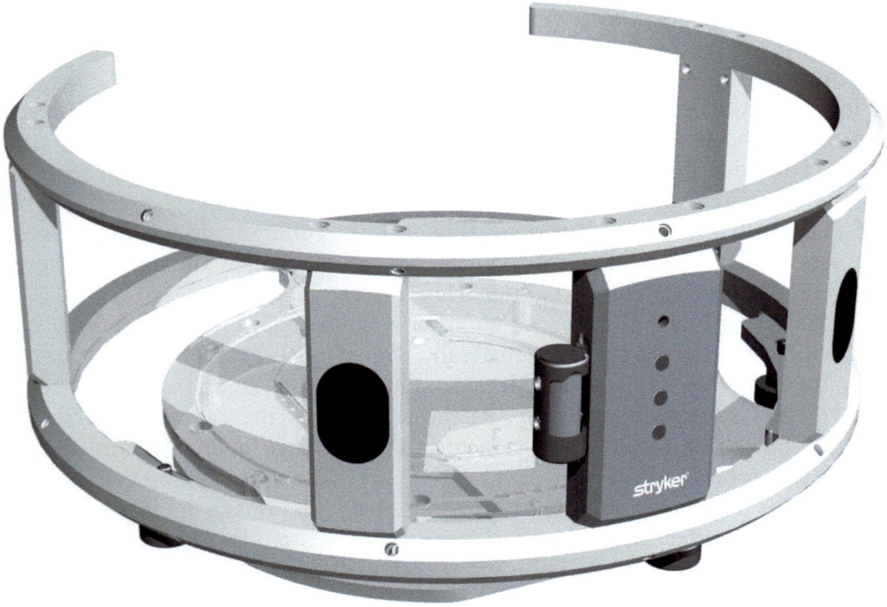

Fig. 6.1.2. Example of a C-arm tracker

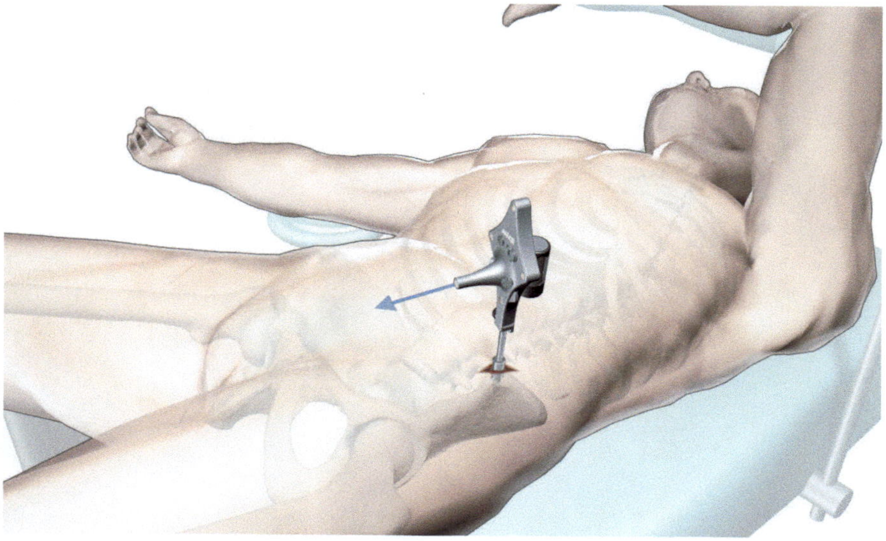

Fig. 6.1.3. Example of a patient tracker attached to the iliac crest

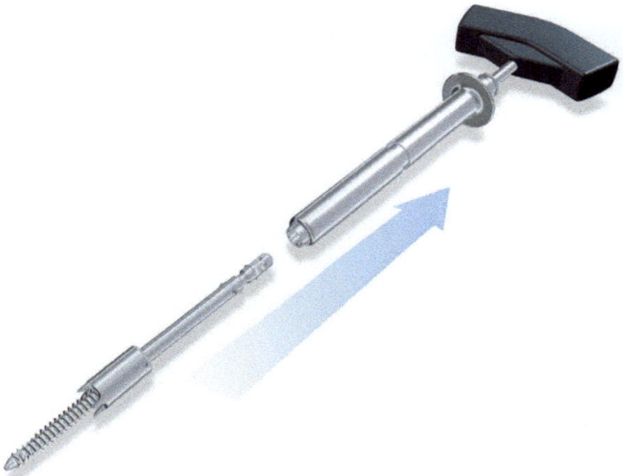

Fig. 6.1.4. Example of an anchoring system based on a rotation safe single screw

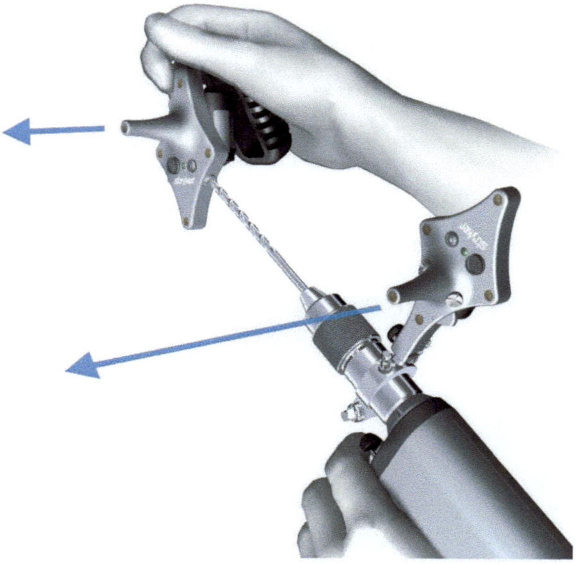

Fig. 6.1.5. Calibration of a navigated power drill

A tracker is attached to the surgical instrument followed by calibration of the assembly (Fig. 6.1.5). Calibration is necessary to determine the instrument's geometry relative to the tracker. The instrument tip is inserted into the calibration device. At the same time the navigation system tracks the position of both devices, determines the position of the instrument tip and stores it either in the instrument itself or in the software. After calibration the position and orientation of the instrument are superimposed simultaneously on all acquired images. The surgical intervention can now be monitored live on the screen (Fig. 6.1.6).

A very important feature of all fluoroscopic navigation systems is the virtual tip elongation. The displayed instrument is extended by a user-defined value. This allows performing on-the-fly planning and measurements.

Fluoroscopic navigation systems also allow tracking and displaying the current position of the image intensifier relative to the acquired images (Fig. 6.1.7). By this the C-arm can be quickly maneuvered to the targeted field of interest without the need for taking extra shots.

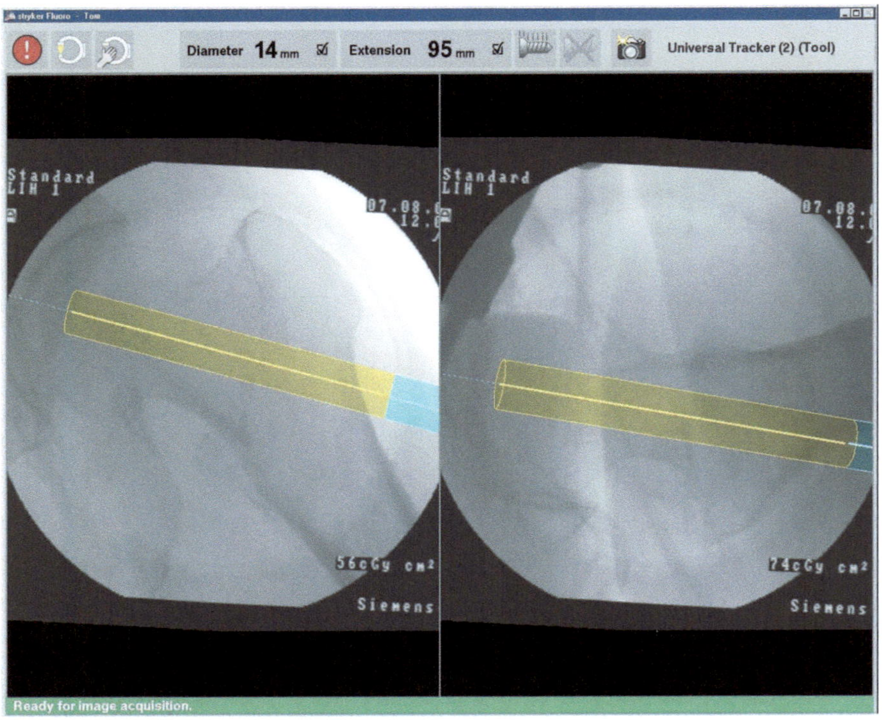

Fig. 6.1.6. Example of hip screw navigation on a frontal and a lateral view. The blue element represents the actual position of the instrument while the yellow element represents the virtual tip extension

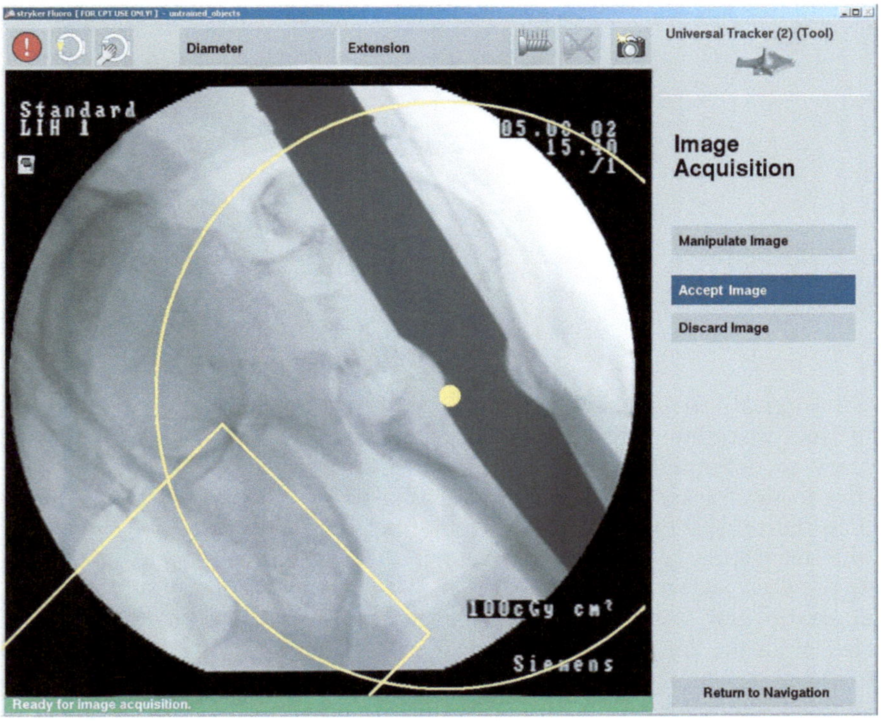

Fig. 6.1.7. C-arm guidance: the yellow circle represents the actual position of the image intensifier

Future Challenges

One of the main challenges of fluoroscopic navigation is to reduce the invasiveness of bone anchoring devices and the time to prepare and attach them.

To bring current fluoroscopic navigation systems to the next level, dedicated application workflows are needed, which guide the surgeon step by step through the application.

Current navigation systems focus on instrument navigation only. The ability also to navigate bone fragments will close an important gap in trauma surgery. In addition implant databases are needed optimally to select and position implants.

Smart instruments will eliminate the need for instrument calibration and will reduce user interaction with the navigation software. Those instruments will contain integrated RF-ID tags, which store information about their geometry and functionality. The moment the surgeon starts using a navigated instrument, the software automatically progresses to the corresponding screen and the instrument's geometry is loaded.

Recently, new navigation systems have been developed to be coupled to three-dimensional C-arms to fully explore the advantages of intraoperative three-dimensional imaging.

All future development must improve the integration of navigation into the operating room environment to achieve a quick setup, an intuitive usage and a high robustness.

References

1. Hofstetter R, Slomczykowski M, Sati M, Nolte LP (1999) Fluoroscopy as an imaging means for computer-assisted surgical navigation. Computer Aided Surgery 4:65–76
2. Suhm N, Jacob AL, Nolte LP, Regazzoni P, Messmer P (2000) Surgical navigation based on fluoroscopy – clinical application for computer-assisted distal locking of intramedullary implants. Computer Aided Surgery 5: 391–400

New Technology: Image-Guided Navigation in Orthopaedic Trauma Surgeries

K.-S. Leung

Introduction

The fluoroscope is very common piece of equipment in the operating theatre and is very familiar to most trauma surgeons. Fluoroscopic control is commonly employed in orthopaedic trauma surgery. By providing two-dimensional images, it helps the surgeon to locate the fracture fragments, the patient's anatomy, the implants and the instruments during operation. During the operative treatment of fractures, fluoroscopic control is essential for the closed reduction of fractures and many of the minimally invasive procedures of modern orthopaedic trauma surgery. However, the disadvantages of its use are many. These include the radiation exposure to all personnel, including the patient, in the operating room, the images provided are of quality nature only and non-interactive, most machines can only provide real-time images in one plane and maximally two planes, frequent repositioning of the C-arm is needed during surgery and it has always to be in the operation field.

Computer-aided orthopaedic surgery (CAOS) has been applied to many different types of orthopaedic surgery in recent years [5]. In orthopaedic trauma, due to the diversities of fracture patterns, which continue to change until the patient is anaesthetised and the fractures are reduced and stabilised on the operating table, it is therefore essential to have the fluoroscopic image-based system to achieve accurate automatic registration of the fluoroscopic images, which can be used to navigate the surgical instruments, the C-arm as well as the bone fragments during surgery. Furthermore, the C-arm is a very common piece of equipment in almost all operating rooms and familiar to most orthopaedic surgeons; fluoroscopic images are also readily interpreted by orthopaedic surgeons. Combining fluoroscopy and the navigation system will not impose additional major difficulty during surgery.

While navigating the real-time fluoroscopic images taken intraoperatively, fluoro-navigation will thus help to minimise exposure to X-rays for surgeons, operating room personnel and patients, provide multiplanar views for monitoring and accurate positioning of implants, provide real-time interactive quantitative data of the images, expand the application of minimally invasive surgery and remove the C-arm from the operation field.

Operation Principles

With the spatial co-ordinates of a standard X-ray fluoroscope and the skeleton, on which the surgical procedures are going to be carried out, registered into the system, X-ray fluoroscopic images obtained intraoperatively are transferred to the navigation system with automatic scale and distortion corrections. The graphical user interphase then allows the surgeon to navigate with stereotactic tools on the registered biplanar, tri-planar and multi-planar images. As these images are almost the same as those obtained from the standard C-arm, the interpretation of the anatomical features for navigation is simple and straightforward for most surgeons. Surgical procedures can thus be carried out with the virtual fluoroscope (Fig. 6.2.1).

Technical Notes

The fluoroscopy-based navigation system allows the tracking of a surgical instrument and the superimposing of its contour onto fluoroscopy images [2]. This enables the surgeon to know precisely the position of the surgical instrument at any time of the procedure without the need to take additional X-ray shots. When an image is taken it is automatically transferred to the navigation system and the position of the image intensifier of the C-arm is localized. Distortion of the fluoro-images is common and is caused by the flexibility of the C-arm, the magnetic field of the earth as well as the interference of the other

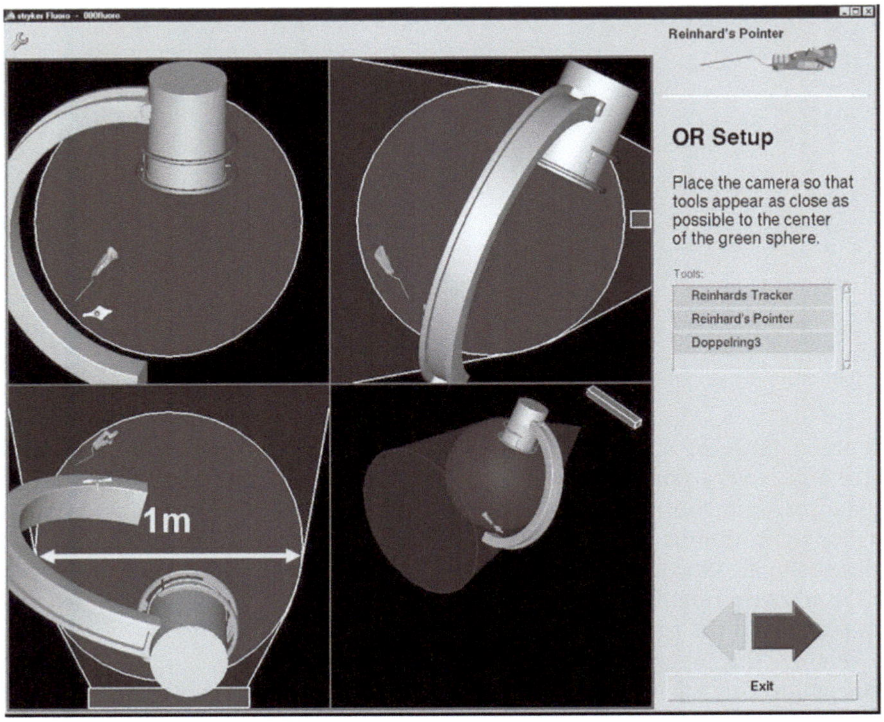

Fig. 6.2.1. Virtual fluoroscopy on the computer monitor

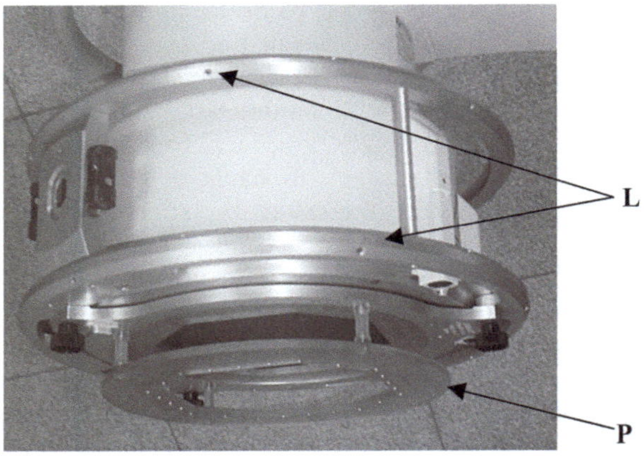

Fig. 6.2.2. Phantom attached on the C-arm tracker to correct image distortion (*P*). The C-arm tracker is located with the light-emitting diodes (*L*)

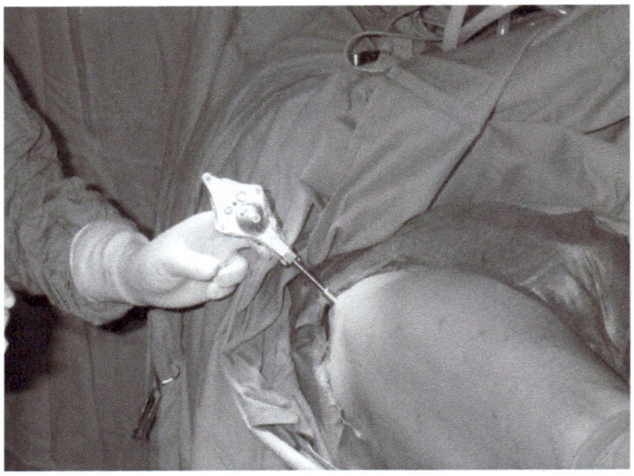

Fig. 6.2.3. A patient tracker is attached to the anterior iliac crest where the image is referred for navigation

equipment in the operating room. The distortion is thus corrected by the use of the metal markers attached to the C-arm (commonly known as the phantom) (Fig. 6.2.2). With the distortion corrected, the image is referenced to the patient's bone, which is localized by a further tracker (Fig. 6.2.3). This allows the removal of the C-arm from the operation field while keeping the registration of the image and visualizing the actual position of the surgical instrument.

For tracking a tool, two basic technologies are available: infra-red based and electromagnetic based. Infra-red technology is very robust and boasts a high localization accuracy, but with problems of line of sight. Line-of-sight problems are not present in the case of electromagnetic systems, which also have distortion problems affecting the accuracy. A new generation of multiple camera-based navigation systems using infra-red technologies will combine the advantages of both technologies.

The first generation of tracking devices was characterized by cable-based active trackers. The second-generation trackers were based on passive infra-red reflecting objects, which had the problem of limited number of tractable objects and visibility when the reflecting surfaces were not clean. The third generation of trackers is based on wireless battery-powered active technology and overcomes the limitations of the first two generations. In addition, these trackers are equipped with on-board electronics communicating with the navigation system, which allows automatic instrument detection and software remote control.

Operating Procedures

The first step of the operation is to set up the system. The patient tracker is anchored to the part of the bone that is going to be operated, and is activated (Fig. 6.2.3). The C-arm tracker is also activated and the position of the devices is orientated to the optimal position for operation (Fig. 6.2.4). In some systems, the accuracy and reliability of the system is validated by either mapping the image of the tracker or confirmed by the position of the tool tracker and the patient tracker.

The calibration of the surgical tool is thus carried out by attaching a tool tracker on the instrument that the surgeon is going to use. The calibration can either be done by tip calibration, which means that only the tip of the instrument (Fig. 6.2.5) will be monitored or by tip and axis calibration, where both the tip and the axis are monitored during navigation (Fig. 6.2.6). The calibration can be a factory default one, or can be done during surgery with a calibration station (Fig. 6.2.7). The latter provides versatility for the application of different surgical instruments. However, for the calibration of axis of the tool, the instrument has to be straight, while for tip calibration, the tool can be of any geometry. With a specifically designed axis adaptor for common instruments in orthopaedic trauma, e.g., screw driver, awl, power drill, the calibration will be much easier with a hand-held calibration device where both the axis and the tip calibration can be done (Fig. 6.2.8). This facilitates surgery and minimises the duration of the procedure.

The next step is to acquire the fluoroscopic image for navigation. With the C-arm positioned (Fig. 6.2.9) to take the images of the skeleton where surgery will carried out, the image taken will be automatically transferred to the system with distortion correction. The images can thus be stored or assigned to different layouts for navigation (Fig. 6.2.10).

In the navigation, the position of the instrument is depicted by the numeric data on the monitor. The virtual tip and the axis thus enable the measurement of the paths (Fig. 6.2.11). This helps to plan the screws that are going to be in-

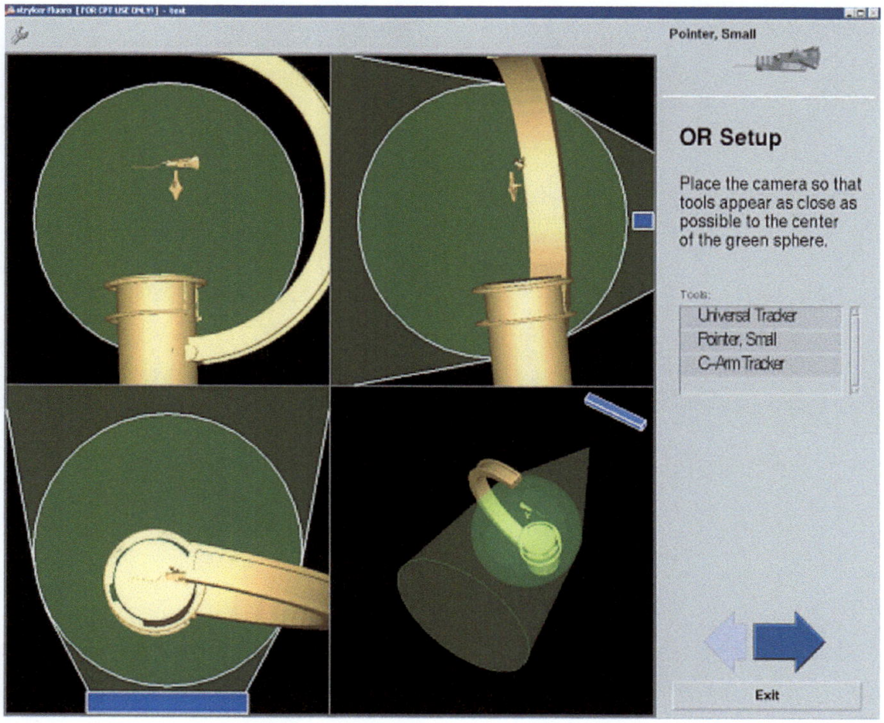

Fig. 6.2.4. C-arm tracker is activated

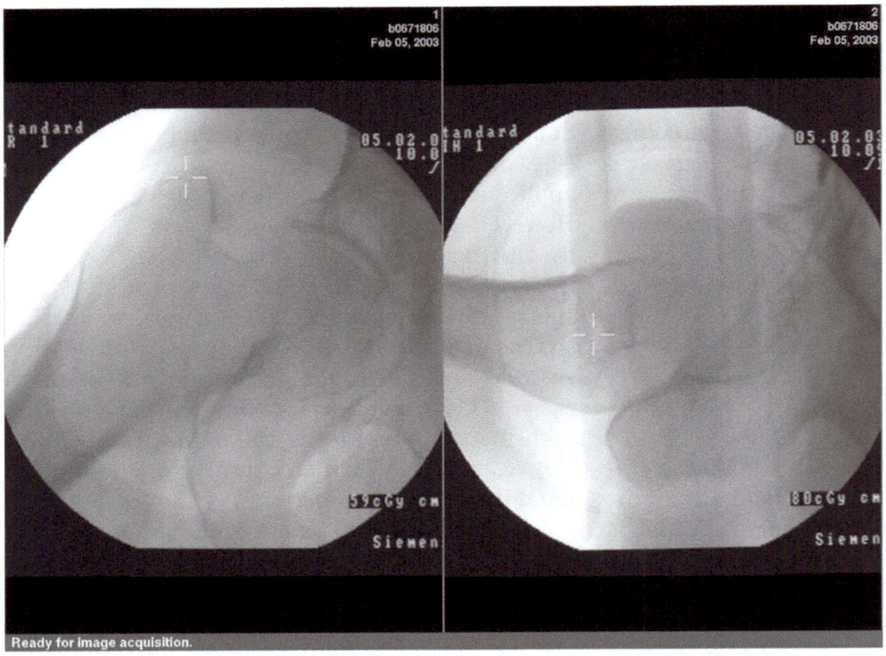

Fig. 6.2.5. Point calibrated instrument is monitored during navigation

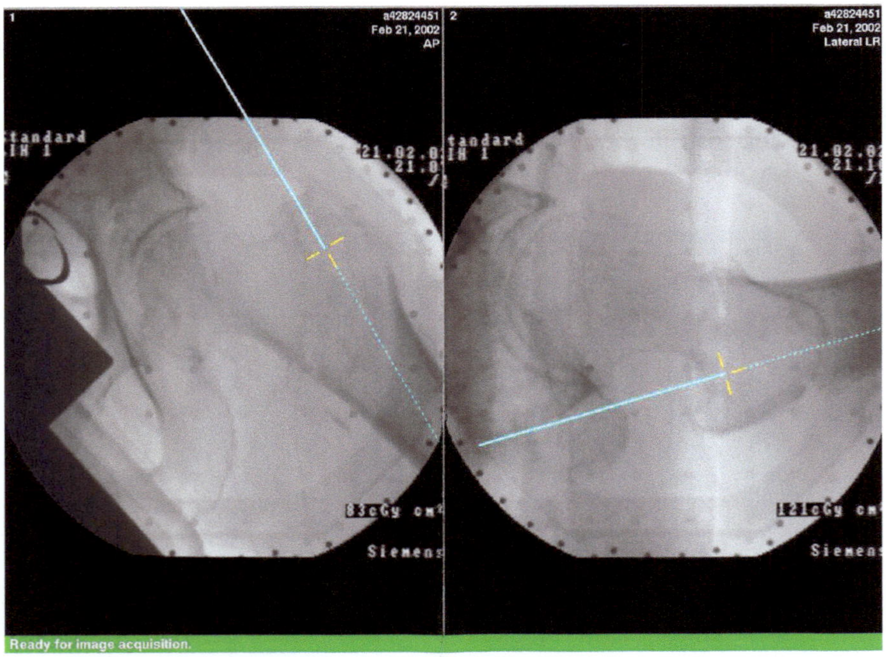

Fig. 6.2.6. The axis and the tip can be monitored if the instrument is calibrated with axis and tip

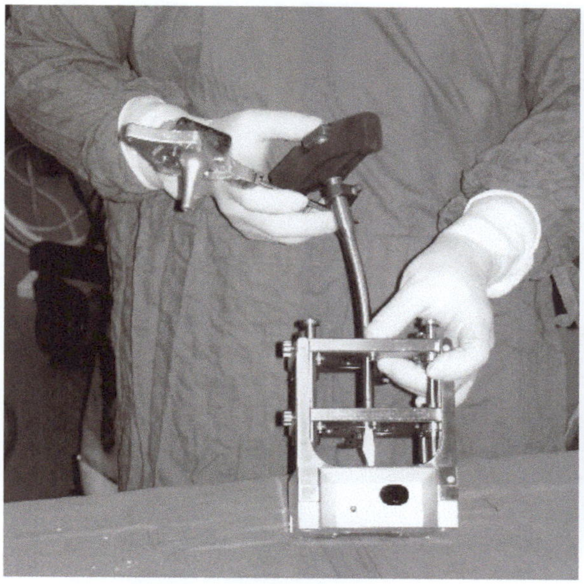

Fig. 6.2.7. A curved awl with the tool tracker attached is being calibrated in the calibration station

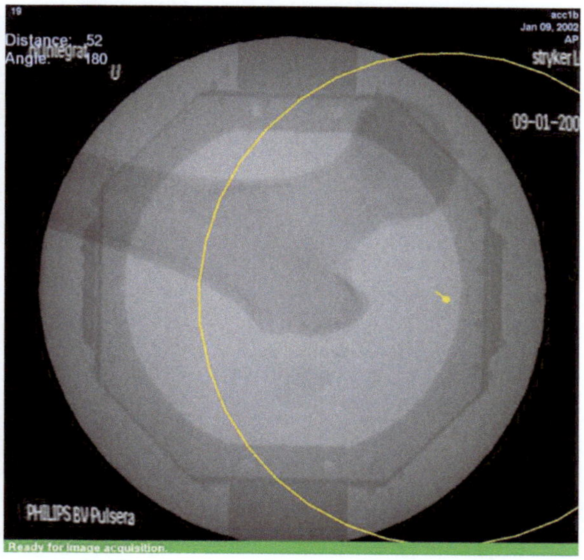

Fig. 6.2.9. Positioning of the C-arm to take images. The *yellow dot* indicates the centre of the C-arm beam

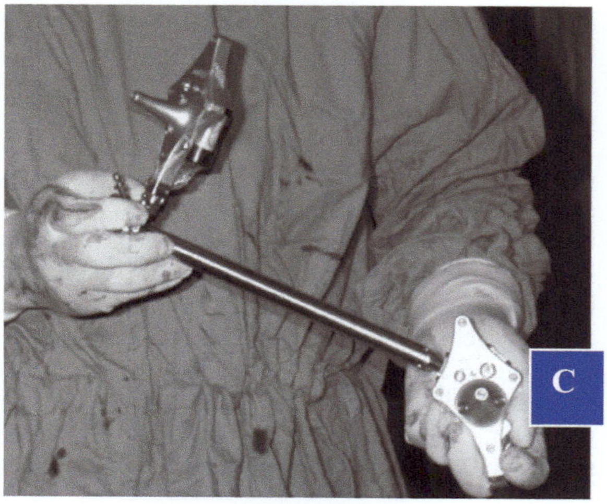

Fig. 6.2.8. A hand-held calibration device (*C*) for calibrating an instrument

serted with the diameter and the length shown on the monitor and superimposed on the images of the bone. The C-arm guidance mode helps to visualise the position of the C-arm in case further images are needed for navigation and thus decreases the number of shots for positioning (Fig. 6.2.12). More intervention can be carried out by modification of the procedures and instruments.

The Applications

Fluoro-navigation is particularly important for orthopaedic trauma as the fracture fragments are mobile and the orientations are not fixed before surgery. It is only possible to navigate the images obtained during the operation after fracture reduction or manipulation is completed [3].

With the fluoro-navigation system, many procedures that require intraoperative fluoroscopic control can now be done without continuous monitoring with the fluoroscope. These procedures include the following.

Fixation of Femoral Neck Fractures with Percutaneous Cannulated Screws (Fig. 6.2.13)

With the fracture closely reduced and stabilised with traction on a traction table, both the frontal and lateral images of the proximal femur are taken and registered in the system. The insertion of screw guide wires can be navigated with the patient tracker anchored on the anterior iliac crest and the power drill as the navigated tool. Two or three screws can thus be planned and inserted with a small incision (Fig. 6.2.14).

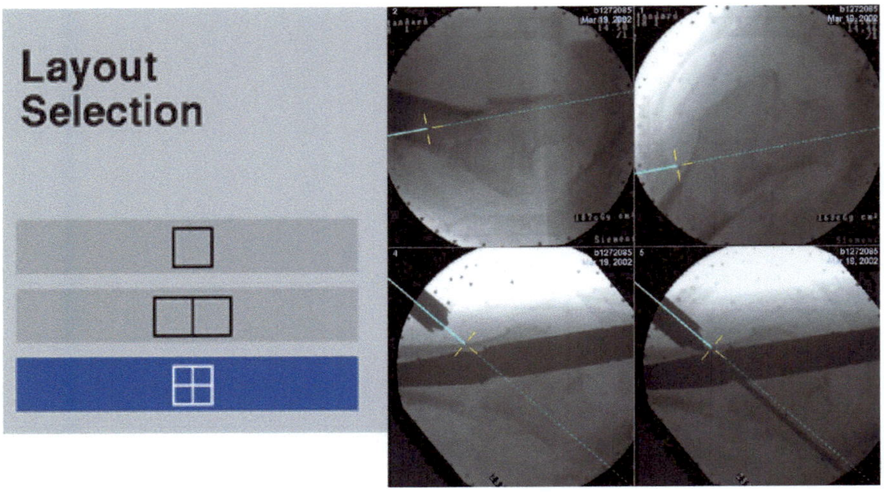

Fig. 6.2.10. Different layouts of the images for navigation

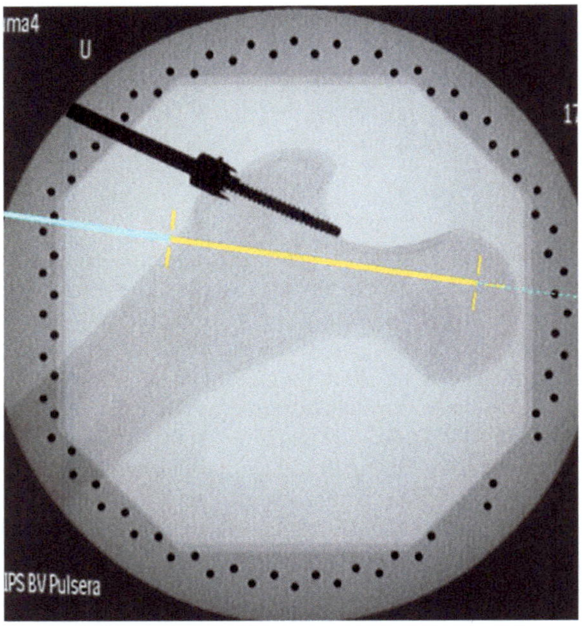

Fig. 6.2.11. Position of the instrument can be shown by the tip and its axis

Intramedullary Locked Nails for Long Bone Fractures

Entry to the medullary canal can be navigated with the proximal femoral frontal and lateral images. The awl is the navigated tool and the patient tracker can be inserted onto the anterior iliac crest when a traction table is used or onto the lateral part of the greater trochanter when a traction table is not used in the nailing procedure.

Insertion of distal locking screws (Fig. 6.2.15) is the commonest procedure applied in the navigation during intramedullary nailing [9, 10]. With the current technology [12], the distal locking screw insertion still requires perfect frontal and lateral fluoroscopic images. With the patient tracker anchored to the proximal nail holding device (Fig. 6.2.16), the power drill with the corresponding drill bit can be calibrated and thus navigated for screw insertion without further fluoroscopic control. Both the length and the diameter

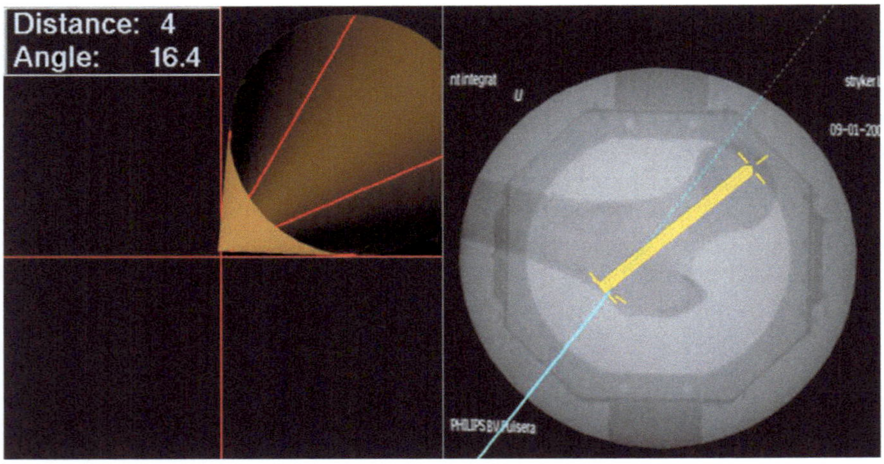

Fig. 6.2.12. Planning of the implants before insertion

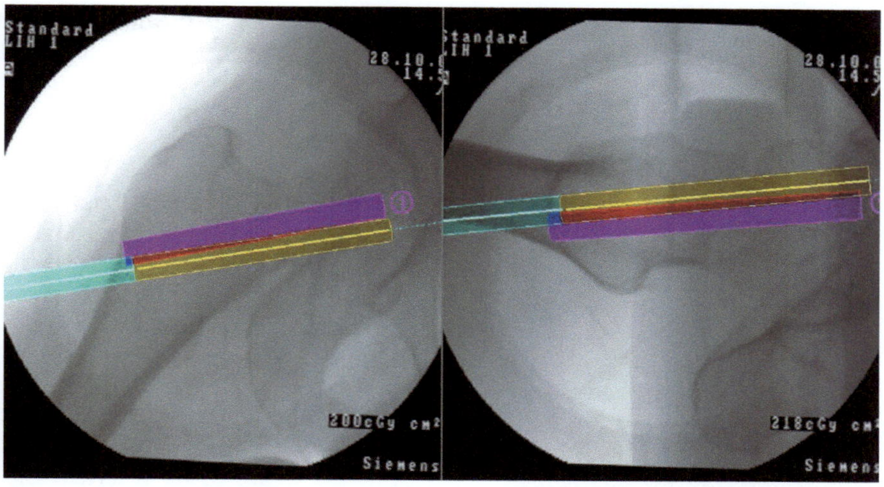

Fig. 6.2.13. Percutaneous cannulated screws fixation of femoral neck fracture under navigation

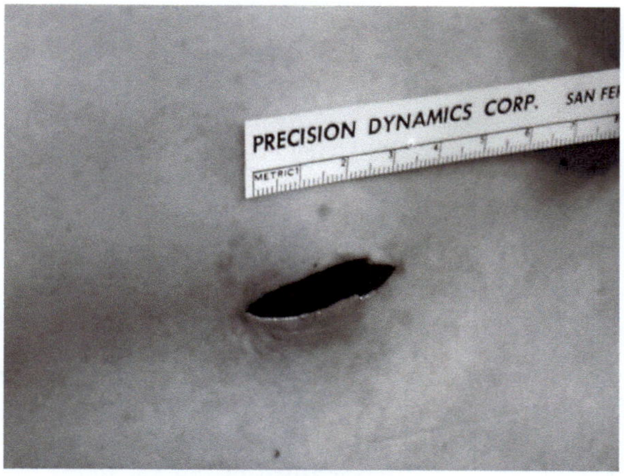

Fig. 6.2.14. Surgical incision for percutaneous screw fixation of femoral neck fracture

of the screws to be inserted can thus be planned. The insertion of the drill bit can thus be navigated (Fig. 6.2.17).

Intramedullary Fixation of Trochanteric Fractures (Gamma Nails) [7] (Fig. 6.2.18)

Entry to the medullary canal is similar to that in the intramedullary nails. Lag screw position and planning are perhaps the best illustrations of the advantages of fluoro-navigation. With the same set of images of the proximal femur (provided there is minimal movement of the fracture fragment after femoral component insertion), the position of the lag screw can be planed on both the frontal and sagittal planes simultaneously without the need of further fluoroscopic control. After insertion of the guide wire with navigation assis-

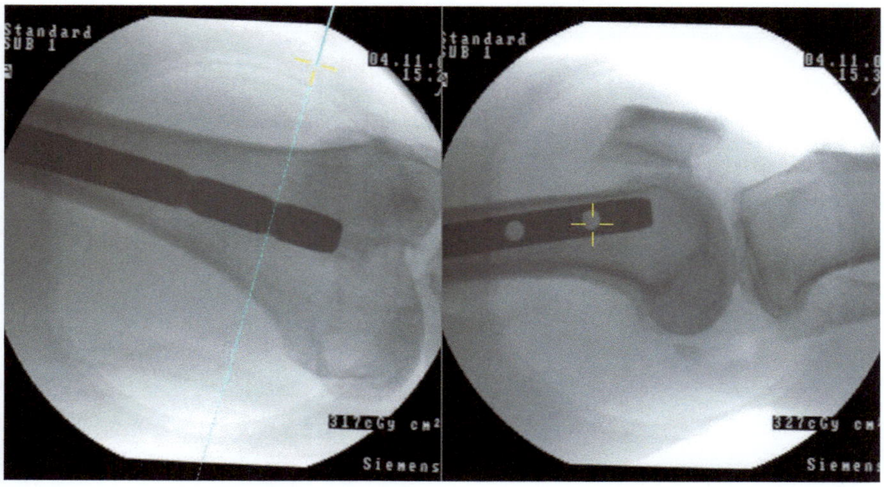

Fig. 6.2.15. Distal locking in intramedullary locked nail with the fluoro-navigation

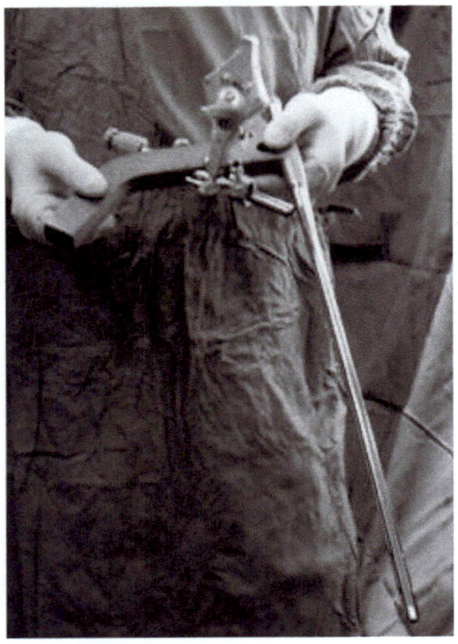

Fig. 6.2.16. Patient tracker is attached to the proximal nail-holding jig to ensure accurate navigation of the distal locked screws

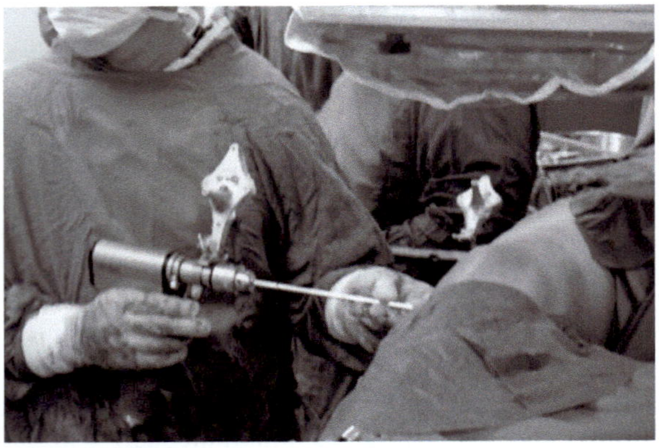

Fig. 6.2.17. Navigation of a power drill for distal locking

tance, the lag screw can thus be inserted accurately. In addition, distal locking screws can be inserted, similar to those in the intramedullary locked nails.

Percutaneous Fixation of Sacro-iliac Fracture Dislocations (Fig. 6.2.19)

This is indicated in unstable fracture dislocation of the sacro-iliac joints where the stability can be restored by trans-iliac sacral screw fixation [1, 11]. With fluoro-navigation, the insertion of the screws can be done with a small incision. As the first sacral body is the bone in which the screws are to be inserted, the patient tracker should be inserted onto the anterior iliac crest of the uninjured side. If an anterior external fixator is inserted during the resuscitation phase, the patient tracker can also be anchored onto the frame. At least three images of the sacro-iliac complex are required for proper navigation: inlet view, outlet view and the sagittal view of the sacrum. Either the drill sleeve or the power drill can be the tool that is to be navigated. We recommend navigation of the drill sleeve as it provides a more rigid position and accurate trajectory for the guide wire insertion. With the images registered in the system, the entry point of the guide can be monitored on the sagittal image of the sacrum. The trajectory of the screws can thus be planned with the inlet and outlet views so that the first screw is to be inserted into the anterior third of the S-1 body and the second screw goes inferior and into the centre of the S-1 body. Both screws go through the sacral pedicle mass superior to the S-1 foramen, which is best monitored with the outlet view.

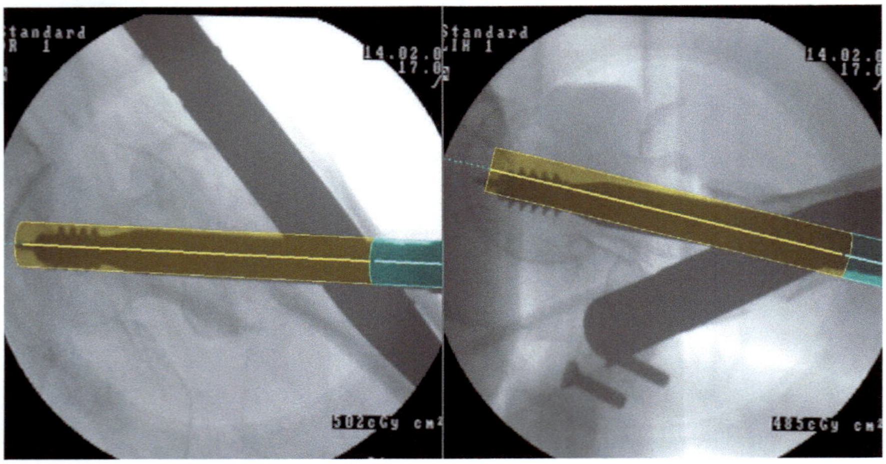

Fig. 6.2.18. Gamma nailing under fluoro-navigation

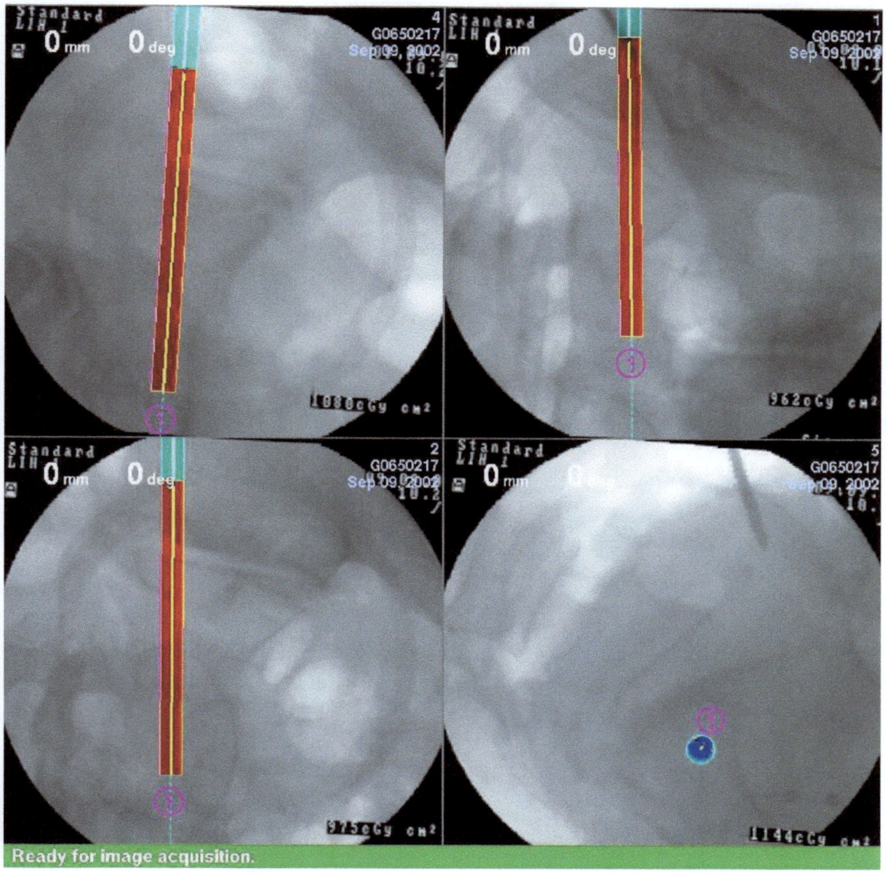

Fig. 6.2.19. Percutaneous screw fixation of sacro-iliac fracture dislocation under fluoro-navigation

Percutaneous Fixation of Iliac Wing Fractures [8] (Fig. 6.2.20 a)

Fixation of iliac wing fractures is indicated when the fracture causes instability of the pelvis. The images that are needed in the navigation are obturator oblique view and iliac oblique view, assisted with outlet-iliac oblique view and inlet-iliac oblique view. With the patient tracker on the iliac crest of the uninjured side or on the external fixator, a drill sleeve is calibrated to provide steady and rigid guidance. The screw is inserted in retrograde manner through a 1.5-cm incision, just below the AIIS, targeting towards the PIIS, vertically and 5–10° towards medially. The screw trajectory is along the roof of the acetabulum from AIIS to PIIS (Fig. 6.2.20 b).

Percutaneous Fixation of Acetabulum Fractures [8] (Fig. 6.2.21)

This is possible in fractures that can be reduced closely by traction. These fractures may include the high transverse fracture [13], central fracture dislocation, particularly in old patients with a degree of osteopenia. A traction table is preferred and the reduction of the fracture under traction is confirmed by fluoroscopy in standard oblique views. With the patient in a lateral decubitus position, the patient tracker is anchored on the ipsilateral ASIS, with fluoroscopic images according to the column where the screws are going to be inserted.

For the anterior column screw, inlet-iliac oblique view, ensure the pin does not go into the pelvis; for the outlet-obturator oblique view, ensure the pin does not go into the acetabulum; assisted with standard inlet and outlet views. Again, a calibrated drill sleeve providing rigid and steadying positioning is navigated. The screw can be inserted antegrade (Fig. 6.2.21 a) via the midpoint between the iliac tubercle and the greater trochanter or retrograde through an incision in the pubic symphysis. The retrograde screw is best inserted with the patient in a supine position.

For the posterior column screw, navigation can be done with the standard iliac oblique and ob-

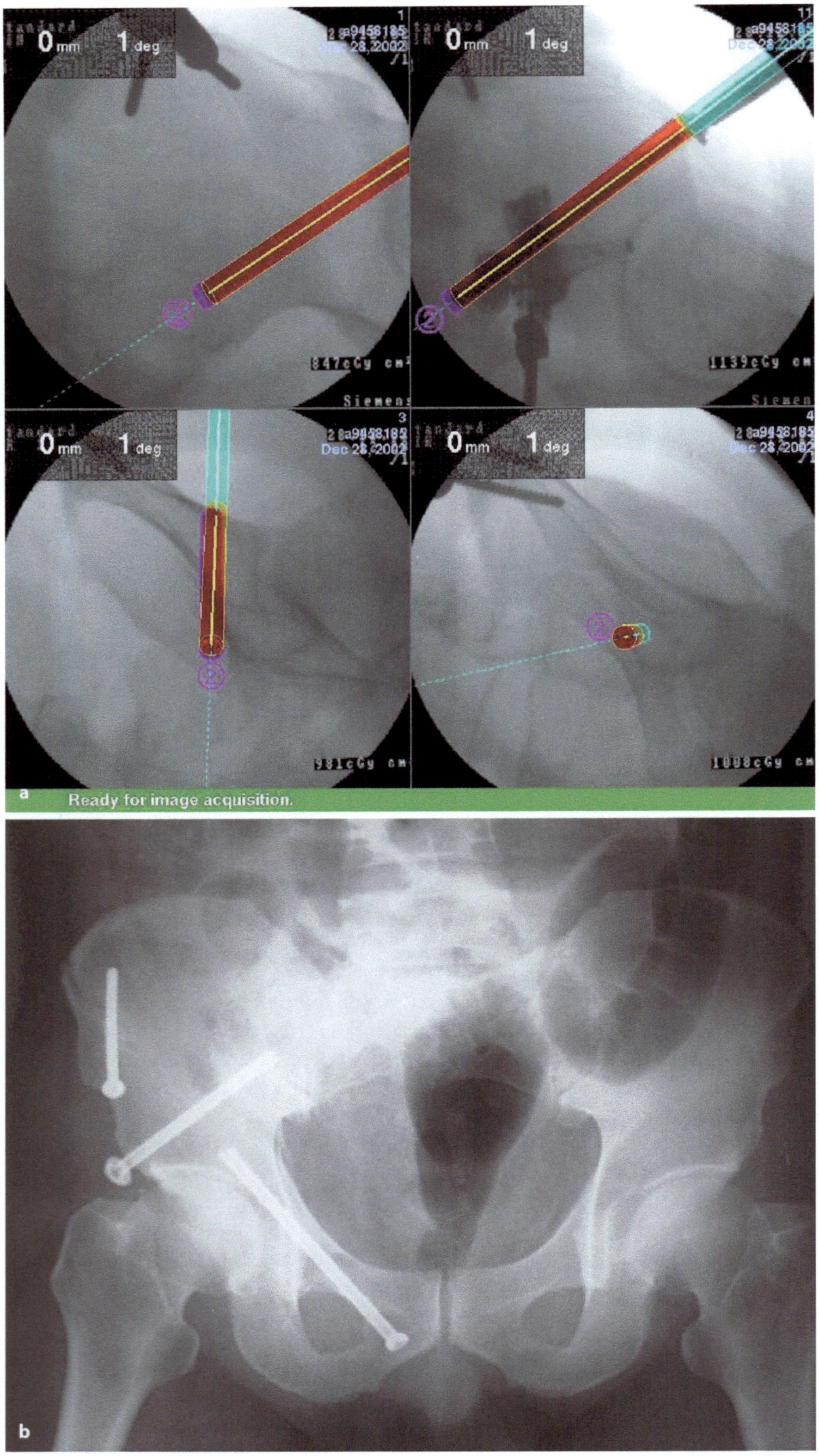

Fig. 6.2.20. Percutaneous fixation of iliac fracture: a planning, b screw positions

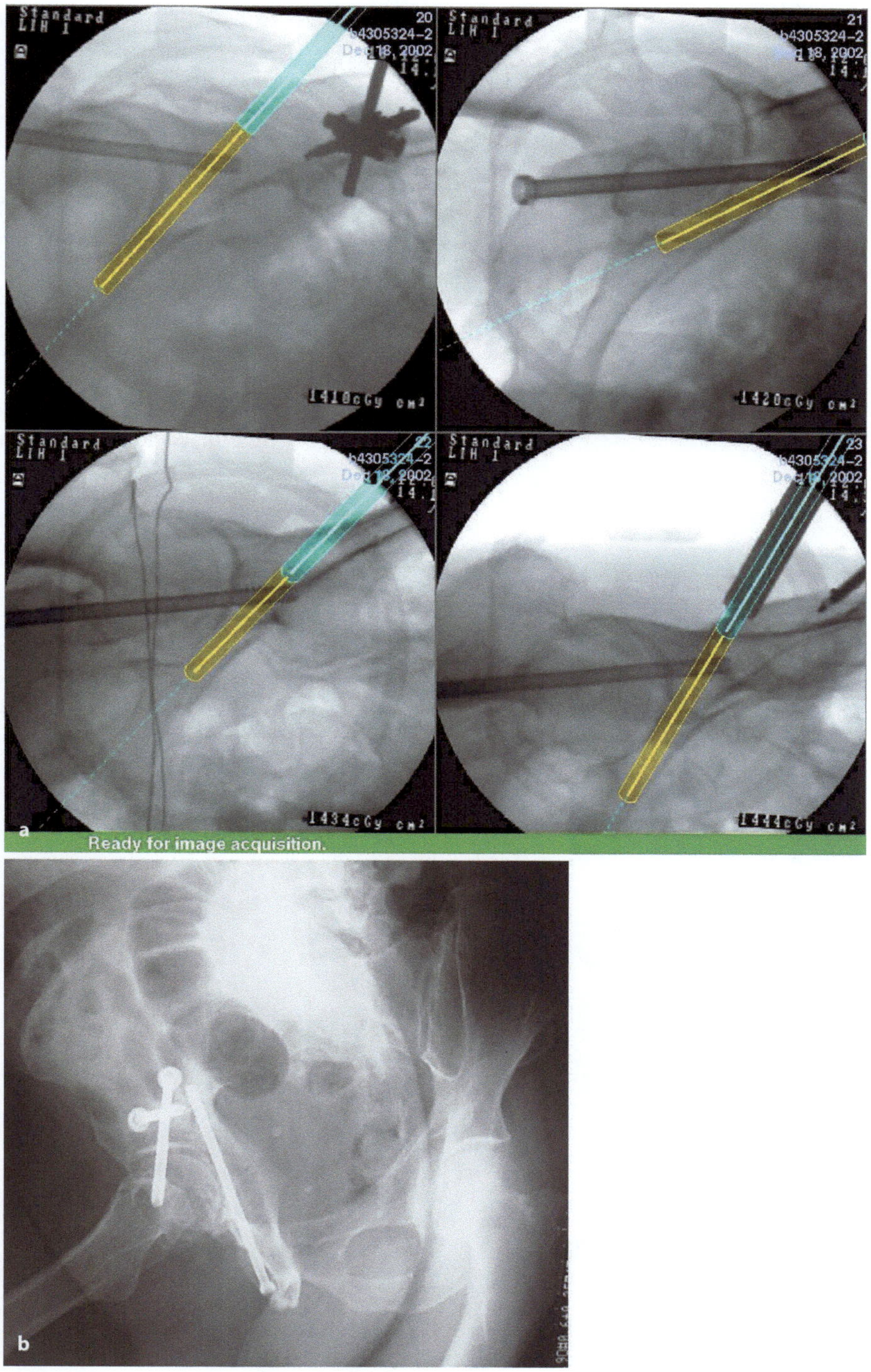

Fig. 6.2.21. Percutaneous fixation of acetabular fractures: a screw planning, b screw positions

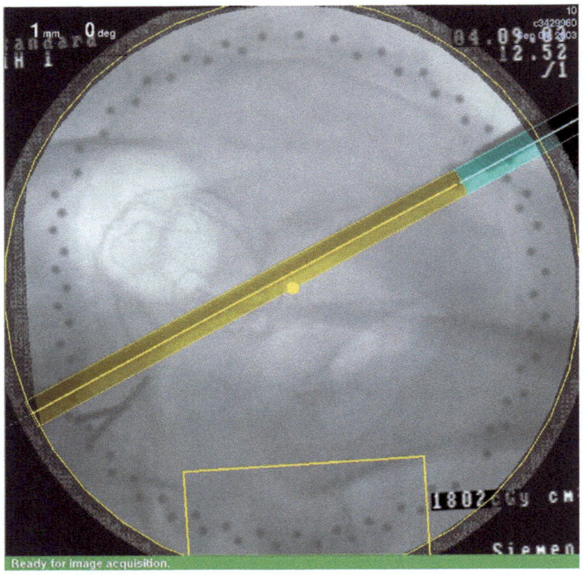

Fig. 6.2.22. Posterior column screw insertion during an open reduction surgery

turator oblique views, assisted with outlet-obturator oblique view (Fig. 6.2.20 b). The entry point is through an incision on the centre of the ischial tuberosity. The knee should be flexed and the hip externally rotated to relax the sciatic nerve. The trajectory of the screw should be along the medial side of the posterior column and directed proximally in the posterior column to the centre of the dome of the acetabulum on the iliac oblique view.

This technique is also applicable in open surgery where screw insertion can be done in a precise manner (Fig. 6.2.22), e.g. posterior column screw through ilio-inguinal approach, anterior column screw through posterior approach.

Insertion of Ilizarov Tension Wires for Complex Articular and Peri-articular Fractures (Fig. 6.2.23)

This can be done after the fracture is reduced by longitudinal traction. With the images of the fracture taken in frontal, lateral and two oblique views, the tension wires can be inserted by navigating the calibrated drill sleeve or power drill. This has the advantages of better planning and positioning of the wires. Additional procedures of screw insertion can also be done with the same technique (Fig. 6.2.24).

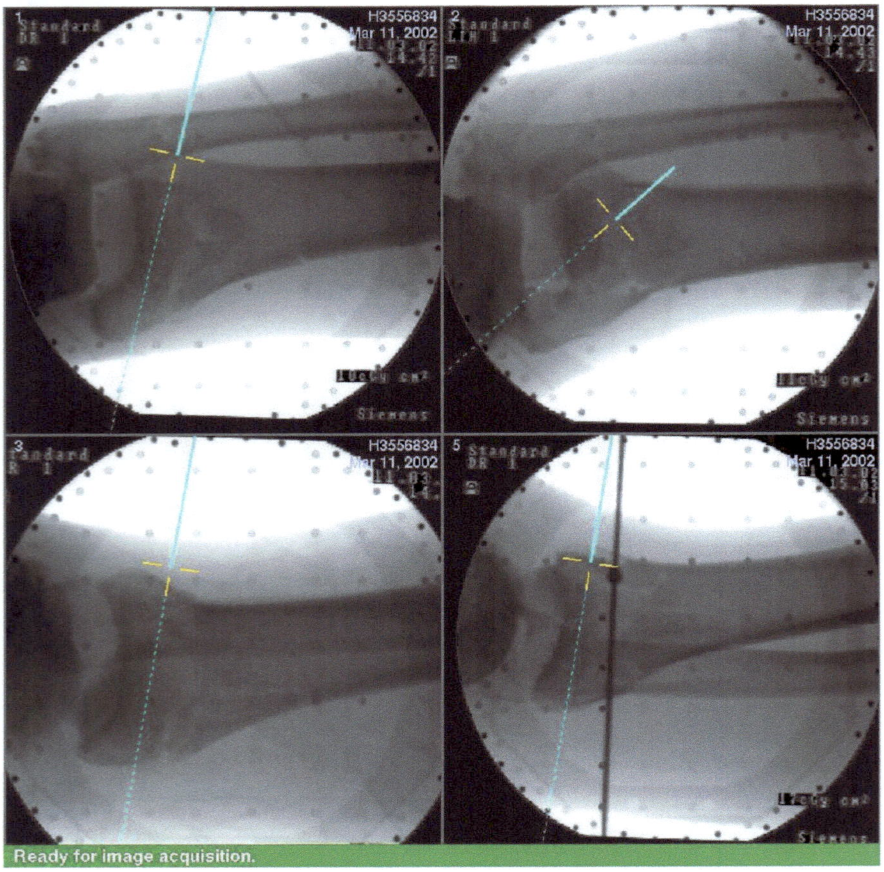

Fig. 6.2.23. Insertion of tension wires under fluoro-navigation of a pilon fracture

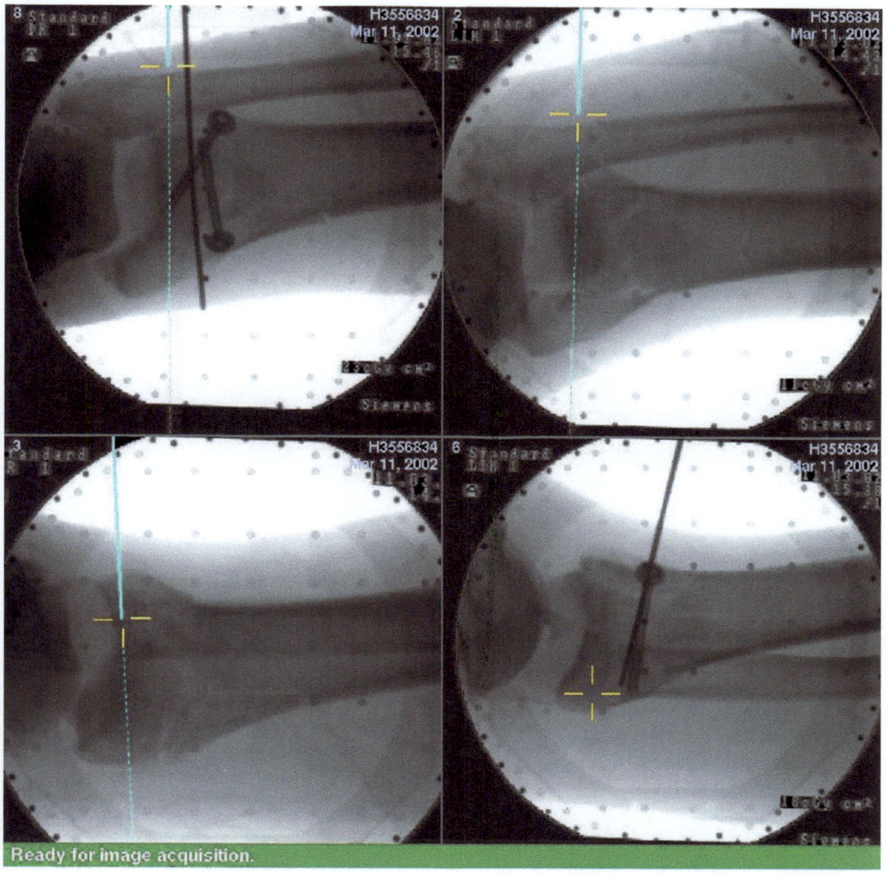

Fig. 6.2.24. Insertion of cannulated screws for fixation of pilon fractures under navigation

Other Applications

Many percutaneous fixation procedures that need fluoroscopic control can also be done with the same principle.

In all these applications, navigating the instruments with great accuracy and real-time quantitative display greatly facilitates the surgical procedures without frequent use of the fluoroscope [4]. The navigation of the C-arm also helps to decrease the radiation exposure and guide the position of the C-arm whenever an image needs to be taken.

The interactive and quantitative data from the navigation system help in implant planning: the position of the implant with the axis defined by two to four planes, the length and the diameter can be clearly depicted with a high degree of accuracy. Early clinical experience has confirmed that the advantages and the extended applications of this technique will benefit many of our patients. The simultaneous monitoring of the trajectory of the instruments in two to four views facilitates the accurate positions of implants and instruments without the need of frequent exposure to X-ray. The adaptation of specific trauma instruments further facilitates the practice of minimally invasive surgery. At this stage, the accuracy of the system is very acceptable and the system is also stable for most operative procedures, as mentioned above. We have been using the system for the past one and a half years and the success rate is above 96% in all the procedures. It has become standard operative equipment in many common orthopaedic trauma surgeries in our department. We anticipate that as the experience accumulates and with improvements in both the hardware and software, the applications will increase.

The Future

Fluoro-navigation, like all applications in computer-aided surgery, is a developing technology. It is therefore expected that further improvements in the hardware and software of the system for quicker image acquisition and accurate registration will be possible in the near future. With improvement of the image quality, more precise positioning and more interactivity will be possible

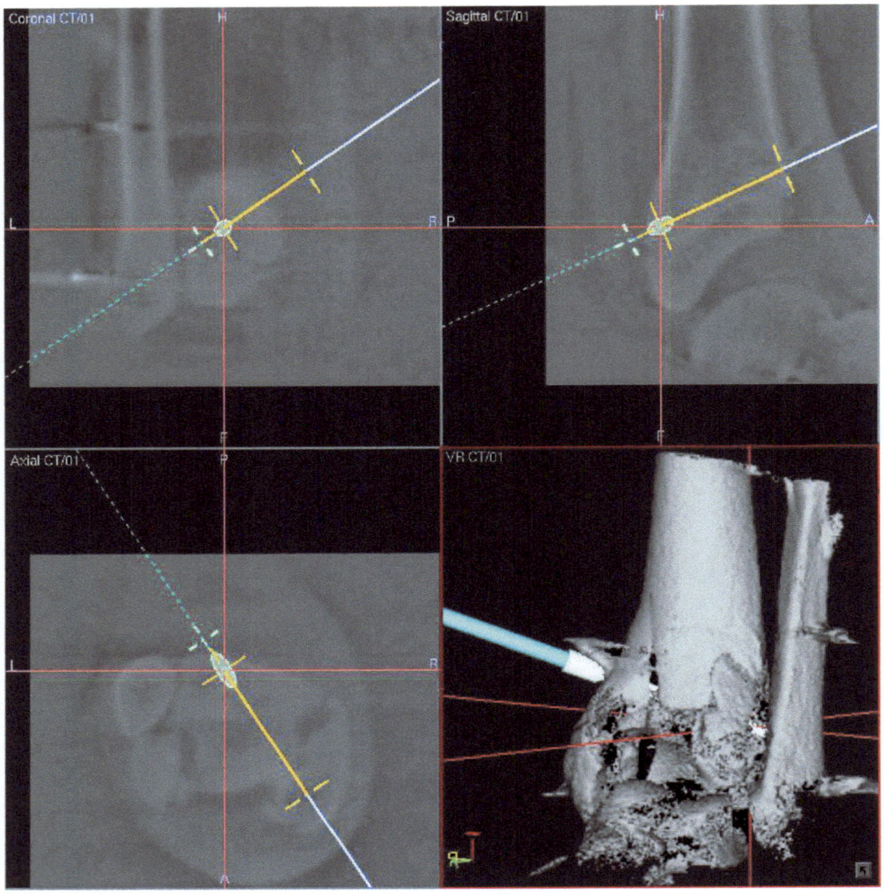

Fig. 6.2.25. Fluoro-navigation with intraoperative three-dimensional fluoro-images

between the system and the surgeons. The development of dedicated surgical instruments for orthopaedic trauma surgery in line with the further improvement of the navigation system will be another major direction of research.

With the establishment of image libraries for instruments, implants and skeleton, it will be possible to minimise further the need for standard X-ray. This is applicable in procedures where instruments and images of the implants are navigated. One good example is the distal locking of the intramedullary locked nails, where the image of the distal nail is navigated and not the bone. As the dimensions of the nails are standardised for each system, the image library of the implants can thus be used in navigation without further acquiring the fluoroscopic images, provided there is minimal deformity of the implant after insertion. Thus the distal locking procedure can be done without the use of the C-arm.

The combination of intraoperative three-dimensional fluoroscopy and the navigation will be another technique for further development [6]. The registration of these three-dimensional fluoroscopic images into the navigation system allows the application of the CT-based navigation system in orthopaedic trauma surgery with fluoro-navigation. The application is particularly useful in minimally invasive surgery for intra-articular and juxta-articular fractures where the fractures can be reduced by closed technique and the fixation by percutaneous screw fixation. With this technique, depressed osteochondral fragments can also be approached and reduction done with a navigated instrument. However, at this stage, fluoroscopic assistance is still needed during the procedure where fracture fragment movement is expected. With expected further improvement in the software and the image acquisition, the combination of fluoroscopy and three-dimensional fluoro-navigation will improve percutaneous fixation of these articular fractures (Fig. 6.2.25). Another direction of development is to explore the possibility of navigating on each individual fracture fragment. This will extend the technique even more to real-time fracture reduction, which at the present moment still needs fluoroscopic control.

The development of virtual fluoroscopy in fluoro-navigation has progressed rapidly in the past few years. The application of virtual fluoroscopy in surgical training needs further exploration. With the image libraries of bone and implants, surgical training, evaluation and assessment can also be possible with the virtual environment. A laboratory for virtual fluoroscopy training has been set up to help the surgeon in preoperative planning, practice of surgical techniques and assessment of surgical competence. This represents one more step towards surgical training in a complete virtual environment.

Conclusion

The development of fluoro-navigation in orthopaedic trauma represents one of the applications of computer-aided surgery. Its development is exciting and challenging. While many of these developments are from the engineers, many applications in surgery were considered impossible in the past. As a result of the innovative thinking and perhaps endless imagination of those who are devoted to perfection in patient care, these applications have become possible and their effects have been proven. There is a great need for closer collaboration between engineers and clinicians in future developments.

Acknowledgements

I would like to thank the CAOS team of the Department of Orthopaedics and Traumatology of the Chinese University of Hong Kong for their assistance in the surgeries and the preparation of this manuscript.

References

1. Hinsche AF, Giannoudis PV, Smith RM. Fluoroscopy-based multiplanar image guidance for insertion of sacroiliac screws. Clin Orthopaed Rel Res 395:135–144, 2001.
2. Hofstetter R, Slomczykowski M, Sati M, Nolte LP. Fluoroscopy as an imaging means for computer-assisted surgical navigation. Computer Aided Surgery 4(2):65–76, 1999.
3. Joskowicz L, Milgrom C, Simkiin A, Tockus L, Yaniv Z. FRACAS: a system for computer-aided image-guided long bone fracture surgery. Computer Aided Surgery 3(6):271–288, 1998.
4. Kahler DM, Mallik K. Computer assisted iliosacral screw placement compared to standard fluoroscopic technique. Abstract from CAOS/USA 1999, p 348.
5. Leung KS. The role of fluoro-navigation in orthopaedic trauma. Symposium CC: New Techniques in Fracture Care: Minimally Invasive Surgery and Enhancement of Bone Healing, AAOS 2003, New Orleans.
6. Leung KS, Yung SHP, Tsui HF, Tang N, Sarvestani A. 3-D Fluoro-navigation for articular fractures – a report of early experience. In: Langlotz F, Davis BL, Bauer A (eds) Proceedings of 3rd International Annual Meeting of CAOS: 204–205, 2003.
7. Leung KS, Yung SHP, Tang N, Kwok KO, Yue HY. Clinical experience of gamma nailing with fluoro-navigation. In: Langlotz F, Davis BL, Bauer A (eds) Proceedings of 3rd International Annual Meeting of CAOS: 206–207, 2003.
8. Leung KS, Tsui HF, Tang N, Yung SHP, Yue HY. Percutaneous screw fixation of pelvi-acetabular fractures under fluoro-navigation guidance. In: Langlotz F, Davis BL, Bauer A (eds) Proceedings of 3rd International Annual Meeting of CAOS: 208–209, 2003.
9. Slomczykowski MA, Hofstetter R, Sati M, Krettek C, Nolte LP. Novel computer-assisted fluoroscopy system for intraoperative guidance: feasibility study for distal locking of femoral nails. J Orthopaed Trauma 15(2): 122–131, 2001.
10. Suhm N. Intraoperative accuracy evaluation of virtual fluoroscopy – a method for application in computer-assisted distal locking. Computer Aided Surgery 6:221–224, 2001.
11. Tsui HF, Griffith JF, Kwok KO, Yung SHP, Leung KS. Accuracy of three-dimensional positions of the sacro-iliac screws under fluoro-navigation system. In: Langlotz F, Davis BL, Bauer A (eds) Proceedings of 3rd International Annual Meeting of CAOS: 374–375, 2003.
12. Viant WJ, Phillips R, Griffith JG, Ozanian TO, Mohsen AM, Cain TJ, Karpinski MR, Sherman KP. A computer assisted orthopaedic surgical system for distal locking of intramedullary nails. Proceedings of the Institution of Mechanical Engineers. Part H. J Eng Med 211(4): 293–300, 1997.
13. Zura RD, Kahler DM. A transverse acetabular nonunion treated with computer-assisted percutaneous internal fixation – a case report. J Bone Joint Surg 82A(2):219–224, 2000.

Review of Existing, Mounted Targeting Devices for Distal Locking of Intramedullary Nails

L. CARDADOR

Introduction

Although intramedullary nailing is one of the most ancient methods for the surgical treatment of fractures, when we speak of closed nailing, meaning endomedullary osteosynthesis of long bones by means of a minimally invasive approach far from and protective of the fracture site, at once we think of Gerhard Küntscher. Nevertheless, his method was restricted to mid-diaphyseal fractures without comminution where proximal and distal fixation by the nail could be obtained by a tight endosteal fit; because, outside of these limits, it could not control rotation, telescoping or angulation. Aware of these restrictions, at the end of his life, he laid down the basis for locked nailing [14] and devised the "detention nail". This concept was later developed in Germany by Klemm and Schellman. But it was in Strasbourg that Kempf and Grosse [9, 11], with their nail design and with the improvements in the image intensifier, developed the modern technique of locked, intramedullary nailing and extended the treatments to more types of fractures and locations that, until then, could not be managed by traditional nailing: comminuted with or without bone loss, long oblique, segmental and with third fragments, and proximal and distal fractures of the femur and tibia. The enthusiasm, based on the benefits of the method, led to the use of locked nails in other long bones, such as the humerus [7, 8, 13, 20, 23, 24], the ulna and radius (see *Practice of Intramedullary Locked Nails*, Vol. 1, Chap. 13 and Vol. 2, Chap. 11), and the development of specific implants for proximal and distal fractures of the femur, like the Gamma and the supracondylar nails.

The Modern Interlocking Nail

Locked nailing, as described by Kempf and Grosse, means locking the nail within the bone by screws, both proximally and distally to the fracture. Proximal locking for the femur or tibia was never difficult, due to insertion system design and its fixation to the proximal tip of the nail. Distal locking presented other problems. The presence of a posterior slot, which gives the nail the required elasticity that allows it to conform to the curves of the bone, sometimes subjects the nail to bending and torsion movements [22], which make it impossible to use a nail-mounted distal targeting device, which could lower the use of irradiation. In Strasbourg a prototype was used for some time but was discarded, due to the great number of failures.

For these reasons, a target device mounted on the image intensifier was devised by Lafforgue and Grosse (see *Practice of Intramedullary Locked Nails*, Vol. 1, Chap. 8) (Fig. 6.3.1). Its use minimizes the amount of irradiation exposure to the operating team and allows distal locking, even with bent and twisted nails, by means of finite adjustments of the image intensifier or even of the patient's position. It has, however, some shortcomings. The need for an experienced X-ray technician is a must, or the procedure can be a headache and long. Its frequent use leads to loss of

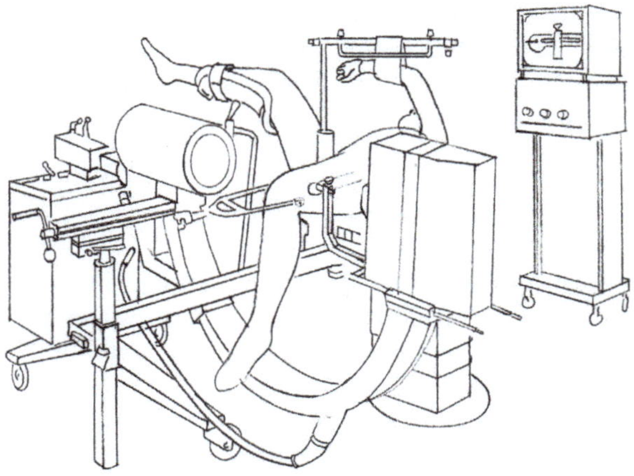

Fig. 6.3.1. Positioning of the patient on the fracture table and the Grosse-Lafforge device mounted onto the image intensifier

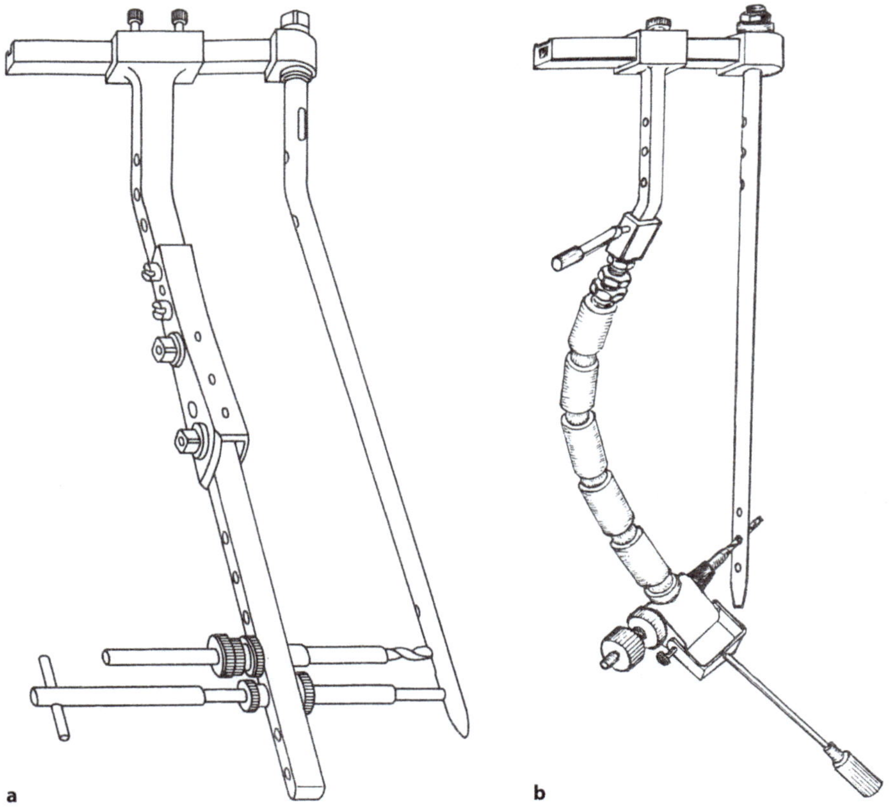

a b

Fig. 6.3.2 a, b. Mechanical jigs by Berentey

proper fixation on the image intensifier and eventual malalignment. Though out of production, it remains a reliable mechanical guide for distal targeting of intramedullary nails.

The enthusiasm for closed intramedullary nailing, the problems of distal locking, and the need to avoid irradiation aroused the imagination of surgeons and engineers world-wide. Some mechanical devices, mainly for use on the femur and tibia – such as those of Steriopoulos [25] and Berentey (Fig. 6.3.2), were tested but never reached the market. Colchero's solid nail [2] had its own targeting devices for distal locking (Fig. 6.3.3), but was designed for open nailing.

Other Fixation/Locking Systems

Parallel to these investigations, efforts were also applied in other directions. Why not design nails with distal fixation capability but without the need for screws?

Some systems, with poor control of the fracture or problems related to insertion or removal, never had great acceptance, while others are widely used. Examples of various techniques for distal locking include: the Brooker-Wills distal locking nail [1, 5, 26], a modified Küntscher nail with distal fixation by means of "wings" deployed from within through a slot in each side of the nail (a system first described by Camargo in 1952) [3], Seidel's humeral (Fig. 6.3.4) and Lefèvre's radial nails – with a distal locking system via the expansion of fins by an internal screw driven by a long screwdriver inserted in the proximal end of the nail, Marchetti-Vicenzi's "universal elastic bundle nail" [19], and de la Caffinière's locked, intramedullary flexible osteosynthesis [4] – using a set of flexible 4- or 5-mm pins with a locking device for their proximal ends, the distal fixation being obtained when they spread out. More recently, the inflatable nail (Fixion) – in which the nail self-locks to the cortices by expansion (Fig. 6.3.5), making any type of interlocking unnecessary – claims good results; but it is expensive and data are still insufficient [15].

The accumulated experience shows that these types of devices usually have problems in dealing with comminuted, distal fractures and osteoporotic bones, and, thus, should only be used in selected cases.

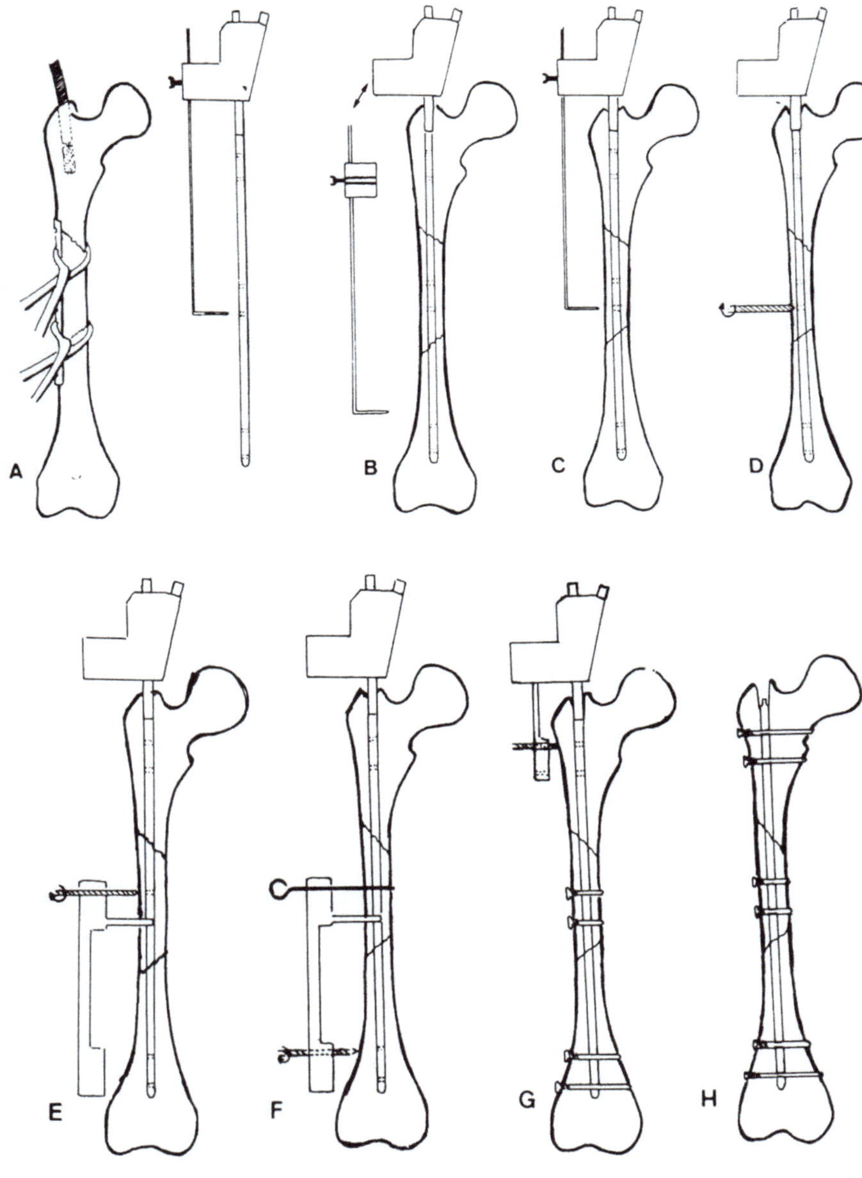

Fig. 6.3.3 A–H. Colchero's surgical technique and targeting devices for locking

Existing Mechanical Jigs

With closed nails with high bending and torsional rigidity, the practical use of mechanical jigs for distal locking becomes possible. They do exist for almost all long bone nailing systems, with the exception of the forearm and for some special procedures.

The standard and trochanteric Gamma nail (Stryker) [12] and later the PFN (AO/ASIF) and others, the SCN (Stryker) and similar devices [17] for retrograde femoral nailing, the ST-Pro for humeral fractures (Fig. 6.3.6) and the ankle arthrodesis nail [6, 18] – both from Biomet-Merck, are typical examples where mounted targeting jigs are in full use. Beyond their rigidity, these nails have in common a short length, so the risk of nail/jig divergence is very small.

These jigs, which act sequentially as introducer and screw-targeting device, consist roughly of a proximal part, designed to fix the nail to the assemblage by means of a screw, and a distal part parallel to the nail, with the same length and coincident holes for locked nailing, although they may be engineered in different ways. Initially made of metal, some are now made of carbon fiber (Fig. 6.3.7), to improve X-ray visualization.

For longer, closed nails, the risk for slight bending exists, and so the need for small adjustments. These are not one-piece jigs. Instead their

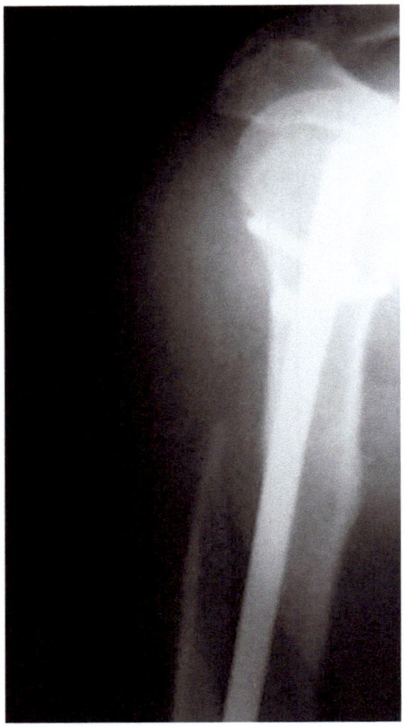

Fig. 6.3.4. Distal part of Seidel's nail showing the expansion of the fins

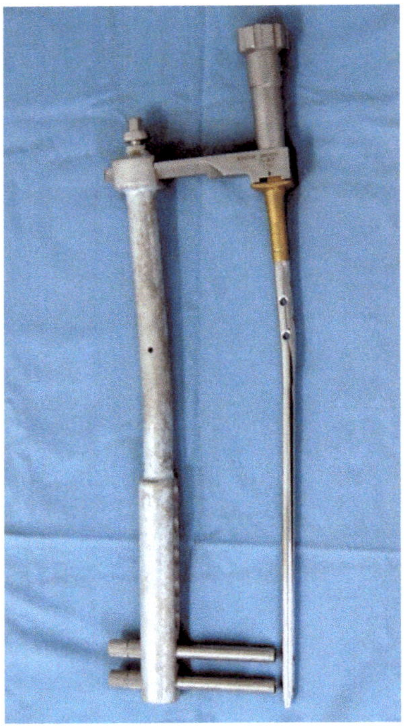

Fig. 6.3.6. The Biomet interlocking humeral nail system

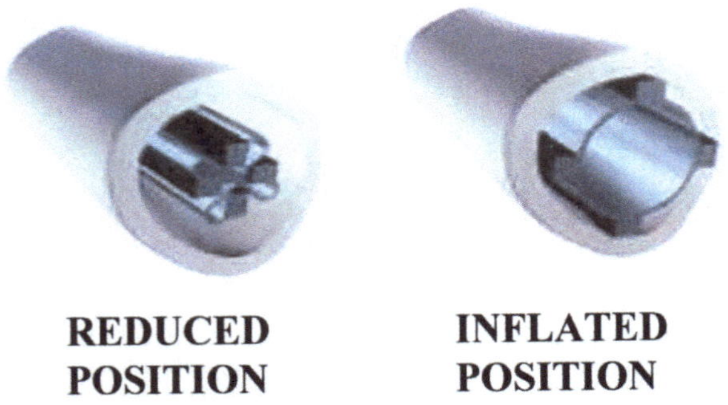

Fig. 6.3.5. Principle of self-locking of the inflatable nail

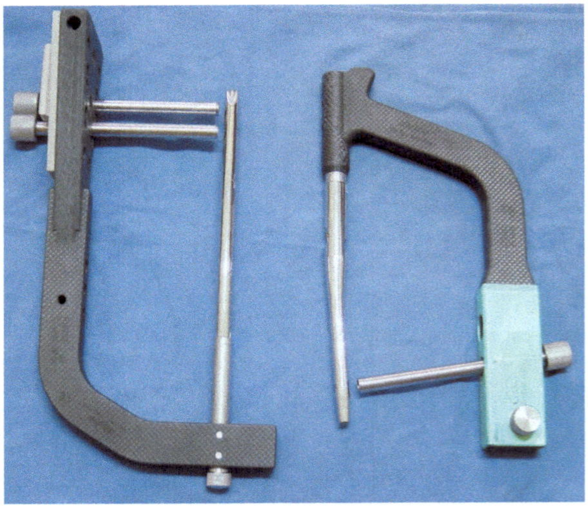

Fig. 6.3.7. The SCN and Gamma nails showing the similarity of their carbon-fiber introducer/targeting devices

design allows some movement to find the distal nail holes intraoperatively, even without the use of an image intensifier.

The new S2 nail (Stryker) employs a "mechanical jig" (see Chap. 6.4), both for the femur and tibia; and the design seems to avoid the problems related to distal locking.

With the use of unreamed, thinner nails, locking the nail becomes vital. The AO/ASIF group proposes a jig for distal locking of their solid UTN nail (Fig. 6.3.8); but its effectiveness remains to be fully proved. Some hand-held, radiolucent targeting devices, like Pennig's [21] and Biomet's (Fig. 6.3.9), are designed for "universal" use, but have not achieved wide acceptance.

Problems Related to Distal Locking

Where problems arose, their causes were fully identified (few were found to be in the jigs themselves), so the careful surgeon could avoid them. Regarding the first Gamma nail, several series [12, 16] showed variable numbers of missed distal screws. This was a fault related to the mismatch

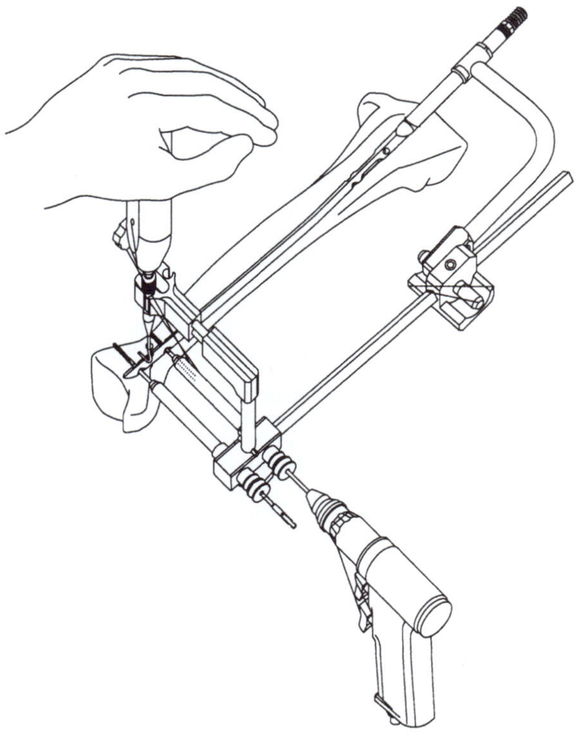

Fig. 6.3.8. The AO/ASIF jig for the UTN nail

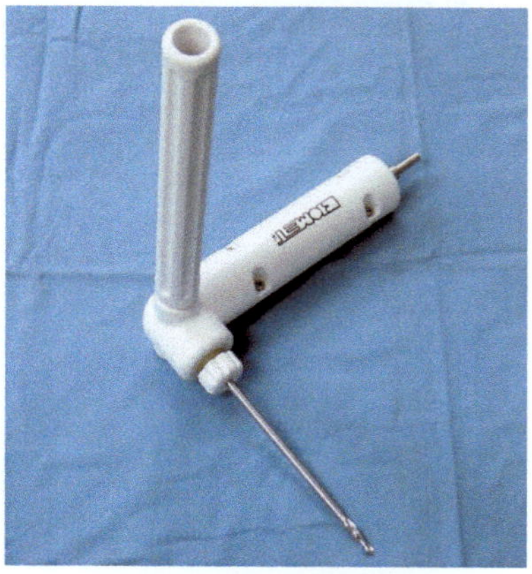

Fig. 6.3.9. Biomet's radiolucent targeting device

of diameter between the drill and the guide sleeve and has been fully corrected.

Another cause for missed screws is the lack of stability between the nail-holding device and the end of the jig. This must always be checked before the introduction of the nail. It is understandable that the greater the distance between the connection point and the screw holes, the easier the miss can occur. That is why one should always begin with the proximal screw, leave the sleeve in situ, and then proceed to the next one.

The tension of the iliotibial tract, if not released, can displace the guide sleeve upward or downward. So, if necessary, make a small cross-incision on the fascia, to allow the sleeve to touch the bone freely.

If the position of the screws is going to fall on a more arced surface of the bone, this can cause the drill to slide over that surface. One must follow the operating technique that suggests using a "pilot-tipped" drill, which makes a small puncture on the bone before the helix of the drill completes the perforation, and without pushing too hard, so it can find its own way through the bone and the holes.

Finally, with the use of locked nails, the tight, endosteal fit that was necessary in Küntscher's technique is dispensable, because control of the fracture is achieved by proximal and distal screws. So, if one anticipates the need for static locking, reaming should be done in a manner such that the nail enters the medullary canal easily, thus avoiding unnecessary stresses to the bone and making the use of a jig more warranted.

The Future

Are mechanical jigs going to disappear? No doubt. But not in the near future. Any system able to replace these devices must be user-friendly and practical for everyday use, achieve better results and be economically competitive. Current investigation on locator devices, based, among others, on laser or radiofrequency systems, and on fluoroscopy-based, computer-assisted navigation (see *Practice of Intramedullary Locked Nails*, Vol. 2, Chap. 11), is still far from producing something that is ready to address the needs not only for selected centers but for a world-wide market.

And remember, at any time, if everything else fails, locking the nailing can still be achieved using the unsophisticated method of direct vision through a cortical window [10], or using the free-hand system with an inexpensive Steinmann pin.

References

1. Brooker AF, Brumback RJ (1998) Brooker-Wills nails in treatment of infra-isthmal injuries of the femur. J Trauma 28: 688–691
2. Colchero F, Orst G, Reboul C, Villalobos F, Vidal J (1983) Enclouage centro-médullaire claveté: étude expérimentale, technique opératoire, résultats. Rev Chir Orthop Reparatrice Appar Mot 69: 547–555
3. De Camargo FP (1952) Osteosíntese intramedular de Kuntscher. Contribuição à técnica e estudo crítico baseado em 240 casos. São Paulo

4. de la Caffinière J-Y, Pelisse F, de la Caffinière M (1994) Locked intramedullary flexible osteosynthesis: a mechanical and clinical study of a new pin fixation device. J Bone Joint Surg Br 76: 778–788
5. Ebraheim NA, Milem CA, Jackson WT (1993) Complicated removal of the distal locking device of Brooker-Wills. Clin Orthop 290: 275–278
6. Gorby PO, Weinfeld GD, Yu GV (2002) Intramedullary nail fixation in rearfoot and ankle: arthrodesis procedures. ACFAS
7. Ikpeme JO (1994) Intramedullary interlocking nailing for humeral fractures: experiences with the Russell-Taylor humeral nail. Injury 25: 447–455
8. Jensen CH, Hansen D, Jorgensen U (1992) Humeral shaft fractures treated by interlocking nailing: a preliminary report on 16 patients. Injury 23: 234–236
9. Kempf I, Grosse A, Beck (1985) Closed intramedullary nailing. Its application to comminuted fractures of the femur. J Bone Joint Surg Am 67: 709–720
10. Kanellopoulos AD, Yiannakopoulos CK, Vossinakis I, Badras LS (2003) Distal locking of femoral nails under direct vision through a cortical window. J Orthop Trauma 17(8): 574–577
11. Kempf I, Grosse A, Lafforge D (1978) L'apport du verrouillage dans l'enclouage centro-médullaire des os longs. Rev Chir Orthop Reparatrice Appar Mot 64: 635–651
12. Kempf I, Grosse A, Taglang G, Favreul E (1993) Le clou gamma dans le traitement à foyer fermé des fractures trochantériennes: résultats et indications à propos d'une série de 121 cas. Rev Chir Orthop Reparatrice Appar Mot 79: 29–40
13. Kempf I, Heckel TH, Pidhorz LE, Taglang G, Grosse A (1994) L'enclouage verrouillé selon Seidel des fractures diaphysaires humérales récentes. Rev Chir Orthop Reparatrice Appar Mot 80: 5–13
14. Küntscher G (1958) The Küntscher method of intramedullary fixation. J Bone Joint Surg Am 40: 17–26
15. Lepore L, Lepore S, Maffuly N (2003) Intramedullary nailing of the femur with an inflatable self-locking nail: comparison with locked nailing. J Orthop Sci 8(6): 796–801
16. Lindsey RW, Teal P, Probe RA, Rhoads D, Davenport S, Schauder K (1991) Early experience with the gamma interlocking nail for peritrochanteric fractures of the proximal femur. J Trauma 31(12): 1649–1658
17. Lucas SE, Seligson D, Henry SL (1993) Intramedullary supracondylar nailing of femoral fractures. A preliminary report of the GSH supracondylar nail. Clin Orthop 296: 200–206
18. Mader K, Pennig D, Gausepohl T, Patsalis T (2003) Calcaneotalotibial arthrodesis with a retrograde posterior-to-anterior locked nail as a salvage procedure for severe ankle pathology. J Bone Joint Surg Am 85 (Suppl 4): 123–128
19. Marchetti PG, Vicenzi G, Impallomeni C (1994) A new nail for elastic intramedullary fixation in fractures and pseudarthrosis of the femur and tibia. Orthopaedics 2: 403–416
20. McKee D (1995) Retrograde locked nailing of humeral shaft fractures. J Bone Joint Surg Br 77: 667
21. Pennig D, Brug E, Kronholz HL (1988) A new distal aiming device for locking nail fixation. Orthopedics 11: 1725–1727
22. Schaffer C, Willinger R, Renault D, Kempf I, Jaeger JH (1986) Theory of induced torsion and intramedullary nailing. In: Saha (ed) Biomechanical engineering V: recent developments. Pergamon, New York, p 367
23. Seidel H (1989) Humeral locking nail: a preliminary report. Orthopedics 12: 219–226
24. Stannard JP, Harris HW, McGwin G, Volgas DA, Alonso JE (2003) Intramedullary nailing of humeral shaft fractures with a locking flexible nail. J Bone Joint Surg Am 85: 2103–2110
25. Steriopoulos KA, Kontakis GM, Katonis PG, Galanakis IA, Dretakis EK (1996) Placement of the distal locking screws of the femoral intramedullary nail without radiation. Arch Orthop Trauma Surg 115(1): 43–44
26. White GM, Healy WL, Brumback RJ, Burgess AR, Brooker AF (1986) The treatment of the femoral shaft with the Brooker-Wills distal locking intramedullary nail. J Bone Joint Surg Am 68: 865–876

CHAPTER 6.4

Distal Locking with Mechanical Jig (Author's Own Technique)

G. Anastopoulos

Objective

This chapter is about a new distal targeting system that addresses the problems and concerns associated with the amount of radiation exposure and difficulties experienced during the distal interlocking procedure of closed intramedullary nailing.

Introduction

Over the past 30 years, closed interlocking nailing has been the method of choice for the management of diaphyseal long bone fractures. Although evolutions and improvements have occurred in the nail design and material in an effort to (a) simplify the technique and (b) accommodate complicated fractures, distal locking remains the most difficult part of the procedure, requiring the greatest learning curve. Undoubtedly, there is demand for a radiation-free, reliable and easy to handle method for distal screw insertion, as techniques currently used for distal interlocking have not managed to reduce operation time and radiation exposure for patients, surgeons and operating room staff [14, 15, 20].

The objective is to describe a technique that would identify the location of the distal holes in intramedullary nails at a long distance. This technique must reproducibly allow the surgeon to drill a hole axially through the bone and nail with a high level of accuracy.

Description of the Targeting System

The main concept for the development of the new targeting system is that if a specific location (a groove) nearby the distal holes could be identified, the exact location of the distal holes could then be easily found.

There are three major elements in the design of the described radiation-independent system. These are:

- A nail with a groove between the two distal holes. The groove is the orientating landmark for the surgeon, as it pinpoints the exact location of the distal holes.
- A bevelled-tip probe. With this probe the groove can be easily felt. In this way the detection of the holes in the nail by the surgeon is facilitated (Fig. 6.4.1).
- A targeting device that matches the nail's geometry (Fig. 6.4.2). It contributes towards accurate drilling of the distal holes and offers guidance for the insertion of the screws through these holes.

The distal targeting device consists of three main components:

- An articulation device, which is connected to the nail adapter and the targeting arm.

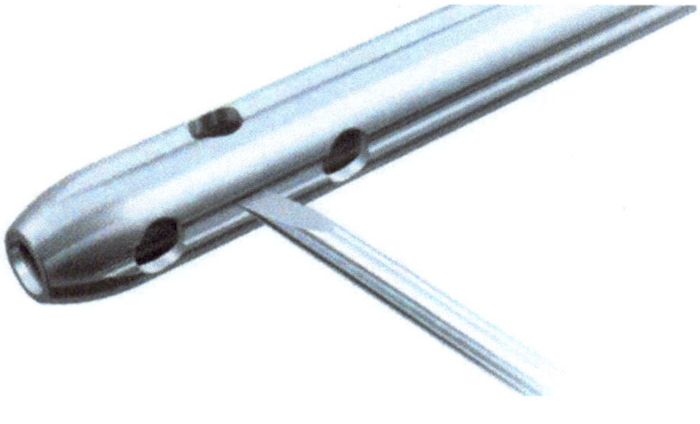

Fig. 6.4.1. The bevelled-tip probe into the longitudinal groove between the distal locking holes of the nail

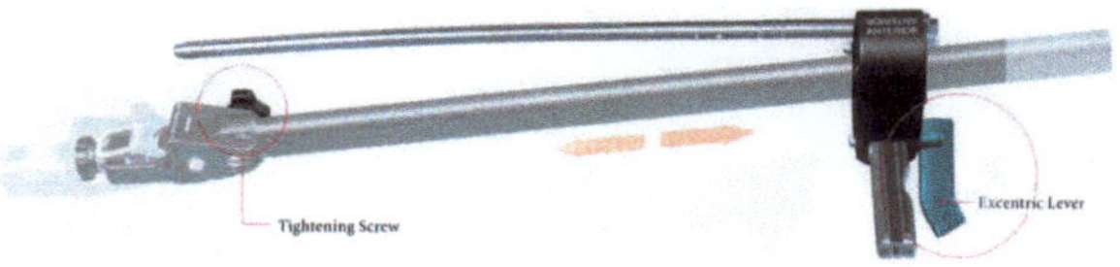

Fig. 6.4.2. The targeting device tightened on the nail adapter

- An arm.
- A targeting clip, which permits additional adjustments for targeting the distal holes. The proximal and the distal holes in the targeting clip are in-line with the distal locking holes in the nail, while the middle hole in the targeting clip is in alignment with the centre of the nail's groove.

Surgical Technique

- Patient positioning, insertion of the guide wire, reaming of the femoral canal and nail selection are performed as usual.
- The selected nail must be calibrated with the distal targeting device prior to its insertion (Fig. 6.4.3).
- The nail is then introduced into the femoral canal with the standard operative technique; however, it must be inserted 10 mm deeper than its final position.
- The distal targeting device is attached to the nail adapter (note: the distal holes must always be locked first).
- A pilot hole is drilled on the lateral cortex only through the central hole of the targeting clip.
- The targeting device is removed from the nail adapter.
- An appropriately sized curette is used to clean the debris from the hole.
- The probe is then introduced through the opened hole until it touches the nail's groove.
- With constant pressure against the probe, the nail is pulled proximally until the probe falls into the distal locking hole (Fig. 6.4.4).
- A fixation sleeve is passed over the probe. The handle of the fixation sleeve is removed (Fig. 6.4.5).

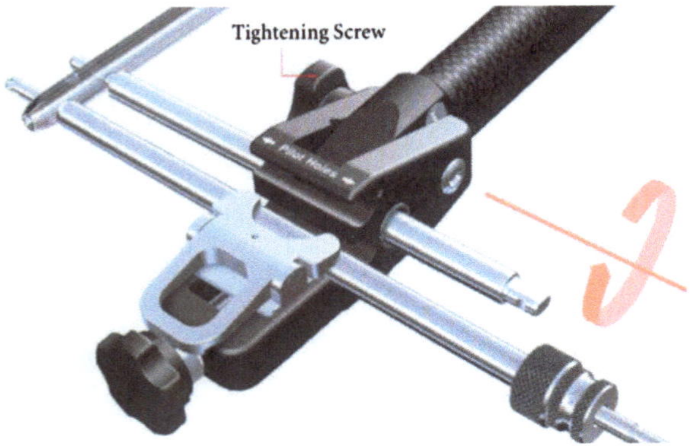

Fig. 6.4.3. Calibration of the distal targeting device to the nail

- The distal targeting device is reattached to the nail adapter and to the fixation sleeve (Fig. 6.4.6).
- The more proximal hole is drilled and the appropriately sized screw is inserted.

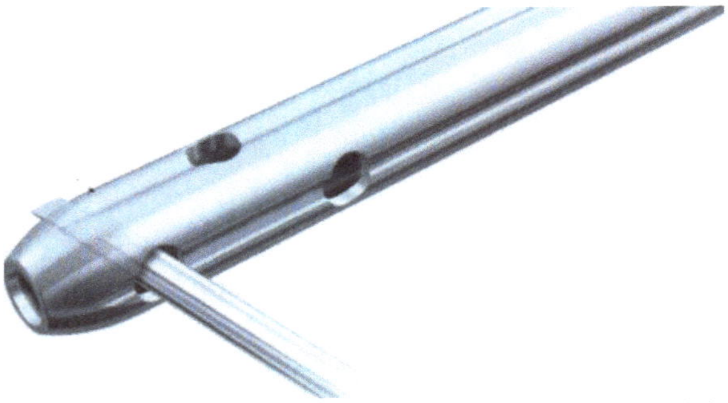

Fig. 6.4.4. By back hammering of the nail the probe is sliding inside the groove of the nail and guided into the most distal locking hole

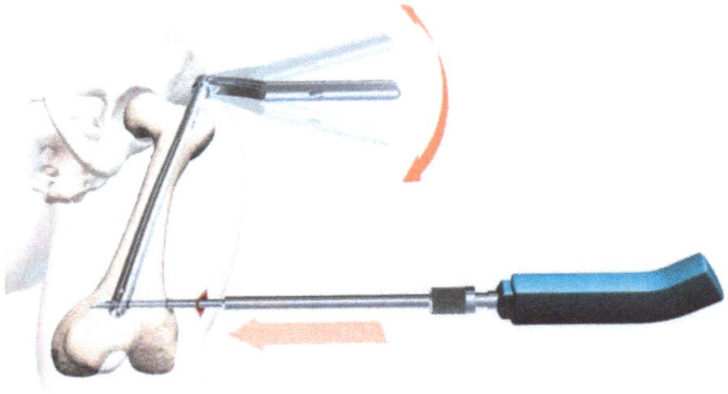

Fig. 6.4.5. The fixation sleeve has passed through the locking hole over the probe (so the system is stable). The handle is then removed

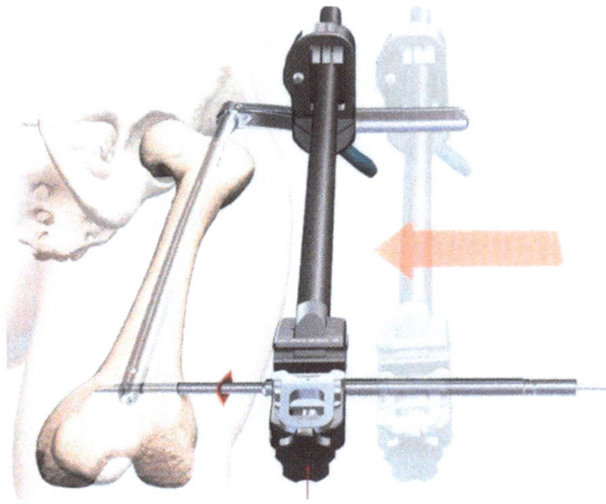

Fig. 6.4.6. The distal targeting device is sliding over the nail adapter and over the fixation sleeve

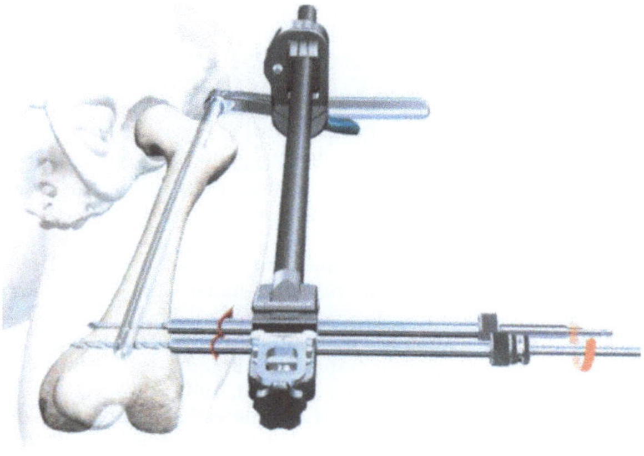

Fig. 6.4.7. Distal locking through the distal targeting device

- The probe and fixation sleeve are removed and the hole is completed by drilling through the medial cortex.
- The appropriately sized screw is inserted (Fig. 6.4.7).
- Proximal locking is performed as usual.

Results from Cadaveric Testing

The distal targeting system was used on 20 femoral and 20 tibial osteotomies in fresh human cadavers over a period of 12 months.

- Distal locking was successful in all cases.
- No C-arm verification was required in any of the cases.
- Average time for distal locking with both screws was 5.3 min.

Discussion

Lafforgue and Grosse in Strasbourg invented the first system for distal locking in 1978 [9]. The system did not achieve widespread use because it was unstable, expensive and it could not be adapted on any image intensifier.

Since then, a variety of methods have been described for facilitating distal locking and reducing radiation exposure [1, 4–8, 11, 16–19, 21]. These methods had inconsistent success mainly because of the final deformation of the nail (axis-pivot phenomenon), which occurs as a result of bending forces in the anteroposterior curvature and also torsion forces that distort the nail, especially in the femur [11]. There has not been a targeting device to address this issue so far. Inevitably, the "free-hand" technique has become the method of choice for distal locking, where the amount of radiation exposure is determined by the surgeon's skill and experience with the technique [2, 3, 10, 12, 13, 22]. Nevertheless, it has been reported that radiation exposure during distal locking of the femur is on average 2.6 times the amount of radiation needed for the actual insertion of the nail [20].

Testing of the new targeting system on cadaveric bones confirmed that the following objectives were met:

- Radiation-independent system.
- Accurate and reproducible.
- Easy to use.
- Safe for the patient.
- Sensitive to deformation of the nail.

These parameters will be validated during the clinical trial that has already begun.

Conclusion

The distal targeting device and the corresponding technique appear to be a significant addition to the current intramedullary nailing procedure, as distal locking is getting simpler and radiation independent. Initial experience with cadaveric bones is encouraging and the usefulness of the device in clinical practice remains to be confirmed in the near future.

References

1. Anastopoulos G, Asimakopoulos A, Exarchou E, Pantazopoulos Th. Closed interlocked nailing in comminuted and segmental femoral shaft fractures. J Trauma 35 (5): 772–775, 1993
2. Brumback RJ. The rationale of interlocking nailing of the femur, tibia, and humerus. Clin Orth Rel Res 324: 292–320, 1996
3. Bucholtz RW, Rathjen K. Concomitant ipsilateral fractures of the hip and femur treated with interlocking nails. Orthopaedics 8: 1402–1406, 1985
4. Conlan DP. Grosse and Kempf locked intramedullary nailing: an improved distal locking screw drill guide. J R Coll Surg Edinb 35: 60–61, 1990
5. Gugala Z, Nana A, Lindsey RW. Tibial intramedullary nail distal interlocking screw placement: comparison of the free-hand versus distally based targeting device techniques. Injury 32: 21–25, 2001
6. Hashemi-Nejad A, Garlich N, Goddard NJ. A simple jig to ease the insertion of distal screws in intramedullary locking nails. Injury 25: 407–408, 1994
7. Hudson I. Locking nailing: an aid to distal targeting. Injury 20: 129–130, 1989
8. Kelley SS, Bonar S, Hussamy OD, Morrison JA. A simple technique for insertion of distal screws into interlocking nails. J Orthop Trauma 9: 227–230, 1995
9. Kempf I, Grosse A, Lafforgue D. L' apport du verrouillage dans l'enclouage centro-medullaire des os longs. Rev Chir Orthop 74: 635–651, 1978

10. Klemm KW, Borner M. Interlocking nailing of complex fractures of the femur and tibia. Clin Orthop 212: 89–100, 1986
11. Krettek C, Mann J, Miclau T, et al. The deformation of slotted and solid femoral nails with insertion: reasons for the failure of distal interlocking screw aiming arms. J Orthop Res 16: 572–575, 1998
12. Krettek C, Miclau T, Konemann B, et al. A new mechanical aiming device for the placement of distal interlocking screws in femoral nails. Arch Orthop Trauma Surg 117: 147–152, 1998
13. Krettek C, Konemann B, Miclau T, et al. A mechanical distal aiming device for distal locking in femoral nails. Clin Orthop Rel Res 364: 267–275, 1999
14. Kwong LM, Johanson PH, Zinar DM, et al. Shielding of the patient's gonads during intramedullary interlocking femoral nailing. J Bone Joint Surg 72-A (10): 1523–1526, 1990
15. Levin PE, Schoen RW, Browner BD. Radiation exposure to the surgeon during closed interlocking intramedullary nailing. J Bone Joint Surg 69A (5): 761–766, 1987
16. MacMillan M, Gross RH. A simplified technique of distal femoral screw insertion for the Grosse-Kempf interlocking nail. Clin Orthop 226: 252–259, 1988
17. Pardiwala D, Prabhu V, Dudhniwala G, Katre R. The AO distal locking aiming device. An evaluation of efficacy and learning curve. Injury 32: 713–718, 2001
18. Penning D, Oppenheim W, Faccioli G, Rossi S. Intramedullary locked nailing of femur and tibia: insertion of distal locking screws without image intensifier. Injury 28 (4): 323–326, 1997
19. Rao JP, Allegra MP, Benavenia J, Dauhajre TA. Distal screw targeting of interlocking nails. Clin Orthop 238: 245–248, 1989
20. Sanders R, Koval KJ, DiPasquale T, Schmelling G, et al. Exposure of the orthopaedic surgeon to radiation. J Bone Joint Surg 75A (3): 326–330, 1993
21. Tyropoulos S, Garnavos C. A new distal targeting device for closed interlocking nailing. Injury 32: 732–735, 2001
22. Wiss DA, Fleming CH, Matta JM, Clark D. Comminuted and rotationally unstable fractures of the femur treated with an interlocking nail. Clin Orthop 212: 35–47, 1986

Section 7 Coating of Implants and Infection Prophylaxis

Rationale for Antibiotic Prophylaxis in Open Fractures

J. Gaudias

It might appear somewhat provocative to raise the question of antibiotics in the treatment of an open fracture, particularly if we refer to current practice. The prescription of antibiotics is in fact the rule, probably based more on habit than on clearly known facts.

Infectious complications, a threat for all open fractures, mobilise surgeons' attention, but individual situations are complex; the situations are as different as the fracture sites, the degree of severity of damage to the soft tissue, the underlying host conditions, and the levels of contamination of the wounds.

Today, stabilisation of the fractures by osteosynthesis is the rule. Whatever fixation used, it will increase the risk of infection. Careful debridement, cleaning of the wounds, immediate or secondary closing of the wounds and antibiotic treatment are the methods of treatment traditionally used to reduce the risk of infection. In this approach, the question of the effectiveness of antibiotic treatment is therefore worth asking. But in view of the complexities of open fractures, in order to try to answer it, we need to reformulate the question by selecting three fields of investigation: the overall effectiveness of antibiotics, assessing their effectiveness according to the type of open fracture, and finally the correlation of their effectiveness and the way the antibiotics are administered, that is the choice of molecule, time when the treatment is started and the length of administration.

Is It Any Use Prescribing Antibiotics to Reduce the Number of Infections After an Open Fracture?

Before examining the clinical work that would enable us to answer this question, it is worth looking at Worlock's experimental model [1]. In this model of an open fracture of the tibia in the rabbit, the osteosynthesis is carried out by an intramedullary pin, and the wound is inoculated with staphylococcus. The effect of a single injection of cefradine is maximally effective when it takes place before the bacteria are inoculated. This corroborates the work of Burke [2], which lays down the foundations of surgical antibiotic prophylaxis for planned surgery. The remainder of the study, on the other hand, covers the real situation of open fractures: the administration of antibiotics only after bacterial inoculation. In these experimental conditions, the effect of this same single dose of antibiotics is more limited, but still persists, decreasing by the order of 40% the infection rate as compared with the control animals.

In the clinical situation with human beings, a placebo effect is required to demonstrate the effectiveness of antibiotic treatment. Three studies of this type are available.

Patzakis [3] compared three groups of patients presenting an open fracture: one group without antibiotics; one group treated with the combination penicillin/streptomycin for 10 days, and one group treated with cefalotine for 10 days. The rates of infection were respectively 13.9, 9.7 and 2.3%. The effectiveness of treatment with antibiotics seems to be proven but is only spectacular when dealing with an antistaphylococcal antibiotic.

The study was not carried out in double-blind conditions, nor was it possible in each group to classify the fractures by type, so that we do not know whether each of the groups includes the same proportion of fractures with high risk of infection (grade III).

In Bergman's study [4], 90 open fractures were randomised in three groups treated with dicloxacillin, benzylpenicillin or placebo. No infection occurred after grade I fractures in any of the groups. With regard to grade II and grade III fractures, 12 patients were treated with dicloxacillin, 10 with penicillin, and 13 with placebo. Two deep infections were observed in the placebo group, and none in the treated groups.

Finally, Braun [5], in a randomised prospective double-blind study comparing placebo and cloxacillin, showed a higher significant reduction of infection rates in the cloxacillin group (2/50 as compared to 12/50 in the placebo group). The fact that there were more grade III fractures in the antibiotic group if anything reinforces this result.

These three studies carried out against placebo give us a first positive answer to the question of the effectiveness of antibiotics in cases of open fracture, at least as an across-the-board response.

The Effectiveness of Antibiotics Depends on the Kind of Open Fracture

Several classifications of increasing complexity have been established to characterise open fractures more precisely. The classification of Gustilo and Anderson [6] seems to be the most widely used; this is in fact the only classification that has been correlated with the risk of infection. In a prospective study covering 240 patients treated for open fracture of the limbs, Dellinger [7] was able to determine the risk of infection from these fractures, by stratifying them on the basis of the Gustilo classification. In a multivariate analysis, three factors appear to be significantly correlated with the risk of infection: in the order of increasing importance they are the grade of the fracture ($p<0.001$), the use of internal or external fixation ($p<0.005$), and its location on the tibia ($p<0.01$).

The risk of infection increases with the gravity of the lesions to the soft tissue. The grade I fractures have a relative risk of 1, the grade II fractures 1.3, and grade IIIA fractures 2.1. Grades IIIB and IIIC are identical and their correlative risk is 23. The increase in the risk of infection when fractures move from grade IIIA to grade IIIB or C is 15 times greater than in the transition from grade I to II or grade II to grade IIIA. In this study, the use of antibiotics was the same whatever the gravity of the lesions of the soft tissue. By definition this transition from grade IIIA to grades IIIB and IIIC indicates a degree of lesions to the soft tissue beyond which it is impossible to obtain cover for the bone structure, as well as an effective means of local defence of the host, and in vivo effectiveness of the antibiotics. In this situation it is possible that the preventive action of the antibiotics may be insignificant in grade IIIB and IIIC fractures.

Methods of Administering Antibiotics in Cases of Open Fracture

Before dealing with the question of the choice of molecule, it is worth raising the question of the usefulness of taking bacteriological samples as a possible guide for secondary adaptation of the antibiotic treatment. If there is any received wisdom in this matter, it is a priori that of original contamination of the wound as the origin of the risk of infection. Let us leave aside the special and very rare situation of heavy groundwater contamination, which might occur with certain wounds, for example in an agricultural environment. In the usual traumatological situation, in countries that have developed effective systems for emergency care, open fractures are immobilised at the accident site, and the wounds are disinfected and covered with sterile dressings. Longstanding data report 70% initial contamination [8, 9]. More recently, the bacteriological analysis of the wounds on admission to hospital shows a low rate of contamination of these wounds of the order of 30% [10, 11]. The isolated bacteria are mainly those from the skin environment. When infection occurs, the infecting bacteria are as a rule different from the initially contaminating bacteria and the infection comes, in most cases, from hospital bacteria. The proportion of infection with negative gram and with relatively resistant bacteria increases with the severity of the lesions of the soft tissue. At the stage of the onset of the infection, this disappearance of the initial contaminating bacteria is a sign of the effectiveness of the initial surgical measures such as debridement and cleaning of the wounds. The fact that the infecting bacteria are hospital bacteria leads us to reflect on the strict compliance with and tightening of the traditional rules of hospital hygiene, which may have been unconsciously neglected in these so-called "emergency" situations.

Choice of the Ideal Antibiotic

The older studies mentioned initially advocated the use of an active molecule to deal with the staphylococci. Randomised prospective clinical trials comparing the molecules with one another are relatively rare.

Vasinius [12], in a comparative study covering 227 patients, compared the effectiveness of clindamycin to that of cloxacillin. The overall rate of infection was 15%. In the fractures treated with clindamycin, infection occurred in 9.3% of cases, as compared to 20% in the group treated with cloxacillin. The effectiveness of the antibiotics was only obvious in the fractures of grade I and II, while the fractures of grade III indicated high rates of infection of 70%, with 45% infection with negative gram bacillus not covered by the spectrum of the two chosen antibiotics.

Gagey [10] and collaborators compared prospectively and randomly the effectiveness of one single dose of 800 mg of pefloxacin and one intravenous treatment with cefazolin for 48 h followed by oxacillin administered orally for 72 h. The groups comprised 300 patients per group and included essentially grade II fractures. Twenty-one infections were described in the group treated with pefloxacin (6.6%), 24 in the cefazolin-oxacillin group (8%); the difference between the two groups was not significant.

Patzakis [13], in a randomised prospective double-blind study, recently compared monotherapy using ciprofloxacin with an associated treatment using cefamandole and gentamicin. The rate of infection for grade I and grade II fractures was 5.8% in the ciprofloxacin group and 6% in the cefamandole-gentamicin group, with no significant statistical difference. The data changed radically for grade III infections: the rate of infection was 31% in the ciprofloxacin group and 7.7% in the cefamandole-gentamicin group. In the study in question, the difference was not statistically significant in view of the low numbers in each group, although the risk of infection was five times higher in the ciprofloxacin group.

Timing and Length of Antibiotic Administration

This data have been studied very little in the literature. The older studies [3–5] mostly refer to 10 days of treatment; the latest development in the literature would favour a shorter treatment. Gagey, using a single dose of pefloxacin, obtained equivalent results to those found in longer treatments [10].

Dellinger [7], in his prospective study concerning the risks of infection, evaluated in parallel two aspects of antibiotic treatment: first, that of the moment of administration in relation to the moment when the fracture occurred and second, the length of administration.

Concerning the first point, no difference appears as regards the risk of infection between the group of patients who had benefited from the administration of antibiotics in the first 3 h following the lesion and those treated more than 3 h after the fracture.

On the second point, the prospective study divided the group up into four categories according to the length of administration of the antibiotics (cefamandole or cefazolin): the shortest treatment consisted of two doses of the antibiotic administered at an 8-h interval; the other groups of patients were treated respectively for 1, 3 and 5 days. The effectiveness of the treatment with antibiotics was the same in this study, whatever the length of administration of the antibiotic.

Practical Conclusion

As things now stand with regard to objective data from the medical literature, it is possible to note the following facts:

- The controlled use of antibiotics is useful in reducing the risk of overall infection after open fracture. This measure is in addition to, but in no case is a replacement of, surgical debridement and debridement of the wounds.
- This beneficial use of antibiotic treatment very likely concerns only fractures of grades I, II and IIIA using the Gustilo and Anderson classification.
- In all cases the antibiotic chosen must have a high rate of effectiveness against staphylococcus. No molecule in the literature has shown greater effectiveness than the others, as long as this criterion is respected.
- A brief administration of antibiotics for 24–48 h is a priori largely sufficient to obtain the optimal effect of the chosen antibiotic while curbing the risk of secondary effects and the pressure of selection.
- Finally, it is crucial to remind all those taking charge of open fractures that the bacteriological data that are obtained once the infection occurs often indicate bacteria of hospital origin and therefore the nosocomial nature of these infections.

These different propositions apply particularly to fractures of grades I, II and IIIA Gustilo classification fractures, which all enable the wound at the fracture site to be closed or at least to be covered by living tissue and properly vascularised. The prognosis for IIIB and IIIC fractures still remains worrying as far as infection is concerned and always raises the question of the optimal treatment. Logically, for grade IIIC fractures, the only prospect for improvement is by shortening the treatment times by removing the ischaemia as early as possible through vascular repair. For grade IIIB fractures, the reduction of the risk of infection is probably far better dealt with in the discussion about the rapid closing of the skin by reconstructing the soft tissue. A few teams have provided reconstructions at the same time, offering attractive prospects in the field of infection [14–16], but these are very short series, and aimed at selected patients, excluding all patients who presented an earlier arteriopathy of any kind or poor host conditions. The practices most used are those of a two-stage treatment, in which the reconstruction of the soft tissue needs to be carried out as soon as possible after the initial debridement phase. In this particular situation, the question of antibiotic treatment arises at the different stages of the operative procedure. If prophylactic antibiotic monotreatment is the rule for fractures of grades I, II, and IIIA, the recent work of Patzakis [13] shows for the first time the interest of an association of antibiotics widening the spectrum in the treatment of high-grade fractures. We must, however, recall that the grade of the fracture can only be confirmed after surgical debridement, which means that widening the spectrum can only be considered at a secondary stage. It is sensible and logical to offer monotherapy using an antistaphylococcal antibiotic, whose effectiveness has been proven across the board to all patients, at least for the first dose.

This being the case, several attitudes could theoretically be discussed:

- Association of antibiotics widening the spectrum, continued until the stage of reconstruction of the soft tissue; possible adaptation of treatment depending on bacteriological sampling carried out during the reconstruction period.
- Short initial antibiotherapy, then resuming wide-spectrum prophylactic treatment, also briefly, during the reconstruction phase, with or without adaptation to the results of the bacteriological sampling results.
- Systemic antibiotic treatment and management of the waiting period before reconstruction of the soft tissue by local antibiotic treatment. The use of gentamicin cement beads in surface application on losses of substance was tested in particular by Moehring, with good results [16].

In all these different examples, the different approaches raise the question of the optimal length of antibiotic treatment, whether continuous or sequential, local or general. No response has been found in the literature and the question still remains to be answered. Since the relatively rare occurrence of high-grade fractures leads each team to offer its own rationale in administering antibiotics, it is rather unlikely that a consensus will emerge in the short term concerning the right attitude for this kind of fracture.

The simplest propositions for the use of antibiotics after open fracture consist in very brief treatment with an active antistaphylococcal agent for all open fractures, administering the first dose as soon as possible. The use of the Gustilo/Anderson classification, the only one to have been correlated with the risk of infection, makes it possible on leaving the operating theatre to identify the fractures for which the risk of infection is particularly high (grade IIIB–IIIC). It is likely that for these fractures the prevention of the infection is essentially in the hands of the surgical team, relying on the quality of the debridement and the possibilities of rapid reconstruction of the soft tissue and of wound closure. To our today's knowledge, the widening of the scope of antibiotic treatment is left to the team's discretion. No factors indicating advantages in prolonging treatment beyond the few days following the achievement of wound closure at the operation site have been found.

References

1. Worlock P, Slack R, Harvey L, Mawhinney R. The prevention of infection in open fractures: an experimental study of the effect of fracture stability. Injury 1994; 25(1): 31–38
2. Burke JF. The effective period of preventive antibiotic action in experimental infections and dermal lesions. Surgery 1961; 50: 161–168
3. Patzakis MJ, Harvey JP Jr, Ivler D. The rôle of antibiotics in the management of open fractures. J Bone Joint Surg Am 1974; 56(3): 532–541
4. Bergman BR. Antibiotic prophylaxis in open and closed fractures: a controlled clinical trial. Acta Orthop Scand 1982; 53(1): 57–62
5. Braun R, Enzler MA, Rittmann WW. A double blind clinical trial of prophylactic cloxacillin in open fractures. J Orthop Trauma 1987; 1: 12–17
6. Gustilo RB, Mendoza RM, Williams DN. Problems in the management of type III (severe) open fractures: a new classification of type III open fractures. J Trauma 1984; 24: 741–746
7. Dellinger EP, Miller SD, Wertz MJ, Grypma M, Roppert B, Anderson PA. Risk of infection after open fracture of the arm or leg. Arch Surg 1988; 123: 1320–1327
8. Gustilo RB, Merkow RL, Templeman D. Current concept review: the management of open fractures. J Bone Joint Surg 1990; 72A: 299–304
9. Patzakis MJ, Wilkins J, Moore TM. Considerations in reducing the infection rate in open tibial fractures. Clin Orthop 1983b; 178: 36–41
10. Gagey O, Doyon F, Dellamonica P, Carsenti-Etesse H, Desplaces N. Prophylaxie des infections dans les fractures ouvertes de jambe. Rev Chir Orthop 1999; 85: 328–336
11. Valenziano CP, Chattar-Cora D, O'Neill A, Hubli EH, Cudjoe EA. Efficacy of primary wound cultures in long bone open extremity fractures: are they of any value? Arch Orthop Trauma Surg 2002; 122(5): 259–261
12. Vasenius J, Tulikoura I, Vainionpaa S, Rokkaken P. Clindamycin versus cloxacillin in the treatment of 240 open fractures. A randomized prospective study. Ann Chir Gynaecol 1998; 87(3): 224–228

13. Patzakis MJ, Bains RS, Lee J, Schepherd L, Singer G, Ressler R, Harvey F, Holtom P. Prospective randomized, double blind study comparing single agent antibiotic therapy, ciprofloxacin, to combination antibiotic therapy in open fracture wounds. J Orthop Trauma 2000; 14(8): 529–533
14. Tropet Y, Garbuio P, Obert L, Jeunet L, Elias B. One stage emergency treatment of open grade IIIB tibial shaft fractures with bone loss. Ann Plast Surg 2001; 46(2): 113–119
15. Hertel R, Lambert SM, Muller S, Ballmer FT, Ganz R. On the timing of soft tissue reconstruction for open fractures of the lower leg. Arch Orthop Trauma Surg 1999; 119 (1/2): 7–12
16. Moehring HD, Gravel C, Chapman MW, Olson SA. Comparison of antibiotic beads and intravenous antibiotics in open fractures. Clin Orthop 2000; 372: 254–261

Active Coating of Implants used in Orthopedic Surgery

M.-J. Raschke, T. Fuchs, R. Stange, M. Lucke, F. Kandziora, B. Wildemann, G. Schmidmaier

Complications still occur in trauma and orthopedic surgery in spite of improvements in operating techniques and optimization of implants. These complications include delayed fracture healing, non-unions and extensive osseous infections. This may be explained by more complex patterns of injuries, the shift of the population pyramid bringing increased frequencies of complex fractures linked to osteoporosis and more intricate operating procedures.

Growth factors for local application (bone morphogenetic protein [BMP]-2, BMP-7) have been approved by the FDA and CE-marked in Europe, but have not become widely accepted. Reasons may be that, although these proteins are expensive and of limited availability, considerable quantities have to be implanted locally. Furthermore, local release from a bovine collagen carrier in tissue is not evident.

The use of coated implants incorporating active ingredients could release drugs locally and thereby generate a high concentration directly in the area of interest without systemic side-effects. Compounds that could be used in this way include growth factors for the improvement of fracture healing and antibiotics for prophylaxis of implant-related infections.

The coating of implants with biodegradable poly(D,L-lactide) (PDLLA) can facilitate the local controlled release of incorporated growth factors directly into the fracture. The coated implant thus serves both as a fracture stabilization device and as a carrier for active components.

This review presents different models (fracture healing, intervertebral fusion, infection model) demonstrating the efficiency of the coating technology. These findings seem to justify the transfer of this technology into clinical settings.

In a preliminary study, gentamicin-coated intramedullary tibial nails were implanted in six patients exhibiting fractures with severe soft tissue damage. The preliminary findings do not allow conclusions to be drawn in respect of therapy of fractures with severe soft tissue damage or revision surgery. However, the coating seems to be suitable as a "key technology" for the incorporation of active ingredients. In addition, this technology could be helpful in endoprosthetic revisions.

The proper choice of growth factors or suitable antimicrobial substances will require extensive clinical investigations.

Introduction

In spite of improvements in operating techniques and the use of optimized implants in trauma and orthopedic surgery, complications continue to occur. These may result from complex injury patterns, the shift of the population pyramid increasing the occurrence of complex fractures involving osteoporosis and more intricate operating procedures [4]. The complications range from delayed healing and non-union of fractures to extensive bone infections.

Disturbances of fracture healing can be traumatically, mechanically or biologically caused.

Many of the complications are directly correlated with the total duration of treatment, as well as with potential risks such as blood loss, infections, injuries to blood vessels or nerves, compartment syndrome and lasting loss of function. Depending on the duration of the hospital stay, infections resulting from hospital pathogens may also occur, sometimes with lethal consequences [23]. Fractures of the long tubular bones bring the risk of development of proximal deep leg vein thromboses in 30–50% of patients as a result of the prolonged immobilization. In up to 5% of these patients this can lead to a clinically significant lung embolism [2]. Up to 5% of fractures of the lower extremities are affected by delayed healing or remain as non-unions [3]. As the population grows older, fractures related to osteoporosis make up a high proportion of cases involving complications.

For many years attempts have been made to speed up the healing of fractures using either locally or systemically acting substances. The problems listed above could be reduced by stimulation of fracture healing. The use of hormones or growth factors represents a potential starting point. In vitro and in vivo studies have demonstrated that substances such as parathyroid hormone, growth hormone, and growth factors like insulin-like growth factor-I (IGF-I), transforming growth factor-β1 (TGF-β1) and BMPs, possess a stimulating effect on osteogenic and chondrogenic cells and could thus stimulate bone healing [19, 26]. The exact mechanism by which growth factors exert this positive effect, and their interaction during the course of fracture healing, has not yet been fully clarified. Animal experiments have already demonstrated positive effects with the systemic use of growth hormone in distraction osteogenesis and healing of bone defects [15, 16]. The use of systemically administered growth hormone in fracture healing is currently being investigated in a clinical study. For patients the use of growth hormone or growth factors and the resulting acceleration of fracture healing could reduce the need for subsequent fracture-related operations and bring a reduction in the treatment period with earlier return to work, as well as reducing limitation of working ability and early retirements. This would represent a major gain in quality of life. At the same time the costs for health services (hospital stays, follow-up treatment and aids) could be reduced.

Coating Process

Systemic treatment with substances such as growth factors and antibiotics can be problematic. It therefore seems useful to progress the development of suitable systems for delivering them locally. Local delivery leads to high local concentrations of the substance without subjecting the whole organism to high systemic doses.

To provide optimal conditions for the action of the substances, and to ensure sufficient biological activity for optimal effects, these local delivery systems need to possess the following qualities. The carrier materials must be bioresorbable and replaced by bone [3]. They must also be biocompatible so that immune reactions, toxicity and side-effects are reduced. Neither locally induced inflammatory reactions, nor physical blocking due to incomplete breakdown, can be allowed to inhibit bone growth. The carrier material must also be sterilizable and must permit the substances to be delivered in variable amounts. The incorporated substances must be released in a continuous and controlled way so that they are not resorbed before they can exert their effects. A high level of user-friendliness and easy handling for the operating surgeon are desirable qualities [10]. It should also be possible to apply the substances in closed fractures to avoid incurring the risks associated with the opening of fractures.

The collagen sponges already in clinical use for the local delivery of growth factors and antibiotics, most of them based on bovine collagen, do not adequately fulfill these requirements. The uncontrolled release can lead to very high substance concentrations and allergic reactions to the collagen can occur.

The process being described in the present review uses a bioresorbable polylactide coating (PDLLA). It can be applied to metallic surfaces in a "cold" coating process, rendering them "biological". The osteosynthetic implant itself can thus act as a substance carrier.

The coating process is carried out under clean room conditions at room temperature, which means that thermolabile substances can also be incorporated without their activity being affected. In the investigations presented here, the thickness of the layer, which can be altered, was about 10 µm. Tests of the stability of the coating on metallic surfaces show that it can survive high levels

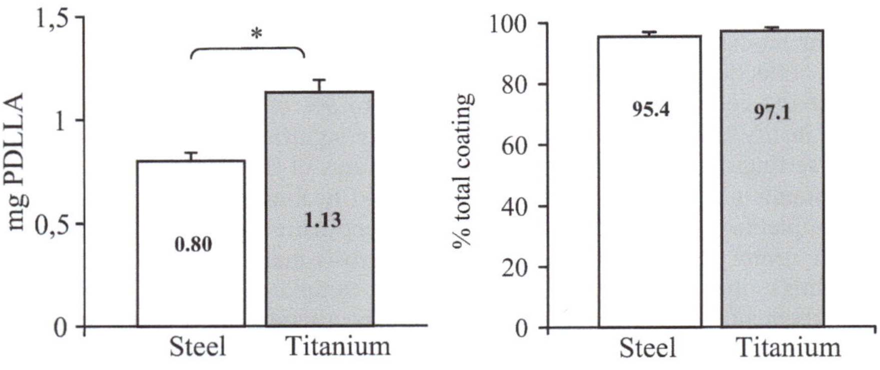

Fig. 7.2.1. Coating properties on steel and titanium. Significantly more PDLLA can be applied to titanium than to steel implants under the same conditions. After implantation and explantation of the Kirschner wires, the abrasion of the coating mass was shown to be below 5%

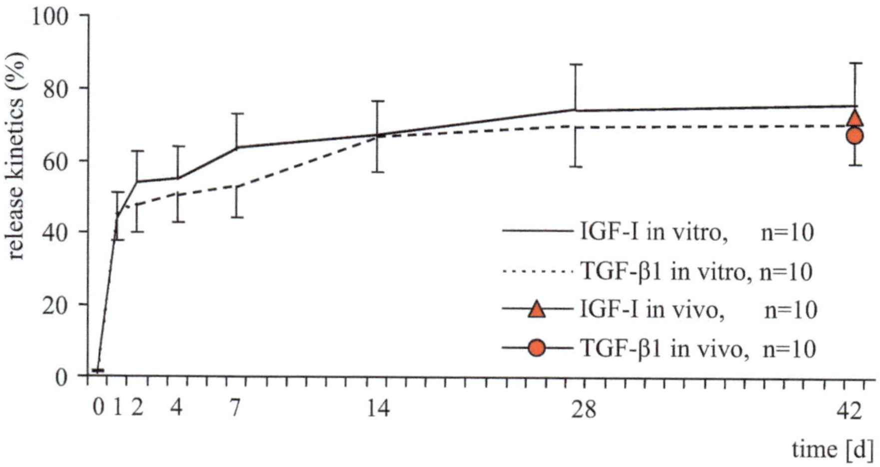

Fig. 7.2.2. Kinetics of in vivo and in vitro release of incorporated growth factors from a bioresorbable PDLLA coating, taking IGF-I and TGF-β1 as examples

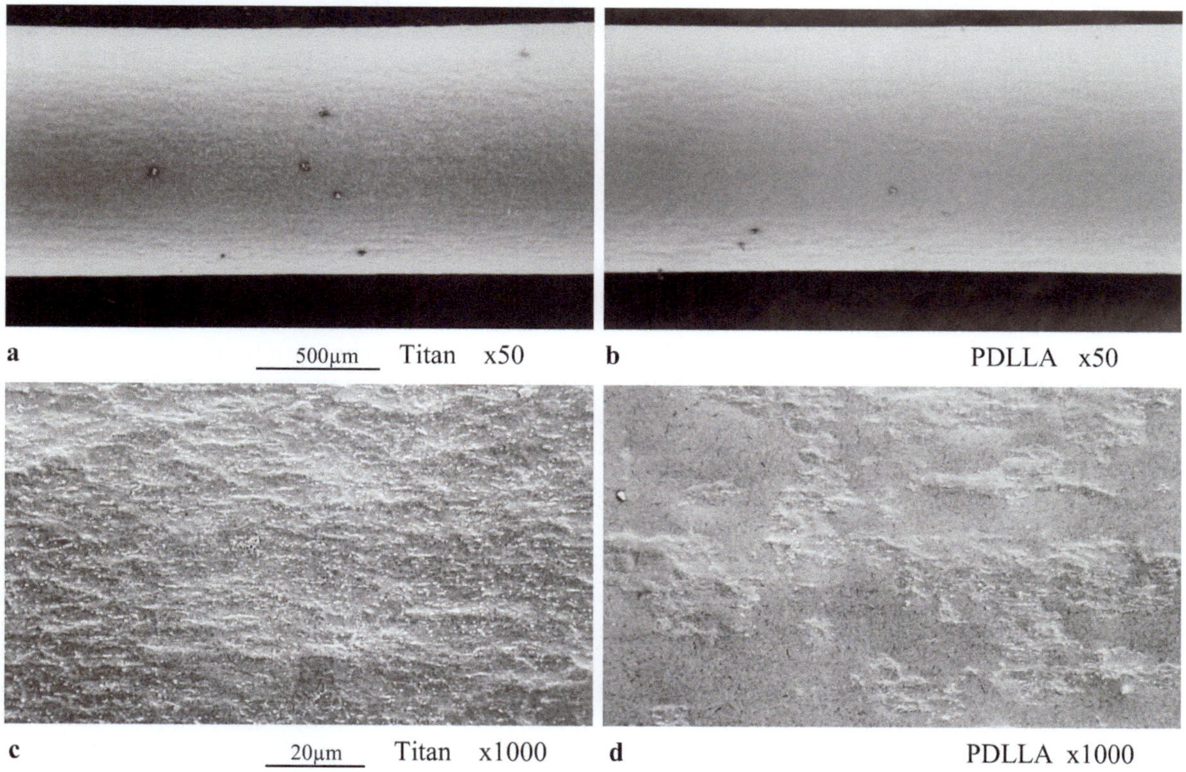

Fig. 7.2.3. a, c Raster electron microscopic images of titanium implants by comparison with PDLLA-coated implants b, d. The smoother, evenly coated surface of the PDLLA-coated implants is clearly apparent

of mechanical wear, such as occur in the implantation of an intramedullary load-bearing element in a tubular bone, without suffering damage. The loss of coating material observed was $<5\%$, with titanium surfaces demonstrating more favorable properties than steel implants (Fig. 7.2.1). In vitro and in vivo investigations showed that the biodegradable coating released bioactive substances continually, after an initial peak, over a period of 6 weeks [19] (Figs. 7.2.2, 7.2.3).

Implants coated with antibiotics can be sterilized using γ-radiation. Neither the mechanical nor the antibacterial properties are damaged by γ-radiation. In vitro investigations did not reveal any differences in activity between irradiated and nonirradiated implants. Implants coated with antibiotics could be used prophylactically to reduce the rate of implant-associated infections [12].

The biodegradable PDLLA coating of implants can also be used for the controlled local release of incorporated growth factors directly at the fracture. The coated implant thus serves both as a stabilizer for the fracture and as a carrier for active substances [14, 19]. The growth factors keep their biological activity when incorporated into the coating and are released locally in a controlled manner.

Growth factors are important in controlling the metabolism of bone cells. In the course of fracture healing, numerous growth factors, cytokines and transmitter substances are released in and around the fracture. They can have endocrine, paracrine or autocrine actions and can act either systemically or locally. Many studies have demonstrated that various growth factors have osteoinductive effects and exert a positive influence on fracture healing [5, 26, 27]. In vivo studies have shown that some of these growth factors, such as IGF-I, TGF-β1 and BMP-2, have a stimulating effect on osteogenic and chondrogenic cells [14] and thus stimulate bone healing [26].

The growth factors exert stimulating effects on bone healing even at very low effective concentrations. For this reason they lend themselves for use in implant coatings for local delivery [5, 21]. The quantity of growth factors incorporated into the coating, and their release, can be kept so low in relation to the whole organism that no systemic side-effects occur. High concentrations can be delivered at their site of action with a low level of systemic stress side-effects. The amount of growth factors incorporated into the coating is less by a factor of about 100 than the dose normally delivered using collagen sponges, although the effectiveness is the same.

The principle of indirect stabilization of the fracture by the implant is supported and the fracture does not need to be opened to introduce the active substances [18, 19].

Animal Experiments

The Effect of Local Delivery of Growth Factors IGF-I and TGF-β1 on Osteotomy Healing in a Pig Model

This large-animal study investigated the effect of local application of a combination of IGF-I (300 µg) and TGF-β1 (60 µg) on osteotomy healing in pigs.

An osteotomy of the tibial shaft of Yucatan minipigs was stabilized using titanium intramedullary tibial nails with static locking. The nails were either coated or uncoated.

Progress was evaluated by means of X-ray examination, analysis of blood parameters (including serum IGF-I concentration and IGF-I binding proteins) and determination of body weight and temperature. After 28 days both tibiae were removed, biomechanically tested and histomorphometrically analyzed.

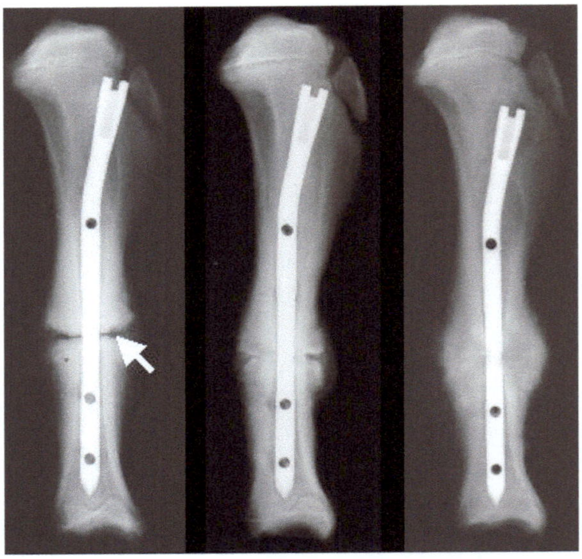

Fig. 7.2.4. Lateral X-ray pictures of tibiae 28 days after osteotomy. Comparison of bone regeneration in the osteotomy cleft in the groups: controls, PDLLA and PDLLA + growth factors. The *arrow* marks the osteotomy cleft. In the PDLLA + growth factors group, bony consolidation of the osteotomy cleft has taken place, whereas in the cleft is still visible

The results showed no differences between the two groups with respect to the blood parameters investigated, body weight or temperature. As had already been found using a small-animal model [18], the large-animal model did not reveal either local or systemic undesirable effects of the growth factors or the carrier material PDLLA. X-ray examinations showed that osteotomy healing was significantly faster in the growth factors group than in the control groups (Fig. 7.2.4) with significantly higher torsional stability (Fig. 7.2.5) and histomorphometrically advanced healing of the break (Fig. 7.2.6). As in the small-animal model, the PDLLA coating without incorporated growth factors exerted a stimulating effect on healing processes [14].

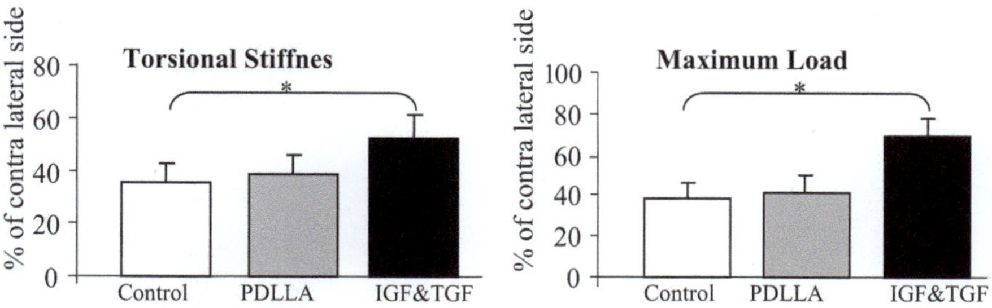

Fig. 7.2.5. Biomechanical testing of the osteotomized tibiae in comparison with the opposite side. The tibiae treated with growth factors show significantly higher values than the control and PDLLA groups for both torsional stiffness and maximal torque

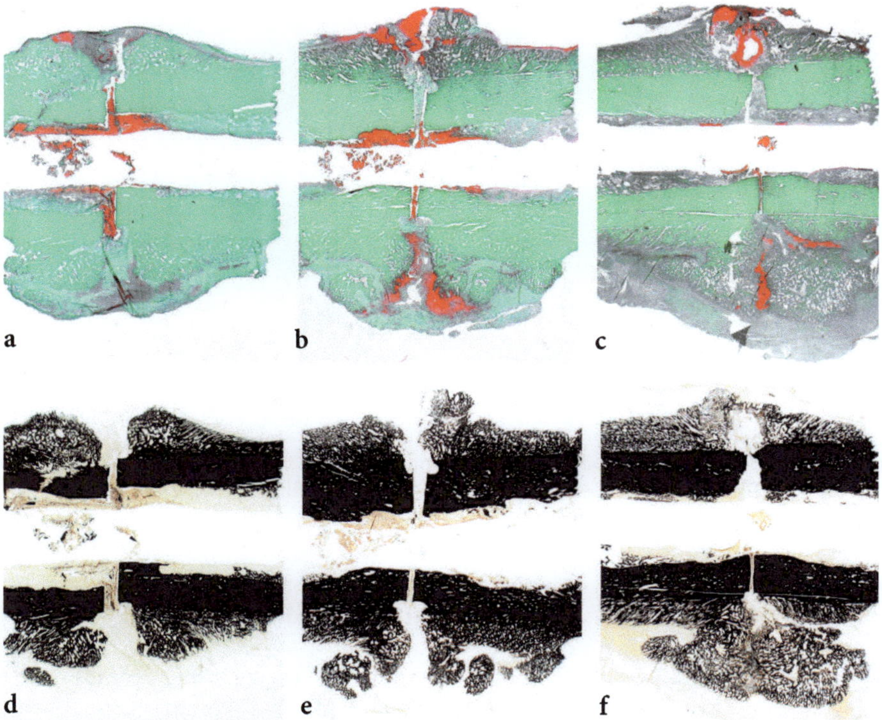

Fig. 7.2.6. a–c Histological sections stained with Safranin O/light green and d–f van Kossa. Comparison of bone regeneration in the osteotomy cleft in the groups: controls (a, d), PDLLA (b, c) and PDLLA + growth factors (c, f). The histological results support the biomechanical values. Here, too, healing is clearly further advanced in the animals treated with growth factors than in the controls

Local Delivery of Growth Factors for the Optimization of Intervertebral Cervical Spinal Fusion in a Sheep Model

The aim of further studies, as well as stimulating fracture and osteotomy healing, was to investigate the effect of growth factors delivered locally from PDLLA-coated cages on intervertebral spinal fusion in sheep. This was intended to create conditions that would optimize fusion of the cervical spine. In several in vivo studies it was found that the biodegradable PDLLA coating of intervertebral implants ensures reliable, simple and effective delivery of IGF-I, TGF-β1 and BMP-2 in the intervertebral area. It was also shown that the effectiveness of the PDLLA carrier is significantly superior to that of a collagen carrier. No side-effects of the PDLLA coating were detected in this study. Combined delivery of IGF-I and TGF-β1 using a PDLLA-coated cage was evaluated in a dose escalation study. Intermediate and high doses of IGF-I and TGF-β1 demonstrated a significant osteoinductive effect. The intermediate dose of 150 µg IGF-I (5% w/w) plus 30 µg TGF-β1 (1% w/w), in

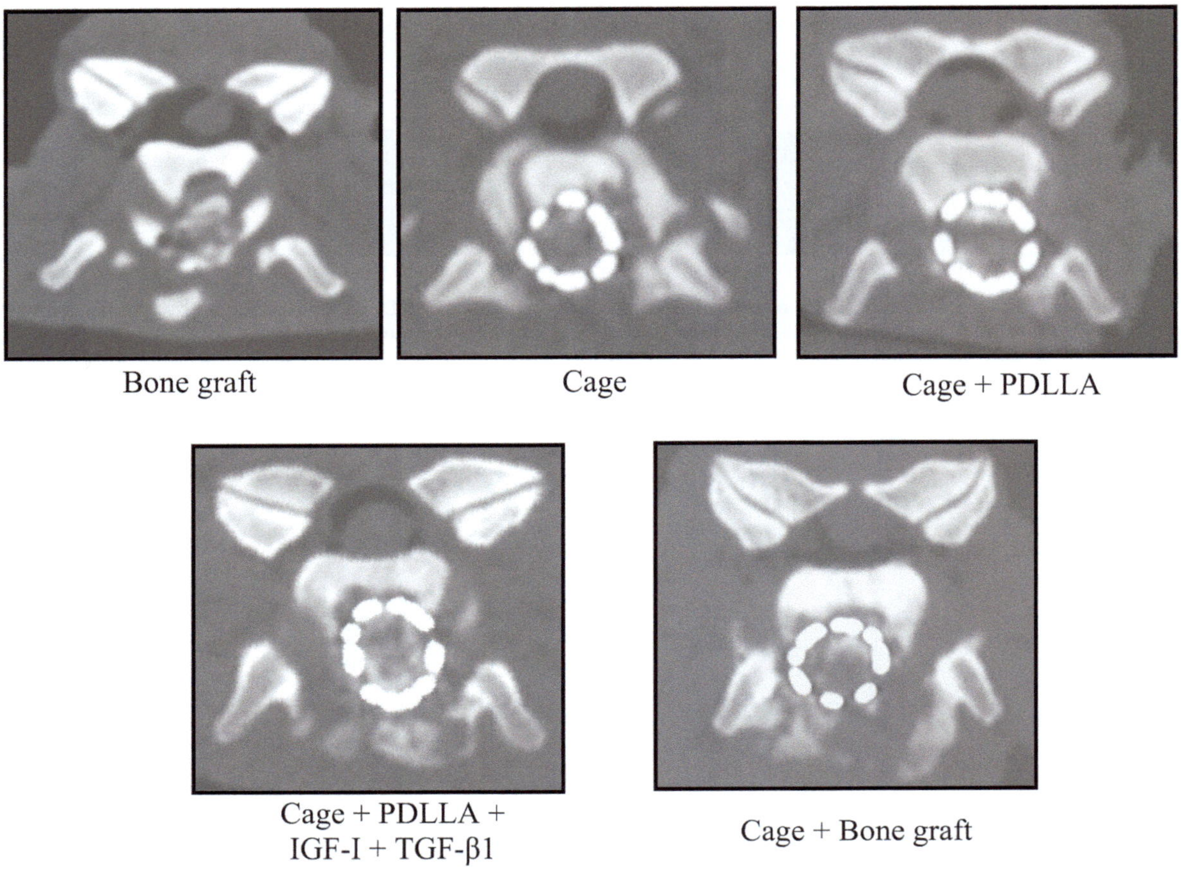

Fig. 7.2.7. Axial computed tomography pictures 12 weeks after cervical spinal fusion (C3 and C4). In the group with growth-factor-coated implants, new bone growth within the cage is clearly increased by comparison with the other groups

particular, exerted the greatest effect: at lower doses the osteoinductive effect was absent and at higher doses no increase was induced in bone matrix formation. Furthermore no undesirable effects on laboratory parameters, body weight or body temperature were detected at any of the doses of IGF-I and TGF-β1. Delivery of IGF-I and TGF-β1 using PDLLA-coated cages was able to cause significant stimulation of intervertebral spinal fusion. It was also shown that the growth factors used, either BMP-2 or IGF-I and TGF-β1, allowed a significant improvement in intervertebral fusion by comparison with autologous bone material and at the same time rendered the harvesting of such bone material unnecessary. The delivery of IGF-I and TGF-β1 using a PDLLA carrier yielded significantly better fusion results than BMP-2 delivered using a collagen carrier, the previously accepted experimental "gold standard" [7–9] (Figs. 7.2.7, 7.2.8).

Gentamicin-Coated Implants for Prophylaxis Against Implant-Associated Infections

Infections represent a very serious complication in orthopedic surgery. When combined with large foreign bodies such as prostheses or other implants, bone infections are very hard to treat. In some cases the implant supports the infection and, as a result, has to be removed [1, 17, 23], often making it necessary to carry out multiple revision operations and give long-term treatment with antibiotics [20, 22, 24, 25].

Staphylococcus aureus and coagulase-negative staphylococci (*Staph. epidermidis*) can be isolated in 70–90% of deep wound infections [17, 22].

These pathogens possess a high affinity for bone and are able to protect themselves from systemic antibiotics by means of glycocalix production [6, 11].

Preliminary studies showed that coating implants with PDLLA significantly reduces the adhesion of microorganisms to the implant surface (see Fig. 7.2.1) [18]. Like growth factors, gentami-

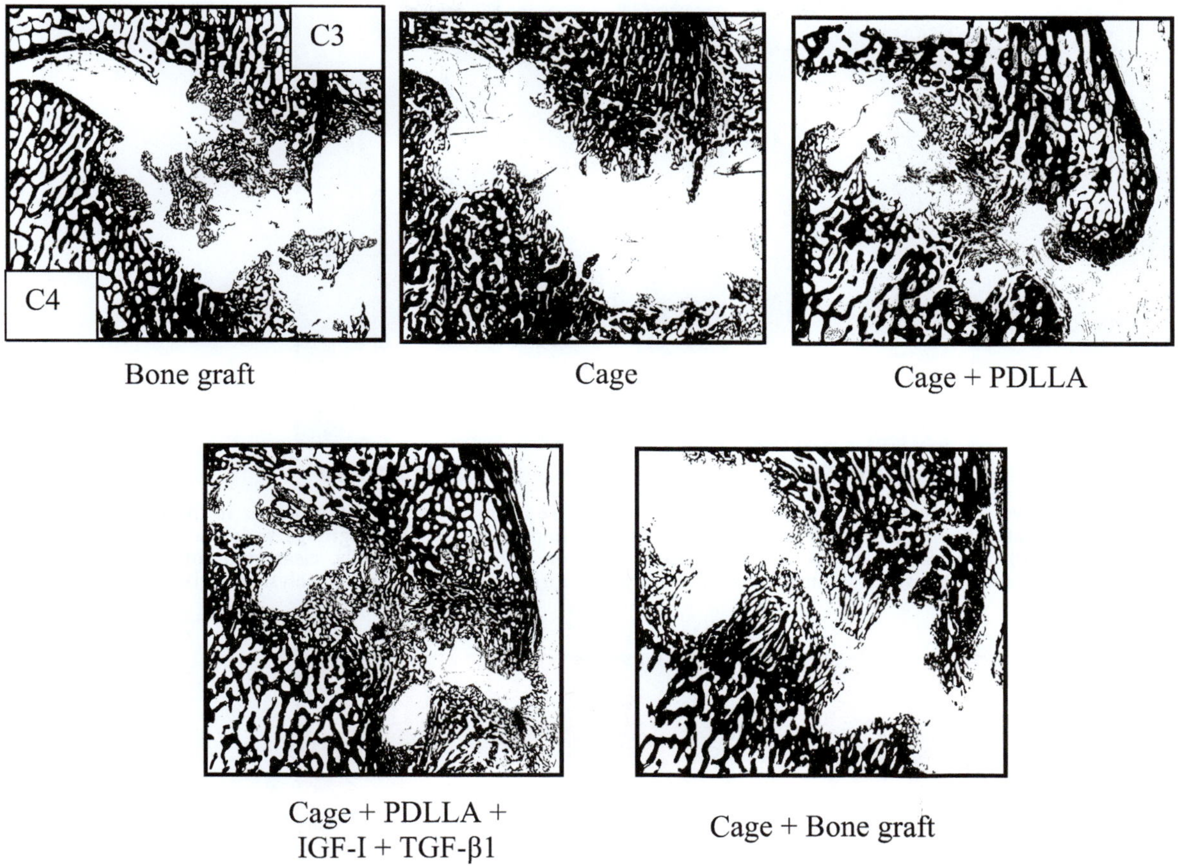

Fig. 7.2.8. Sagittal histological sections stained with van Kossa. Bony fusion of the vertebral bodies C3 and C4 is only apparent in the group with growth-factor-coated cages. No bone regeneration is apparent in the comparison groups

cin can be incorporated into a PDLLA coating for implants.

The effect of a gentamicin-containing PDLLA coating for implants was investigated using an infection model [13]. In this model, *Staph. aureus* was introduced into the tibial medullary cavity at three different concentrations with a Kirschner wire. Controls received sterile PBS solution. Routine radiological examinations indicated bony destruction characteristic of osteomyelitis after as little as 2 weeks (Fig. 7.2.9). After 6 weeks the Kirschner wire was removed and rolled across the surface of an agar plate, which was then incubated at 37 °C. At evaluation the growth of *Staph. aureus* was found to be markedly less for the PDLLA + gentamicin-coated implants than for the controls (Fig. 7.2.10). Histological examination of the tibiae after 6 weeks confirmed the radiological findings (Fig. 7.2.11). There were clearly less colony forming units (CFU) in the infected bones treated with antibiotic-coated devices compared to the control groups.

This antibiotic-containing coating was able to reduce the rate of implant-associated infections significantly in a rat model [12, 13].

First Human Application

The promising results from experimental studies using animals provided grounds for applying this technology in humans. Gentamicin-coated intramedullary nails were implanted into humans in particularly critical clinical situations. Since July 2003, six coated tibial intramedullary nails (UTN, Synthes) have been implanted in patients with complicated fractures of the lower leg. Implantation of antibiotic-coated nails is particularly indicated in the case of grade III open fractures as these have an up to 30% greater risk of developing osteomyelitis compared to patients with closed fractures. Their use is also indicated in cases of re-osteosynthesis as these patients are also known to be at increased risk of bone infection.

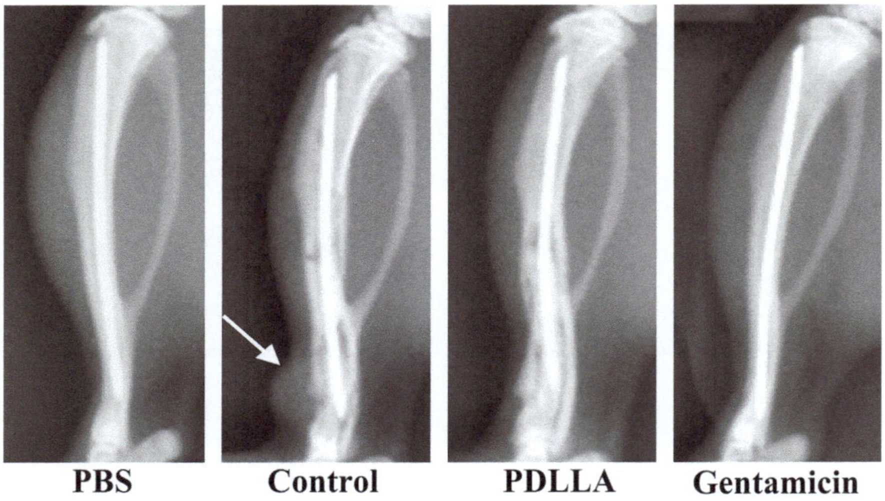

Fig. 7.2.9. X-rays 6 weeks after the operation. The PBS group was inoculated with sterile PBS solution. In the other three groups, 10^3 CFU *Staph. aureus* was introduced into the medullary cavity. No signs of infections or osteolysis are apparent in the PBS group or in the gentamicin-coated implant group. In the groups with titanium wire (controls) or PDLLA coating only, clear signs of infections, abscess formation (*arrow*) and osteolysis are visible

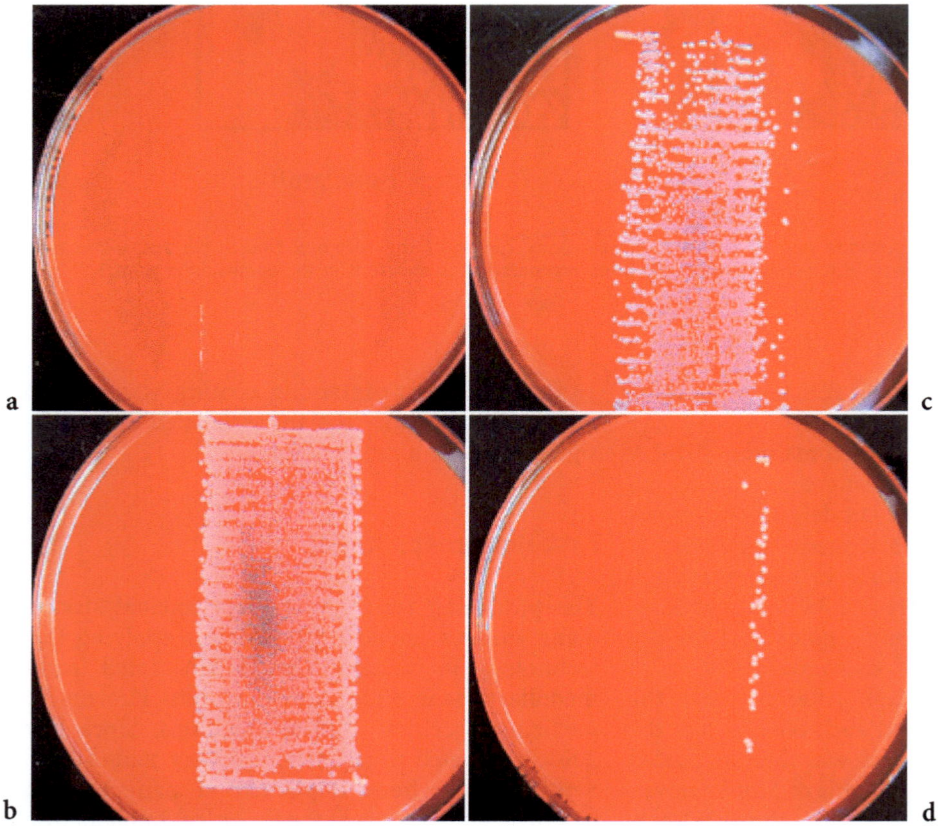

Fig. 7.2.10. Streak cultures from Kirschner wires 6 weeks after implantation. a The wires for the PBS group and the d gentamicin coating group show no formation of bacterial colonies and formation of bacterial colonies only in the distal area of the nail respectively. b, c A thick lawn of colonies is apparent for the control and PDLLA groups

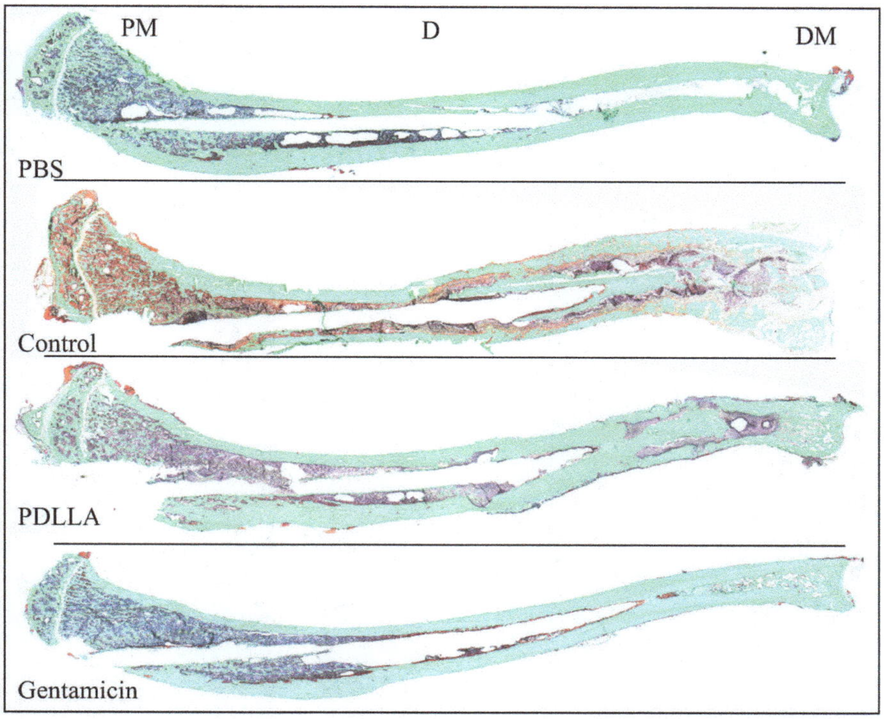

Fig. 7.2.11. Masson-Goldner-stained sections 6 weeks after the operation. *PM* proximal epiphysis and metaphysis, *D* diaphysis, *DM* distal epiphysis and metaphysis. **a, d** The sections of the PBS and gentamicin groups show no signs of destruction of the bone structure. **b** In the control group, considerable destruction and extension of the cortices are apparent. **c** Sequestration and bone destruction are also clearly apparent in the section of the PDLLA group

Case Report: UTN Protect

A 17-year-old male pedestrian was hit by a car. The following pattern of injuries was found: cerebral contusion 1°, thoracic trauma with serial fractures of the ribs on both sides, vertebral body fracture of C7, lesion of the right cervical plexus and a grade IIIB open fracture of the lower leg.

Initial treatment consisted of a Philadelphia collar, thoracic drainage and external fixation of the right lower leg. Final treatment of the right lower leg using a gentamicin-coated intramedullary nail (UTN Protect 9 mm×380 mm, Synthes) was performed on the fifth day after the trauma (Figs. 7.2.12–7.2.15).

The postoperative course was without complications and all wounds healed primarily (Figs. 7.2.16, 7.2.17). From the second day after the operation the patient was mobilized with a partial load of 15 kg. On day 25 after the operation he was discharged from hospital fully mobilized, with normal inflammation parameters and no signs of an allergic reaction to the implant. Because of his plexus lesion he was then transferred to a neurological rehabilitation establishment. The gentamicin levels found in the drainage fluid and in the serum over the course of 4 weeks were less than 0.3 µl/ml.

Discussion

The coating of implants enables them to function as carriers for biological substances as well as giving mechanical stabilization. In the studies presented here it has been shown that coating titanium implants with bioresorbable polylactide provides an appropriate way of delivering active substances locally, and at effective concentrations, for a variety of indications. The coating does not alter the implant's proven biomechanical properties. In animal experiments both titanium cages coated with growth factors for intervertebral cervical spinal fusion and tibial nails coated with growth factors achieved improved fusion results or bone healing compared to replace control groups. In spinal surgery this could the harvesting of additional bone material, for example from the iliac crest. Fractures with severe soft tissue damage, situations in which perfusion is reduced, critical size defects, osteoporotic fractures and non-un-

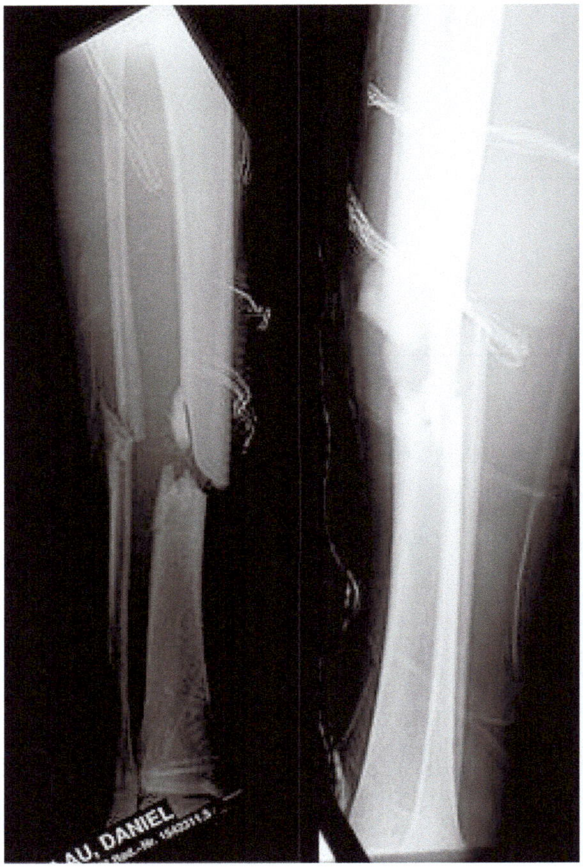

Fig. 7.2.12. X-ray of grade IIIB open tibia fracture

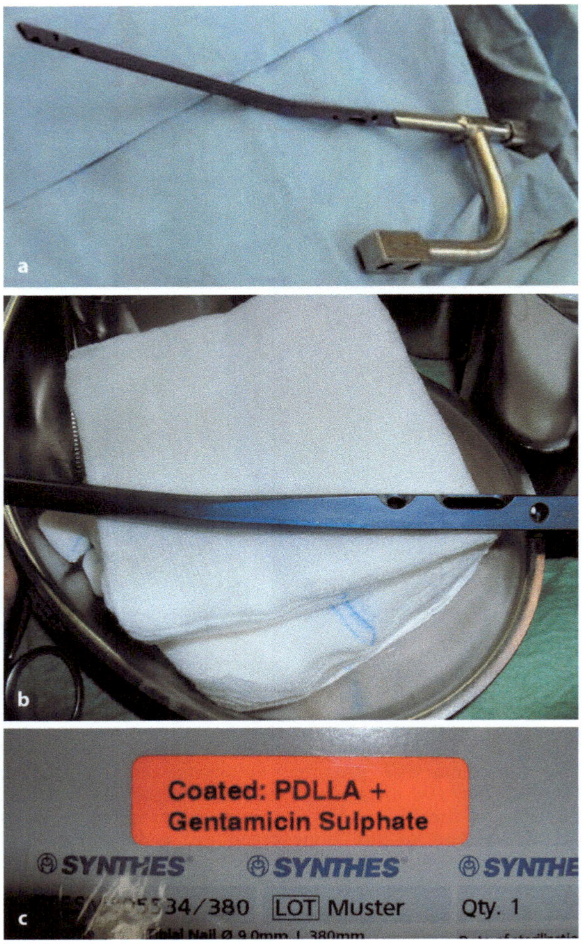

Fig. 7.2.13 a–c. Gentamicin-coated UTN Protect. The UTN Protect is manufactured by Synthes. The 10-µm thick PDLLA coating is bioresorbable. Gentamicin is incorporated in the coating

ions are difficult problems. Tibial nails coated with growth factors could stimulate fracture healing and promote bony regeneration.

In an animal infection model it was demonstrated that active substances other than growth factors can also be incorporated into the bioresorbable PDLLA coating of a titanium implant for local release. Antibiotics were delivered locally in this way and the usefulness of gentamicin-coated tibial nails for infection prophylaxis was also demonstrated. Open fractures are at a particularly high risk of infection and, as a result, of implant-associated osteomyelitis.

The first gentamicin-coated tibial nails have already been used in humans. In a pilot study gentamicin-coated intramedullary nails were implanted in six patients with fractures of the lower leg including severe soft tissue damage. No undesirable side-effects occurred and the systemic gentamicin level in serum was below the detection limit. Although the preliminary results do not yet permit conclusions to be drawn about their significance in the treatment of fractures with severe soft tissue damage or revision operations, this key technology appears to be appropriate for the incorporation of active substances. Its use could also be considered in endoprosthetic revision and for patient groups with increased risk profiles as well as with fractures involving severe soft tissue damage. Extensive clinical trials will be required to show which factors or substances should be used for the improvement of treatment.

In summary, the coating process presented here should be seen as a key technology. A wide variety of implants made from different materials can be coated. The appropriate active substance can be delivered locally in a targeted and individual manner according to the indication or the range of pathogens present. Local delivery makes it possible to avoid subjecting the organism to high systemic doses and also enables local support for

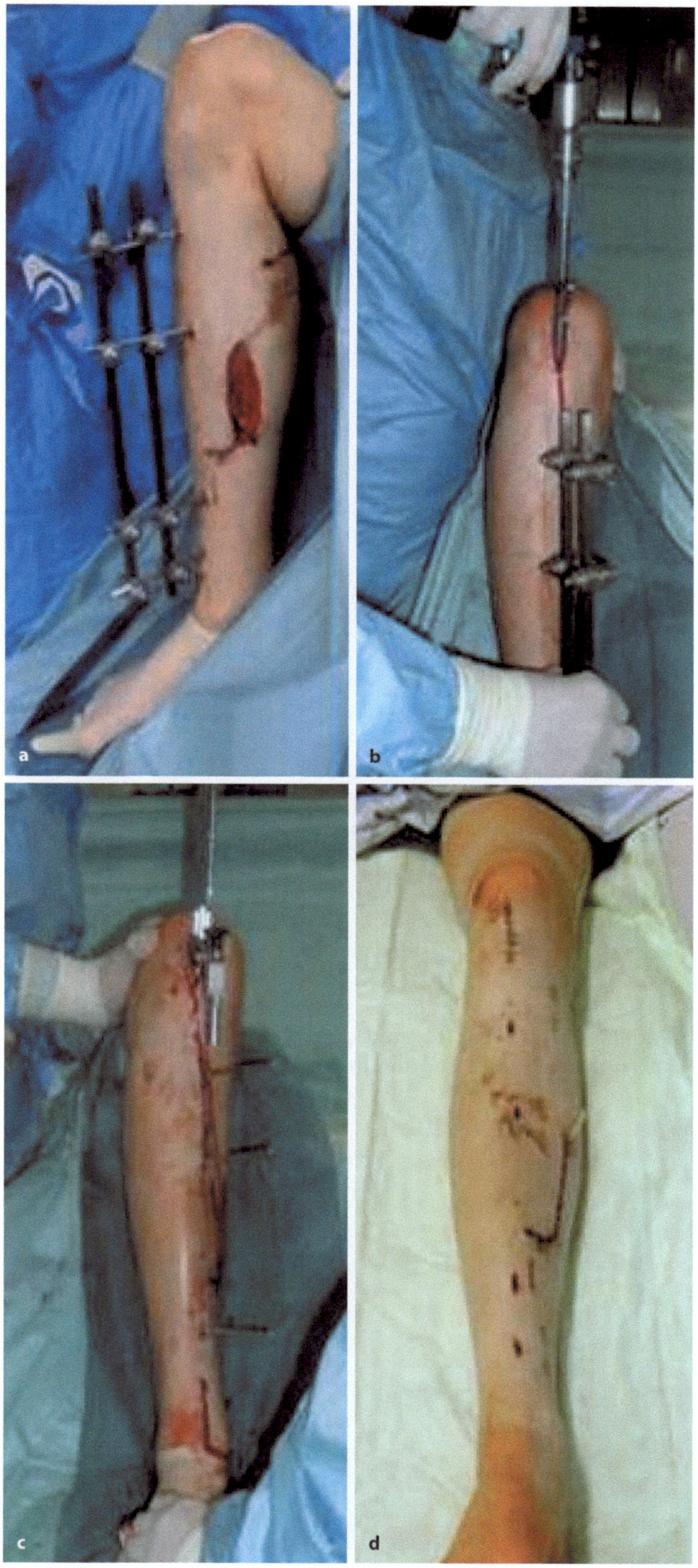

Fig. 7.2.14 a–d. a On the day of the accident the right tibia was stabilized by an AO fixator for damage control. On the fifth day after the accident a UTN Protect was implanted. **b** Implantation of the UTN. **c** Implantation of the coated nail. **d** Image of the right leg after surgery. The open wound of the grade IIIB open tibia fracture was drained by an easy-flow drain and closed in the same operation after removal of the external fixator

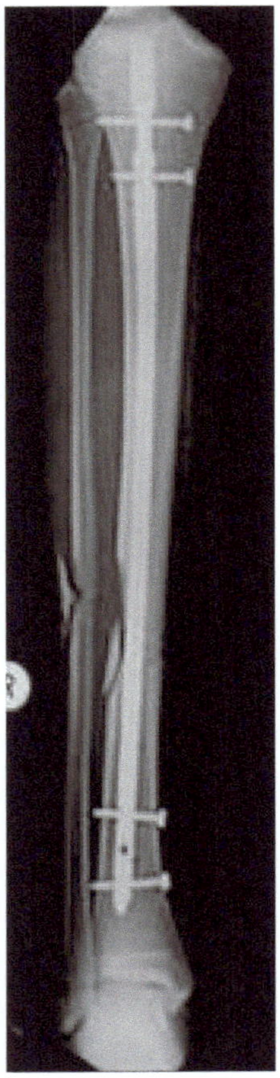

Fig. 7.2.15. The postoperative X-ray showed a good anatomic alignment of the fractured tibia

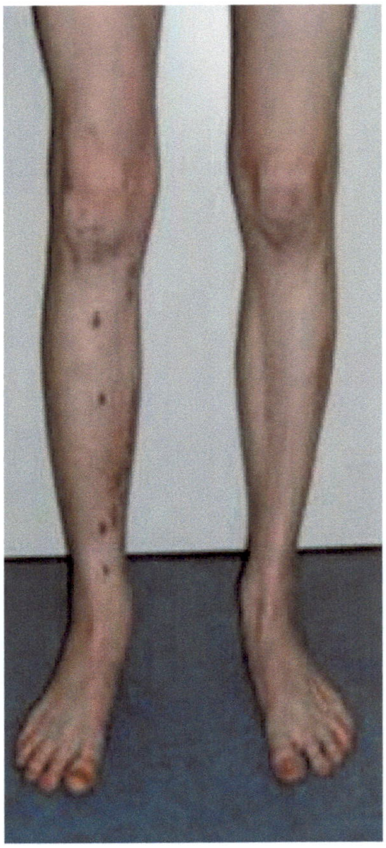

Fig. 7.2.16. Four months after surgery all wounds were healed. There were no signs of inflammation. The patient was mobilized with full weight-bearing

the systemic action of substances, e.g. i.v. delivered autobiotics.

The use of coated implants in traumatology is of course not a standard procedure, yet. However, experimental studies and the first clinical applications are promising. Alongside continued development of implants and operating techniques, this technology could help to further reduce the rate of complications in orthopedic and trauma surgery.

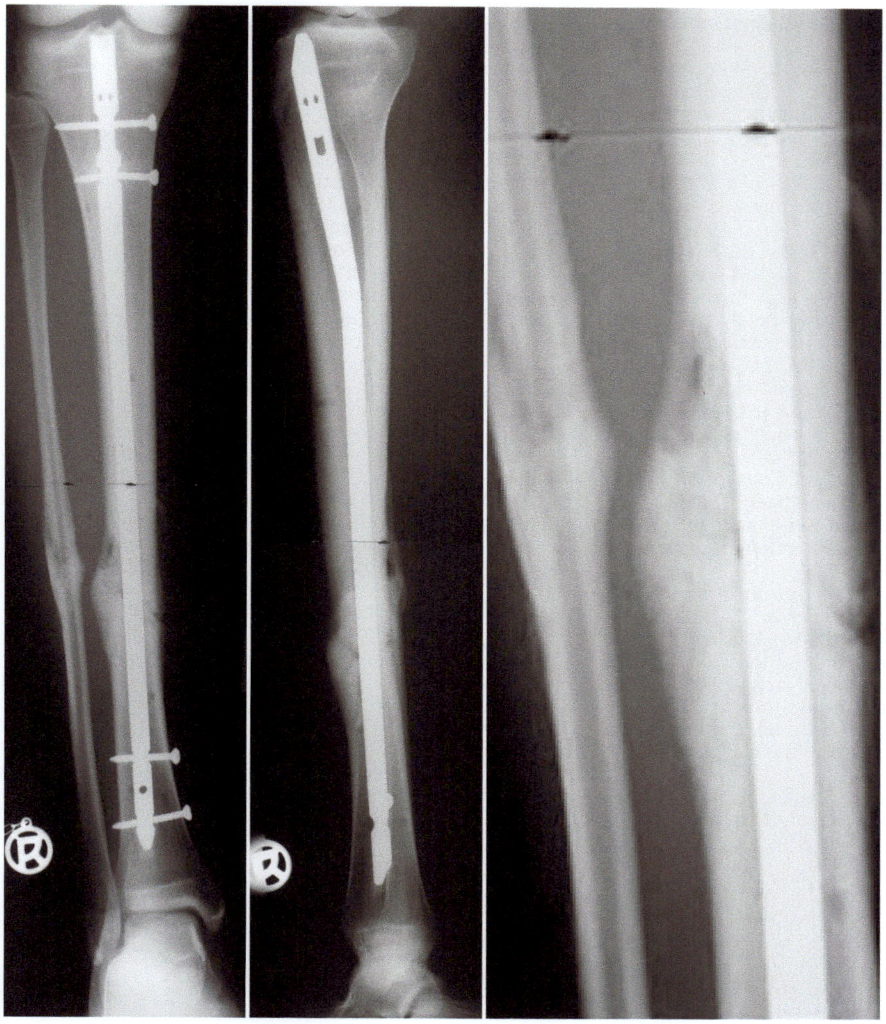

Fig. 7.2.17. X-ray 4 months after injury showed a healed tibia fracture with good alignment. No signs of loosening of the nail were seen. Removal of the UTN Protect is planned 18 months after injury

References

1. Beck A, Kinzl L, Bischoff M (1999) [Antibiotic prophylaxis and therapy in trauma surgery]. Unfallchirurg 102: 955–966.
2. Coventry M, Nolan D, Bukenbauch R (1973) "Delayed" prophylactic anticoagulation: a study of results and complications in 2,012 total hip arthroplasties. J Bone Joint Surg 55: 1487–1492.
3. Einhorn TA (1995) Enhancement of fracture healing. J Bone Joint Surg Am 77: 940–956.
4. Einhorn TA, Lane JM (1998) Significant advances have been made in the way surgeons treat fractures [editorial]. Clin Orthop S2–S3.
5. Fujimoto R, Tanizawa T, Nishida S, Yamamoto N, Soshi S, Endo N, Takahashi HE (1999) Local effects of transforming growth factor-beta1 on rat calvaria: changes depending on the dose and the injection site. J Bone Miner Metab 17: 11–17.
6. Gristina AG, Costerton JW (1985) Bacterial adherence to biomaterials and tissue. The significance of its role in clinical sepsis. J Bone Joint Surg Am 67: 264–273.
7. Kandziora F, Pflugmacher R, Scholz M, Schäfer J, Schollmeier G, Schmidmaier G, Duda G, Raschke M, Haas NP (2003) Dose-dependent effects of combined IGF-I and TGF-β1 application in a sheep cervical spine fusion model. Eur Spine J 12: 464–473.
8. Kandziora F, Bail H, Schmidmaier G, Schollmeier G, Scholz M, Knispel C, Hiller T, Pflugmacher R, Mittlmeier T, Raschke M, Haas NP (2002) Bone morphogenic protein-2 application by a poly(D,L-lactide)-coated interbodycage: in vivo results of a new carrier for growth factors. J Neurosurg (Spine 1) 97: 40–48.
9. Kandziora F, Schmidmaier G, Schollmeier G, Bail H, Pflugmacher R, Gorke T, Wagner M, Raschke M, Mittlmeier T, Haas NP (2002) IGF-I and TGF-beta1 application by a poly-(D,L-lactide)-coated cage promotes intervertebral bone matrix formation in the sheep cervical spine. Spine 27: 1710–1723.
10. Li RH, Wozney JM (2001) Delivering on the promise of bone morphogenetic proteins. Trends Biotechnol 19: 255–265.
11. Littlewood EA, Hattenberger M, Zak O, O'Reilly T (1997) Effect of combination therapy of rifampicin and azithromycin on TNF levels during a rat model of

chronic osteomyelitis. J Antimicrob Chemother 39: 493–498.

12. Lucke M, Schmidmaier G, Sadoni S, Wildemann B, Schiller R, Haas N, Raschke M (2003) Gentamicin coating of metallic implants reduces implant related osteomyelitis in rats. Bone 32: 521–531.
13. Lucke M, Schmidmaier G, Sadoni S, Wildemann B, Schiller R, Stemberger A, Haas N, Raschke M (2003) A new model of implant related osteomyelitis in rats. J Biomed Mater Res 67B: 593–602.
14. Raschke M, Wildemann B, Inden P, Bail H, Flyvbjerg A, Hoffmann J, Haas NP, Schmidmaier G (2002) Insulin-like growth factor-1 and transforming growth factor-beta1 accelerates osteotomy healing using polylactide-coated implants as a delivery system: a biomechanical and histological study in minipigs. Bone 30(1): 144–151.
15. Raschke M, Kolbeck S, Bail H, Schmidmaier G, Flyvbjerg A, Lindner T, Dahne M, Roenne I, Haas N (2001) Homologous growth hormone accelerates healing of segmental bone defects. Bone 29: 368–373.
16. Raschke MJ, Bail H, Windhagen HJ, Kolbeck SF, Weiler A, Raun K, Kappelgard A, Skiaerbaek C, Haas NP (1999) Recombinant growth hormone accelerates bone regenerate consolidation in distraction osteogenesis. Bone 24: 81–88.
17. Sanderson PJ (1989) Preventing infection in orthopaedic implants. J Antimicrob Chemother 24: 277–280.
18. Schmidmaier G, Wildemann B, Bail H, Lucke M, Fuchs T, Stemberger A, Flyvbjerg A, Haas NP, Raschke M (2001) Local application of growth factors (insulin-like growth factor-1 and transforming growth factor-β1) from a biodegradable poly(D,L-lactide) coating of osteosynthetic implants accelerates fracture healing in rats. Bone 28: 341–350.
19. Schmidmaier G, Wildemann B, Stemberger A, Haas NP, Raschke M (2001) Biodegradable poly(D,L-lactide) coating of implants for continuous release of growth factors. J Biomed Mater Res, Applied Biomat 58: 449–455.
20. Southorn PA, Plevak DJ, Wright AJ, Wilson WR (1986) Adverse effects of vancomycin administered in the perioperative period. Mayo Clin Proc 61: 721–724.
21. Sumner DR, Turner TM, Purchio AF, Gombotz WR, Urban RM, Galante JO (1995) Enhancement of bone ingrowth by transforming growth factor-beta. J Bone Joint Surg Am 77: 1135–1147.
22. Suter F, Avai A, Fusco U, Gerundini M, Caprioli S, Maggiolo F (1994) Teicoplanin versus cefamandole in the prevention of infection in total hip replacement. Eur J Clin Microbiol Infect Dis 13: 793–796.
23. Taylor GJ, Bannister GC, Calder S (1990) Perioperative wound infection in elective orthopaedic surgery [published erratum appears in J Hosp Infect 1991; 17(2): 155]. J Hosp Infect 16: 241–247.
24. Wall R, Klenerman L, McCullough C, Fyfe I (1988) A comparison of teicoplanin and cefuroxime as prophylaxis for orthopaedic implant surgery: a preliminary report. J Antimicrob Chemother 21 (Suppl A): 141–146.
25. Wood MJ (1996) The comparative efficacy and safety of teicoplanin and vancomycin [see comments] [published erratum appears in J Antimicrob Chemother 1996; 38(5): 919 and 1997; 40(1): 147]. J Antimicrob Chemother 37: 209–222.
26. Yasko AW, Lane JM, Fellinger EJ, Rosen V, Wozney JM, Wang EA (1992) The healing of segmental bone defects, induced by recombinant human bone morphogenetic protein (rhBMP-2). A radiographic, histological, and biomechanical study in rats. J Bone Joint Surg Am 74: 659–670.
27. Zheng MH, Wood DJ, Papadimitriou JM (1992) What's new in the role of cytokines on osteoblast proliferation and differentiation? Pathol Res Pract 188: 1104–1121.

Plasma Polymer – High-Porosity Silver Composite Coating for Infection Prophylaxis in Intramedullary Nailing

V. Alt, M. Wagener, D. Salz, T. Bechert, P. Steinrücke, R. Schnettler

Introduction

Infection after intramedullary nailing of fractures is one of the most devastating situations in trauma surgery and can lead to septic non-union and chronic osteomyelitis [1, 2]. Infections can occur in closed fracture treatment [3] but open fractures in particular have a high risk of infection [4]. There has been a long controversial discussion whether open long bone fractures should be treated by a reamed or by an unreamed nail. The theoretical advantage of unreamed nails is the preservation of endosteal blood supply with a lower infection risk and better healing results [5]. However, reduction of infection rates by unreamed nailing could never be proven and a recent systematic literature review showed that there were no differences in infection rates between unreamed and reamed nailing [6]. In contrast to initial hypotheses, several authors found that reamed nailing exhibited lower rates of non-unions, shorter fracture consolidation time and lower incidence of hardware failure [6–8] and advocated reamed nailing also for grade IIIB open fractures [9].

The use of implants for fracture treatment favours infections compared to surgery where no foreign material is implanted into the body [10]. This is mainly related to the adhesion and proliferation of the bacteria on the implant surface [11], often with synthesis of an extracellular polysaccharide matrix called biofilm (Fig. 7.3.1), which has been identified as a crucial step in the pathophysiology of infection and as an important factor of virulency of bacteria [10, 12]. This biofilm formation enables the bacteria to elude host defence and antibiotic treatment [13]. Staphylococci are the most frequent infection-causing strains in bone and joint surgery [14]. *Staph. epidermidis* is found in up to 90% of all bone infections with indwelling devices (osteosynthesis material, joint prostheses, etc.) [16], which is most likely related to the strong biofilm-building capacity of these bacteria [12]. Also certain strains of *Staph. aureus* have been found to produce biofilms [16] and bone infections with *Staph. aureus* are in general more difficult to treat compared to infections with *Staph. epidermidis* [17]. Once biofilm formation is established, only implant removal promises eradication of the infection [18, 19].

Independently from the technique of intramedullary nailing, adequate prophylaxis is the most efficient way to prevent infection. Besides general pre-requirements such as aseptic operating room conditions, mainly soft-tissue management and the use of systemic antibiotics are crucial parameters to reduce infection rates [20]. A comprehen-

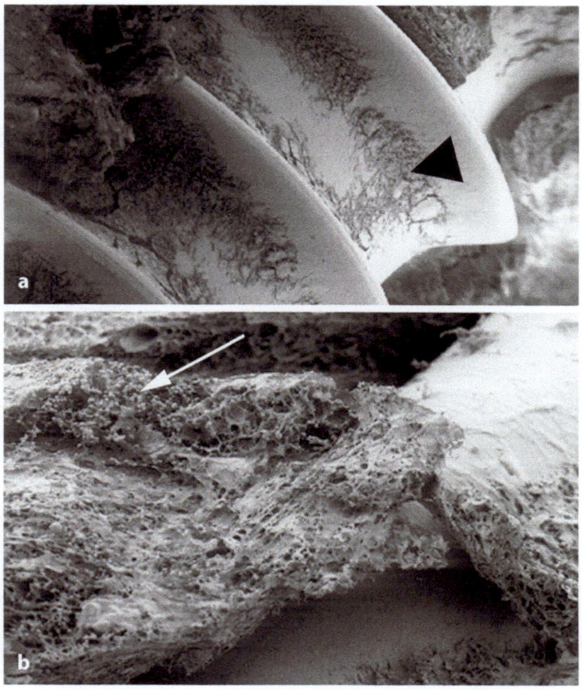

Fig. 7.3.1. Scanning electron microscopy of biofilm-producing *Staph. aureus*. a Biofilm formation of *Staph. aureus* on the thread of a screw. b Higher magnification reveals the round staphylococci embedded in the biofilm. Magnifications: a ×83, b ×521. Source: Laboratory of Experimental Trauma Surgery, Giessen, Germany

sive overview of intravenous antibiotic prophylaxis for open fractures is given in Chap. 7.1.

Furthermore, coating of implants promises prevention of colonisation of the implant's surface with reduction of infection rates. Gentamicin is the most common antibiotic used for loading of bone cements in infection prophylaxis in total joint surgery in Europe [21] due to its good antibacterial activity, excellent biocompatibility, and favourable release kinetics [22]. Recently, gentamicin was used in a poly(D,L-lactide) matrix for coating of osteosynthetic implants in an experimental study [23].

Also metallic silver in the form of high-porosity silver particles was shown to exhibit high antimicrobial activity in bone cements including activity against multiresistant strains, e.g. methicillin-resistant *Staph. aureus* (MRSA) and methicillin-resistant *Staph. epidermidis* [24]. Metallic silver can also be used in combination with a SiO_x plasma polymer for coating of osteosynthetic devices.

Plasma Polymerisation Coating Technique

Plasma polymerisation is a versatile technique for the preparation of functional coatings on various materials and devices. Depending on the precursor material and the processing parameters, films with a thickness well below 100 nm can be obtained. In general these films are chemically inert, insoluble, mechanically and thermally stable and are used as membranes or protective coatings, for example [25]. By using hexamethyldisiloxane (HMDSO) as a precursor material, it is possible to obtain highly biocompatible films due to the formation of a coating that basically consists of a SiO_x plasma polymer.

Plasma Polymers Containing Metal Particles

Small metallic silver particles can be embedded into a SiO_x plasma polymer film in order to achieve an antimicrobial effect with such a coating on orthopaedic implants. Plasma polymer matrices for the embedding of metal clusters were used for the first time by Perrin et al. [26]. The deposition technique developed by these authors is based on the simultaneous deposition of the metal by sputtering and plasma polymerisation. An alternative method is the simultaneous deposition of the metal by evaporation and plasma polymerisation [27–31]. The coatings investigated in this work have been prepared by silver cluster deposition via inert gas evaporation and condensation and subsequent plasma polymerisation. Two different types of coatings have been prepared: for the coating named type A the silver clusters have been directly deposited on the substrate material and were embedded in a plasma polymer film, the coating named type B consists of silver clusters being embedded between two plasma polymer layers so that the silver is not in direct contact with the substrate material (Fig. 7.3.2).

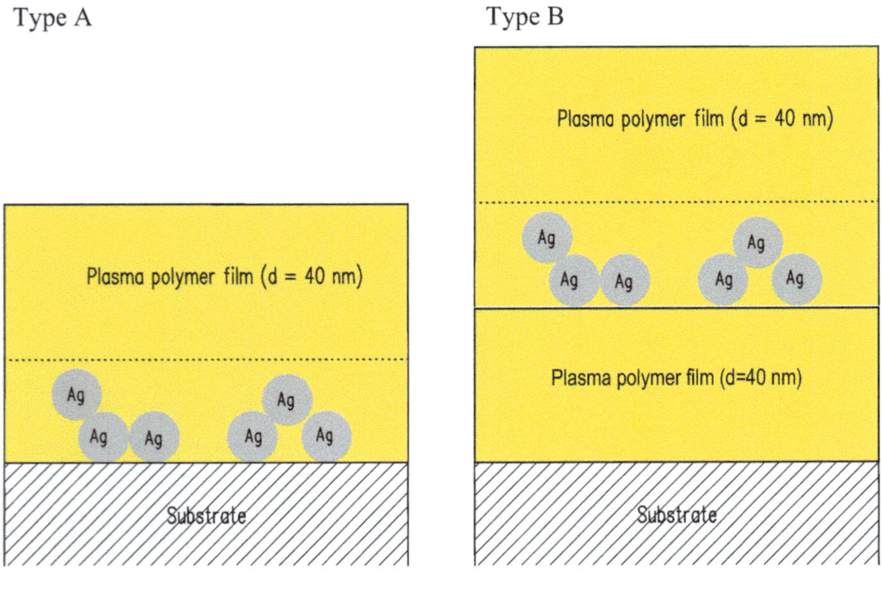

Fig. 7.3.2. Model of the two different coatings prepared in this work

Implants Coated with a Plasma-Polymer-Containing Metallic Silver

As test implant materials, stainless steel and titanium Kirschner wires with trocar points (diameter 2 mm, length 150 mm) were used. The metallic silver clusters were produced using an inert gas evaporation technique. Silver wire (Alfa Products, Karlsruhe, Germany; metal impurities less than 15 ppm) is evaporated from a resistance-heated tungsten crucible in an argon atmosphere at pressures between 5 and 10 mbar. The silver clusters are deposited on the substrate, which is rotated in the metal vapour to achieve a homogeneous silver cluster distribution on the substrate. The evaporation rate can be controlled by the current of the vapour source. The subsequent plasma polymer film was prepared in a microwave discharge from HMDSO monomers at 2500 W and at a process gas flow between 20 and 400 sccm.

For the characterisation of the metal–plasma polymer composites, transmission electron microscopy (TEM) and time-of-flight secondary ion mass spectroscopy (TOF-SIMS) were used. The TEM analysis of the composite coatings showed that the silver forms clusters with a size of approx. 10 nm on the substrate materials (Fig. 7.3.3). The clusters form agglomerates, which are supposed to be porous instead of solid silver islands. Between the agglomerates of silver clusters open channels exist. Therefore, the plasma polymer film that has been deposited on top of the silver clusters has contact with the substrate material. That results in a good adhesion of the plasma polymer onto the substrate.

From the TOF-SIMS analysis (Fig. 7.3.4), it can be seen that the plasma polymer film is approximately 40 nm thick (5000 s of sputtering corresponds to 45 nm polymer film). Only Si and C can be seen during the first 5000 s of sputtering. Below the polymer film, silver is found (see increasing intensity of Ag beyond 5000 s sputtering time). Not only can the principal structure of the film be confirmed by this method, but also the infiltration of the silver agglomerates by the plasma polymer film can be confirmed as the Si signal does not change dramatically when the Ag signal increases. The structural analysis of the film by TEM and TOF-SIMS confirmed the models shown in Fig. 7.3.2.

Antimicrobial Testing

For antimicrobial testing, an in vitro microplate proliferation test was used that has shown its accuracy for bone cement samples [32] and for biomaterials in general [33]. In brief, the samples are tested by three different subsequent incubation steps. During the first step, they are incubated in wells of a 96-well microplate with 10^6 colony-forming units of bacteria per well in a 250-µl cell suspension for 1 h, allowing adhesion of the

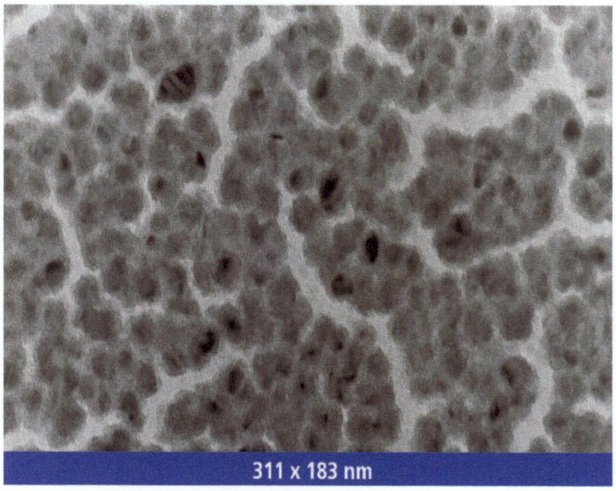

Fig. 7.3.3. Transmission electron microscopy of silver clusters in a plasma polymer film

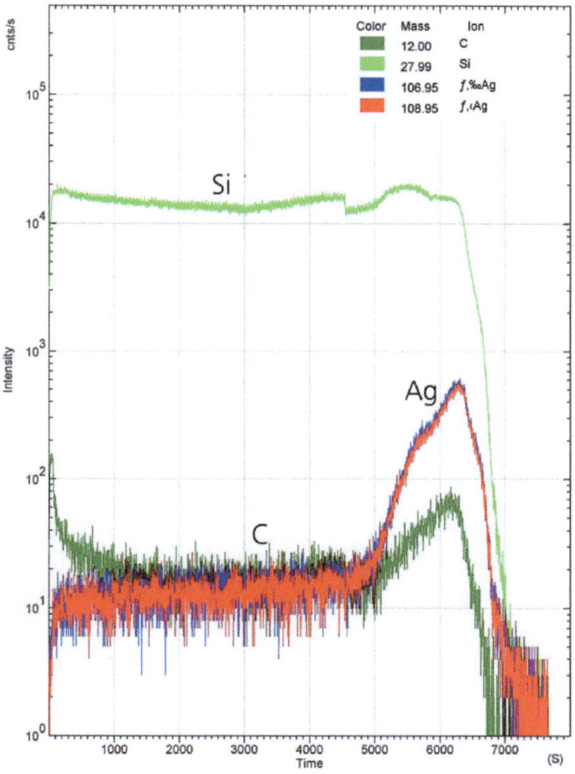

Fig. 7.3.4. TOF-SIMS analysis of silver clusters in a HMDSO plasma polymer film (type A)

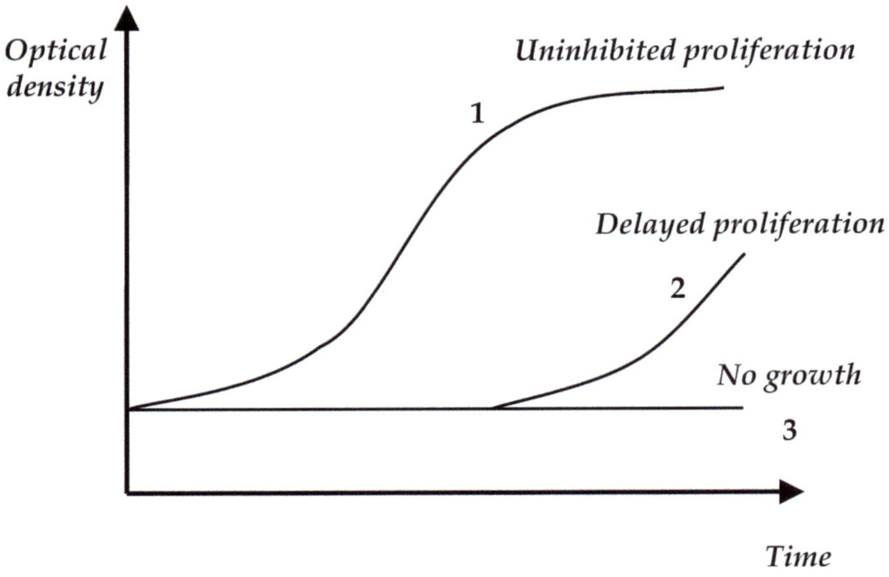

Fig. 7.3.5. *Curve 1* uninhibited bacterial proliferation indicating missing antibacterial properties of the implant; *curve 2* delayed onset of bacterial proliferation indicating slight antibacterial effect of the implant; *curve 3* inhibited bacterial growth indicating bactericidal effect of the implant

strain on the samples. After this first incubation, rinsing of the samples with PBS removes loosely attached cells from the sample surface. In a second step, the remaining adherent bacteria on the implant surface are incubated in minimal medium (PBS with 0.25% glucose, 0.2% $(NH_4)_2SO_4$, and 1% sterile trypticase soy broth) for 18 h in another 96-well microplate. If there is no antimicrobial effect of the implant, attached cells on the surface of the sample start to multiply and to release clonal counterparts into the well. If there is an antimicrobial effect of the implant, the cells are killed and are not able to seed out daughter cells. After removal of the samples the released bacteria were amplified in a final step by adding 50 µl of TSB medium to each well for 36 h, which can be analysed by a microplate reader (VersaMax, Molecular Devices, Sunnyvale, California, USA) system providing time-proliferation curves for each tested sample. These curves allow differentiation between the absence of antimicrobial activity, intermediate antimicrobial, and bactericidal effects of the tested sample (Fig. 7.3.5).

The samples were tested against *Staph. epidermidis*, which is the most common strain in device-associated infections [15].

Antimicrobial Activity of Silver-Coated Implants

Uncoated samples of both stainless steel and titanium wires showed uninhibited proliferation of the tested *Staph. epidermidis* indicating missing antimicrobial properties of the device (Fig. 7.3.6). In contrary to this, coating of the material with high-porosity silver directly on the substrate (type A) showed no bacterial growth for stainless steel and titanium. This means that this coating type of osteosynthetic devices exhibits bactericidal activity both for stainless steel and titanium. If the metallic silver is embedded between two polymer layers (coating type B) on stainless steel there was a delayed onset of bacterial growth indicating intermediate antimicrobial activity for this material-coating combination. However, coating type B exhibited also bactericidal effects on titanium implants.

In summary, coating with direct application of the metallic silver plasma polymer matrix onto the surface of implants showed very promising bactericidal activity on both stainless steel and titanium.

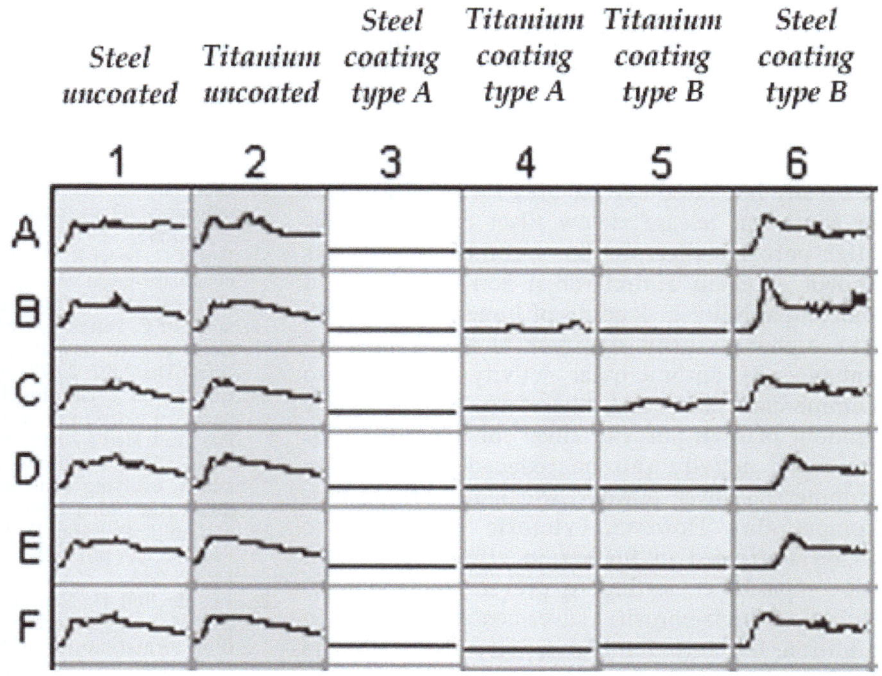

Fig. 7.3.6. Time-proliferation curves for coated and uncoated stainless-steel and titanium implants. Uncoated implants show uninhibited bacterial proliferation for both stainless steel (*lane 1*) and titanium (*lane 2*). Coating type A with direct deposition of the silver cluster coating matrix onto the implant surface exhibits complete inhibition of bacterial proliferation (*lanes 3 and 4*) implicating a bactericidal effect of this type of coating on both materials. Coating type B with silver embedded between two plasma polymer layers also showed a bactericidal effect for titanium implants. For stainless steel this type of coating only led to a delayed onset of bacterial growth indicating intermediate antimicrobial activity of this material-coating combination

Discussion and Conclusion

This investigation showed the high antibacterial activity of metallic silver in a SiO_x plasma polymer coating of osteosynthetic devices. In summary, a suitable technique for metallic silver coating of implants was found, which promises new prophylaxis options in fracture treatment including intramedullary nailing.

The antimicrobial activity of silver is based on different effects on the cells, e.g. binding to and subsequent inactivation of SH-groups of enzymes and other proteins [34, 35], interference with the energy production and energy conservation of the bacterial cell [36]. Silver does not prevent adhesion of the bacteria to the implant surface but kills adherent microorganisms and inhibits their proliferation [33]. This mechanism is the most likely reason for prevention of infection in silver-loaded devices, e.g. in catheters [37] or in bone cement [24]. If bacterial proliferation is inhibited by silver, the formation of biofilm will also be avoided.

Compared to gentamicin coating of implants, which has been used in another study with favourable results against *Staph. aureus*, silver has two distinct advantages. First, silver is effective against almost all strains including MRSA and MRSE [24] because silver resistance does not play an important role in the hospital microbial germ flora [38]. A possible explanation for this phenomenon is that silver acts on different metabolic levels in the cell and, therefore, resistance cannot be acquired by single-point mutation as for aminoglycoside antibiotics like gentamicin. With increasing incidences of multiresistant strains in nosocomial infections, the broad antimicrobial activity of silver is a very favourable new option in infection prophylaxis. Second, even if infection occurs in silver-coated implants, there are still all options given for antibiotic treatment of the patient. In cases in which gentamicin is used as infection prophylaxis, the infection-causing strains often acquire gentamicin resistance [39]. This gentamicin resistance is often combined with resistance against other aminoglycosides and excludes the further use of these agents against the infection.

The metallic silver that was used for the coating of the implants clearly differentiates from "commercial silver coatings". The silver is embedded in a plasma polymer film and forms a highly porous film structure consisting of nanoparticles with a size between 5 and 10 nm, which are agglomerated into larger particles in the micrometer range. Compared to a solid silver film with 0% porosity without any enlargement of the active surface, the highly porous film has a dramatically increased surface area resulting in higher silver ion release at low silver concentrations. High-porosity silver in the form of powder has shown excellent antimicrobial activity and good biocompatibility in loading of bone cements [24]. The higher porosity structure of silver seems to enhance its antimicrobial activity compared to commercial silver and, therefore, the necessary amount of high-porosity silver for adequate antimicrobial activity can be reduced compared to commercial silver powder, which favours its biocompatibility. However, cytotoxic concerns have to be addressed in further in vitro and in vivo biocompatibility testing to prevent bioincompatibility of high-porosity silver-coated devices. In addition, the antimicrobial activity also has to be reproduced in animal and human trials.

In conclusion, direct application of high-porosity silver plasma polymer coating matrix onto the surface of implants showed preliminary excellent and promising results for a new strategy of infection prevention in surgical fracture treatment. Further studies have to confirm these observations and have to elucidate biocompatibility of this type of coating for osteosynthetic devices.

References

1. Lortat-Jacob A, Sutour JM, Beaufils P. Infection following centro-medullary nailing of diaphyseal femoral and tibial fractures. Rev Chir Orthop Reparatrice Appar Mot 1986; 72:485–494.
2. Khatod M, Botte MJ, Hoyt DB, Meyer RS, Smith JM, Akeson WH. Outcomes in open tibia fractures: relationship between delay in treatment and infection. J Trauma 2003; 55:949–954.
3. Coles CP, Gross M. Closed tibial shaft fractures: management and treatment complications. A review of the prospective literature. Can J Surg 2000; 43:256–262.
4. Malik MH, Harwood P, Diggle P, Khan SA. Factors affecting rates of infection and nonunion in intramedullary nailing. J Bone Joint Surg Br 2004; 86:556–560.
5. Sanders R, Jersinovich I, Anglen J, DiPasquale T, Herscovici D Jr. The treatment of open tibial shaft fractures using an interlocked intramedullary nail without reaming. J Orthop Trauma 1994; 8:504–510.
6. Kapur R, Misra A, Johnstone AJ, Maffulli N. Intramedullary nailing of the tibia: to ream or not to ream: a systematic review of the literature. CME Orthop 2000; 1:48–54.
7. Court-Brown CM, Will E, Christie J, McQueen MM. Reamed or unreamed nailing for closed tibial fractures. A prospective study in Tscherne C1 fractures. J Bone Joint Surg Br 1996; 78:580–583.
8. Duwelius PJ, Schmidt AH, Rubinstein RA, Green JM. Nonreamed interlocked intramedullary tibial nailing. One community's experience. Clin Orthop 1995; 315: 104–113.
9. Keating JF, Blachut PA, O'Brien PJ, Meek RN, Broekhuyse H. Reamed nailing of open tibial fractures: does the antibiotic bead pouch reduce the deep infection rate? J Orthop Trauma 1996; 10:298–303.
10. Gristina AG. Biomaterial-centered infection; microbial adhesion versus tissue integration. Science 1987; 237: 1588–1595.
11. Peters G, Locci R, Pulverer G. Adherence and growth of coagulase-negative staphylococci on surfaces of intravenous catheters. J Infect Dis 1982; 146:479–482.
12. von Eiff C, Peters G, Heilmann C. Pathogenesis of infections due to coagulase-negative staphylococci. Lancet Infect Dis 2002; 2:677–685.
13. Ciampolini J, Harding KG. Pathophysiology of chronic bacterial osteomyelitis. Why do antibiotics fail so often? Postgrad Med J 2000; 76:479–483.
14. Haas DW, McAndrew MP. Bacterial osteomyelitis in adults: evolving considerations in diagnosis and treatment. Am J Med 1996; 101:550–561.
15. Mahan J, Seligson D, Henry SL, Hynes P, Dobbins J. Factors in pin tract infections. Orthopedics 1991; 14:305–308.
16. van de Belt H, Neut D, Schenk W, van Horn JR, van Der Mei HC, Busscher HJ. Staphylococcus aureus biofilm formation on different gentamicin-loaded polymethylmethacrylate bone cements. Biomaterials 2001; 22:1607–1611.
17. Cunningham R, Cockayne A, Humphreys H. Clinical and molecular aspects of the pathogenesis of Staphylococcus aureus bone and joint infections. J Med Microbiol 1996; 44:157–164.
18. Gristina AG, Oga M, Webb LX, Hobgood CD. Adherent bacterial colonization in the pathogenesis of osteomyelitis. Science 1985; 228:990–993.
19. Habash M, Reid G. Microbial biofilms: their development and significance for medical device-related infections. J Clin Pharmacol 1999; 39:887–898.
20. Templeman DC, Gulli B, Tsukayama DT, Gustilo RB. Update on the management of open fractures of the tibial shaft. Clin Orthop 1998; 350:18–25.
21. Espehaug B, Engesaeter LB, Vollset SE, Havelin LI, Langeland N. Antibiotic prophylaxis in total hip arthroplasty. Review of 10,905 primary cemented total hip replacements reported to the Norwegian arthroplasty register, 1987 to 1995. J Bone Joint Surg Br 1997; 79:590–595.
22. Wahlig H, Dingeldein D. Pharmacokinetic study of gentamicin-loaded cement in total hip replacements. Comparative effects of varying dosage. J Bone Joint Surg Br 1984; 66:175–179.
23. Lucke M, Schmidmaier G, Sadoni S, Wildemann B, Schiller R, Haas NP, Raschke M. Gentamicin coating of metallic implants reduces implant-related osteomyelitis in rats. Bone 2003; 32:521–531.
24. Alt V, Bechert T, Steinrucke P, Wagener M, Seidel P, Dingeldein E, Domann E, Schnettler R. An in vitro assessment of the antibacterial properties and cytotoxicity of nanoparticulate silver bone cement. Biomaterials 2004; 25:4383–4391.
25. Li K, Meichsner J. Gas-separating properties of membranes coated by HMDSO plasma polymer. Surface Coating Technology 1999; 116–119, 841–847.
26. Perrin J, Despax B, Kay E. Optical properties and microstructure of gold-fluorocarbon-polymer composite films. Phys Rev B 1985; 32:719–732.
27. Kampfrath L, Heilmann A, Hamann C. Plasma polymerized thin films containing small silver particles. Vacuum 1988; 38:1–3.

28. Heilmann A, Hamann C. Deposition, structure and properties of plasma polymer metal composite films. Prog Colloid Polym Sci 1991; 85:102–110.
29. Heilmann A, Werner J, Hopfe V. Optical properties of plasma polymer films with encapsulated silver particles. Z Phys D 1993; 26:39–41.
30. Lamber R, Wetjen S, Jaeger N. Size dependence of the lattice parameter of small palladium particles. Phys Rev B 1995; 51:10968–10971.
31. Lamber R, Wetjen S, Schulz-Eckloff G. Metal clusters in plasma polymer matrices: gold clusters. J Phys Chem 1995; 99:13834–13838.
32. Alt V, Bechert T, Steinrucke P, Wagener M, Seidel P, Dingeldein E, Domann E, Schnettler R. In vitro testing of antimicrobial activity of bone cement. Antimicrob Agents Chemother 2004; 48(11):4084–4088.
33. Bechert T, Steinrucke P, Guggenbichler JP. A new method for screening anti-infective biomaterials. Nat Med 2000; 6:1053–1056.
34. Ghandour W, Hubbard JA, Deistrung J, Hughes MN, Poole RK. The uptake of silver ions by Escherichia coli: toxic effects and interactions with copper ions. Appl Microbiol Biotechnol 1988; 28:559–565.
35. Petering HG. Pharmacology and toxicology of heavy metals: silver. Pharmacol Ther A 1976; 1:127–130.
36. Bragg PD, Rainnie DJ. The effect of silver ions on the respiratory chain of Escherichia coli. Can J Microbiol 1973; 20:883–889.
37. Boswald M, Lugauer S, Regenfus A, Braun GG, Martus P, Geis C, Scharf J, Bechert T, Greil J, Guggenbichler JP. Reduced rates of catheter-associated infection by use of a new silver-impregnated central venous catheter. Infection 1999; 27(Suppl 1):S56–60.
38. Gupta A, Phung LT, Taylor DE, Silver S. Diversity of silver resistance genes in IncH incompatibility group plasmids. Microbiology 2001; 147:3393–3402.
39. Thornes B, Murray P, Bouchier-Hayes D. Development of resistant strains of Staphylococcus epidermidis on gentamicin-loaded bone cement in vivo. J Bone Joint Surg Br 2002; 84-B:758–760.

Subject Index

D

E

F

G

H

I

K

L

MIX
Papier aus verantwortungsvollen Quellen
Paper from responsible sources
FSC® C105338

FSC
www.fsc.org

If you have any concerns about our products,
you can contact us on
ProductSafety@springernature.com

In case Publisher is established outside the EU,
the EU authorized representative is:
Springer Nature Customer Service Center GmbH
Europaplatz 3, 69115 Heidelberg, Germany

Printed by Libri Plureos GmbH
in Hamburg, Germany